Introduction to Pharmaceutical Biotechnology, Volume 2 (Second Edition)

Enzymes, proteins and bioinformatics

Online at: https://doi.org/10.1088/978-0-7503-5387-8

Introduction to Pharmaceutical Biotechnology, Volume 2 (Second Edition)

Enzymes, proteins and bioinformatics

Ahmed Al-Harrasi
Department of Organic Chemistry, University of Nizwa,
616 Birkat Al Maus, Nizwa, Oman

Saurabh Bhatia
Natural & Medical Sciences Research Center, University of Nizwa, P.O. Box 33,
616 Birkat Al Mauz, Nizwa, Oman

and

School of Health Sciences, University of Petroleum and Energy Studies, Dehradun,
Uttarakhand, India

Ajmal Khan
Natural and Medical Sciences Research Center, University of Nizwa,
Birkat-ul-Mouz 616, Nizwa, Sultanate of Oman

IOP Publishing, Bristol, UK

ISBN 978-0-7503-5387-8 (ebook)
ISBN 978-0-7503-5385-4 (print)
ISBN 978-0-7503-5388-5 (myPrint)
ISBN 978-0-7503-5386-1 (mobi)

DOI 10.1088/978-0-7503-5387-8

Version: 20240901

IOP ebooks

British Library Cataloguing-in-Publication Data: A catalogue record for this book is available from the British Library.

Published by IOP Publishing, wholly owned by The Institute of Physics, London

IOP Publishing, No.2 The Distillery, Glassfields, Avon Street, Bristol, BS2 0GR, UK

US Office: IOP Publishing, Inc., 190 North Independence Mall West, Suite 601, Philadelphia, PA 19106, USA

Saurabh Bhatia has dedicated this book to his Mother (Mrs Vinod Bala Bhatia), his Father (Mr Ram Lal Bhatia) and his Brother (Mr Sanjay Bhatia).

Contents

Preface

There has been a long-felt requirement for a textbook representing current and recent developments in the field of pharmaceutical biotechnology. The few available books have become out of date, in particular due to the development of new biotechnology from advances in concepts and techniques. This volume has been written with a view to provide background knowledge on the state of the art of the subject and provide a practical view of the developments to date in genes, enzymes and proteins. The book covers several different facets of evolutional progress and achievements in each line of inquiry. Attention is focused on newer perspectives on the roles of genes, enzymes and proteins in the field of pharmaceutical biotechnology. The current volume is organized into three important areas—enzymes, genomics and proteomics—and is comprised of ten chapters. The book begins with the general properties, mechanisms, applications, production, immobilization and purification of enzymes, with some applications in the form of biosensors and biotransformation reactions. This information is followed by characterizations in genomics, genomes sequencing, comparative genomics and genomic evolution. Other highlights pertain to protein engineering. This book will be of interest to biochemists, biologists, microbiologists, biotechnologists, food technologists and others involved in research on the biotechnological applications of proteins and enzymes.

Acknowledgement

We would like to dedicate this book to all students, researchers, academicians, and all the scholars. who have sincerely contributed to the area of Pharmaceutical Biotechnology, depicted in the book, at national as well as international level. We would also like to acknowledge the University of Nizwa, Sultanate of Oman for extending its support in accomplishing this book project successfully. We are grateful to the Natural and Medical Sciences Research Center (NMSRC) housed at the University of Nizwa for providing central resources of advanced analytical instruments for our research work and for promoting interdisciplinary research studies. This centre has given a valuable base to this book project. Thus, authors are thankful to NMSRC for offering excellent facilities required for the completion of this book.

Natural and Medical Sciences Research Center, University of Nizwa

Last, but not least, we show our sincere gratitude to the whole team of IOP Publishing for furnishing their active cooperation and support.

Author biographies

Professor Ahmed Al-Harrasi

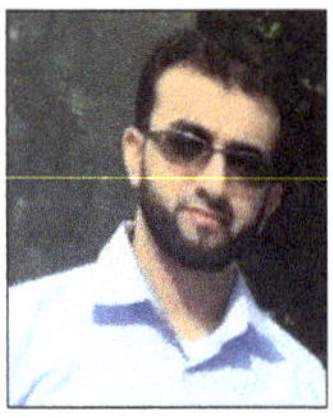

Ahmed Al-Harrasi is a professor of organic chemistry and the vice chancellor for graduate studies, research and external relations at the University of Nizwa. He obtained his BSc in Chemistry from SQU and his MSc and PhD in Organic Chemistry from Free University of Berlin as a DAAD-fellow. Then he received the Fulbright award in 2008 for postdoctoral research in Chemical Biology from Cornell University. He is a founder and chair of the Natural and Medical Sciences Research Center. He is a member of the Scientific Council of UNESCO. He was named on the list of top 2% scientists for the last three years. He has authored over 800 scientific papers and more than 20 books and book chapters. He received the Order of Royal Commendation from His Majesty, The Sultan of Oman as an outstanding Omani individual for his remarkable contribution and active role in research.

Dr Saurabh Bhatia

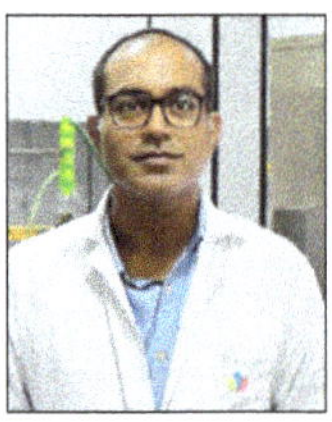

Saurabh Bhatia is an Associate Professor within the Natural and Medical Sciences Research Centre at the University of Nizwa, Oman. He has published 127 referred journal articles and written 94 book chapters. Dr Bhatia has also authored 10 books and is the Associate Editor on several international journals.

Dr Ajmal Khan

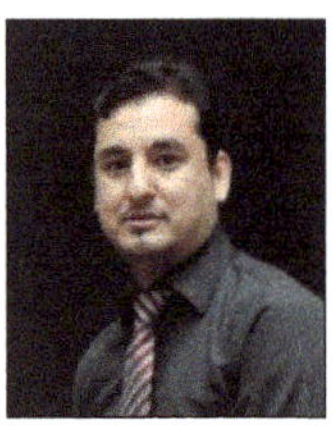

Ajmal Khan is currently working as an Associate Professor in Natural and Medical Sciences Research Centre at the University of Nizwa, Oman. Dr Khan published more than 450 articles in international peer review journals with impact factor of more than 2000 and citation more than 9000. Besides this, he published two US patents, and 3 books and 13 books chapters. Dr Khan is Associate Editor for four journals and in editorial board of three international journals.

IOP Publishing

Introduction to Pharmaceutical Biotechnology, Volume 2
(Second Edition)
Enzymes, proteins and bioinformatics
Ahmed Al-Harrasi, Saurabh Bhatia and Ajmal Khan

Chapter 1

Introduction to enzymes and their applications

1.1 Introduction

The cell is the structural and functional unit of life—the basic building block of living systems. Cells effectively utilize biocatalysts, known as enzymes, which are notable for their high catalytic efficiency and specificity for substrates and reactions. Enzymes have amazing catalytic power and their high level of specificity for their substrate makes them suitable for biological reactions. They are crucial for cellular metabolism. Each and every chemical reaction that takes place in plants, micro-organisms and animals proceeds at a quantifiable rate as a direct result of enzymatic catalysis. Most of the history of biochemistry is directly or indirectly related to the history of enzyme research. Catalysis in biological systems was initially reported in the early 1800s based on research into the digestion of meat. In this report the catalytic activity of secretions from the stomach, the conversion of starch into sugar by saliva, and various plant extracts were reported.

In 1837, Berzelius documented the catalytic nature of fermentation. In the 1850s Louis Pasteur reported that fermentation was a process initiated by living organisms. During this study it was reported that the fermentation of sugar into alcohol by yeast was catalyzed by ferments. He also hypothesized that these ferments are close to the structure of yeast. These ferments were later called enzymes (in yeast). The key breakthrough in the history of enzymes came in 1897 when Edward Buchner isolated, from yeast cells, the soluble active form of the set of enzymes that catalyzes the fermentation of sugar to alcohol. Emul Fischer reported the first systematic studies on enzyme specificity in the early twentieth century [1]. Later, in 1926, James Sumner extracted *urease* in pure crystalline form from jack beans [2]. He also recognized the protein nature of *urease*. In 1930, John Northrop and his co-workers crystallized pepsin and trypsin and established them as proteins [3]. In subsequent years enzymology developed rapidly (table 1.1). The important developments during

doi:10.1088/978-0-7503-5387-8ch1

Table 1.1. Chronology of enzyme studies.

Name	Year	Work
Anfinsen	1956–8	The sequence of an amino acid regulates the folding pattern and activity of a ribonuclease.
Beatle and tatum	1940	'One gene one enzyme' hypothesis.
Bertrand	1896–7	Co-enzyme or co-ferment (currently known as co-factors).
Berzelius	1835	Concept of catalysis.
Berzelius	1837	Exploration of biological catalysis.
Briggs and haldane	1925	Derivation of enzyme rate equations using the steady-state approximation.
Buchner	1897	Isolation of the soluble active form of enzymes from yeast cells.
Chances	1943	Application of spectroscopic techniques for studying enzymes.
Cori and cori	1937–9	Muscle phosphorylase.
Duclaux henri	1898	Nomenclature: substrate plus suffix 'ase'.
Fischer	1894–5	'Lock and key' hypothesis of enzyme specificity.
Harden and young	1901–3	Methods for the derivation of kinetic rate laws; principle of enzyme–substrate complex. 1906 Co-ezymase (NAD).
Jacob, Monod and changeux	1961	Allosterism.
Koshland	1953	'Induced fit' hypothesis.
Kuhne	1878	Explored trypsin catalyzed reactions; introduction of word 'enzyme'.
Michaelis and menten	1913	Extension of the kinetic theory of enzyme catalysis.
Northrop and kunitz	1930–3	Crystallization of proteolytic enzymes.
Pasteur	1850	Fermentation of sugar into alcohol by yeast.
Payen and persoz	1833	Alcohol precipitation of thermolabile 'diastase' from malt.
Phillips, johnson and north	1965	Three-dimensional structure of lysozyme obtained at 1.5 A resolution.
Sumner	1926	Crystallization of urease.
Sutherland	1956	Cyclic AMP adenyl cyclase.
Umbarger, yates and pardee	1956	Regulation of enzyme activity via feedback inhibition.
Wilhelmy	1850	Quantitative evaluation of the rates of sucrose inversion.

this period are: the elucidation of major metabolic pathways, such as the glycolysis and tricarboxylic acid cycle; the detection of numerous biochemical events of digestion, coagulation, muscular contraction and endocrine function, and their roles in the maintenance, control and integration of complex metabolic processes; the kinetic backgrounds to explain the observations of enzyme action and inhibition; and the development of protocols for examining the structures of functionally sensitive proteins. There has been exhaustive research on enzyme-catalyzed reactions and enzymes involved in cell metabolism. At present, 2000 different enzymes have been recognized, each of which catalyzes a different chemical reaction. Currently, more focus is being directed towards the application of enzymes. The high efficiency of enzymes makes them commercially valuable and their specificity of action is offering diverse advantages in clinical medicine.

1.2 Properties of enzymes

Enzymes are the complex protein molecules, often called biocatalysts, which are produced by living cells. They are highly specific both in the reactions that they catalyze and in their choice of reactants, which are known as substrates. An enzyme typically catalyzes a single chemical reaction or a set of closely related reactions [4]. Side reactions resulting in the wasteful formation of by-products are rare in enzyme-catalyzed reactions, in comparison to uncatalyzed ones. Enzymes can also be defined as soluble, colloidal and organic catalysts that are produced by living cells, but are capable of acting independently of the cells [4]. Enzymes are currently being used in diverse areas in the food, feed, paper, leather, agriculture and textiles industries, resulting in major cost reductions. Simultaneously, rapid scientific progress is now encouraging the chemistry and pharmacological industries to embrace enzyme technology, a trend supported by concerns regarding energy, raw materials, health and the environment. One of the most common advantages of enzymes is their ability to function continuously even after their removal or separation from the cells. This means that even after the separation of cells from *in vivo* environments, they continue to work efficiently under *in vitro* conditions; we can conclude that these biocatalysts remain in an active state even after their isolation. Enzymes are primarily non-toxic, biodegradable, and can be produced in large quantities by microorganisms for various industrial applications. In this chapter, the isolation, production, purification, utilization and application of enzymes (in soluble and immobilized or insoluble form) are discussed in detail. Procedures such as recombinant DNA technology and protein engineering are frequently used to produce more efficient and beneficial enzymes. The industrial production and utilization of enzymes is an important part of industry. Interdisciplinary collaboration between areas such as chemistry, process engineering, microbiology and biochemistry is required to develop the best possible enzyme technology, and eventually to achieve increased production and maintain the enzyme's physico-chemical properties under *in vitro* environments.

For catalytic action, small quantities of an enzyme are sufficient, where this quantity of enzyme is much smaller in comparison to its substrates. The overall concentration of substrate transformed per mass of enzyme is often very large. Without exception, all enzymes are proteinaceous and exhibit all the properties of a protein. The treatment of enzymes by extreme temperature or extreme pH, or by treatment with other denaturing agents, results in the complete loss of catalytic activity. Structural configurations such as the primary, secondary, tertiary and quaternary structures of enzyme proteins are essential for their catalytic activity. The degree of catalytic activity chiefly depends on the integrity of the enzyme's structure as a protein. As per reports, enzymes have molecular weights ranging from about 12 000 to over 1 million Da. A number of enzymes consist only of polypeptides and contain no chemical groups other than amino acid residues, e.g. pancreatic ribonuclease. Numerous enzymes require a specific, heat stable, low molecular weight organic molecule, known as a co-enzyme. Moreover, a number of enzymes require both a co-enzyme and one or more metal ions for activity. A complete biochemically active compound is formed by the combination of a catalytically active enzyme (also called the protein part) with a co-enzyme or a metal ion—this is called a holoenzyme. The protein part of a holoenzyme is called an apoenzyme. In this arrangement a co-enzyme may bind covalently or noncovalently to the apoenzyme. In certain enzymes the co-enzyme or metal ion is only loosely and transiently bound to the protein. However, in others it is tightly and permanently bound, in which case it is known as a prosthetic group. A prosthetic group signifies a covalently bound co-enzyme. According to reports, co-enzymes and metal ions are stable under heating, while the protein part of an enzyme (the apoenzyme), is denatured by heat.

$$\underset{\text{(Total enzyme)}}{\text{Holoenzyme}} = \underset{\text{(Protein)}}{\text{Apoenzyme}} + \underset{\text{(Non-protein)}}{\text{Prosthetic group}}$$

Prosthetic groups may be classified functionally into two major classes: co-enzymes and co-factors. Co-enzymes may be considered to be biosynthetically related to the vitamins, such as the co-enzyme nicotinamide adenine dinucleotide (NAD) which is vital for cellular energy metabolism and integrates the vitamin niacin into its chemical makeup. Moreover, a co-enzyme may be considered as a co-substrate, experiencing a chemical transformation throughout the enzyme reaction (NAD is reduced to NADH), the reversal of which requires a separate enzyme, perhaps from a different cellular site. Co-enzymes might thus travel intra-cellularly between apo-enzymes and, by transferring chemical groupings, integrate several metabolic processes. Table 1.2 shows a list of the more common co-enzymes and their functions. In contrast to co-enzymes, co-factors, such as pyridoxal phosphate or hem groups, remain with one enzyme molecule and in conjunction complete a cycle of a chemical change brought about by one enzyme turnover [5]. Other enzymes, such as carboxypeptidase, require metal ions as co-factors, the divalent

Table 1.2. Several co-enzymes employed in the transfer of specific atoms or functional groups.

Co-enzyme	Entity transferred
Thyamin pyrophosphate	Aldehydes
Tetrahydrofolate	Other one-carbon groups
Pyridoxal phosphate	Amino groups
Nicotinamide adenine dinucleotide	Hydrogen atoms (electrons)
Flavin adenine dinucleotide	Hydrogen atoms (electrons)
Co-enzyme A	Acyl groups
Biocytin	CO_2
3′-Deoxyadenorylcohalamine (co-enzyme B12)	H atoms and alkyl groups

Table 1.3. Several enzymes and their co-factors.

Enzyme	Co-factor(s)	Enzyme	Co-factor(s)
Pyruvate kinase	K^+ and Mg^+	Urease	Ni^{++}
Nitrate reductase	Mo	Peroxidase	Fe^{++} or Fe^{+++}
Glucose 6-phosphatase		Hexokinase	Mg^+
DNA polymerase	Zn	Glutathione peroxidase	Se
Cytochrome oxidase	Cu**	Cytochrome oxidase	Fe^{++} or Fe^{+++}
Carbonic anhydrase	Zn^{++}	Catalase	Fe^{++} or Fe^{+++}
Arginase	Mn	Alcohol dehydrogenase	Zn^{++}

cations Mg^{2+}, Zn^{2+} and Mn^{2+} being the most common; these are often called enzyme activators [6]. Table 1.3 lists several enzymes and their respective co-factors.

1.3 Catalysis

The role of a catalyst is to increase the speed of a chemical reaction. When the rate of a chemical reaction is governed by a soluble catalyst, which may result in a further increase in the rate of chemical reaction, it is called homogeneous catalysis. In this case catalysis occurs in a solution. When the catalyst is in a separate phase from the reactants, or when catalysis occurs on a insoluble surface or an immobilized matrix, it is known as heterogeneous catalysis. Enzymes are also called biological catalysts. These biological catalysts generally have the properties of homogeneous catalysts, however, a number of enzymes present in membranes are insoluble, and thus are called heterogeneous catalysts. Enzyme specificity is the absolute specificity of protein catalysts to identify and bind to only one or a few molecules. In this process the enzyme carries a defined arrangement of atoms in their active site to bind with the substrate. This active site on the enzyme should have a shape that accurately matches the substrates. Thus specificity is achieved when an enzyme with an active site binds with the chemical reactants (the substrates) at their active sites via weak bond interactions. To undergo a chemical reaction, this active site carries certain residues that form a temporary bond with the chemical reactants, termed the binding site, whereas the catalytic site carries the residues that are responsible for catalysis. Specificity is achieved when a substrate binds to an enzyme that has a defined arrangement of atoms in the active site. An enzyme always catalyzes a single type of chemical reaction, which involves the formation and breakdown of covalent bonds. Since they are specific to one particular reaction, this feature of enzymes is called reaction specificity, also known as absolute reaction specificity, i.e. no by-products are formed.

1.4 The structure of enzymes

Enzymes always act as catalysts and small quantities compared to their substrate are required to considerably increase the rate of chemical reactions, wherein the enzymes themselves experience no overall change [7, 8]. In contrast to all true catalysts, an enzyme does not alter the ultimate equilibrium position of a reaction, which is thermodynamically determined, thus merely the rate of completion of equilibrium of a feasible reaction is augmented. In addition to catalytic properties, enzymes exhibit the physico-chemical behavior of proteins: their solubility, electrophoretic properties, electrolytic behaviors and chemical reactivity [7, 8]. The primary structural configuration and catalytic action of enzymes is determined by the linear chain of amino acid residues linked via peptide bonds, which constitute a protein molecule. Localized folding of the primary structure is called a secondary structure, whereas the complete folding of the molecule is known as a tertiary structure. In contrast to these structural configurations, a quaternary structure is the agglomeration of several folded chains. The structural features of enzymes are shown in figures 1.1 and 1.2. In contrast to traditional chemical catalysts, e.g. hydrogen ions,

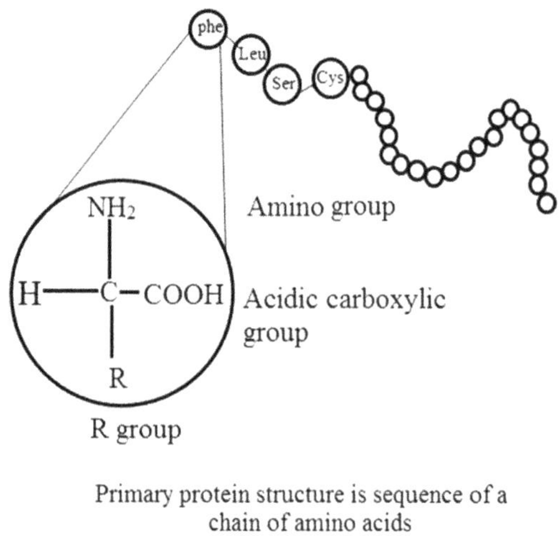

Figure 1.1. Structural features of enzyme.

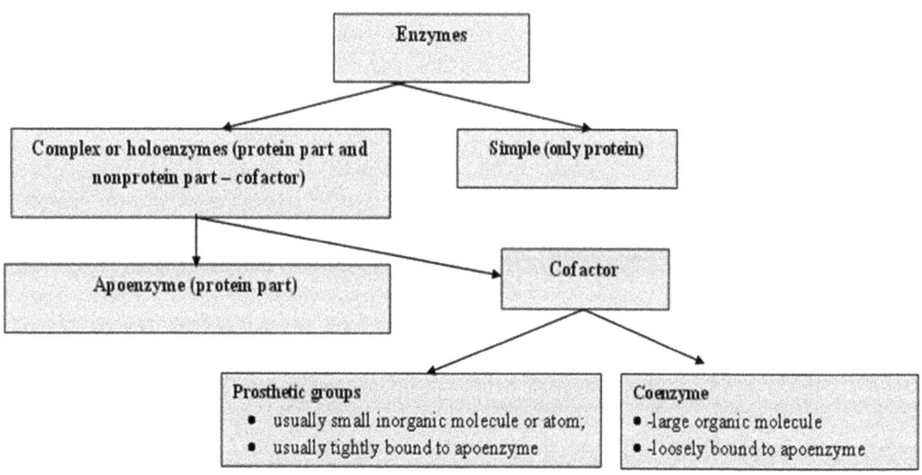

Figure 1.2. Principle components of an enzyme.

heavy metals or metal oxides, which are most effective in organic solvents, at very high temperatures or at extreme pH values, enzymes operate most efficiently under very mild conditions. When using enzymes, there are certain issues that require attention, such as deviation from homogeneous aqueous solutions, physiological pH and temperature, which can rapidly destroy enzyme activity. However, under normal conditions the increase in reaction rate is rarely matched by their non-protein counterparts.

1.5 Structural features: primary and secondary structures

Three-dimensional analysis of the amino acid sequence of lysozyme of hen's egg white has demonstrated some features essential for primary structure [9, 10]. These are:

- Molecules derived from a similar source have a similar order of amino acid residues and appear to be random with no obvious predictability.
- Even though numerous enzymes are intramolecularly crosslinked via disulfide bridges of cysteine, no branching occurs.

Current databases suggest that a small number of amino acids are extra and most are 'functional', i.e. the majority of them co-operatively control the higher orders of structural organization and therefore the catalytic activity. When comparing the primary structures of enzymes performing similar functions, wide structural homologies are detected in their sequence, mainly in the patterns of their nonpolar residues. For example, pancreatic juice contains five inactive precursors (zymogens), namely chymotrypsinogen A, B and C, trypsinogen and proelastase; all of these are activated to the respective proteases by proteolytic cleavage [11].

1.6 Nomenclature and classification

By 1950, many enzymes had been found; however, there was a lack of a systematic approach to their classification [12, 13]. The naming of numerous enzymes was characterized by misleading and uninformative names, leading to confusion around their nomenclature [14]. Following the guidance of the International Union of Biochemistry, formal recommendations were subsequently formulated. The interdependence of nomenclature and classification necessitates joint consideration and examination (figure 1.3) [15]. The suffix '-ase' is assigned to individual enzymes, which refer to single catalytic entities. Conversely, systems that consist of multiple enzymes are termed based on the overall reaction they catalyze, followed by the term 'system.' For instance, the fatty acid synthase system [16]. Enzymes are categorized based on the specific chemical reactions they catalyze, differentiating them from other enzymes [17]. Enzymes are categorized into several groups based on the specific sort of reaction they catalyze and the name(s) of the substrate(s) involved. This also serves as the foundation for numerical codes [18]. The first Enzyme Commission, established in 1961, developed a systematic approach to categorizing enzymes by assigning a unique numerical code to each enzyme. The code numbers, commonly utilized and identified by the prefix EC, consist of four distinct elements delineated by periods. Each element carries a specific significance as follows:

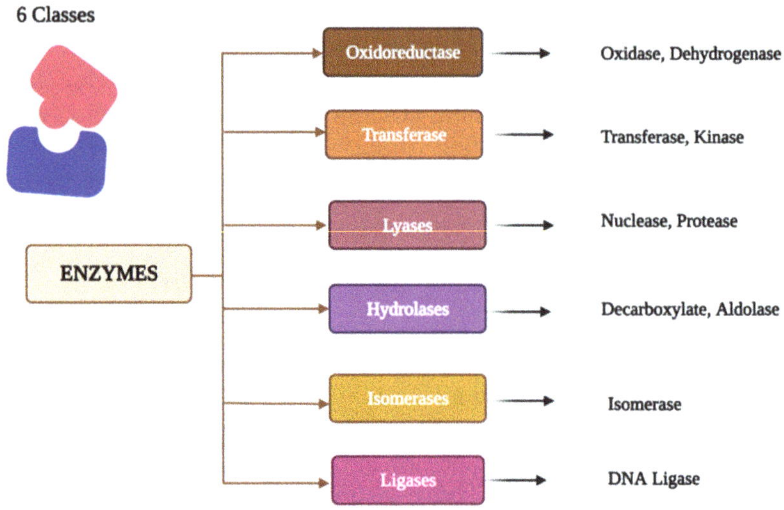

Figure 1.3. Educational diagram depicting the six major classes of enzymes with examples of their functions.

(1) The initial numeral indicates the specific central division or class to which the enzyme is categorized within the six primary divisions [19].
(2) The subsequent numeral denotes the subclassification of the enzyme.
(3) Denotes the sub-subclass.
(4) The digit denotes the enzyme's serial number within its sub-subclass.

1.6.1 Class 1—oxidoreductase

Enzymes, which facilitate oxidoreduction processes through catalysis, are categorized within this class [20]. The substance that undergoes oxidation is commonly referred to as the hydrogen donor. Pyruvate dehydrogenase is an excellent example of catalysts' outstanding role in facilitating oxidation and reduction reactions [21]. Catalysts are of the utmost importance in the process of enabling these reactions. The enzymatic activity of this enzyme is highly efficient in facilitating the oxidation reaction of pyruvate, leading to the production of acetyl co-enzyme A [22]. The group within the hydrogen (or electron) donor molecule that goes through oxidation is denoted by the second digit of the code number assigned to oxidoreductases. For example, the digit 'I' indicates the oxidation of a group with the formula -CHOH-[21].

1.6.2 Class 2—transferase

Enzymes belonging to the class known as transferases are responsible for facilitating the movement of certain groups from one chemical molecule to another [23]. Examples of such groups include methyl groups or glycosyl groups. This transfer occurs between a donor component and an acceptor compound [24].

$$X{-}Y + Z{-}H = X{-}H + Z{-}Y$$

The next digit in the code assigned to transferases denotes the group transferred during enzymatic reactions. For instance, a one-carbon group is transferred, whereas an aldehydic or ketonic group is transferred. The third digit provides more details regarding the specific group being transferred. For instance, subclasses are further separated into methyltransferases (EC 2.1.1), hydroxymethyl- and formyl transferase, and so forth [25].

1.6.3 Class 3—hydrolases

These enzymes facilitate the process of hydrolyzing substrates of high molecular weight. The mentioned cleaved bonds include C–O, C–N, and C–C and phosphoric anhydride bonds [26]. The classification of hydrolysis as transferases can be justified by considering it as the transfer of a particular group to water, which acts as the acceptor [27]. However, it is worth noting that the reaction involving water as the acceptor was usually identified before other reactions and is often regarded as the primary physiological function of the enzyme. This is why enzymes of this nature are categorized as hydrolases instead of transferases. The code number of hydrolases includes a second figure that denotes the hydrolyzed bond type [28]. For instance, enzymes with EC 3.1 code are classified as esterases, whereas those with EC 3.2 code are classified as glycosylases, and so on. For instance, the case of esterases includes carboxylic ester hydrolases, thioester hydrolases, and phosphoric monoester hydrolases. Similarly, in the context of glycosylases, it encompasses O-glycosidases, among others. In peptidyl-peptide hydrolases, the third parameter is mainly determined by the catalytic method, which is elucidated through investigations of the active center or the influence of pH [29].

1.6.4 Class 4—lyases

Lyases include a set of enzymes that help add or delete groups of chemicals from a substrate by methods that do not entail oxidation, reduction, or hydrolysis [30]. Transferases and hydrolases differ regarding the fate of the chemical group involved. Hydrolases are enzymes that catalyze the release of a chemical group in its unbound state, whereas transferases allow the transfer of a chemical group from one molecule to another [31]. Transferases are 'enzymes that facilitate the transfer of a chemical group from one molecule to another.' These enzymes catalyze the cleavage of C–C, C–O, C–N, and other bonds through an elimination reaction, forming double bonds or rings [32]. Alternatively, they can facilitate adding functional groups to existing double bonds. Decarboxylase, aldolase, and dehydratase are enzymatic catalysts that facilitate the removal of carbon dioxide, aldehyde, and water. The second digit within the code number denotes the specific bond that has been broken. For instance, carbon–carbon lyases correspond to carbon–oxygen lyases, and so on [33].

1.6.5 Class 5—isomerases

Enzymes are biological catalysts that facilitate the interconversion of isomers. The nomenclature of these enzymes is based on the specific form of isomerism they exhibit, which includes epimerases, racemases, cis–trans-isomerases, isomerases, tautomerizes, mutases, and cyclo-isomerases [34]. An intramolecular oxidoreduction process, classified occasionally, facilitates the substrate's interconversion. No oxidized product is formed when the hydrogen source and acceptor are the same molecule. Nevertheless, they can include tightly bound NAD(P) [35]. Hence, these enzymes do not fall under the category of oxidoreductases. The specific type of isomerism determines the formation of subclasses, while the sub-subclasses are determined by the specific type of substrates [36].

1.6.6 Class 6—ligases

Ligases represent a category of enzymes that help in the amalgamation of two different compounds by the hydrolysis of a diphosphate bond in adenosine triphosphate (ATP) or a related triphosphate molecule [37]. For instance, C–O bonds are associated with enzymes that acylate tRNA. Similarly, C–S bonds are formed by acyl-CoA derivatives. Subclasses are exclusively employed within the context of C–N ligases. Certain enzymes have been removed periodically, while others have undergone renumbering [38]. The responsibility for the naming and reclassifying of biological entities is exclusively entrusted to the International Union of Biochemistry. In instances where reclassification leads to the removal of an enzyme, the previous numerical designation remains not reassigned to a new enzyme but is forever removed. The repositioning of re-classified enzymes is accompanied by a note identifying their previous numerical designation for referencing [39]. The BRENDA enzyme database was established in 1987 and classifies enzymes based on the Enzyme Commission's list of enzymes and subsequent updates. The EC numbers encompass a total of 8423 distinct enzymes [40]. It is common for a wide range of enzymes with distinct characteristics to be classified under a single EC number. In incorporating fresh data into the database, a blend of computer-based and human controls is employed to uphold rigorous data quality. The present databank thoroughly compiles information about each enzyme [41]. The nomenclature of enzymes encompasses various details, including the EC number, systematic name, suggested name, synonyms, and CAS Registration Number. Likewise, the inclusion of reaction and specificity data offers comprehensive insights into various aspects of catalyzed reactions, including reaction type, natural substrate, substrate spectrum, product spectrum, inhibitors, co-factors, prosthetic groups, metal compounds/salts, turnover number, specific activity, K_m value, pH optimum and range, as well as temperature optimum and range [33]. The information about enzyme structure encompasses its molecular weight, subunit composition, and the presence of glycoprotein and lipoprotein components. The present inquiry seeks to elucidate pertinent details regarding the isolation and preparation of a particular substance [42].

1.7 The mechanism of action of enzymes

The mechanism of action is based on a chemical reaction, in which the enzyme binds to the substrate and finally forms an enzyme–substrate complex. This reaction take place in a relatively small area of the enzyme called the active or catalytic site. In other words, the mechanism of enzyme action is based on the nature of the enzyme–substrate interaction, which accounts for the reaction specificity of the biological catalysts. The active or catalytic site of an enzyme is constituted by several amino acids, located at some distance from each other in the peptide chain. These amino acids are brought close together by the folding resulting from the secondary and tertiary structure of the enzymes. Side chains of amino acid residues at the catalytic site provide groups for binding with specific groups of the substrate. Co-factors assist the catalysis. The substrate forms bonds with amino acid residues in the substrate binding domain of the active site. The binding induces a conformational reaction in the active site. During the reaction, the enzyme forms a transition-state complex. As the products of the reaction disassociate, the enzyme returns to the original state. Two different models postulated for the mechanism of enzyme action are given below.

1.7.1 The fisher template model (lock and key model)

This is a rigid model of the catalytic site, proposed by Emil Fischer in 1894 [43]. The model explains the interaction between a substrate and an enzyme in terms of a lock and key analogy. In this model, the catalytic site is presumed to be preshaped. The substrate fits as a key fits into a lock. The drawback of this model is the implied rigidity of the catalytic site. The model cannot explain changes in enzyme structure in the presence of allosteric modulators.

1.7.2 Induced fit model

In contrast to the above method, this model suggests a flexible mode for the catalytic site. To overcome the problems of the lock and key model owing to the rigid catalytic site, Koshland [44–46] suggested an induced fit model in 1963. The important feature of this procedure is the flexibility of the active site. In the induced fit model, the substrate induces a conformational change in the active site of the enzyme so that the substrate fits into the active site in the most convenient way so as to promote the chemical reaction. This method suggests competitive inhibition, allosteric modulation and inactivation of enzymes on denaturation.

The Michaelis–Menten theory of enzyme action [47] offers the basis for most current research on the mechanism of enzyme action. This concept of the enzyme–substrate complex scheme assumes the combination of the enzyme and substrate in phase one (occasionally known as the transition phase) of the enzyme activity and liberation of the enzyme and the products of the catalysis in phase two of the reaction.

$$\text{Enzyme} + \text{Substrate} \rightarrow \text{Enzyme} - \text{Substrate Complex} \rightarrow \text{Enzyme} + \text{Substrate}$$

Table 1.4. Various enzymes exhibiting covalent catalytic behavior.

Enzyme	Reactive group	Typical covalent enzyme–substrate intermediate
Chymotrypsin, trypsin, thrombin, esterase	Serine $HO–CH_2–CH–$	Acylserine
Phosphoglucomutase, alkaline phosphatase	Serine $HO–CH_2–CH–$	Phosphorylserine
Glyceraldehyde-3-phosphate dehydrogenase papain	Cysteine $HS–CH_2–CH–$	Acylcysteine

1.7.3 Covalent catalysis

Covalent catalysis is evidenced in enzymes capable of forming covalent bonds between the substance and the catalytic group of the active site [48]. A number of enzymes react with their substrates to form very unstable, covalently joined enzyme–substrate complexes, which undergo further reaction to yield products much more readily than in an uncatalyzed reaction. Several of the enzymes that exhibit covalent catalytic behavior are listed in table 1.4.

1.8 Catalysis via chymotrypsin

Hummel and Kalnitzky suggested an enzyme mechanism through the depiction of the sequential transition states experienced by the enzyme–substrate complex during catalysis [49]. Chymotrypsin is a digestive enzyme, responsible for proteolysis (breakdown of proteins and polypeptides) in the duodenum. Chymotrypsin favorably breaks peptide amide bonds (the carboxyl side of the amide bond is a large hydrophobic amino acid). These amino acids contain an aromatic ring in their side chain that fits into a 'hydrophobic pocket' of the enzyme. It is stimulated in the presence of trypsin. Trypsin and chymotrypsin are both serine proteases with high sequence and structural similarities, but with different substrate specificity [50, 51].

1.8.1 Intermediary stages of chymotrypsin

As discussed above, chymotrypsin is a protease enzyme that cuts on the C-terminal phenylalanine, tryptophan and tyrosine on peptide chains [52]. Additionally, it is more specific for aromatic amino acids because of its hydrophobic pocket. Comparable to other serine proteases, chymotrypsin also catalyzes the hydrolysis of certain esters [53]. The molecular events involved in catalysis are called intermediary enzymology. Chymotrypsin, a protease, favorably accelerates breakdown of peptide bonds in which the aromatic amino acid (Phy, Try, or Trp) or bulky nonpolar R group (Met) contribute a carboxyl group. The synthetic substrate p-nitrophenyl acetate allows colorimetric analysis of chymotrypsin activity, as hydrolysis to p-nitrophenol, which is alkali, changes into the chromophore anionic forms.

1.8.2 Kinetic behavior of α-chymotrypsin

The kinetics of chymotrypsin of p-nitrophenyl acetate can be considered in a 'stop-flow' apparatus. This procedure utilizes substrate quantities of enzymes and measures the events in the first few milliseconds [54]. The use of p-nitrophenyl acetate as a substrate offers the prospect of investigating solvent effects on both the acylation of the enzyme and the hydrolysis (deacylation) of the acyl enzyme [54]. The significant features of the slow-flow kinetics of chymotrypsin are:

- Release of p-nitrophenyl anion with chymotrypsin. Hydrolysis of p-nitrophenyl acetate occurs in two different phases: a burst phase featuring rapid liberation of an anion.
    - a subsequent 'steady-state' phase, with slower release of extra anion.
- In catalysis by chymotrypsin, the slow stage is hydrolysis of the chymotrypsin–acetate (CT–Ac) complex. When all the existing chymotrypsin has been converted to CT–Ac, no further release of p-nitrophenyl acetate anion can take place until more free chymotrypsin is released by the slow, hydrolytic elimination of acetate anion from the CT–Ac complex [55, 56]. The free chymotrypsin then is presented for further formation of chymotrypsin–p-nitrophenyl acetate complexes (CT–PNP) and CT–Ac complexes with attendant liberation of PNP. The development and decay of the enzyme–substrate complex, based on the Michaelis–Menten kinetics can be represented as [55, 56]:

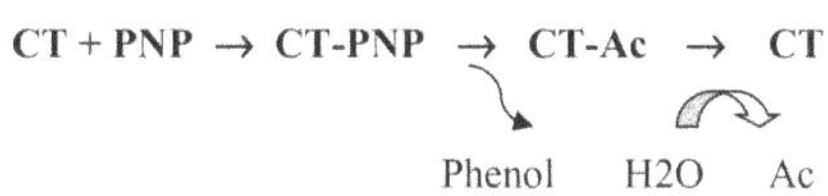

  where CT = chymotrypsin, PNP = p-nitrophenyl acetate, CT–PNP = chymotrypsin–p-nitrophenyl acetate complex and CT–Ac = chymotrypsin–acetate complex. In comparison to the hydrolysis of the CT–Ac complex, the formation of CT–PNP and CT–Ac complexs is relatively fast.
- A 'charge relay network' acts as a proton shuttle during catalysis by chymotrypsin. The charge relay network of chymotrypsin encompasses three aminoacyl residues that are far apart in a primary structural sense, but close together in a tertiary structural sense. While most of the charged residues of chymotrypsin are present at the surface of the molecule, those of the charge relay network are hidden in the otherwise nonpolar inner side of the protein. These charges transmit residues which activate sequential proton shifts that

shuttle protons in the opposite direction. An equivalent series of proton shifts is assumed to accompany the hydrolysis of the physiologic chymotrypsin substrate, e.g. a peptide.

1.8.3 Selective proteolysis in creation of the catalytic sites of enzymes

Various enzymes, hormones and other physiologically active proteins are produced as inactive precursors (zymogens) that are further transformed to the active form by selective enzymatic cleavage (limited proteolysis) of peptide bonds. The final step to activating enzymatic function is limited proteolysis, either in a single activation step or in a consecutive series (cascade). The specificity of each activation reaction is evaluated by the complementarity of the zymogen substrate and the active site of the attacking protease. The arrangement of successive activation reactions is controlled by the specificity of each enzyme, while the extent of amplification of the initial stimulus is evaluated by the effectiveness of each activating step. Zymogen activation produces a prompt and irreversible response to a physiological stimulus, and is capable of initiating new physiological functions. Classical examples are the processes of hormone production, fibrinolysis, complement activation, blood coagulation, supra-molecular assembly, metamorphosis, fertilization and digestion. The zymogens of the pancreatic serine proteases, in particular, have functioned as models for detailed studies of the nature of the molecular changes that are involved in the intense increase in enzymatic activity that results upon incomplete proteolysis of the zymogen.

Specific proteolysis is a common means of activating enzymes and other proteins in biological systems. A number of proteins are manufactured and released in the form of inactive precursor proteins called proproteins. Various enzymes attain full enzymatic activity as they suddenly fold into their characteristic three-dimensional forms. In contrast, other enzymes are produced as inactive precursors that are successively activated by breakdown of one or a few specific peptide bonds. The inactive precursor is known as a zymogen (or a pro-enzyme). In other words, when the proteins are enzymes, the proteins are called pro-ezymes or zymogens (table 1.5). An energy source (ATP) is not required for cleavage [11]. Thus, in comparison to reversible regulation by phosphorylation, even proteins sited outside cells can be triggered by this means. An additional noteworthy difference is that proteolytic activation, in comparison with allosteric control and reversible covalent modification, occurs just once in the life of an

Table 1.5. Gastric and pancreatic zymogens.

Active enzyme	Zymogen	Site of production
Chymotrypsin	Chymotrypsinogen	Pancreas
Trypsin	Trypsinogen	Pancreas
Carboxypeptidase	Procarboxypeptidase	Pancreas
Elastase	Proelastase	Pancreas
Pepsin	Pepsinogen	Stomach

enzyme molecule. Transformation of a proprotein to the mature protein includes selective proteolysis. This transforms the proproteins by one or more consecutive proteolytic clips to a arrangement in which the individual activity of the mature protein (its enzymatic activity) is expressed, e.g. the hormone insulin (proinsulin), the digestive enzyme chymotrypsin (chymotrypsinogen), a number of factors for blood clotting and for the blood clot dissolution cascades, and the connective tissue protein collagen (procollagen). Chymotrypsinogen consists of 245 amino acid residues, and is practically devoid of enzymatic activity. As the reaction starts, it is converted into a fully active enzyme. This occurs when the peptide bond joining arginine 15 and isoleucine 16 is cleaved by trypsin. The subsequent active enzyme, known as π-chymotrypsin, then acts on other π-chymotrypsin molecules. Two dipeptides are eliminated to form α-chymotrypsin (the stable form of the enzyme) [11]. The three subsequent chains in α-chymotrypsin remain interconnected to each another by two interchain disulfide bonds. The outstanding feature of this process is that cleavage of a single specific peptide bond alters the protein from a catalytically inactive form into one that is fully active. The transformation of prochymotrypsin (Pro-CT), a 2,4,5-aminoacyl residue polypeptide, to the active enzyme α-chymotrypsin includes three proteolytic clips and the formation of an active intermediate called π-chymotrypsin (π-CT) and consequently to the mature catalytically active enzyme α-chymotrypsin (α-CT). Examples of gastric and pancreatic zymogens are listed in table 1.5.

1.8.4 Kinetic models for enzymes

Generally, enzyme kinetics is defined as the study of the rate of reactions, i.e., how the substrate concentration impacts the velocity of the reaction. Enzyme kinetics involves optimization of bio-catalytic reactions to allow process design and scaling up processes to further increase the production and minimize the overall overhead costs of various procedures. Kinetic investigations in the branch of biochemistry concerned with enzymes can be categorized into three types:

- *Transient-state kinetics*: This is the stage of reaction before the steady or rapid-equilibrium state, and involves quick reactions between the enzymes and substrate. These sudden changes in the reaction mixture when the substrate and enzymes are mixed require advance equipment to monitor the reaction before it changes into the steady state. The mechanisms of the reaction are associated with the enzyme structural configuration. Basic steps are involved during an enzyme-catalyzed reaction, which allow the direct study of the intermediates and products formed during a single enzyme cycle, which may further help in direct analysis of individual reaction steps for short times. In this type of reaction a sufficient concentration of enzymes is used to witness the intermediate and product formation.
- *Steady-state kinetics*: This is the phase in which the rate of formation of intermediates and the rate of decomposition remain the same, and thus the concentrations of reactive intermediates remain the same. During this reaction substrate concentration is greater than enzyme concentration. The

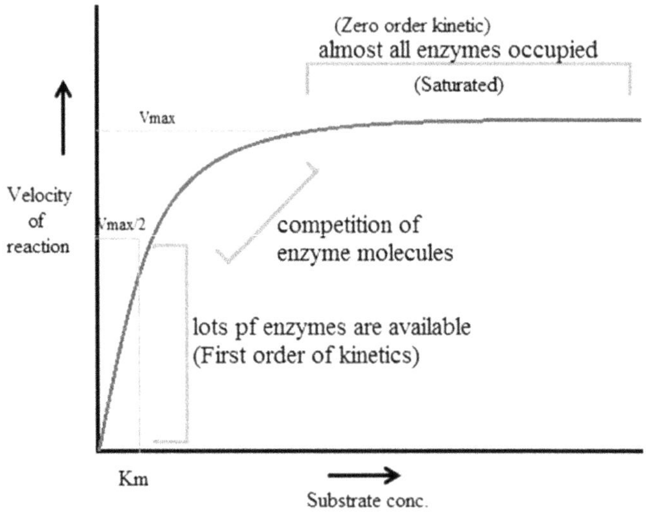

Figure 1.4. The Michaelis–Menten enzyme kinetic.

Michaelis–Menten enzyme kinetic (figure 1.4) can be considered as the most often studied reaction for several enzymes. For example, chymotrypsin (protease) with a high concentration of substrate achieves maximum velocity of the reaction (called the first order of reaction) but at a certain point the substrate occupies all binding sites of the enzyme, after which further addition of substrate does not increase the rate. This is called the zeroth order of reaction (the steady state). It is the phase in which the enzyme and substrate concentrations cannot be determined using the dissociation constant. Thus steady-state enzyme kinetics is based on the theory that a catalytic reaction remains constant if the reaction is not exposed to continuous changes.

- *Rapid-equilibrium kinetics*: This the phase in which both the enzyme and substrate concentrations can be determined using the dissociation constant. During this procedure total enzyme concentration remains constant during the reaction and the concentration is very small compared to the amount of substrate. In this reaction, before the rate-determining reaction, the reactions are in equilibrium with their components, thus this stage is called rapid-equilibrium kinetics.

According to reports, factors that affect enzyme-catalyzed reactions also affect the velocity of a reaction. These factors are called modifiers of enzyme-catalyzed reactions. These modifiers can be divided into two classes: inorganic modifiers (enzyme activators) and organic modifiers (enzyme inhibitors). These factors can have different types of effects on the velocity of the reaction; nevertheless the most vital effect is that they offer many pathways to products, e.g. when one modifier is bound to an enzyme, it alters the rate of reaction and thus forms two rate constants.

However, when two modifiers participate, there are five self-regulating equilibria, resulting in three paths for making products.

There are two mechanisms, single-substrate and multiple-substrate, that are helpful in studying the different stages of enzymatic reactions. Understanding these stages helps in understanding the properties of enzymes. Certain enzymes have single substrates (a single-substrate binding site), e.g. triosephosphate isomerase, whereas certain enzymes have multiple substrates molecules (multiple binding sites), such as dihydrofolate reductase, and bind with multiple substrates. After the exploration of specific RNA sequences required for RNA replication, new biocatalysts in the form of ribozymes have emerged with the potential to catalyze specific biochemical reactions. There is a misconception about biological catalysts that all biological catalysts are made up of proteins, which is not true; some are RNA-based catalysts (ribozymes and ribosomes). Both are important for many cellular functions. A major difference between enzymes and ribozymes is that RNA-based catalysts are restricted to only a few reactions; however, their reaction mechanisms and kinetics can be studied and classified by similar procedures. Enzyme-based mutation, in particular site-directed mutagenesis, is an important approach to alter genes and investigate the functional and structural features of enzymes, e.g. mutation of the enzyme present in *Coprinus cinereus* peroxidase offers an understanding of its increased thermostability. Challenges involved in studying cascades of reactions catalyzed by a multi-enzyme, e.g. proteasome involved in the ubiquitin–proteasome pathway, can be overcome by establishing understanding of the complex structure and the respective biochemical reactions. This understanding allows exploration of active sites, intermediate compounds, final products and their interrelation with complex machinery, as well as biochemical reactions. It has been well understood that enzymes that accelerate complex reactions have numerous substrates and involve complex enzyme kinetic mechanisms. As discussed above, most of the biochemical reactions occurring in the body are multi-substrate reactions. In such reactions two substrates are involved and yield two products (figure 1.5). These types of reactions involve the transfer of a compound from one compoment to another, e.g. when glucose reacts with ATP in the presence of hexokinase it forms glucose 6-phophaste and ADP. Here, phosphate from ATP is transfered to glucose to form glucose 6 phosphate. The mechanism of catalysis involves two types of reactions: sequential and non-sequential reactions. Sequential reaction results in the formation of a ternary complex. This means that both of the substrates involved in the reaction bind with an enzyme to form the product (figure 1.5). Sequential reaction is further divided into two types: the random and compulsory order mechanisms. As the name suggests, in a 'random' mechanism, either substrate can bind first and any product can leave first. In contrast to the random order mechanism, in the compulsory order mechanism the order of binding of the substrate and order of release of the product is specific; this is also called the Theorell–Chance mechanism (figure 1.5). In a non-sequential reaction, also called the 'ping-pong' mechanism, formation of ternary complex does not take place. In these types of reactions, when the first substrate binds with enzyme its product is released, and then the second substrate binds and its product is released. Such a reaction is called a double placement reaction. Thus only

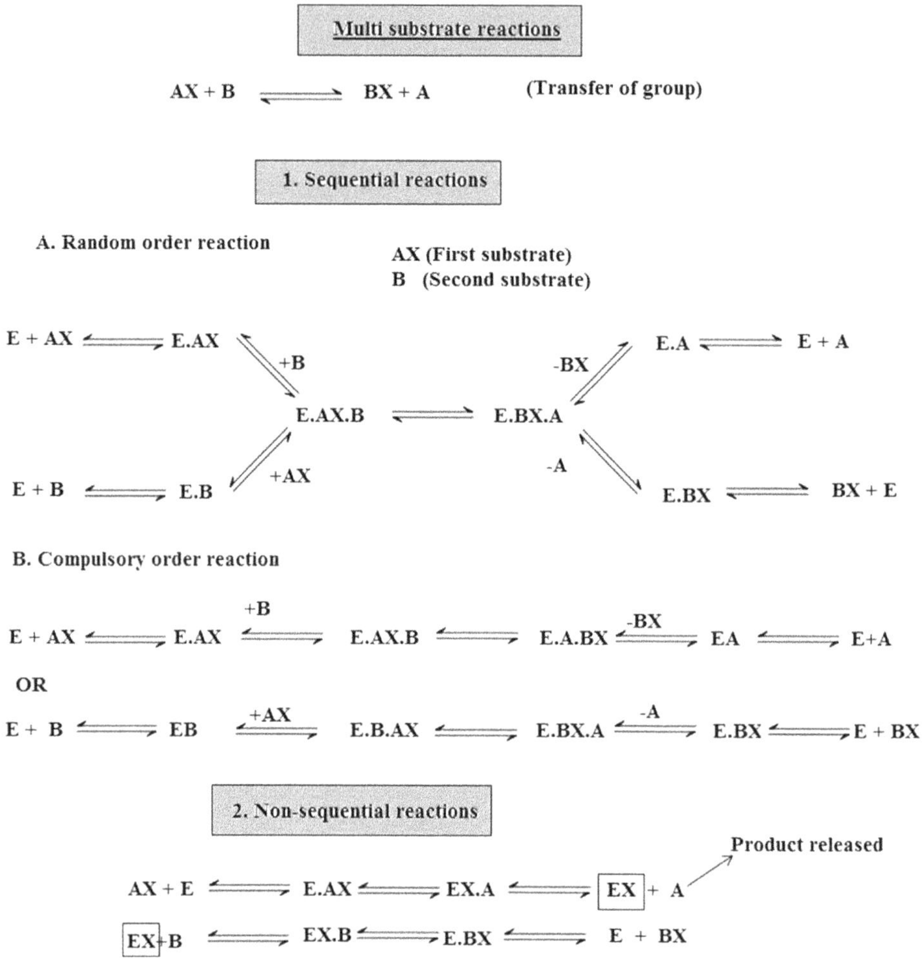

Figure 1.5. Multi-substrate reactions.

a single substrate binds at a time; this may be due to the presence of a single binding site on the enzyme. Major differences between the sequential and non-sequential reactions are that the formation of a ternary complex takes place only in the sequential reaction, and that in the sequential reaction both substrates bind to the enzyme and release products, while in the non-sequential mechanism the substrates bind and release their products one after the other (figure 1.5).

Another type of sequential mechanism is the systematic mechanism, which involves the addition of substrates and formation of products in a specific order.

1.8.5 Enzyme mediated acid–base (general) catalysis

Several protein enzymes use general acid–base catalysis as a way to increase reaction rates [57]. The amino acid histidine is optimized for this function because it has a pK_a (where K_a is the acid dissociation constant) near physiological pH [57].

When the substrate has been bound at the catalytic site, the charged functional groups of the side chains of neighboring aminoacyl residues may contribute in catalysis by behaving as acidic or basic catalysts. There are two extensive groups of acid–base catalysis by enzymes: general and specific (acid or base) catalysis. Specific acid or specific base catalysis are those reactions in which the reaction rates fluctuate under the influence of changes in H^+ or H_3O^+ concentration, but are independent of the concentrations of the other acids or bases present in the solution. In contrast to specific catalysis, general acid or general base catalysis are the reactions whose rates are very reactive to all acids (proton donors) or bases (proton acceptors) present in the solution. To examine whether a given enzyme-catalyzed reaction is a general or specific acid or base catalysis, the rate of reaction is determined under two sets of circumstances:

- at different pH values at a constant buffer concentration, and
- at constant pH values but at different buffer concentrations. Against this background, if the degree of the reaction deviates as a function of pH at a constant buffer concentration, the reaction is specific base/acid catalyzed if the pH is above/below 7.0. If the reaction rate at a constant pH rises as the buffer concentration increases, the reaction is general base/acid catalysis, if the pH is above/below 7.0.

1.8.6 Metallozymes

Almost 25% of all enzymes include tightly bound metal ions or need them for activity. The major role of these metal ions is investigated using techniques such as x-ray crystallography, magnetic resonance imaging (MRI) and electron spin resonance (ESR). A metalloprotein is a protein that contains a metal ion co-factor. Metallozymes contain a certain amount of functional metal ion that is retained during the course of purification [58]. A metal-activated enzyme binds with metals less firmly, but needs to be activated by addition of metals. Four types of complexes are possible for the tertiary complexes of the catalytic site (Enz), a metal ion (M) and substrate (S) that exhibit 1:1:1 stoichiometry:

Enz--S--M

Substrate-bridge complex

M--Enz--S

Enzyme-bridge complex

Enz--M--S

Simple metal-bridge complex

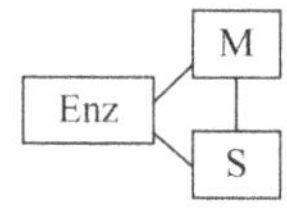

Cyclic metal-bridge complex

All of these complexes are possible for metal-activated enzymes. Metallozymes cannot form the EnzSM complex (substrate–bridge complexes), as the purified enzyme exists as Enz–M. Three generalization can be made:

- The majority of the kinases (ATP: phosphotransferases) form substrate–bridge complexes of the type enzyme–nucleotide–M.
- Phosphotransferases (phosphoenolpyruvate or pyruvate used as the substrate), enzymes catalyzing other reactions of phosphoenolpyruvate and carboxylases, form metal bridge complexes (Enz–M–S).
- A particular enzyme may form one type of bridge complex with one substrate and a different type with another.

The metal ions participate in each of the four mechanisms by which the enzymes are known to accelerate the rates of chemical reaction:

- Approximation of reactants.
- Covalent catalysis.
- General acid–base catalysis.
- Induction of strain in the enzyme or substrate.

Metal ions are electrophiles (attracted to electrons) and share an electron pair forming a sigma bond. They may also be considered as super acids as they exist in neutral solutions, frequently having a positive charge which is greater than their quantity. Mn^{2+}, Ca^{2+} and Mg^{2+} are the metal ions that are most commonly used in enzymatic catalysis. Two metal ions, iron and manganese are used in the form of haemprotein. Metal ions have the potential to accept electrons via sigma or pi bonds to successively activate electrophiles or nucleophiles. By means of donating electrons, metals can activate nucleophiles or act as nucleophiles themselves. The co-ordination sphere of a metal may bring together the enzyme and substrate or form chelate-producing distortion in either the enzyme or substrate [59]. A metal ion may also mask a nucleophile and thus avoid an otherwise probable side reaction. Metals can also function as three-dimensional templates for the co-ordination of basic groups on the enzyme or substrate.

1.9 Enzyme inhibition

Enzyme inhibition decreases the activity of an enzyme without significantly disrupting its three-dimensional macromolecular structure. Inhibition is therefore distinct from denaturation and is the result of a specific action by a reagent directed or transmitted to the active site region. When low molecular weight compounds interfere with the activity of enzymes by partially reducing or completely inhibiting the enzyme activity either reversibly or irreversibly, it is known as enzyme inhibition. The compounds responsible for such inhibition are called enzyme inhibitors. To protect the enzyme catalytic site from any change, a ligand binds with a critical side chain in the enzyme. Chemical modification can be performed to test the inhibitor for any drug value. Studies of enzymes can yield much information about the following:

- A number of drugs useful in medicine, which seem to function because they can inhibit certain enzymes in malfunctioning cells.
- The convenience of elucidating metabolic pathways in cells.
- The mechanism of the catalytic activity.
- The nature of the functional group at the active site.
- The substrate specificity of the enzyme.

The pharmacological action of drugs is mainly based on enzyme inhibition, e.g. sulfonamides and other antibiotics. In the majority of cases the enzyme inhibited is known. The development of nerve gases, insecticides and herbicides is based on enzyme inhibition studies. There are two major types of enzyme inhibition: reversible and irreversible.

Reversible inhibitors efficiently bind to enzymes by forming weak non-covalent interactions, e.g. ionic bonds, hydrophobic interactions and hydrogen bonds. Reversible inhibitors do not form any strong chemical bonds or reactions with the enzyme, they are formed quickly and can easily be removed, in contrast to irreversible inhibitors. Reversible inhibition includes competitive inhibition, uncompetitive inhibition and noncompetitive inhibition. Irreversible inhibition includes group specific inhibition (reacts only to a certain chemical group), reactive substrate analogs (affinity label) and inhibitors that are structurally similar to the substrate and will bind to the active site, and mechanism-based inhibitors (enzymes transform the inhibitor into a reactive form within the active site).

Table 1.6. Industrially produced enzymes from plant sources and their applications.

Enzyme	Source(s)	Application(s)
β-Amylase	Barley, soy bean	Baking, preparation of maltose syrup
Bromelain	Pineapple	Baking
Esterase	Wheat	Ester hydrolysis
Ficin	Fig meat	Tenderizer
Papain	Papaya	Meat tenderizer, tanning, baking
Peroxidase	Horse radish	Diagnostic
Urease	Jack bean	Diagnostic

1.10 Pharmaceutical applications

Currently, enzymes are often utilized for a broad range of applications such as: washing powders (e.g. proteases, lipases, amylases); textile manufacture (amylases and catalase to remove the starch); the leather industry (proteases to hydrolyze proteins); the paper industry; improvement of the environment; food production (enzyme-modified cheese/butter), processing (glucose oxidase for dough strengthening) and preservation; and medical applications. According to current reports, several enzymes are produced industrially and there are significant applications in the food industry (45% of use), detergent industry (35%), textiles industry (10%) and leather industry (3%). Details on the applications of individual enzymes are provided in table 1.6.

1.10.1 Diagnostic applications of enzymes

Enzymes have been used widely in diagnostic applications varying from immunoassays to biosensors. Enzyme immunoassay methods hold great promise for application under a wide variety of conditions. Under laboratory conditions they can be as sensitive as

Table 1.7. Diagnostically significant enzymes.

Enzyme and abbreviation	Tissue source[a]	Reaction
γ-Glutamyl transferase GGT	K L	γ-Glutamyl peptide to γ-glutamylamino acid
Ornithine carbamoyltransferase	L	Carbamoyl-P to citrulline
OCT triacylglycerol lipase	Pa	Triacylglycerol to diacylglycerol and fatty acid
Lactate dehydrogenase LD	H L M K	Lactate to pyruvate
Isocitrate dehydrogenase ICD	L	Isocitrate to oxoglutarate
Hydroxybutyrate dehydrogenase HBD (LD I)	H	2-Hydroxybutyrate to 2-oxybutyrate
Fructose-biphosphate aldolase ALD	M H	Fructose-1,6-biphosphate to triosephosphate
Creatine lipase CPK	M H B	Creatine to creatine phosphate
Chymotrypsin CT	Pa	Proteins to polypeptides
Cholinesterase CHE	L	Acylcholine to fatty acid and choline
Aspartate aminotransferase GOT (AST)	H L M K B	Aspartate to glutamate
Alkaline phosphatase AP	B I L Pl K	Phosphate monoester to alcohol and Pi (pH 8–10)
Alanine aminotransferase GPT (AAT)	L	Alanine to gultamate
Acid phosphatase SP	Pr E	Phosphate monoester to alcohol and Pi (pH 8–10)
Acetylcholinesterase ACHE	B E	Acetylcholine to acetate and choline
α-Amylase	Pa S	Starch to maltose
5′-Nucleosidase 5.N	Ht Pa	5′-Ribonucleotide to ribonucleoside

[a] B, brain; E, erythrocytes; H, heart muscle; Ht, hepatobiliary tract; I, intestinal mucosa; K, kidney; L, M, skeletal muscle; Pa, pancreas; P1, placenta; Pr, prostate gland; S, saliva.

radio-immunoassays, but they can also be adapted as simple field screening procedures [60, 61]. The examination of enzyme quantity in the extracellular body fluids (blood plasma and serum, urine, digestive juices, amniotic fluid and cerebrospinal fluid) are vital aids to the clinical diagnosis and management of disease. Most enzyme-catalyzed reactions occur within living cells, however, when an energy imbalance occurs in the cells because of exposure to infective agents, bacterial toxins, etc, enzymes 'leak' through the membranes into the circulatory system. This causes their fluid level to be raised above the normal cell level. Estimation of the type, extent and duration of these raised enzyme activities can then furnish information on the identity of the damaged cell and indicate the extent of injury. Enzyme assays can make an important contribution to the diagnosis of diseases, as a minute change in enzyme concentration can easily be measured. Determination of the changes in enzyme level thus offers a greater degree of organ and disease differentiation in comparison to other possible clinico-chemical parameters, e.g. albumin or gamma globulin. Currently, the diagnostic specificity of enzyme tests is such that they are limited primarily to confirming diagnosis, offering data to be weighed alonside other clinical reports, owing to lack of disease specific enzymes. Table 1.7 includes a number of diagnostically important enzymes which are most often examined in clinic laboratories [60–62].

1.10.1.1 Enzyme examinations in diseases of the liver and biliary

The diseases of the liver and gastrointestinal tract were among the first to which serum enzyme tests were applied. They have proved to be most effective owing to the large size of the organs and the wide range and abundance of enzymes [63–66]. The liver-based enzymes GOT, GPT and AP are examined to evaluate the site and nature of liver disease. LD, GGT, OCT and CHE are also examined. Several enzymes employed in the diagnosis of liver diseases along with their respective levels are listed in table 1.8.

1.10.1.2 Enzyme applications in heart disease

According to previous reports, no single enzyme has yet been reported to cure myocardial damage. The discovery of serum glutamine oxalacetic acid transaminase determination (GOT) in 1954 was considered a significant step forward in the diagnosis of acute myocardial infarction. A mixture of results from assays of CPK

Table 1.8. Liver diseases and enzymes used in diagnosis [32–36].

Disease	Enzyme used	Enzyme level
Solvent poisoning of liver	GOT, GPT and LD	GOT:GPT:LD 6500:3000:10 000 (U ml^{-1})
Hepatobiliary disease (obstructive jaundice)	GOT and GPT	5–10 times normal level
Fatty liver	GPT	2 times normal level
Chronic hepatitis and cirrhosis	All liver transaminases	3–12 times normal level and inflammation of the liver
Acute hepatitis	GOT and GPT	20–50 times normal level

(creatine phosphokinase), HBD (α-hydroxybutyrate dehydrogenase) and GOT (glutamine oxalacetic acid transaminase)—each of which has been shown to be elevated in more than 90% of cases—is used for diagnostic purposes [67, 68]. The level of CPK starts rising three to four hours after the initial onset of pain, followed in order by GOT and AST (HBD) which appear after approximately eight hours. The maximum levels are reached in the same sequence, CPK after 24 h, LD 1 after 36 h and AST after about two days. The rise in enzyme levels is fairly moderate, AST and CPK increase by four to ten times their respective normal levels and LD 1 is approximately five-fold higher than normal. An enzyme known as hyaluronidase (hyaluronate hydrolysis) has been reported to cure heart attack [68]. The activity of many enzymes including aldolase, malic dehydrogenase, isomerase and ICD may increase following myocardial infarction [67, 68].

1.10.1.3 Diagnosis of muscle disease

Skeletal muscle disorders include diseases of the muscle fibers (myopathies) or of the muscle nerves (neurogenic disorders) [69]. In myopathies CPJ, LD, ALD, GOT and GPT levels are raised. In the case of neurogenic diseases and hereditary diseases, CPK is occasionally raised (2–3 fold) [69]. Damage to the muscle may be due to extensive muscular exercise, drugs, physical trauma, inflammatory diseases, microbial infection or metabolic dysfunction, or it may be genetically predisposed. In muscular disorders the level of CPK is elevated in serum with the highest frequency and is assayed in the diagnosis of these disorders. An additional useful assayed enzyme is acetylcholinesterase (AChE), which is significant in regulating certain nerve impulses [70]. Various pesticides affect this enzyme, so farm labors are frequently tested to be sure that they have not received accidental exposure to significant agricultural toxins. There are number of enzymes that are characteristically used in the clinical laboratory to diagnose diseases. There are highly specific markers for enzymes active in the pancreas, red blood cells, liver, heart, brain, prostate gland and many of the endocrine glands [70]. From the time when these enzymes became comparatively easy to examine using automated techniques, they have been part of the standard blood tests that veterinarians and medical doctors are likely to need in the diagnosis and treatment/management of diseases.

1.10.2 Enzymes in therapeutics

Enzymes have two significant features that differentiate them from all other types of drugs. First, enzymes frequently bind and act on their targeted sites with high affinity and specificity. Second, enzymes are catalytic and convert numerous target molecules to the desired products. These two important features make enzymes specific and potent drugs that can achieve therapeutic biochemistry in the body that small molecules cannot. These features have resulted in the development of many enzyme-based drugs for a wide range of disorders [71]. Currently, numerous enzymes are used as therapeutic agents, owing to the following features:

- High specificity to their substrates.
- Proficient in producing the desired effect without provoking any side effects.

Table 1.9. Therapeutically important enzymes.

Enzyme preparation	Source	Therapeutic application
Aspargenase	*Escherichia coli*, guinea pig serum	Cytotoxic agents
Bromelain	*Ananas comosus*	Inflammation, edema
Chymotrypsin	Bovine pancreas	Inflammation edema ophthalmology and upper respiratory tract diseases
Deoxyribonuclease (DNA hydrolysis)	Bovine pancreas	Reduces viscosity of pulmonary secretions
Dextranase (dextran hydrolysis)	*Penicillium funiculosum*	Dental plaque restriction
Diastase (starch hydrolysis)	Malt	Amylaceous dyspepsia
Galactosidase (lactose hydrolysis)	*Aspergillus niger*	Inherited β-galactosidase deficiency
Hyaluronidase (mucopolysaccharide hydrolysis)	Animal testes	Increase absorption rate, increase effectiveness of local anesthetics
Pancreatin	Animal pancreas	Pancreatitis
Papain (protease)	*Carica papaya*	Dyspepsia and gastritis
Penicillinase	*Bacillus cereus*	Penicillin allergy
Plasmin (protease)	Plasminogen	Thrombotic disorders anticoagulation
Streptodornase (DNAase)	Streptococci	Depolymerization of DNA in purulent exudates
Streptokinase (protease)	Streptococci	Thromboemolic diseases
Tissue plasminogen activator (protease)	Recombinant DNA technology	Thromboeniolic diseases
Trypsin (protease)	Animal pancreas	Cleaning necrotic tissue
Urokinase (protease)	Human urine	Thromboemolic diseases

- Water soluble.
- Extremely effective in a biological environment.

Enzymes as therapeutic agents also have some serious disadvantages which restrict their application. Their bulky structure, due to their large molecular weight, excludes them from the intracellular domain. Owing to their high proteinaceous nature they are highly antigenic and are rapidly cleared from blood plasma. Extensive purification from pyrogens and toxins is essential for parenteral enzymes, which increases the cost. Table 1.9 lists some therapeutically important enzymes.

1.10.2.1 Enzyme therapy of cancer

In traditional medicine, proteolytic enzymes derived from plant extracts have been used for a long time In addition to proteolytic enzymes from natural resources such as plants, 'modern' enzyme therapy includes pancreatic enzymes. Therapeutically, the use of proteolytic enzymes is partly based on scientific reports and is partly empirical [72]. Clinical evidence of the use of proteolytic enzymes in cancer studies has typically been obtained with an enzyme preparation comprising a combination of papain, trypsin and chymotrypsin. Earlier reports proved that enzyme therapy can reduce the adverse effects caused by radiotherapy and chemotherapy. There is also a report available that, in some types of tumors, survival may be sustained. The positive effects of systemic enzyme therapy appear to be based on its anti-inflammatory potential. Nevertheless, the exact mechanism of action of systemic enzyme therapy remains unsolved. The proportion of proteinases to antiproteinases, which is regularly used as a prognostic marker in cancer studies, is likely to be influenced by the oral administration of proteolytic enzymes, most likely via induction of the synthesis of antiproteinases. In addition, there are many alterations of cytokine composition during treatment with orally administered enzymes, which might be a sign of the efficacy of enzyme therapy [73].

Proteases and their inhibitors have long been studied in several tumor systems. However, out of numerous promising serine and metalloproteinase inhibitors, not a single one is included in oncology at present. The present exploration for active antiproteolytic agents is in contrast to the traditional approach, as evidenced by John Beard, who proposed the management of advanced cancer using fresh pancreatic extracts whose antitumor activity was based on their proteolytic potential.

The enzymatic treatment of tumors is based on the idea of denying the abnormal cells their essential metabolic precursors such as amino acids, nucleic acids and folates. A number of enzymes have been examined and evidenced as antitumor agents. l-serine dehydratase, l-arginase, carboxypeptidase G (folate depletion), l-asparaginase, l-methioninase, l-phenylalanine ammonia lyase, l-glutaminase, l-tyrosinase and xanthine oxidase have been studied for their anticancer activity. Enzyme preparations such as asparaginase (amidase), bromelain (protease) and chymotrypsin (protease) have also been studied as cancer treatments (table 1.9) [74].

l-asparaginase is the most widely investigated enzyme. It has been reported in treatment against three neoplastic diseases, acute lymphoblastic leukemia, leukemic lymphosarcoma and myeloblastic leukemia. It deprives the cancerous cells of their nutritional asparagine supply. Asparagine is essential for protein synthesis, which takes place inside the cell, and decreased protein synthesis perhaps accounts for the immunosuppression and toxic effects of asparaginase-based treatment [75].

$$\text{L-Asparagine} + \text{PPi} + \text{AMP} \xrightleftharpoons{\text{Aspargenase}} \text{L-Aspartate} + \text{NH3} + \text{ATP}$$

The prospects of enzyme-based treatment against cancer are very bright, but the difficulties of antigenicity and short circulation time remain to be overcome.

1.10.2.2 Enzymes in thrombolytic treatment

Activation of the blood clotting mechanism during inflammation is part of the body's defense mechanism which requires therapeutic intervention. Under normal physiological conditions there is an equilibrium between blood coagulation (clotting) and fibrinolysis (the process of dissolving the clotted blood) [76]. Biocatalysts such as enzymes, ribozymes, pro-enzymes, activators and pro-activators are responsible for maintaining equilibrium between clot formation and fibrinolysis. Imbalances in the concentration of these bio-activators may disturb physiology. In the biological process of fibrogenesis, clot formation takes place due to the plasma protein (soluble fibrinogen), which is ultimately converted to insoluble fibrin by the enzyme thrombin. This process is dependent on the conversion of thrombin from prothrombin. This bio-conversion takes place after the cascade of enzymatic reactions which involved certain key biological compounds called clotting factors. A blood clot dissolving enzyme known as plasmin is present in the blood as the pro-enzyme plasminogen. During clot dissolution activators convert the plasminogen to plasmin. This biological process is well regulated by certain process such as vasoconstriction, formation of a fibrin and clot platelet aggregation [75].

As the body utilizes enzymes in conserving this key balance of homeostasis, in a similar way we can utilize enzymes to repair or restore the homeostatic balance once it is lost. Several reports have shown that one of the best approaches for treating such clinical conditions is the administration of enzymes capable of converting plasminogen to plasmin (the enzyme which dissolves the clot) via intraveneous injection. This type of treatment is called therapeutic thrombolysis or thrombolytic therapy. In this treatment, pharmacological agents are used to medically induce clot breakdown [76]. Various novel thrombolytic agents have been derived from different sources for therapeutic use, such as from bacteria (streptokinase), the venom of the Malayan pit viper (Arvin), a filamentous fungus Koji mold *Aspergillus oryzae* (brinase), a South American snake (reptilase) and human urine (urokinase) [76].

Current advancements in thrombolytic therapy are more focused on the treatment of occlusions (blockages) of blood vessels. These types of therapy can be considered as life-saving and emergency medicine for life-threatening conditions such as myocardial infarction and massive pulmonary embolism, which are the most common reasons for cardiac arrest. This life-saving treatment is more reliable in preventing the blockages of vessels in the lungs and heart. Artery blockage conditions such as pulmonary embolism in the lungs by the formation of a clot creates tension on the right side of the heart, resulting in shortness of breath and chest pain mainly upon breathing in. Enzyme-based thrombolysis for treating massive pulmonary embolism has been considered as an effective approach to dissolving clots in these large vessels. Since surgical removal raises the chances of new blood clot formation that can cause another pulmonary embolism at the same or a different site, it is considered a dangerous practice and thrombolytic therapy is considered the more effective treatment [76]. Nevertheless, reoccurrence of clot formation or clot re-formation is very common in patients who have undergone enzyme-based thrombolytic treatment. Researchers from various organizations (1971) determined the effectiveness of streptokinase over heparin in reducing the chances of death in acute myocardial infarction patients. Significant results were obtained during this experiment. As discussed above, re-formation of the clot is one of the major concerns in fibrinolytic therapy. Most clinicians start treatment with a high dose of fibrinolytic agents, which is reduced later on. This approach may reduce disease progression for some time, but often increases the chances of clot re-formation. Even after the dissolution of the clot it is very difficult to maintain the same physiologically balanced environment (homeostasis) at the site of damaged tissues and the chance of new clot formation at that particular location is very high. Therefore, fibrinolytic based treatment is always accompanied by anticoagulants, such as heparin [75].

Major concerns associated with streptokinase therapy are fever, a tendency for bleeding, antigenicity (as with any foreign protein) and the difficulty of determining the proper dose [76]. Post-enzymatic treatment bleeding is one of the major concerns and it is also a concern when anticoagulants are used alone. According to current research, urokinase (produced in the kidneys and obtained from human urine) is considered safer than streptokinase. For the production of urokinase, 2300 l of urine is required to yield only 29 mg of purified urokinase, thus considering the expense involved in its manufacture, its clinical utilization has been restricted. Other examples are Arvin and reptilase. Utilization of these has been restricted for several reasons, but they are still considered as potential replacements for heparin as anticoagulants. Some researchers have noticed that optimum dose plays an important role and is one of the key factors in determining re-clot formation. Thorough investigation is required to overcome any shortcomings and increase the acceptance of these enzymes in therapeutic use [76].

1.10.2.3 The role of enzymes in digestive disorders and inflammations

Enzymes play an essential role in the management of various digestive disorders, such as exocrine pancreatic insufficiency [77]. Supplementation with enzymes may also be advantageous for other conditions associated with poor digestion, such as lactose intolerance. Generally, pancreatic enzymes such as porcine and bovine have been the preferred form of supplementation for exocrine pancreatic insufficiency [77]. Utilization of microbe-derived lipase has presented promise with reports showing benefits alike to pancreatic enzymes, but with a lower dosage concentration and a broader pH range. The safety and efficacy of enzymes derived from microbial species in the treatment of conditions such as malabsorption and lactose intolerance is promising. Plant-derived enzymes, e.g. bromelain from pineapple, serve as active digestive aids in the breakdown of proteins. Synergistic properties have also been reported using a combination of animal-based enzymes and microbe-derived enzymes or bromelain. Buccal administration of pancreatin (derived from an alcoholic extract of animal pancreas) enhances the enzymatic digestion of starch and proteins in patients with pancreatic cysts and pancreatitis. Pancreatin in combination with lipase is used to treat patients with fatty stools. Hydrolytic enzymes such as papain and fungal extracts (*Aspergillus niger* and *Aspergillus otyzae*) are used to enhance absorption from the small intestine [78]. These fungal extracts comprise amylases and proteases along with cellulases, which support the breakdown of the otherwise indigestible fibers of cabbages, etc, and thus reduce dyspepsia and flatulence [79]. Currently, microorganisms are used at a large scale for the production of therapeutic enzymes. Among various microorganisms *Saccharomyces cerevisiae*, *Saccharomyces fragilis*, *Bacillus subtilis* and two *Aspergillus* species are considered safe by the FDA (USA) for obtaining oral β-galactosidase (from *A. oryzae*) which is often used by patients suffering from inherited intestinal disease lactose deficiency [80]. Children with this genetic disorder children are incapable of digesting milk lactose. Enzymatic preparations such as β-galactosidase catalyze the conversion of lactose to glucose and galactose, which are quickly absorbed by the intestine. Other enzymatic preparations, e.g. penicillinase (from *B. subtilis*) are often used to treat hypersensitivity reactions caused by the antibiotic penicillin [81]. This enzyme catalyzes the conversion of penicillin to penicillanic acid, which is non-immunogenic. In addition, microbial and plant hydrolases are also used to decrease inflammation and edema [82]. Thrombin, trypsin, chymotrypsin, papain, streptokinase, streptodornase and sempeptidase are under clinical trial investigation. These enzymatic preparations are administered orally and have considerable proteolytic activity in the serum. Streptodornase has also displayed pain-relieving action on systemic injection [83]. Preparations have also been used to clean dirty wounds and necrotic tissue and to remove debris from second and third degree burns.

1.11 Plants and algae enzyme systems

Plant based foods are usually consumed in their raw form. This eases the main concern with animal-based enzymes by preserving the integrity of the enzymes themselves. Moreover, plant-based digestive enzymes are effective over a broad scope of pH levels. This range is usually between 3.0 and 9.0, which is highly well-matched with the human gastrointestinal environment. Thus plant-based enzymes are compatible for supporting comprehensive digestive health. Protease, amylase, lipase and cellulose are the important enzymes and are present in plants. Protease breaks down protein that can be present in meat, fish, poultry, eggs, cheese and nuts. Amylase assists your body with the breakdown and subsequent absorption of carbohydrates and starches. Lipase aids the digestion of fat. When your diet includes lipase-rich foods, it eases the production burden on the gall bladder, liver and pancreas. *Cellulase* is present in many fruits and vegetables, and it breaks down food fibers, which increases their nutritional value to our bodies. The presence of *cellulase* in plant-based sources is important, because it is not naturally present in the human body. Fruits and vegetables are an ideal source for enzymes. They are enzyme-rich and easily consumed without needing to be cooked or processed, ultimately preserving the full functionality of the enzymes. By using plant biotechnology several enzymes can be produced from plants as well algal resources. During algal photosynthesis various proteins and enzymes are produced which can be utilized in economic development and environment management, such as in wastewater treatment, production of fine chemicals, and biodiesel production. Due to their potential to capture and fix carbon dioxide using solar energy, photosynthetic marine algae are considered as potential models for the production of proteins. It has been recently observed that algal chloroplasts can be transformed for the production recombinant proteins [84]. Five different classes of recombinant enzymes; *xylanase*, α-galactosidase, phytase, phosphate anhydrolase, and β-mannanase, Dunaliella *tertiolecta or C. reinhardtii* were in the plastids of *D. tertiolecta* or *C. reinhardtii.* Similar strategies should allow for recombinant protein production in many species of marine algae [84].

1.12 Enzyme safety

Ensuring the safety of enzymes utilized in various industries, such as food, pharmaceuticals, textiles, and detergents, is vital. Safety encompasses several factors, including the non-pathogenic nature of the creatures and the lack of toxicity in both the enzymes and the product of the enzyme's chemical reaction that they catalyze because there are no antibiotics available and there are comparatively few microbial pollutants [85]. Enzymes originating from non-approved species require comprehensive evaluation for a range of toxicity assessments. There is currently no evidence to suggest that any enzyme possesses inherent toxicity, mutagenicity, or carcinogenicity, even though these properties may be anticipated due to their protein-based composition [86]. Nevertheless, the safety of enzyme formulations is not without concern since they may contain pollutants derived from the enzyme source, generated during processing or storage, or arising from secondary micro-organism metabolites such as mycotoxins and aflatoxins. Enzymes have significantly fewer potential adverse effects and unknown reactions than other substances, supplements, or pharmaceuticals. Because of this, they are incredibly secure [87]. Several enzymes are considered GRAS (Generally Regarded As Safe) foods in the United States. Examples of these enzymes are amylase, α-amylase, bromelain, catalase, cellulase, ficin, a-galactosidase, glucoamylase, glucose isomerase, glucose oxidase, invertase, lactase, lipase, papain, pectinase, pepsin, rennet, and trypsin. The Food and Drug Administration (FDA) neither approves nor disapproves of enzymes. Hence, there is no clear status for specific digestive enzyme blends [88]. Immobilized enzymes can potentially eliminate some of the risks associated with free enzymes. This is a very secure method as long as the materials employed are appropriate and neither they nor

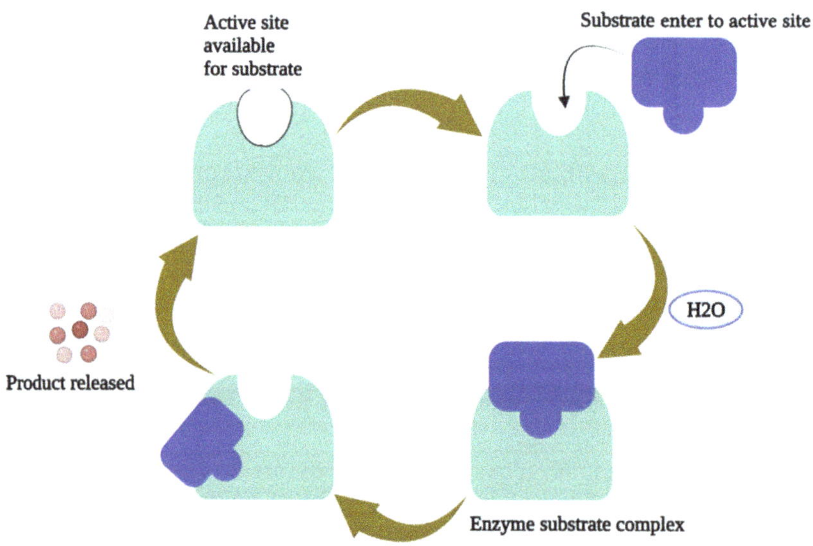

Figure 1.6. Graphical depiction of the catalytic cycle of an enzyme, showcasing the substrate to product transformation.

the immobilized enzymes leak into the product stream. Many enzymes have undergone safety assessments over the past few years, with results showing that enzyme preparations are safe to use. Among the enzymes that have undergone safety testing are *Trichoderma reesei*-derived, xylanase enzyme (SP 628) from *Thermomyces lanuginosus*, and xylanase enzyme (SP 578) from *Aspergillus aculeatus*. Fusarium xylanase expressed by *Thermomyces lanuginosus*, *Aspergillus niger* amino peptidase enzyme preparation, Kluyveromyces lactis lipase produced by *Rhizopus oryza*, and glucanase preparation designed for use in food [89].

1.13 Enzyme structure determination

Learning the enzyme's three-dimensional structure is like studying the blueprint for a magnificent building. Understanding the mechanisms contributing to their remarkable catalytic powers helps direct the development of precision medicines and other biotech applications (figure 1.6).

1.13.1 X-ray crystallography

The atomic and molecular structure of crystalline materials, including enzymes, can be determined with great precision using x-ray crystallography. This technique has been game-changing in structural biology since it permits the first direct imaging of molecular structure [90]. Enzyme structure, active site architecture, and substrate, co-factor, and inhibitor interactions can all be better understood with the help of x-ray crystallography. Because of its near-atomic resolution, super-high-quality x-ray crystallography has the potential to disclose the precise locations of individual atoms within the enzyme [91]. The catalytically active location of an enzyme may be seen by x-ray crystallography. To design effective inhibitors, one needs to have a thorough understanding of enzyme chemistry. Enzyme structure in the presence of substrates and inhibitors can be seen via x-ray crystallography [92]. These structures are functional for drug design because they reveal details about how enzymes and ligands interact. Enzymes undergo conformational changes during their catalytic cycles. To observe metabolic processes in real-time, x-ray crystallography offers the ability to record enzymes in their active conformations. The substance, known as an enzymatic protein found in saliva and tears, is employed in x-ray crystallography due to its significant function in preventing bacterial illnesses [93]. In 1965, Dorothy Hodgkin made an essential advancement in crystallography when she found the structure of lysozyme by applying x-ray crystallography. Her insight completely altered the dynamics. In 1964, she received the Nobel Prize in Chemistry due to her notable contributions to the field. Following this, researchers have used their comprehension of the structural attributes of lysozyme to create antibiotics and other therapeutic therapies that specifically target bacterial ailments [94].

1.13.2 NMR spectroscopy

Nuclear magnetic resonance (NMR) spectroscopy is a widely used and adaptable scientific method utilized to analyze enzymes and several other chemicals at the atomic level [95]. This technology enables the investigation of their structural characteristics, dynamic properties, and intermolecular associations. This technique is founded on the principles of nuclear electromagnetic resonance, which investigates how atomic nuclei are influenced by radiofrequency energy and a magnetic field from the outside. NMR spectroscopy has emerged as a crucial instrument in investigating enzymes, enabling a deeper comprehension of their tridimensional configuration, catalytic efficacy, and relationship to surfaces, co-factors, and inhibition [96]. It is possible to study enzymes in their native habitat, which is the solution that allows one to see the enzymes' dynamic action. NMR spectroscopy may examine the dynamic interactions between ribonuclease and its substrate in a solution. Thus, novel treatment possibilities have been revealed by our improved understanding of how this enzyme detects and destroys RNA molecules [97].

1.13.3 Cryo-electron microscopy

Our capacity to visualize the intricate three-dimensional structures of biomolecules like enzymes has been substantially enhanced by advances in cryo-electron microscopy (Cryo-EM) and other current structural biology techniques [98]. Cryo-EM allows materials to be preserved in a nearly natural state by freezing them at very low temperatures (cryogenic conditions) instead of the fixed, stained, and dehydrated state they are in for conventional electron microscopy. By not altering the samples too much, we can learn more about how they functioned in their original form. Cryo-EM has recently advanced to the point that it can compete with x-ray crystallography and NMR spectroscopy for atomic or near-atomic resolution. This degree of precision makes a deeper understanding of the mechanics behind enzymatic operations possible [99]. Unlike x-ray crystallography, cryo-electron microscopy (Cryo-EM) can investigate large and complex molecular assemblies without crystallization. Membrane and massive macromolecular complexes are just two of the sample contexts that can be explored with Cryo-EM. It can record the many molecular structural states, which could shed light on the molecules' plasticity and reactivity. The enzyme ATP synthase is responsible for synthesizing the cellular energy molecule adenosine triphosphate (ATP). The rotor-stator mechanism of ATP synthase and the specifics of its energy conversion during ATP synthesis have recently been revealed by Cryo-EM, providing fresh insights into the complex molecular machinery of this enzyme [100].

1.14 Enzyme engineering and design

To improve the catalytic activity, substrate selectivity, stability, and other features of enzymes, scientists have turned to a field known as enzyme engineering. This strategy entails altering the molecular structure of enzymes to broaden their applications beyond their native capabilities [101].

1.14.1 Directed evolution of enzymes

The principles of natural selection inspired the powerful technology of directed evolution. Mutation and selective breeding mold enzymes to perform specific functions [102]. Consider an enzyme that aids in the digestion of hazardous substances in the wild. Directed evolution allows scientists to create novel enzyme varieties by manipulating their genetic code. We will need to do further testing to determine whether or not these versions are more effective than the possibly dangerous chemical. In future rounds, only enzymes that have proven to have improved catalytic function are subjected to mutation and testing. The enzyme improves its ability to degrade pollutants over time, making it a more eco-friendly and long-term solution to environmental degradation [103].

1.14.2 Rational design of enzymes

Think of an enzyme that only requires one specific substance to accomplish its task. Researchers may be able to predict which amino acids will be needed for substrate recognition and catalysis by analyzing the enzyme's active site and learning how it interacts with substrates [104]. Enzyme substrate selectivity can be broadened through the substitution of single amino acids or the introduction of mutations. The rational design approach is essential to build targeted enzymes for numerous biotech applications. The enzyme acetylcholinesterase (AChE) degrades the neurotransmitter acetylcholine, which has an essential role in the neurological system. Neuronal function may be impaired by the accumulation of harmful chemicals that block AChE in certain neurological diseases [105]. Using rational design, researchers have altered AChE's active site to make the enzyme more resistant to various inhibitors without compromising its capacity to break down acetylcholine. Modifying this variant of acetylcholinesterase may one day be critical to effective treatment of neurological illnesses [106].

1.14.3 Applications of engineered enzymes

Because of their many applications in biotechnology and industry, modified enzymes have become indispensable in the modern world. Plastic trash is one of the leading causes of ecosystem decline [107]. Polyethylene terephthalate (PET) enzymes have been created by scientists in order to facilitate their disposal. These synthetic enzymes make plastic trash more amenable to recycling and biodegradation, lessening its adverse effects on the environment and paving the way for future innovations in environmentally friendly materials. The pharmaceutical industry can also benefit from enzyme engineering because it allows for the environmentally sound production of complex therapeutic compounds. Designed enzymes help turn biomass into usable energy for making biofuels. They have potential use in the kitchen, medicine, and lab where new chemicals are being created [108].

1.15 Enzymes in medicine and healthcare

Enzymes have a crucial role in drug delivery and as therapeutic action targets. We will also discuss the advantages and disadvantages of using enzymes as the basis for pharmaceutical products. Because enzymes are involved in many different bodily activities, they are being examined as possible therapeutic targets. Enzymes present an opportunity to develop novel drug delivery strategies that maximize therapeutic advantages while minimizing unwanted consequences [109].

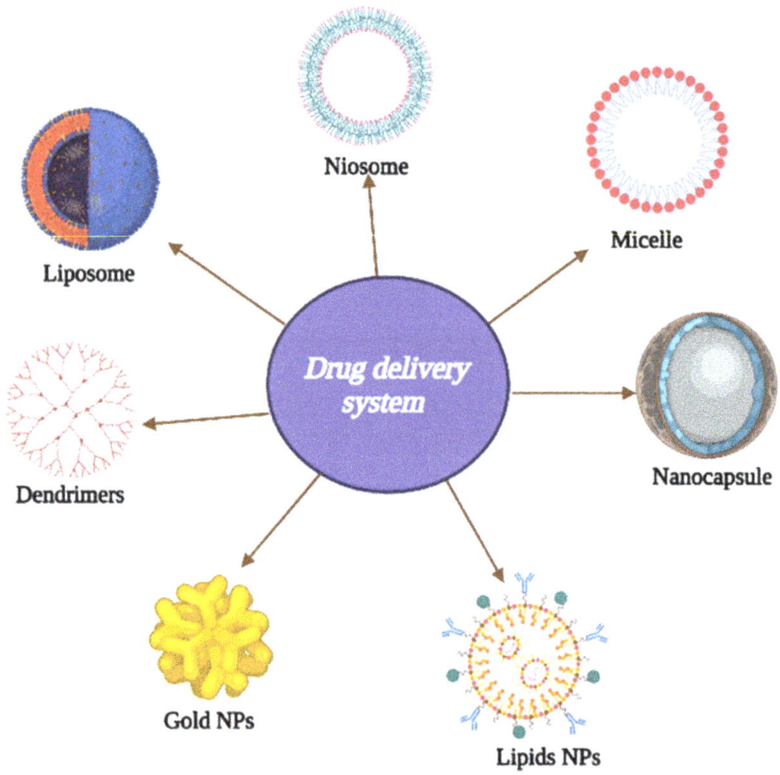

Figure 1.7. Overview of various nanotechnology-based drug delivery systems, highlighting liposomes, nanoparticles, and other carriers.

1.15.1 Enzyme-targeted drug delivery

By delivering medications more selectively to particular cells or tissues, enzyme-targeted drug delivery systems boost medication concentrations at the site of action. Enzyme-activated prodrugs use inert drug molecules that become active when they touch certain enzymes at the site of action. The therapy's upbeat benefits are amplified while its negative ones are mitigated. For instance, specific anticancer prodrugs become very effective anticancer treatments when specifically triggered by enzymes that are overexpressed in tumor cells (figure 1.7) [110].

1.15.2 Enzymes as drug targets

Enzyme-targeted drug delivery methods allow for more precise drug administration, perhaps leading to higher local concentrations of the active ingredient in the required cells or tissues. Enzyme-activated prodrugs are a type of prodrug intended to be converted into active forms by enzymes already present at the site of action [111]. This method minimizes harmful consequences while maximizing therapeutic gain. For instance, specific anticancer prodrugs are transformed into particular and potent anticancer drugs when they are selectively activated by overexpressed enzymes in tumor cells [112].

1.15.3 Challenges and opportunities in enzyme drug discovery

Finding potent and specific enzyme inhibitors, being aware of the potential for off-target effects and guaranteeing drug stability and pharmacokinetics are some of the difficulties inherent in enzyme-based drug research. Thanks to the development of computational tools and structural biology, researchers now better understand how enzymes function. By applying this knowledge to rational drug design and computational tools for screening, novel enzyme-targeted medicines can be produced more rapidly [113].

1.15.4 Enzymes in gene therapy

Incorporating, altering, or suppressing specific genes is the basis of gene therapy, which tries to treat genetic illnesses. Therapeutic drug development, specific gene delivery, and precise gene editing are just a few examples of the many applications of enzymes in gene therapy [114]. The Cas (CRISPR-associated) and CRISPR (Clustered Regularly Interspaced Short Palindromic Repeats) proteins have been developed as game-changing gene editing methods. Cas enzymes are guided to their targets in the genome by guide RNAs, where they make precise cuts in the DNA [115]. CRISPR-Cas has the potential to accurately fix mutations that cause genetic illnesses like sickle cell anemia and cystic fibrosis. By putting the CRISPR-Cas system into cells to correct genetic flaws, researchers may be able to treat hereditary illnesses at their origin [116]. People with certain genetic illnesses lack enough essential enzymes due to inherited abnormalities. Enzyme replacement therapy (ERT) treats enzyme deficiency by replacing the missing enzyme with one given to the patient. Gaucher disease and Pompe disease are two examples of lysosomal storage disorders brought on by deficiencies in specific lysosomal enzymes. The new enzyme will not do any good unless introduced into normal cells. The treatment plan for lysosomal storage disorders has substantially slowed the progression of the disease and improved the quality of life for those affected [117]. Scientists utilize viral vectors, engineered viruses, to deliver therapeutic genes to the patient's cells. In order to create and improve viral vectors that can efficiently convey genes, enzymes are needed. Due to their efficiency in delivering genes to their target recipients without provoking strong immune reactions, AAV vectors are widely used in gene treatments [118]. AAV vectors are enzyme-modified to remove viral genes and replace them with therapeutic genes of interest. This method is vital in gene therapy because it guarantees therapeutic genes' efficient and secure delivery [119].

1.15.5 Enzymes in personalized medicine

The objective of personalized healthcare is to offer individualized therapies customized to suit the specific biological, environmental, and psychological characteristics of every person receiving treatment. To achieve this goal, enzymes are crucial because of the information they provide for disease diagnosis, the role they play in guiding the selection of medicines based on individual genetic variability, and the capacity they provide for the development of treatments that precisely address the underlying molecular causes of disease [120].

1.15.6 Enzyme biomarkers in disease diagnosis

Enzymes are frequently used in various medical diseases' diagnostic procedures because they serve as measurable indicators of biological processes or disease states. Cardiac troponins are enzymes that are released into the bloodstream in reaction to injury to heart muscle cells (myocardial infarction), and they are crucial markers for diagnosing heart attacks. High levels of cardiac troponin in the blood can be used to diagnose and treat acute myocardial damage [121].

1.15.7 Pharmacogenomics and enzyme variability

Pharmacogenomics studies how an individual's genetic makeup affects their response to drugs. The metabolism and effectiveness of medications are profoundly affected by enzyme variability. The CYP enzyme family metabolizes many different medications. Variations in the CYP genes may affect the capacity to metabolize certain drugs. Differences in CYP might cause slower medication metabolism, which can increase blood drug levels and increase the risk of adverse drug reactions in some persons. Knowing a patient's CYP enzyme profile could help clinicians choose the best treatment and dose for that individual [122].

1.15.8 Enzyme-based therapies for personalized treatment

Those genetically predisposed to lack certain enzymes may benefit from ERT, which entails giving them therapeutic enzymes. The severity of enzyme deficits in lysosomal storage diseases can vary widely between different mutations. Determining the precise enzyme deficiency of each patient is crucial for providing successful, tailored enzyme replacement medication. This customized approach guarantees that each patient receives the most effective enzyme and dosage possible [123].

1.16 Enzymes in bioremediation

Bioremediation is a sustainable method for restoring contaminated environments. Enzymes are essential to improving bioremediation systems due to their catalytic characteristics. When enzymes are added to wastewater, organic molecules, and contaminants degrade more quickly, producing less harmful by-products or becoming harmless altogether. Lipases are enzymes that metabolize fats and oils into their constituent fatty acids and glycerol. Lipases could be used to hydrolyze fats and oils in domestic and industrial wastewater, decreasing the risk of clogged pipes and easing some harmful impacts of these discharges on the environment [124]. Enzymes can catalyze the conversion of hazardous compounds, hydrocarbons, and other organic contaminants into less toxic molecules. Enzymes called alkane hydroxylases hydrolyze alkanes, making up most of crude oil. When applied to oil-stained areas, these enzymes speed up the natural recovery process. The breakdown of the hydrocarbons makes this possible [125]. Soil bioremediation is aided by enzymes, which speed up the breakdown of organic molecules and the removal of contaminants. Phytoremediation is a method that uses plant roots and the microorganisms that live in them to detoxify soil from toxins. The enzyme phytase can remediate polluted soils by promoting plant phosphorus absorption and mobilization from organic molecules [126].

1.17 Enzymes in agriculture and crop production

Enzymes are natural catalysts that help plants speed up their metabolism. The many benefits of employing them in agriculture include improved nutrient absorption, insect and disease resistance, post-harvest convenience, and longer shelf life [127]. The availability of enzymes and nutrient absorption may improve plants' resistance, development, and growth. Phosphatases are enzymes that break down organic matter in the soil, freeing up phosphate for plant uptake. By increasing the amount of phosphate available to the plant, phosphatases improve germination rates, root growth, and general plant health. This is especially useful because plants may have problems receiving adequate phosphate from the soil in low-phosphate

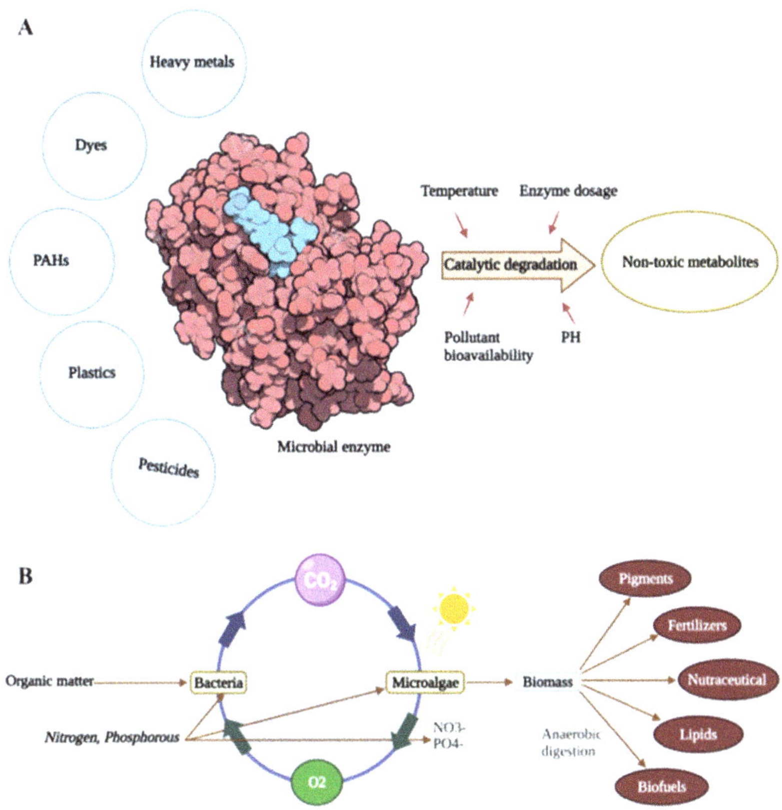

Figure 1.8. (A) Conceptual diagram outlining the role of microbial enzymes in the catalytic degradation of environmental pollutants to non-toxic metabolites. (B) Schematic representation of the microalgal biomass production cycle illustrating nutrient recycling and bioresource applications.

environments [128]. Reduced reliance on chemical pesticides results from cutting-edge strategies that use enzymes to shield crops against pests, illnesses, and environmental stressors. Chitinases are digestive enzymes that break down insect and arthropod exoskeletons made of the protein chitin. Chitin-eating insects and pests have no chance against plants that express the chitinase gene. This enzymatic method can help protect crops from pests while decreasing the need for chemical pesticides [129]. Post-harvest handling and storage with the help of enzymes could help keep harvested crops fresh and usable for longer. Polygalacturonate is an enzyme that helps ripen fruit. Manipulating this enzyme's activity may lengthen or reduce the post-harvest storage duration. Inhibiting polygalacturonate activity may extend the freshness of some fruits, such as tomatoes, throughout storage and shipping [130].

1.18 Enzymes in waste management

Enzymes are necessary for biodegradation and energy generation from a wide variety of waste, making waste management an essential aspect of environmental sustainability. Compost, rich in nutrients that can be used to improve soil, is produced more quickly by adding enzymes to the natural decomposition process of organic waste. Plant cell walls contain cellulose, an essential structural component that can be degraded by enzymes known as cellulases. The composting process can be sped up with cellulases, which help decompose organic waste such as food scraps, yard debris, and leaves [131]. High-quality compost is produced by this method, and it can be utilized as a fertilizer in sustainable farming by increasing soil fertility with natural means [132]. Enzymes are used to break down plastic waste into simpler molecules to lessen plastic pollution and its negative impacts on the environment. PETase can break down polyethylene terephthalate (PET), a standard plastic. We now know which bacteria manufacture PETase naturally, and thanks to genetic engineering, we can make the enzyme more effective. An enzymatic method shows promise for efficiently recycling PET plastic, which could help keep plastic trash out of landfills and waterways [133]. Enzymes are used in waste-to-energy conversion systems to convert organic waste into biogas and biofuels. With the help of bacteria and enzymes, organic waste such as food scraps and agricultural leftovers can be broken down in anaerobic digestion even when oxygen is unavailable. Biogas, which is primarily methane, is created by this method and represents a renewable energy source. Using biogas to fuel vehicles, heat homes, or generate electricity helps minimize emissions of greenhouse gases caused by waste breakdown (figure 1.8) [134].

References

[1] Franzen R and Tois J 2003 Purine and sugar chemistry on solid phase-100 years after the Emil Fischer's chemistry Nobel Prize 1902 *Comb. Chem. High Throughput Screen.* **6** 433–44

[2] Simoni R D, Hill R L and Vaughan M 2002 Urease, the first crystalline enzyme and the proof that enzymes are proteins: the work of James B. Sumner *J. Biol. Chem.* **277** e1–2

[3] Northrop J H 1930 Crystalline pepsin: I. Isolation and tests of purity *J. Gen. Physiol.* **13** 739–66

[4] Berg J, Tymoczko J and Stryer L 2002 *Biochemistry* 5th edn (New York: NCBI)
[5] Percudani R and Peracchi A 2003 A genomic overview of pyridoxal-phosphate-dependent enzymes *EMBO Rep.* **4** 850–4
[6] Fischer J D, Holliday G L and Thornton J M 2010 The CoFactor database: organic cofactors in enzyme catalysis *Bioinformatics* **26** 2496–7
[7] Agarwal P K 2006 Enzymes: an integrated view of structure, dynamics and function *Microb. Cell Fact.* **5** 1–12
[8] Lee H C 2006 Structure and enzymatic functions of human CD38 *Mol. Med.* **12** 317–23
[9] Rodriguez R *et al* 1985 Amino acid sequence of pigeon egg-white lysozyme *Biochem. Int.* **11** 841–3
[10] Canfield R E 1963 The amino acid sequence of egg white lysozyme *J. Biol. Chem.* **238** 2698–707
[11] Berg J M, Tymoczko J L and Stryer L 2002 *Biochemistry* 5th edn (New York: NCBI)
[12] Fredholm B B *et al* 1994 VI. Nomenclature and classification of purinoceptors *Pharmacol. Rev.* **46** 143
[13] Webb E C 1992 *Enzyme nomenclature 1992. Recommendations of the Nomenclature Committee of the International Union of Biochemistry and Molecular Biology on the Nomenclature and Classification of Enzymes* (New York: Academic)
[14] Boyce S and Tipton K F 2001 Enzyme classification and nomenclature *Encyclopedia of Life Sciences* (Wiley)
[15] McDonald A G and Tipton K F 2014 Fifty-five years of enzyme classification: advances and difficulties *FEBS J.* **281** 583–92
[16] McDonald A G, Boyce S and Tipton K F 2015 Enzyme classification and nomenclature *Encyclopedia of Life Sciences* (Wiley) pp 1–11
[17] King J 1969 The nomenclature of enzymes and methods of expressing results *Br. J. Anaesth.* **41** 222–6
[18] Rawlings N D 2020 Twenty-five years of nomenclature and classification of proteolytic enzymes *Biochim. Biophys. Acta Proteins Proteom.* **1868** 140345
[19] Montville T J and Kaiser A L 1993 Antimicrobial proteins: classification, nomenclature, diversity, and relationship to bacteriocins *Bacteriocins of Lactic Acid Bacteria* (Amsterdam: Elsevier) pp 1–22
[20] Schomburg D and Stephan D 2013 *Enzyme Handbook 9: Class 1.1: Oxidoreductases.* (Berlin: Springer Science & Business Media)
[21] Chou K-C and Elrod D W 2003 Prediction of enzyme family classes *J. Proteome Res.* **2** 183–90
[22] Chou K C and Cai Y D 2004 Predicting enzyme family class in a hybridization space *Protein Sci.* **13** 2857–63
[23] Strange R C *et al* 2001 Glutathione-S-transferase family of enzymes *Mutat. Res. /Fundam. Mol. Mech. Mutagenesis* **482** 21–6
[24] Sinning I *et al* 1993 Structure determination and refinement of human alpha class glutathione transferase A1-1, and a comparison with the Mu and Pi class enzymes *J. Mol. Biol.* **232** 192–212
[25] Watson M A *et al* 1998 Human glutathione S-transferase P1 polymorphisms: relationship to lung tissue enzyme activity and population frequency distribution *Carcinogenesis* **19** 275–80

[26] Holmquist M 2000 Alpha beta-hydrolase fold enzymes structures, functions and mechanisms *Curr. Protein Pept. Sci.* **1** 209–35
[27] Fretland A J and Omiecinski C J 2000 Epoxide hydrolases: biochemistry and molecular biology *Chem. Biol. Interact.* **129** 41–59
[28] Adibekian A *et al* 2011 Click-generated triazole ureas as ultrapotent *in vivo*–active serine hydrolase inhibitors *Nat. Chem. Biol.* **7** 469–78
[29] Shrivastava S 2020 Introduction to glycoside hydrolases: classification, identification and occurrence *Industrial Applications of Glycoside Hydrolases* (Singapore: Springer) pp 3–84
[30] Modolo L V, Reichert A I and Dixon R A 2009 Introduction to the different classes of biosynthetic enzymes *Plant-Derived Natural Products: Synthesis, Function, and Application* (New York: Springer) pp 143–63
[31] Xu F *et al* 2018 Diversity of three-dimensional structures and catalytic mechanisms of alginate lyases *Appl. Environ. Microbiol.* **84** e2040–17
[32] Hegemann J D and Süssmuth R D 2020 Matters of class: coming of age of class III and IV lanthipeptides *RSC Chem. Biol.* **1** 110–27
[33] Cai Y-D and Chou K-C 2005 Using functional domain composition to predict enzyme family classes *J. Proteome Res.* **4** 109–11
[34] Cuesta S M *et al* 2014 The evolution of enzyme function in the isomerases *Curr. Opin. Struct. Biol.* **26** 121–30
[35] Kuddus M 2019 Introduction to food enzymes *Enzymes in Food Biotechnology* (Amsterdam: Elsevier) pp 1–18
[36] Qiu J-D *et al* 2010 Using the concept of Chou's pseudo amino acid composition to predict enzyme family classes: an approach with support vector machine based on discrete wavelet transform *Protein Pept. Lett.* **17** 715–22
[37] Holliday G L *et al* 2014 Exploring the biological and chemical complexity of the ligases *J. Mol. Biol.* **426** 2098–111
[38] Maculins T *et al* 2016 Bacteria-host relationship: ubiquitin ligases as weapons of invasion *Cell Res.* **26** 499–510
[39] Zheng N and Shabek N 2017 Ubiquitin ligases: structure, function, and regulation *Annu. Rev. Biochem.* **86** 129–57
[40] Dobson P D and Doig A J 2005 Predicting enzyme class from protein structure without alignments *J. Mol. Biol.* **345** 187–99
[41] Kouidmi I, Levesque R C and Paradis-Bleau C 2014 The biology of Mur ligases as an antibacterial target *Mol. Microbiol.* **94** 242–53
[42] Sharma B and Taganna J 2020 Genome-wide analysis of the U-box E3 ubiquitin ligase enzyme gene family in tomato *Sci. Rep.* **10** 9581
[43] Lemieux R U and Spohr U 1994 Concept for enzyme specificity 1 *Adv. Carbohydr. Chem. Biochem.* **50**
[44] Csermely P, Palotai R and Nussinov R 2010 Induced fit, conformational selection and independent dynamic segments: an extended view of binding events *Trends Biochem. Sci.* **35** 539–46
[45] de Koshland J 1995 The key–lock theory and the induced fit theory *Angew. Chem. Int. Ed. Engl.* **33** 2375–8
[46] Boehr D D, Nussinov R and Wright P E 2009 The role of dynamic conformational ensembles in biomolecular recognition *Nat. Chem. Biol.* **5** 789–96

[47] Johnson K A and Goody R S 2011 The original Michaelis constant: translation of the 1913 Michaelis–Menten paper *Biochemistry* **50** 8264–9
[48] Cooper G M 2000 *The Central Role of Enzymes as Biological Catalysts* (Sinauer Associates)
[49] West E *et al* 1966 *Textbook of Biochemistry* 4th edn (Delhi: Oxford and IBH)
[50] Gutfreund H and Sturtevant J 1956 The mechanism of chymotrypsin-catalyzed reactions *Proc. Natl Acad. Sci.* **42** 719–28
[51] Ma W, Tang C and Lai L 2005 Specificity of trypsin and chymotrypsin: loop-motion-controlled dynamic correlation as a determinant *Biophys. J.* **89** 1183–93
[52] Fink A L 1976 Cryoenzymology of chymotrypsin: the detection of intermediates in the catalysis of a specific anilide substrate *Biochemistry* **15** 1580–6
[53] Brandt K G, Himoe A and Hess G P 1967 Investigations of the chymotrypsin-catalyzed hydrolysis of specific substrates: III. Determination of individual rate constants and enzyme-substrate binding constants for specific amide and ester substrates *J. Biol. Chem.* **242** 3973–82
[54] Kezdy F J and Bender M L 1962 The kinetics of the α-chymotrypsin-catalyzed hydrolysis of p-nitrophenyl acetate *Biochemistry* **1** 1097–106
[55] Neurath H and Walsh K A 1976 Role of proteolytic enzymes in biological regulation (a review) *Proc. Natl Acad. Sci.* **73** 3825–32
[56] Ulusu N N 2015 Evolution of enzyme kinetic mechanisms *J. Mol. Evol.* **80** 251–7
[57] Nakano S-i, Chadalavada D M and Bevilacqua P C 2000 General acid-base catalysis in the mechanism of a hepatitis delta virus ribozyme *Science* **287** 1493–7
[58] Vallee B L and Williams R 1968 Metalloenzymes: the entatic nature of their active sites *Proc. Natl Acad. Sci.* **59** 498–505
[59] Shook R L and Borovik A 2010 Role of the secondary coordination sphere in metal-mediated dioxygen activation *Inorg. Chem.* **49** 3646–60
[60] Bodansky O 1959 Diagnostic applications of enzymes in medicine: general enzymological aspects *Am. J. Med.* **27** 861–74
[61] Voller A, Bidwell D and Bartlett A 1976 Enzyme immunoassays in diagnostic medicine: theory and practice *Bull. World Health Organ.* **53** 55
[62] Robinson P K 2015 Enzymes: principles and biotechnological applications *Essays Biochem.* **59** 1
[63] Wolf P L 1999 Biochemical diagnosis of liver disease *Indian J. Clin. Biochem.* **14** 59–90
[64] Ellis G *et al* 1978 Serum enzyme tests in diseases of the liver and biliary tree *Am. J. Clin. Pathol.* **70** 248–58
[65] Giannini E G, Testa R and Savarino V 2005 Liver enzyme alteration: a guide for clinicians *Cmaj* **172** 367–79
[66] Wieme R and Demeulenaere L 1970 Enzyme assays in liver disease *J. Clin. Pathol. Suppl. (Ass. Clin. Path.)* **4** 51
[67] Agress C M 1965 Ischemic heart disease—use of serum enzyme determinations in diagnosis *Calif. Med.* **103** 21
[68] Chowdhury B *et al* 2017 Hyaluronidase 2 deficiency causes increased mesenchymal cells, congenital heart defects, and heart failure *Circ.: Cardiovasc. Genet.* **10** e001598
[69] Sobel B E and Shell W E 1972 Serum enzyme determinations in the diagnosis and assessment of myocardial infarction *Circulation* **45** 471–82
[70] Plebani M 2001 Enzymes and muscle diseases *Reumatismo* **53** 158–65
[71] Vellard M 2003 The enzyme as drug: application of enzymes as pharmaceuticals *Curr. Opin. Biotechnol.* **14** 444–50

[72] Gurung N *et al* 2013 A broader view: microbial enzymes and their relevance in industries, medicine, and beyond *BioMed Res. Int.* **2013** 329121
[73] Leipner J and Saller R 2000 Systemic enzyme therapy in oncology: effect and mode of action *Drugs* **59** 769–80
[74] Novak J F and Trnka F 2005 Proenzyme therapy of cancer *Anticancer Res.* **25** 1157–77
[75] Collen D and Lijnen R H 2005 Thrombolytic agents *Thromb. Haemost.* **93** 627–30
[76] Cichoke A 1990 Enzymes in thrombolytic therapy *Dynamic Chiropractic* **8** 17
[77] Roxas M 2008 The role of enzyme supplementation in digestive disorders *Altern. Med. Rev.* **13** 307–14
[78] Rao M B *et al* 1998 Molecular and biotechnological aspects of microbial proteases *Microbiol. Mol. Biol. Rev.* **62** 597–635
[79] Fieker A, Philpott J and Armand M 2011 Enzyme replacement therapy for pancreatic insufficiency: present and future *Clin. Exp. Gastroenterol.* **4** 55–73
[80] Montalto M *et al* 2006 Management and treatment of lactose malabsorption *World J. Gastroenterol.: WJG* **12** 187
[81] Blumberg P M and Strominger J L 1974 Interaction of penicillin with the bacterial cell: penicillin-binding proteins and penicillin-sensitive enzymes *Bacteriol. Rev.* **38** 291–335
[82] Ricciotti E and FitzGerald G A 2011 Prostaglandins and inflammation *Arter. Thromb. Vasc. Biol.* **31** 986–1000
[83] Miller R R, De Young D V and Paxinos J 1970 Enzymes for trauma *Postgrad. Med. J.* **46** 154–6
[84] Georgianna D R *et al* 2013 Production of recombinant enzymes in the marine alga Dunaliella tertiolecta *Algal Res.* **2** 2–9
[85] Pariza M W and Johnson E A 2001 Evaluating the safety of microbial enzyme preparations used in food processing: update for a new century *Regul. Toxicol. Pharm.* **33** 173–86
[86] Amine A *et al* 2006 Enzyme inhibition-based biosensors for food safety and environmental monitoring *Biosens. Bioelectron.* **21** 1405–23
[87] Ladics G S and Sewalt V 2018 Industrial microbial enzyme safety: what does the weight-of-evidence indicate? *Regul. Toxicol. Pharm.* **98** 151–4
[88] van Dijck P W, Selten G C and Hempenius R A 2003 On the safety of a new generation of DSM Aspergillus niger enzyme production strains *Regul. Toxicol. Pharm.* **38** 27–35
[89] Pariza M and Foster E 1983 Determining the safety of enzymes used in food processing *J. Food Prot.* **46** 453–68
[90] Blow D and Steitz T 1970 X-ray diffraction studies of enzymes *Annu. Rev. Biochem.* **39** 63–100
[91] James M N 1980 An x-ray crystallographic approach to enzyme structure and function *Can. J. Biochem.* **58** 251–71
[92] Abad M C *et al* 2002 The x-ray crystallographic structure of *Escherichia coli* branching enzyme *J. Biol. Chem.* **277** 42164–70
[93] Ladd M F C, Palmer R A and Palmer R A 1977 *Structure Determination by X-Ray Crystallography* (Berlin: Springer) vol 233
[94] Eisenberg D 1970 X-ray crystallography and enzyme structure *The Enzymes* (Amsterdam: Elsevier) pp 1–89
[95] Gauto D F *et al* 2019 Integrated NMR and cryo-EM atomic-resolution structure determination of a half-megadalton enzyme complex *Nat. Commun.* **10** 2697

[96] Lisi G P and Loria J P 2016 Using NMR spectroscopy to elucidate the role of molecular motions in enzyme function *Prog. Nucl. Magn. Reson. Spectrosc.* **92** 1–17

[97] Chen J L *et al* 2016 3D structure determination of an unstable transient enzyme intermediate by paramagnetic NMR spectroscopy *Angew. Chem.* **128** 13948–52

[98] Bartesaghi A *et al* 2014 Structure of β-galactosidase at 3.2-Å resolution obtained by cryo-electron microscopy *Proc. Natl Acad. Sci.* **111** 11709–14

[99] Oosterheert W and Gros P 2020 Cryo-electron microscopy structure and potential enzymatic function of human six-transmembrane epithelial antigen of the prostate 1 (STEAP1) *J. Biol. Chem.* **295** 9502–12

[100] Zhou Z H 2008 Towards atomic resolution structural determination by single-particle cryo-electron microscopy *Curr. Opin. Struct. Biol.* **18** 218–28

[101] Victorino da Silva Amatto I *et al* 2022 Enzyme engineering and its industrial applications *Biotechnol. Appl. Biochem.* **69** 389–409

[102] Dalby P A 2011 Strategy and success for the directed evolution of enzymes *Curr. Opin. Struct. Biol.* **21** 473–80

[103] Johannes T W and Zhao H 2006 Directed evolution of enzymes and biosynthetic pathways *Curr. Opin. Microbiol.* **9** 261–7

[104] Chica R A, Doucet N and Pelletier J N 2005 Semi-rational approaches to engineering enzyme activity: combining the benefits of directed evolution and rational design *Curr. Opin. Biotechnol.* **16** 378–84

[105] Otten L G, Hollmann F and Arends I W 2010 Enzyme engineering for enantioselectivity: from trial-and-error to rational design? *Trends Biotechnol.* **28** 46–54

[106] Noble C G and Shi P-Y 2012 Structural biology of dengue virus enzymes: towards rational design of therapeutics *Antivir. Res.* **96** 115–26

[107] Jemli S *et al* 2016 Biocatalysts: application and engineering for industrial purposes *Crit. Rev. Biotechnol.* **36** 246–58

[108] Lin C, Ballinger K R and Khetani S R 2015 The application of engineered liver tissues for novel drug discovery *Expert Opin. Drug Discovery* **10** 519–40

[109] van Beilen J B and Li Z 2002 Enzyme technology: an overview *Curr. Opin. Biotechnol.* **13** 338–44

[110] Han H-K and Amidon G L 2000 Targeted prodrug design to optimize drug delivery *Aaps Pharmsci.* **2** 48–58

[111] Shi Y and Burn P 2004 Lipid metabolic enzymes: emerging drug targets for the treatment of obesity *Nat. Rev. Drug Discovery* **3** 695–710

[112] Opperdoes F R and Michels P A 2001 Enzymes of carbohydrate metabolism as potential drug targets *Int. J. Parasitol.* **31** 482–90

[113] Renaud J-P *et al* 2016 Biophysics in drug discovery: impact, challenges and opportunities *Nat. Rev. Drug Discov.* **15** 679–98

[114] Aghi M, Hochberg F and Breakefield X O 2000 Prodrug activation enzymes in cancer gene therapy *J. Gene Med.* **2** 148–64

[115] Hupfeld M *et al* 2018 A functional type II-A CRISPR–Cas system from *Listeria* enables efficient genome editing of large non-integrating bacteriophage *Nucleic Acids Res.* **46** 6920–33

[116] Glass Z *et al* 2018 Engineering the delivery system for CRISPR-based genome editing *Trends Biotechnol.* **36** 173–85

[117] Kang T S and Stevens R C 2009 Structural aspects of therapeutic enzymes to treat metabolic disorders *Hum. Mutat.* **30** 1591–610

[118] Lico C, Chen Q and Santi L 2008 Viral vectors for production of recombinant proteins in plants *J. Cell. Physiol.* **216** 366–77
[119] Warnock J N, Daigre C and Al-Rubeai M 2011 Introduction to viral vectors *Viral Vectors for Gene Therapy: Methods and Protocols* (Humana Press) pp 1–25
[120] Sookoian S and Pirola C J 2015 Liver enzymes, metabolomics and genome-wide association studies: from systems biology to the personalized medicine *World J. Gastroenterol.: WJG* **21** 711
[121] Hemalatha T *et al* 2013 Enzymes in clinical medicine: an overview *Indian J. Exp. Biol.* **51** 777–88
[122] Kirchheiner J and Seeringer A 2007 Clinical implications of pharmacogenetics of cytochrome P450 drug metabolizing enzymes *Biochim. Biophys. Acta (BBA)—Gen. Subj.* **1770** 489–94
[123] de la Fuente M *et al* 2021 Enzyme therapy: current challenges and future perspectives *Int. J. Mol. Sci.* **22** 9181
[124] Aitken M D 1993 Waste treatment applications of enzymes: opportunities and obstacles *Chem. Eng. J.* **52** B49–58
[125] Lim J and Mohamad Z 2022 Enzymes immobilized polymeric supports for wastewater treatment application: a short review *Mater. Today Proc.* **65** 2946–52
[126] Bilal M *et al* 2019 Emerging contaminants of high concern and their enzyme-assisted biodegradation—a review *Environ. Int.* **124** 336–53
[127] Naseri A *et al* 2020 Enzyme-assisted extraction and characterization of protein from red seaweed Palmaria palmata *Algal Res.* **47** 101849
[128] Alagawany M, Elnesr S S and Farag M 2018 The role of exogenous enzymes in promoting growth and improving nutrient digestibility in poultry *Iran. J. Vet. Res.* **19** 157
[129] Akhtar K *et al* 2019 Straw mulching with fertilizer nitrogen: an approach for improving crop yield, soil nutrients and enzyme activities *Soil Use Manag.* **35** 526–35
[130] Barletta A 2011 Introduction: current market and expected developments *Enzymes in Farm Animal Nutrition* (CABI) pp 1–11
[131] Stadlmair L F *et al* 2018 Enzymes in removal of pharmaceuticals from wastewater: a critical review of challenges, applications and screening methods for their selection *Chemosphere* **205** 649–61
[132] Facchin S *et al* 2013 Biodiversity and secretion of enzymes with potential utility in wastewater treatment *Open J. Ecol.* **3** 34–47
[133] Taylor K *et al* 1996 Enzyme-based wastewater treatment: removal of phenols by oxidative enzymes *Environmental Biotechnology: Principles and Applications* (McGraw-Hill) pp 524–32
[134] Te Poele S and Van der Graaf J 2005 Enzymatic cleaning in ultrafiltration of wastewater treatment plant effluent *Desalination* **179** 73–81

IOP Publishing

Introduction to Pharmaceutical Biotechnology, Volume 2 (Second Edition)
Enzymes, proteins and bioinformatics
Ahmed Al-Harrasi, Saurabh Bhatia and Ajmal Khan

Chapter 2

Technologies and procedures involved in enzyme production

2.1 Introduction

Enzyme production has become a significant area in the modern biotechnology industry. With advancements in traditional enzyme production methodologies, different industrial sectors can now easily exploit new applications offering novel activities and/or improved stability. Enzymes have been used by human beings since ancient times, either in the form of vegetables rich in enzymes, or in the form of microorganisms. These microorganisms have been used for many purposes, such as in brewing, and the baking industry. In the late nineteenth century numerous biological conversions were attributed to the action of enzymes. Isolation was first introduced by Payen and Persoz in 1833 [1]. They isolated an enzyme complex from malt, which they named 'diastase', that converts gelatinized starch into sugars, primarily maltose. In 1874, the history of modern enzyme production really began when Christian Hansen first synthesized rennet by isolating it from dried calves' stomachs with saline solution [2]. This was the first enzymatic preparation of relatively high purity used for commercial purposes. The Christian Hansen Company is still developing rennet today, in an almost identical way. In 1896, the utilization of the mold fungus koji in the production of certain foodstuffs and flavor additives based on soya protein and fermented beverages was the basis on which the Japanese researcher Takamine established a fermentation process for the industrial production of fungal amylase.

This process involves culturing of *Aspergillus oryzae* on moist rice or wheat bran, and the product is called 'Takadiastase' which is currently used as a pharmaceutical agent to cure digestive disorders [3]. The market value of the industrial enzymes market was estimated as approximately \$2 billion, and has increased at an average annual rate of 3%–5% in the last decade. Several enzyme production based

doi:10.1088/978-0-7503-5387-8ch2

companies have emerged, such as Novozymes dominating with 45% sales, followed by Danisco which holds a 20% share of the market. Bulk enzymes, such as proteases, amylases, lipases, etc, which are required in large quantities have, however, an intrinsically low unit value, so they demand significantly lower manufacturing costs. In contrast, the therapeutics sector includes enzymes such as urokinase, which are produced in lower quantities and at greater manufacturing cost. The technologies involved in the production of enzymes unite the disciplines of microbiology, genetics, biochemistry and engineering. Requirements for new enzymes can be achieved by the development of new procedures or the development of new procedures to address the unsatisfactory performance of known enzymes. Recent developments in gene technology have had a large impact on the enzyme industry. Genetic engineering tools have allowed enzyme manufacturers to synthesize adequate amounts of any enzyme irrespective of source, whereas protein engineering facilitates alteration of the enzymes before production. This chapter offers an outline of enzyme production procedures beginning from raw materials to the finished product, and also offers an understanding of the different alternative technologies existing for different phases of production.

2.1.1 Sources of enzymes

These enzymes are used for applications in industries on commercial scales [4]. There are various applications of these enzymes, for example, softening hides by using the feces of dogs and pigeons before tanning. A German researcher named Otto Rohm reported in 1905 that extracts from animal organs (pig and cow pancrease) could be used as the source of the enzyme protase, for leather softening [4]. The utilization of enzymes (mainly proteases) for cleaning laundry began in 1915. However, this was not initially successful due to allergic reactions to impurities in the enzymes. Currently, advance techniques are available for purification and the use of enzymes in washing powders (without allergic reactions) is common. A real boom in the large-scale industrial production of enzymes from microorganisms occurred after the 1950s. From the industrial point of view, enzymes can be derived from different sources, however, microbes act as an active source for unique biological enzymes and thus most enzymes are derived from microbial sources [4]. A wide variety of living organisms can serve as sources of enzymes, as depicted in figure 2.1.

2.1.1.1 Enzymes from animal and plant sources

A few decades ago, plants and animals were considered the major sources for enzymes. Even today, they are still major sources of certain enzymes [4], such as lipases, esterases and protease. Hen's eggs and human milk contain high amounts of lysozyme. This lysozyme with bovine lactoferrin offers innate immunity to an infant by killing gram-negative bacteria. Certain plants such as papaya (papain) and pineapple (bromelain) are excellent sources of enzymes. The following lists a few recent breakthroughs and discoveries:

- Enzymes present in herbivore gut fungi and their potential applications in fuels and chemical industry [5].

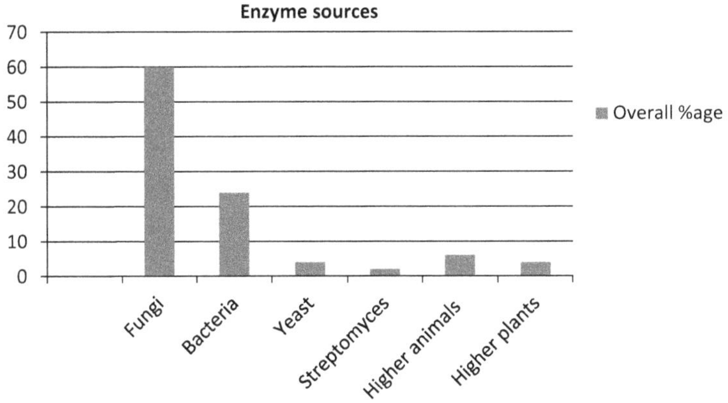

Figure 2.1. Enzyme sources.

- Bacterial enzymes responsible for human infection [6].
- Gro3P phosphatase responsible for the conversion of glucose and fats into other compounds (i.e., regulate how your body converts sugar and fats) [7].
- A class of DNA repair enzymes (DNA glycosylase) [8].
- An enzyme (reductive aminase) that will make a drug used to treat Parkinson's disease [9].

Enzyme production involves many critical steps which present major challenges in the production of enzymes from different sources. Lack of suitable isolation and purification procedures, low yield and high cost of overall process are the major challenges facing enzyme-based industries. Certain enzymes are more closely associated with cell walls and face certain problems such as low concentration, insolubility and maintaining biological activity. Offering an optimal pH and isoelectric point during extraction is an important factor in determining the biological activity of these enzymes. Thus selection of the purification procedure and the correct physical and chemical conditions also helps to retain the biological activity of an enzyme. Certain enzymes are very sensitive to variation in environmental factors, and can immediately lose activity, so their catalytic activity needs to be maintained by using a continuous process to accelerate the purification process. One of the recent developments for purification is a miniaturization automated approach that not only accelerates but also optimizes and statistically analyzes the enzymes during purification. The utilization of chromatographic techniques (aided by the development of new resins) and ultrafiltration are the main approaches to enzyme purification. The contamination and toxicity of enzymes are again major challenges that can be minimized during the production procedure, e.g. enzymes derived from bovine sources involve a high risk of contamination with bovine spongiform encephalopathy (an illness caused by the ingestion of abnormal proteins called prions). These prions can be carefully heat-inactivated at a certain temperature which will not affect the enzyme properties. Due to these serious concerns, microbial sources are generally preferred over plant- and animal-based enzymes [10, 11].

2.1.1.2 Enzymes derived from mammalian cell cultures

Mammalian cell cultures offer a continuous supply of enzymes that are commercially important (table 2.1), however, a major constraint is the cost, which can be extremely high [12]. With more advancements in tissue culture, in particular in the mass cultivation of cells and the availability of cheaper culture media, it is now possible to affordably produce many therapeutic enzymes such as urokinase. Further advancements in mammalian cell culture are exploring the application of cell immobilization, capillary culture, large-scale suspension culture and perfusion techniques. By using such approaches it is now possible to produce therapeutic enzymes, such as tissue plasminogen activator, at a large scale.

2.1.1.3 Microbial enzymes

Enzymes derived from microbes are referred to as microbial enzymes. Microbial enzymes were exploited for many decades without a complete understanding of how they work. Microbes are considered as the most reliable source for the production of commercial enzymes. In fact, many such enzymes are already being used on a commercial scale (table 2.2).

Since the rate of cell growth and proliferation in microbes is very high, a large amount of enzymes can be produced by culturing microorganisms under controlled *in vitro* environments. The media and other facilities involved in culturing microbes are economical in comparison to using plants and animals [4]. Moreover, plant and animal cells are more susceptible to contamination than microorganisms. Recombinant DNA technology can be utilized to increase the production of a desired protein in microorganisms, which is more challenging in plant and animal cells because of their high genetic complexity as eukaryotes compared to prokaryotes. This notion is based on the sexual mode of reproduction in eukaryotes which offers more genetic variation then prokaryotes (asexual reproduction).

To satisfy industrial demands, microbial sources must allow the proper recovery, isolation and purification of enzymes. The production procedure for enzymes is described in figure 2.2. The initial step in isolation is to select the best source that allows easy production of the enzyme within the shortest amount of time. Since microbial strains can grow rapidly and can be manipulated with the help of genetic

Table 2.1. Commercially produced enzymes from animal sources and their applications.

Enzyme(s)	Source(s)	Application(s)
Amylase, esterase	Lamb, calf	Digestive aids, preparation of cheese
Pepsin, trypsin	Bovine	
Lipase, rennin (chymosin) phospholipase, phytase	Porcine	
Lysozyme	Hen eggs	Cell wall breakage in bacteria
Human urine	Urokinase	For dissolution of blood clots

Table 2.2. Selected list of industrially (microbially) produced enzymes, their sources and applications.

Enzyme	Source(s)	Application(s)
α-amylase	*Aspergillus oryzae*, *Aspergillus niger*, *Bacillus subtilis*, *Bacillus licheniforms*	Production of beer and alcohol; preparation of glucose syrups; as a digestive aid; removal of starch sizes
Amyloglucosidase	*A. niger*, *Rhizopus niveus*	Starch hydrolysis
Cellulase	*A. niger*, *Tricoderma koningi*	Alcohol and glucose production
Glucoamylase	*A. niger*, *Bacillus amyloliquefaciens*	Production of beer and alcohol; starch hydrolysis
Glucose isomerase	*Arthrobacter* spp., *Bacillus* spp.	Manufacture of high fructose syrups
Glucose oxidase	*A. niger*	Antioxidant in prepared foods
Invertase	*Saccharomyces cerevisiae*	Sucrose inversion; preparation of artificial honey; confectionaries
Keratinase	*Streptomyces fradiae*	Removal of hair from hides
Lactase	*Kluyveromyus* spp., *Saccharomyces fragilis*	Lactose hydrolysis; removal of lactose from whey
Lipase	*Candida lipolytica*, *A. niger*	Preparation of cheese; flavor production
Pectinase	*Aspergillus* spp., *Sclerotina medina*	Clarification of fruit juices and wines; alcohol production; coffee concentration
Penicillin acylase	*Escherichia coli*	Production of 6-aminopenicillanic acid
Penicillanase	*B. subtilis*	Removal of penicillin
Protease, acid	*A. niger*	Digestive aid; substitute for calf rennet
Protease, neutral	*B. amyloliquefaciens*	Fish and meat tenderizer
Protease, alkaline	*A. oryzae*, *Streptomyces griseus*, *Bacillus* spp.	Meat tenderizer; detergent additive; beer stabilizer
Pollulanase	*Klebsiella aerogens*	Hydrolysis of starch
Takadiastase	*A. oryzae*	Bread supplement; digestive aid

engineering, i.e., rDNA and gene editing tools, they are considered as the best sources for the production of a large variety of enzymes. Several therapeutic enzymes have been successfully produced from different microbial sources, as shown in table 2.2.

2.1.1.3.1 Aspergillus niger for the production of bulk enzymes

Enzymes derived from fungal sources such as *Aspergillus*, *Rhizopus* and *Penicillium* are considered as safe. These sources all produce extracellular enzymes which can be conveniently recovered. Although various microorganisms produce extracellular enzymes, the most frequently utilized in industrial applications is *Aspergillus niger*. *A. niger*, a filamentous fungi, produces significant amounts of extracellular enzymes and citric acid, which are widely used for industrial purposes. So far, more than 50 enzymes have been isolated from this source, including various commercial enzymes

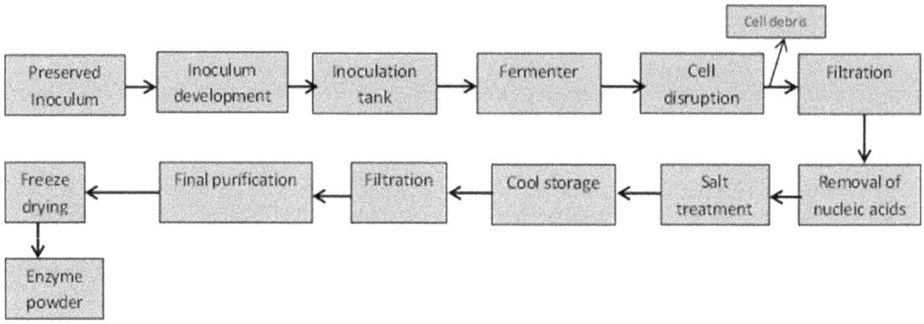

Figure 2.2. Schematic representation of the production of enzymes by microorganisms.

that are conveniently produced by *A. niger*. Some of the key enzymes are protease, insulinase phytase, catalase α-amylase, lipase, pectinase and cellulase [4]. This acid tolerant microorganism has significant hydrolytic potential in the production of α-amylase, and it also prevents bacteria-mediated contamination [13].

2.2 Enzyme production technology

Generally, the procedures used for microbial production of enzymes are equivalent to the methods used for the production of other industrial products. The significant features are, briefly [4]:

- Selection of organisms.
- Formulation of medium.
- Production process.
- Recovery and purification of enzymes.

A flow chart for enzyme production by microorganisms is depicted in figure 2.3.

2.2.1 Selection of microorganisms

Appropriate selection of microorganisms allows a high rate of production of enzymes. Selection can be achieved using different approaches, such as mutagens and radiation, in particular UV rays. The selection procedure for microorganisms is described in figure 2.4. The most significant factor in selecting microorganisms is that the organism should produce a high amount of the desired enzyme in a very short time, while the quantities of other metabolites produced should be low. After selecting the organism, strain improvement to optimize enzyme production can be achieved using suitable methods (as above, using mutagens or UV rays). After selection of the microorganisms, inoculum can be prepared in a liquid medium.

In enzyme research, the identification of enzymes is an important goal. The classical selective microbial screening method helps in discovering enzymes in populations of microorganisms. During this procedure organisms are selected and then individually isolated to develop pure cultures. A pure culture can be propagated to a higher level, however, only few colonies are obtained from this pure culture. Due to syntrophic benefits (interspecies interaction) it is again challenging to isolate

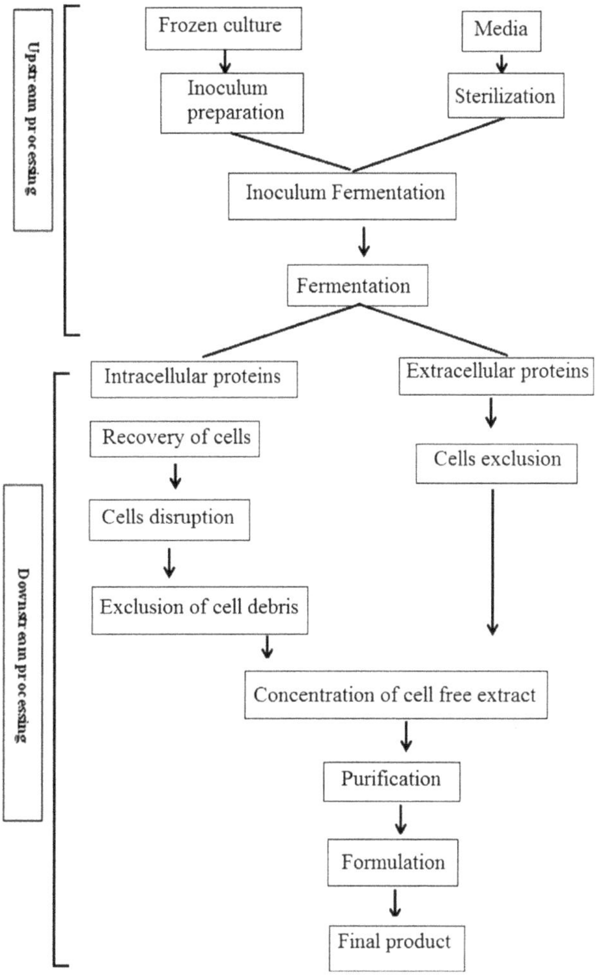

Figure 2.3. Enzyme production at an industrial scale.

pure colonies under standard conditions. Thus only 1% of pure culture can be derived from this classical selection method [14].

However, if pure cultures are only considered for enzyme isolation, then the maximum potential of the microorganisms, which are capable of producing other novel enzymes, will be ignored. There are vast numbers of microorganisms present in nature and it is challenging to cultivate all of them using classical microbiological techniques. The arrival of metagenomics allowed the retrieval of genetic material from the microbial environment without using any cultivation methods. At present, metagenomics are extensively used as a technique to isolate and identify enzymes with unique properties from the uncultivable part of microbial populations. These techniques allow researchers to establish the relationship between the genetic material (the genes responsible for enzyme production), the enzyme utilized (or whether an enzyme is utilized or not) and their properties. Recent developments in the field of

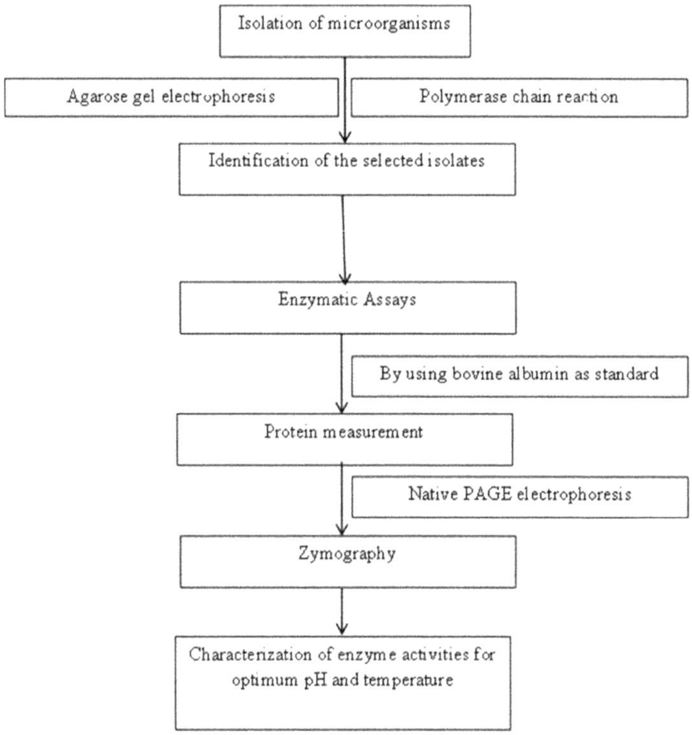

Figure 2.4. Microorganism selection for enzyme production by the classical method.

enzyme technology allow the exploration of new approaches, such as metaproteomics. Most importantly, using metagenomics it is possible to discover the genetic potential required by a cell to produce enzymes, i.e., identification of those particular genes that are responsible for the synthesis of the desired enzyme. After identification of the gene, there remains the challenge to discover whether the enzyme is synthesized under a particular environment and also whether the enzyme produced will carry all the desired properties. To further improve the selection process, the study of symbiotic environments (consortiums) was suggested, by integrating various omics-techniques, such as metagenomics (shotgun sequencing methods), metatranscriptomics and metaproteomics (extensive characterization of the whole protein complement of one microbiota condition at a particular time) [15, 16]. 'At a particular time' is significant, as the protein expression at different times helps in understanding protein dynamics. Consequently, metaproteomics allows temporal interpretation studies of protein expression, in comparison to the observational studies of the static metagenome.

2.2.2 Medium selection

In the classical approach, a suitable culture medium with defined composition is selected that contains all the vital components to encourage the growth of only those microorganisms that are capable of producing relatively large amounts of enzymes. The nutritional component of the culture medium should be available at a low price and should be safe. For the growth of anchorage-dependent microorganisms, a number of substrates in the medium have been explored, such as yeast extract, whey, starch hydrolysate, corn steep liquor, molasses and soybean meal. In traditional approaches of fermentation, cereals (wheat) and pulses (peanut) have been utilized as substrates. Optimal pH is required for significant microbial growth and also plays an important role in enzyme production.

2.2.3 Production process

The production of enzymes is often performed at larger scales using fermentation techniques, in particular submerged fermentation (the development of microorganisms in a liquid broth) and solid-substrate fermentation (the development of microorganisms on a solid substrate, e.g. rice bran or wheat bran). In submerged fermentation a liquid broth is utilized to offer nutrients that result in the production of industrial enzymes, antibiotics or other products. At the industrial scale, submerged liquid fermentation procedures are classically employed for the production of enzymes from microbial sources, whereas solid-substrate fermentation is rarely used for this purpose. This is because submerged liquid fermentation offers a number of advantages, such as ease of handling and greater control of environmental factors (such as temperature and pH). However, the solid-substrate fermentation method can also be utilized to improve the yield and decrease the cost of enzyme production [17, 18].

Solid-substrate fermentation is an alternative approach to submerged fermentation which is often employed for the production of fungal enzymes such as cellulases, amylases, proteases and pectioases [19]. During this process microorganisms are developed under a controlled environment to produce enzymes, fuel and nutrients. Sterilization is not essentially required for solid-substrate fermentation, as the fermentation substrate starts sterilization and the microbes inhibit the growth of micro-flora. It has been reported that both approaches (submerged and solid-substrate fermentation) are considered as effective techniques to produce several valuable products. Due to advancements in fermentation technology, particularly in solid-substrate fermentation, bioreactors of different sizes have now been designed. The design of bioreactors is based on the principles of biochemical engineering, including mathematical modeling, which is important in defining the cellular development of microorganisms. Several problems, such as heat and mass transfer, can be overcome using such bioreactors.

For fermentation (if required), batch and continuous sterilization techniques can be employed to sterilize a suitable medium. Afterwards the medium is inoculated with a suitable microorganism to initiate the fermentation process. The culture's environmental conditions, such as pH, temperature, O_2 and nutrient supplementation are initially optimized and later maintained to achieve the desired growth of microorganisms. The addition of an antifoaming agent is required to inhibit surface tension. Production also involves fermentation kinetics, the mathematical analysis of certain factors that helps in designing or improving the batch and continuous process. It has been observed that continuous fermentation processes give a lower enzyme yield, thus enzyme production is often conducted using batch fermentation, and only rarely using the continuous process. The vessel should be sterile during the fermentation process. Aseptic conditions can be maintained by effective management of vessel design, operating procedures, continuous monitoring and maintenance, and skilled technicians. Usually, the duration of the fermentation process varies from 2 to 7 days. Certain additional metabolites are also produced in the medium which can interfere with recovery of the desired enzyme, however, only desired enzyme(s) should be recovered and purified.

2.2.4 Recovery and purification of enzymes

After developing the selected microorganisms or establishing a pure culture, the recovery of suitable extracellular enzymes is again a challenge, since the culture medium can be full of unwanted end-products released by the stationary phase of the microorganisms. These unwanted substances can interfere with the recovery of suitable enzymes. Since the recovery of extracellular enzymes is easier than that of intracellular enzymes, based on the recovery process used, commercial enzyme preparations are available in crude or highly purified form. However, other factors such as the form of medium (solid or liquid), viscosity, the nature of the enzyme and the degree of purity desired, etc, affect the recovery of enzymes. As discussed, downstream processing, which involves recovery and purification steps for extracellular enzymes, is easier compared to intracellular enzymes which require more advance techniques for cell lysis. The selection of a suitable hydrolyzing agent for intracellular enzyme recovery is a crucial step. It requires a basic understanding of cell membrane physiology and should be carried out such that the enzyme properties are not affected. Different physical, chemical and enzymatic hydrolyzing agents have been reported to break the cell wall and release their intracellular material [20]. However, the recovery of enzymes closely associated with the membrane is challenging. Cell lysis is always followed by differential centrifugation which allows the separation of cytoplasmic particles on the basis of size and specific gravity. For recovery from microbial sources, the cell membrane can be lysed by physical means, such as sonication, high pressure and glass beads. Lysozyme is often used as a hydrolyzing agent for the lysis of the bacterial cell wall. For cell wall breakdown in yeasts, the carbohydrate enzyme β-glucanase is used to break down the glycosidic bonds within beta-glucans, which allows the release and solubilization of these polymers from the cell walls. However, enzymatic procedures have the disadvantage of their high cost. Cellulose-degrading enzyme methods are often employed for intracellular enzyme recovery. The methodologies utilized for both intracellular and extracellular enzyme extraction always remain same, however, the hydrolyzing agents often differ. The objective of both procedures is to decrease the loss of the anticipated enzyme and its activity [20].

2.2.5 Cell debris removal

Procedures such as cross-flow microfiltration with rapid back pulsing and differential centrifugation can be employed to remove cell debris. For thermostable enzymes, a more convenient method is to denature the unwanted proteins by heating, then cooling the solution, and finally unwanted proteins can be removed by centrifugation.

2.2.6 Nucleic acid removal

Non-proteinaceous contamination, such as nucleic acids, restricts recovery and purification of enzymes. These contaminants can be removed by precipitation processes using polyamines, streptomycin and polyethyleneimine [21]. The presence of DNA/RNA contaminants can be examined by blotting techniques and simple wavelength scan assessment of DNA/RNA.

2.2.7 Precipitation of enzymes

In a solution, salt concentration generally determines the protein solubility. During the process called salting-in, the concentration of salts is low, which can stabilize several charged groups over the protein molecule, and which can ultimately increase the solubility of the protein. In contrast, an increase in salt concentration increases the solubility to a particular point, afterwards a further increase in the salt concentration increases precipitation of proteins as water molecules are now replaced with salt concentration, so insufficient water molecules for solubilization of the protein are available. Precipitation of protein in the presence of a surplus amount of salt is called salting-out. Various salts can be utilized for this phenomenon. Ammonium sulfate is often used for this purpose as it has high solubility and is comparatively inexpensive. Ammonium sulfate reduces the solubility of proteins and enhances the precipitation, which may further increase the stability of the native conformation. Precipitation is very beneficial in downstream processing, as the precipitated enzyme can be solubilized in a minimal volume to concentrate the enzyme [22].

2.2.8 Liquid–liquid partition

The desired enzymes can be obtained by liquid–liquid chromatography using polyethylene glycol or polyamines. Liquid–liquid partition chromatography can also be utilized to identify conformational changes in well-characterized enzymes [23]. Various advanced liquid–liquid fractionation techniques have emerged, such as the aqueous two-phase system, which was initially accidently utilized by Martinus Willem Beijerinck (1896) by mixing an aqueous solution of starch and gelatin [24, 25]. The influence of organic solvents on the partitioning of enzymes in aqueous two-phase systems was studied in 1987 [24]. As per this report, partition coefficients for alkaline phosphatase decrease with ethylene glycol, glycerol, sucrose and urea. In 1996, the effects of low temperature (−18 °C) on glycolytic enzymes (e.g. phosphofructokinase) were investigated in terms of the stability and partitioning within an aqueous two-phase system [26]. It was found that the presence of ethylene glycol, phase polymers and low temperature stabilized enzyme activities.

This technique has now gained much attention because of its great potential for the extraction, separation, purification and enrichment of proteins, in particular enzymes, nucleic acids and other biomolecules. This complex partition behavior is formed by mixing a variety of components in water. As water is the main component of both phases in aqueous two-phase systems, it offers a protected environment to biomolecules for their separation and polymers to stabilize their structure and biological activities. In contrast, other liquid–liquid extraction methods containing organic solvents can cause severe damage to biological products [27].

One of the more reliable systems for enzymes is the PEG–salt aqueous two-phase systems. This system is an excellent and useful liquid–liquid extraction approach for the downstream processing of proteins and enzymes.

Several enzymes have been purified using liquid–liquid extraction. For purification using liquid–liquid partition, a novel, efficient and economical extraction method with a high purification factor, composed of surfactant and acetonitrile, has recently been developed to purify polygalacturonase from *Durio zibethinus* [28].

2.2.9 Chromatographic separation

Various chromatographic procedures for separation and purification of enzymes are available such as:

- *Ion-exchange chromatography*: A pH-dependent process which is governed by the enzyme structure and isoelectric point. The enzymes' charge becomes positive (they bind to cation exchangers) when present in a solution with pH less than the isoelectric point and becomes negative when present in a solution of pH greater than the isoelectric point (they bind to anion exchangers).
- *Size exclusion chromatography*: In this process enzymes in a solution are separated by their size, and in some cases molecular weight.
- *Hydrophobic interaction*: Proteins are not denatured in hydrophobic interaction chromatography, and the enzymes eluted from the column retain their enzymatic activity. Hydrophobic interaction is performed to separate the amylase, lipase and trypsinogen present in dog pancreatic juice through high-performance liquid chromatography [29].
- *Dye ligand chromatography*: A unique and selective purification technique in which ligands may act as substrate analogs, offering affinity interactions with their corresponding enzymes, e.g. the interaction of Cibacron blue F3GA with proteins and enzymes. Another example of synthetic affinity ligands is chlorotriazine dyes, often used as affinity-based protein purification methods for a number of reasons, such as their low cost, easy chemical immobilization of the dyes to the matrix and the fact that the final product dye-adsorbents are resistant to chemical and biological degradation.

Among all of these, ion-exchange chromatography is the most frequently used for enzyme purification. Many fractionation issues have been faced in the separation of certain enzymes, such as cellulolytic enzymes. For separation of such enzymes ion-exchange chromatography and isoelectric focusing (chromatofocusing) are considered beneficial [30].

2.2.10 Drying and packing

Drying is the most suitable method to obtain a concentrated form of an enzyme. This step is crucial in preserving the original properties and function of an enzymatic preparation. Drying can be achieved using several evaporators or dryers, e.g. film evaporators, freeze dryers (lyophilizes) and spray dryers. The dried enzyme can be packed and marketed. For some enzymes, stability can be attained by keeping them in ammonium sulfate suspensions.

Most of the enzymes used in foods or medical treatments should be of high-grade purity, and must meet the required specifications set by the regulatory bodies. These enzymes must be completely free from toxic materials, harmful microorganisms and should not cause any allergic reactions.

Based on a recent breakthrough, the innate bacterial system for the formation of outer membrane vesicles can be used to protect the enzyme function. This type of packing prevents the degradation of the enzyme and protects its natural integrity. Thus outer membrane vesicle packing provide the enzyme with increased stability across a extensive range of storage conditions [31].

The drying of enzymes has usually been achieved by spray-drying and freeze-drying. In a recent study, two traditional methods of α-amylase drying were studied. The product derived from both procedures showed high enzymatic activity, however, spray-drying can be considered as more economical, because in freeze-drying the process duration can be considered as a limiting factor [32].

2.2.11 Regulation of microbial enzyme production

Fermentation conditions such as nutrients, pH, O_2, temperature, etc, can be optimized to obtain the maximum production of therapeutic proteins such as microbial enzymes. To achieve maximum production, a deep understanding of the genetic elements responsible for the regulation of enzyme synthesis is required. Enzyme synthesis can be repressed by regulatory proteins. These proteins actively bind with DNA and increase or inhibit the function of RNA polymerase. Thus these proteins can act as repressors or activators. The regulation of microbial enzyme synthesis and the genetic elements involved are briefly discussed here.

2.2.12 Induction

Enzyme induction is defined as an increase in the production of enzymes as a result of any stimulus, whereas repression can be defined as the decrease in enzyme production after a stimulus [33]. The process of induction is often present in bacteria and other microbes, whereas it is more rarely observed in animal metabolism, e.g. cholesterol synthesis and regulation of gluconeogenesis provide examples of enzyme induction and repression [33].

Several inducers should be explored to make the enzyme more efficiently. These inducers are available in different forms: substrate, product and intermediate. Sucrose, starch and galactosides are examples of substrates, whereas fatty acid, phenylacetate and xylobiose are products or intermediates. These inducers selectively and efficiently allow the expression of gene coding for a particular enzyme and hence exert the opposite action to an enzyme repressor. Some examples of enzymes and their respective inducers are listed in table 2.3. The high cost of these inducers and their treatment (sterilization, addition at specific time) has restricted their utilization. Thus recently several efforts have been made to produce mutants of

Table 2.3. Selected examples of inducible enzymes along with the inducers.

Enzyme	Inducer
β-Galactosidase	Galactosides
Amylase	Starch
Invertase	Sucrose
Lipase	Fatty acids
Penicillin G amidase	Phenylacetate
Xylanase	Xylobiose

microorganisms in which inducer dependence is eliminated. There are certain proteins that are responsible for mutation, and reports suggest that it is the proteins responsible for induction of the stress response pathways that allow mutation [34, 35].

2.2.13 Feedback repression

During feedback repression, repression of the synthesis of an enzyme (required at an initial stage of the pathway) takes place, e.g. the supplementation of a higher concentration of addition of such an end-product (usually a small molecule) to the culture medium leads to the inhibition of the enzymes synthesis of the specific pathway. This type of end-product addition significantly affects the enzyme production. In this method the desired organisms are cultured to achieve large-scale production of desired enzymes. Feedback inhibition takes place once the reaction end-product inhibits the enzyme that helped in their production. Thus feedback regulation by the end-product significantly affects enzyme synthesis. This takes place when the end-product accumulates in large quantities. The synthesis of feedback regulated enzymes in the laboratory is somewhat challenging. However, mutants that do not carrying feedback repression can be produced to prevent this issue. Mitchell *et al* reported feedback repression of ornithine decarboxylase synthesis mediated by an antizyme [36].

2.2.14 Nutrient repression

Overproduction of microbial metabolites is linked to the growth phases of microorganisms. Different types of overproduction are caused by inducers, effectors, inhibitors and various signal molecules. In microbial cells, the biosynthesis of enzymes catalyzing metabolic reactions is regulated by distinct positive and negative mechanisms, such as induction, nutritional regulation (carbon or nitrogen source regulation), feedback regulation, etc [37]. The native metabolism of the microorganism is so developed that no production of unnecessary enzymes occurs. In other words, the microorganisms do not produce enzymes that are not required by them, as this is a wasteful exercise. The inhibition of surplus enzyme production is achieved by nutrient repression. The nutrients can be carbon, nitrogen, phosphate or sulfate suppliers in the growth medium [37]. For large-scale synthesis of enzymes, nutrient repression must be overcome. In using carbon sources and energy from artificial media, certain microorganisms, in particular heterotrophic bacteria, can utilize an extensive range of sugars, organic acids and other organic compounds. Usually, glucose is considered as the ideal carbon source for *B. subtilis*. The presence of a large amount of glucose supports the strong repression of genes encoding the enzymes for the utilization of alternative carbon sources in the presence of glucose [38, 39]. Some other carbohydrates such as malate also act as a second preferred carbon source for *B. subtilis*. Malate is also responsible for causing a strong catabolite repression of transporters for alternative carbon sources [40]. This strong catabolite repression allows the cells to select suitable carbon sources. Generally, it involves the regulation of gene expression to prevent transcription of catabolic genes, which permits the cells to select among several available carbon sources. Regulation of gene expression allows the regulation of protein activity to avert the formation of specific inducers.

Glucose repression is a type of nutrient-based repression which prevents the production of certain enzymes that are required for metabolism. To prevent glucose repression carbohydrate can be supplemented to the fermentation medium in such a manner that the amount of glucose becomes almost zero at any given time. To date, many efforts have been made to explore mutants that are resistant to catabolize repression by glucose, e.g. development of mutants of *Trichoderma reesei* that are resistant to catabolite repression [41].

Moreover, many other carbon sources such as succinate, citrate, lactate and pyruvate act as catabolite repressors for some microorganisms. Several examples of nitrogen sources as repressors are also present in microorganisms. It is already known that not all nitrogen sources support growth equally. Thus yeast chooses its nitrogen sources to allow the best growth through a mechanism referred to as nitrogen catabolite repression. As per the literature, two nitrogen sources, ammonia and glutamine (due to presence of ammonium ions or amino acids), are considered to elicit nitrogen catabolite repression. Thus inexpensive ammonium salts are often utilized as nitrogen sources. By developing mutants resistant to this nitrogen source, repression by ammonium salts can be prevented [42].

2.3 Procedures involved in enzyme production

2.3.1 Source and location of enzymes

Every cell synthesizes enzymes, thus they can be derived from plant tissues, animal tissues and microorganisms. The amount of enzymes produced on an industrial scale from plants and animal sources is significant, nevertheless microbial enzymes have gradually overtaken them for both technical and commercial reasons. Plant-based enzymes need a large amount of plant material and the amount of enzyme recovered is very small. Animal-based enzymes are end-products of the meat industry. The only animal enzyme to be produced in quantities greater than 2 ton/year is rennet or chymosin, obtained from the calf stomach. Most plant-based enzymes are hydrolytic enzymes, e.g. α- and β-amylases, β-glucanase, and papain. Most of these enzymes are used by the food industry. Therefore, initially, plant and animal enzymes were preferred over microbial enzymes mainly for considerations of safety and the fear of contamination through microorganisms, toxins, etc. However microorganisms have received significant attention during the last three decades. According to the literature, microbial enzymes are not subjected to any of the production and supply limitations of plant and animal enzymes. The production size of microbial enzymes may be expanded and the types of enzymes accessible from microorganisms are almost limitless. Microbes offer the following advantages over other sources of enzymes:

- Microorganism growth is very fast and they can be cultured on a medium comprising a cheap raw material.
- Genetic engineering and manipulation of microbial cells can be achieved in the research laboratory to enhance the final yield of enzymes.
- Enormous quantities of enzymes can be produced from microbes.
- Animal sacrifice can be stopped.

In a living cell (plant or animal), the mitochondria have a highly organized structure and contain a large number of enzymes, such as glutamate dehydrogenase. Cellular organelles, e.g. granular microsomes, lysosomes and ribosomes, also contain key enzymes; ribosomes are the site of protein biosynthesis and lysosomes contain many hydrolases. The soluble portion of the cytoplasm includes enzymes responsible for glycolysis. In the bacterial cell, certain structures of plant and animal cells are not present. In the cytoplasm, outside the nucleus, the cell is filled with a granular cytoplasm. Enzymes are present in the granules, the soluble cytoplasm and adsorbed on the cell membrane.

Enzymes produced by hyperthermophiles (bacteria and archaea with optimal growth temperatures of >80 °C), also known as hyperthermophilic enzymes, are characteristically thermostable (i.e., resistant to irreversible inactivation at high temperatures) and are optimally active at high temperatures. These enzymes share the same catalytic mechanisms with their mesophilic counterparts. These thermophilic and hyperthermophilic enzymes can be potentially utilized as research reagents and as catalysts for industrial processes [43].

2.3.2 The variety of microorganisms

Selection of a microorganism for enzyme production is performed on the following basis [4]:

- Fermentation duration should be low.
- The microorganisms must adapt themselves to the physical and chemical properties of the culture medium, e.g. temperature, pH, the availability of substrates, etc. Currently, two genera, *Aspergillus* and *Bacillus*, are used for the large-scale production of enzymes.
- The microorganisms must be nonpathogenic.
- The microorganisms must cultivate on an economical raw material.
- The microorganisms must offer high yields of enzymes.

- The microorganisms should synthesize extracellular enzymes, as their isolation and separation is simple and economic, however, only hydrolases have been found extracellularly.
- The strain must not synthesize end-products which hinder the growth of microorganisms.

2.3.3 Media for fermentation

The enzyme production medium should include sources of carbon, nitrogen, energy, minerals, macro-nutrients and micro-nutrients. Growth factors are required in the case of auxotrophic microorganisms. If an inducible enzyme is to be synthesized, the inducer should be supplemented to the medium. At times, co-enzymes act as an inducer or sometimes constituents of the medium may have an induction effect. Enzyme-catalyzed reaction end-products may also act as inductors. Catabolic enzyme fermentation is inhibited by the direct or indirect effect of products on their activity, such as the production of proteases in *Bacillus* species by amino acids. Different sources of carbon, nitrogen and other growth substances are mentioned in table 2.4.

2.3.4 Fermentation

There are several measures available for fermentation; however, for the synthesis of enzymes only three methods are used [44]:

- Submerged culture.
- Solid-substrate culture.
- Deep-bed cultivation.

2.3.4.1 Submerged culture

Submerged fermentation is the cultivation of microorganisms in liquid nutrient broth. In submerged cultures, the synthesis usually takes place in mechanically stirred bioreactors with capacities ranging from 20 000 to 100 000 l batch fermentation [44]. Usually the main fermentation persists for 50–200 h depending upon the enzyme and microorganism used. Continuous fermentation has some limitations due to the difficulty in sterilization of the nutrient media, and instability of highly mutated production strains. On a large scale, continuous fermentation has

Table 2.4. Fermentation medium constituents and their sources.

Constituents	Various sources
Source of carbon and energy	Cereal meal, soybean meal, potato starch, wheat or rice bran, molasses
Source of nitrogen	Fish meal, gelatin, casein, soybean meal, bran, distillers' solubles' peptones
Source substances and trace elements	Yeast extract, corn steep liquor, plant oil, meal of oil-bearing seed bran

been utilized for the production of glucose isomerase. The overall yield of enzyme depends upon the degree of enzyme synthesis during different growth phases. Maximum enzyme production is frequently derived in the stationary phase in an inducible system with catabolic repression, when the microorganism has fallen to zero. Currently, the process is carried out in a two-stage cascade, in which a high quantity of cell mass is first synthesized and then the synthesis of the enzyme takes place in a second reactor under different conditions. Additionally, factors such as nutrient medium, pH, temperature, partial pressure of oxygen and aeration must be taken into consideration. The final yield of extracellular enzymes can be improved by the supplementation of surfactants. Once fermentation is completed, the ferment is cooled and the cell mass is separated. Extracellular enzymes are present in the culture filtrate and therefore the biomass is discarded, however, for intracellular enzymes the biomass contains the enzymes and thus the culture filtrate is discarded [44].

While isolating enzymes from the fermentation medium one must eliminate insoluble products, e.g. microbial cells. This is usually achieved by centrifugation. As most industrial enzymes are extracellular (secreted by cells into the external environment), they remain in the fermented broth after the biomass has been removed. The biomass can be reused as a fertilizer, but it must be treated with lime to inactivate the microorganisms and stabilize it during storage. The enzymes in the rest broth are then concentrated by evaporation, membrane filtration or crystallization, depending on their intended application. If pure enzyme preparations are required, they are usually isolated by gel or ion-exchange chromatography. Some applications require solid enzyme products, so the crude powder enzymes are converted into granules to make them more suitable to use. Occasionally liquid formulations are selected as they are easier to handle and dose along with other liquid ingredients. Enzymes employed during starch conversion to convert glucose into fructose are immobilized, usually on the surfaces of inert granules held in reaction columns or towers. This is done to extend their working life as these enzymes usually go on working for over a year.

2.3.4.2 Solid-substrate culture

Solid-substrate fermentation is currently used in a variety of applications, e.g. antibiotic and enzyme production, recently developed products such as bioactive compounds and organic acids, new trends regarding bioethanol and biodiesel as sources of alternative energy, and biosurfactant molecules with environmental purposes of utilizing unexploited biomass [45]. Solid-substrate fermentation is primarily used for traditional food processing and also for fungal enzyme production. During this process, the microorganism is propagated on a solid substrate supplemented with a high concentration of nutrients, micro-nutrients and minerals and with a large surface area, e.g. cereal meal, wheat bran and/or rice bran. This process is an alternative to the production of enzymes in liquid by submerged fermentation. This process is suitable for the extraction of enzymes from fungi, such as *Penicillium, Aspergillus*, etc [45]. The moisture content of the medium is low which hinders the growth of bacteria. There are two procedures available for growths of fungi: the drum process and tray process. In the drum process horizontally rotating drums are utilized for the propagation of fungi. In the tray process, the fungi are propagated in trays of size 2 × 40 cm. The substrate is spread in a thin layer (thickness 1–10 cm). The microorganisms, in the form of spores, are inoculated and then the trays are incubated in an air-conditioned room. A method called the high-heap process has also been used, in which a constant stream of air is enforced through the nutrient substrate. This ensures a supply of oxygen as well as elimination of the heat of reaction. The growth phase continues for 1–7 days. After completion of growth and fermentation, the fungi are homogenized and dried (moisture content 10%–15%). For this process, homogenized powder can be used directly or the fungal mycelium is extracted with water. There are numerous substrates that can be utilized for the production of enzymes by solid-substrate fermentation such as wheat bran, rice bran, sugar beet pulp, and wheat and corn flour. The selection of the substrate depends on several factors, chiefly related to cost and the availability. Additional factors such as particle size and the level of moisture also play an important role. Smaller substrate particles have a larger surface area for the proliferation of the microorganisms, however, if the surface is too small the efficiency of respiration will be obstructed and poor development and hence poor synthesis of enzymes will result. Larger particles offer more effective aeration and respiration, although there is a reduction in the surface area. Solid-substrate fermentation needs moisture to be present on the substrate for the microorganisms to synthesize enzymes. Therefore, the water content of the substrate must also be optimized, as a higher or lower presence of water may badly affect the microbial activity. Water also has effects on the physico-chemical properties of the solid substrate. Some of the enzymes of industrial importance which have been produced by solid-substrate fermentation are proteases, pectinases, glucoamylases and cellulases. Revankar *et al* reported solid-substrate fermentation for enhanced production of laccase using indigenously isolated *Ganoderma* spp. [46].

2.3.4.3 Deep-bed cultivation

The deep-bed or pile cultivator method process was initially developed to meet the huge demand for enzymes for soya fermentation [46]. During this procedure the microorganisms are allowed to cultivate in rectangular vessels of dimensions 18 × 200 inches. The nutrient medium is added into the vessels up to a height of 2 feet. In deep-bed cultivation, cereal meal, wheat bran, rice bran, soybean, potato flakes, etc are used as the medium. The medium is sterilized and then inoculated with the organism. The nature of the culture vessel is maintained to increase the growth of the organism. At desirable growth, the microbes are used in the extraction of enzymes. This process solves most of the problems related to the traditional process. It uses substrate layers up to 2–6 feet. The deep-bed process is a modification of solid-substrate fermentation and it is fully automated.

2.3.5 Enzyme extraction

The extraction of enzymes can be defined as the liberation of enzymes from cells or cellular constituents. Extraction is done by mechanical, physical, chemical, or a combination of these procedures to disrupt the cell wall or membrane. To enable extraction of either intra- or extracellular enzymes, it may be essential to modify the nature of the liquid medium to complete the dissociation. Down-streaming of enzyme fermentation through drying of the substrate is simple, although it can be complicated depending on whether a crude or high-grade enzyme is to be produced, or whether the enzyme is extracellular or intracellular [46]. For fungal enzymes, centrifugation or filtration are the two procedures which are most often used to separate enzymes, however, bacterial enzymes are difficult to concentrate and purify [46]. Certain enzymes necessitate the presence of a co-factor, lipid or carbohydrates to preserve their activity during extraction.

2.3.5.1 Animal and plant tissue breakdown

Most animal enzymes are confined in a particular organ or in muscles. In this procedure, these organs are initially minced in a vertical cutter mixer after removal of fat [47]. Freezing the animal tissue frequently supports grinding and prevents blockage by wet tissue. For this purpose frozen meat grinders are used. The pulverized tissues are then allowed to pass through a colloid which produces maximum cell disintegration. Grinding of certain plant tissues is a major concern, e.g. seeds which contain more enzymes than green tissues. Grinding of green tissues can be achieved by a process called maceration, in which the plant material is macerated by grinding in a hammer mill or some other chopper mill, and the pulp is pressed. Lytic enzymes can also be used to disrupt the cell wall [48].

There are several ways of extracting enzymes from animal tissue. Initially, aqueous phase separation was proposed for extracting and purifying proteins from animal tissue [49]. Boland *et al* reported the purification of enzymes from animal tissue using aqueous two-phase systems in pilot scale studies.

2.3.5.2 Disruption of microbial cells

Microbial cells synthesize both extracellular and intracellular enzymes. Extracellular enzymes do not require cell disruption, but the release of intracellular enzymes from microorganisms requires a more vigorous method of cell breakage [50–53]. The different methods of microbial cell disruption are illustrated in figure 2.5.

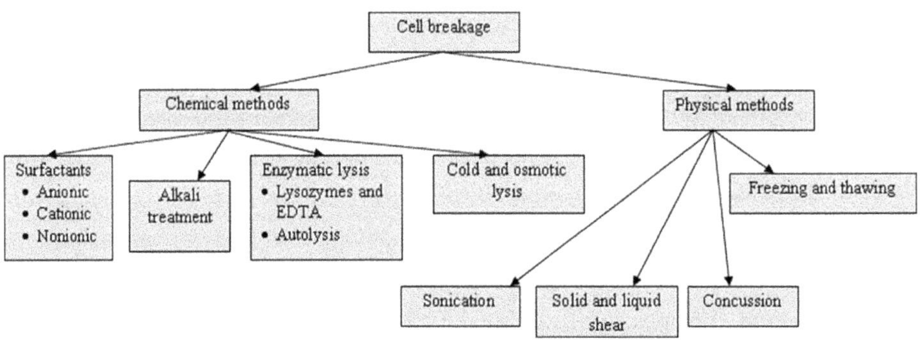

Figure 2.5. Various methods of microbial cell disruption.

For industrial scale cell disruption, the mechanical procedures of disruption seem to be the most popular [50–53]. Of these, the high-pressure homogenizer and the bead mill are the most frequently used. The high-pressure homogenizer is best suited to some bacteria and yeasts, whereas the bead mill is more appropriate for the disintegration of yeast cells and for mycelial organisms and algae. There is sufficient evidence to demonstrate that mechanical cell disruption methods do not harm most intracellular enzymes and proteins; membrane-associated enzymes and multi-enzyme complexes may be the exceptions. Additional techniques which may have potential large-scale applications are ultrasonication, freeze-pressing and enzymatic lysis. An arrangement of two or more disruption techniques for disruption of more resistant organisms may have economic advantages [50–53].

2.3.5.2.1 Disruption by chemical methods

Surfactants. Among surfactants, ionic (cationic and anionic) and nonionic surfactants are used to lyse microbial cells. Surfactants have the potential to solubilize the microbial cell wall. Frequently used surfactants are sodium dodecyl sulfate, cetyl triethyl ammonium bromide, triton X-100, various tweens, etc. Selective extraction of cholesterol oxidase from *Nocardia rhedocrous* by cell permeabilization, using the surfactant Triton X-100, has been evidenced [51]. This surfactant is quite costly, however, and industrial scale use may not be possible. Additionally, contamination of the product with the surfactant is another disadvantage.

Enzymatic lysis. During large-scale operations autolysis is the most frequently used method for the extraction of enzymes. A suspension of cells is maintained at high temperature (23 °C–37 °C) for several hours. After cooling, the cell extract is harvested by centrifugation [52]. This procedure is used in the extraction of transaldolase from frozen *Candida utilis*, invertase from baker's yeast, and glucose-6-phosphate dehydrogenase from yeast. Autolysis is also used for the extraction of intracellular enzymes. The procedure has a risk of thermal denaturation of enzymes or their damage by cellular proteases. Microbial cell lysis can also be achieved by using lysozymes, e.g. egg white lysozyme. Lysozyme hydrolyzes the glycosidic bonds in the glycopeptide component of the bacterial cell wall, releasing intracellular enzymes [52].

Enzyme cell lysis is an attractive tool in terms of its delicacy and specificity to just the cell wall structure, but is restricted by the high cost of the enzyme, which is usually lost into the extract [52]. This can be prevented by the use of an immobilization technique in which soluble immobilized enzymes in ultrafilter reactors are used. Reduction in the cost of cell lytic enzymes may also be possible by increasing the scale of production [50, 52, 54]. The sensitivity of microorganisms against various lytic enzymes changes significantly with the development phase and fermentation conditions. In certain cases, autolysis of microbial cells without any foreign enzyme may be possible.

Cold and osmotic shock. In this procedure, the normal growth temperature is reduced to 0 °C, resulting in loss of viability of the microorganisms. This technique is not applicable to large-scale production, as cell suspensions with a density greater than 10^8 ml^{-1} show no effect of osmotic shock and bacteria are more vulnerable to cold shock.

Some degradative enzymes such as alkaline phosphatase, cyclic phosphodiesterase, 5′-nucleotidase, acid phosphatase, and ribonucleic acid inhibited endonuclease are explicitly released from exponentially growing *E. coli* by osmotic shock [55]. Cell disruption by osmotic shock involves the following steps:

- Bacteria washing to remove growth medium by a buffer solution.
- Resuspending the washed cells in a 20% buffered sucrose solution.
- Removal of cell by centrifugation. After following these steps, the final paste is then suspended in water. The rapid increase in osmotic pressure inside the cells causes the release of cell constituents.

Alkali treatment. A rapid increase in pH will cause the lysis of the bacterial cell wall. This method is used in the large-scale extraction of l-asparaginase from *Erwinica chrysantheme* [55]. The effectiveness of this method depends upon the pH stability of the desired enzyme. If the desired enzyme is inactivated by alkaline pH, then this method is not applicable [55, 56].

2.3.5.2.2 Disruption by physical methods

Sonication. Sonication of proteins results in the formation of aggregates that resemble amyloids. In addition, sonication is often used to break aggregates into smaller pieces for seeding new batches. At the pilot scale, ultrasonic waves are often used for cell lysis. The ultrasonic or sonic waves passing via a liquid consist of alternate compression and rarefaction. If the wave amplitude is high, then a cavity is produced, which leads to the formation and breaking of bubbles. The formed bubbles or cavities create many cycles, generating high local pressures of about 20 000 atmospheres. The mechanical shocks are sensed at a distance of a few microns. Ultrasonic waves have been used successfully in a number of extraction methods [57], in particular in the extraction of enzymes and proteins at small scales.

Freezing and thawing. The reason for the disruption of cells caused by freezing and thawing is still unclear, although the plasma membrane is often considered the primary site for freezing injury [58]. Tansey (2006) reported freeze–thaw lysis for extraction of proteins from mammalian cells [59]. This efficient method for mild solubilization of inclusion bodies uses a freeze–thaw process in the presence of a low concentration of urea. The extraordinary effects of freezing and thawing are very similar to those reported during cold and osmotic shock [60]. Despite the differences in osmotic pressure between intra- and extracellular fluids, intra- and extracellular crystal formation further damages the cell wall. For this procedure 10% of available soluble protein release has been reported.

Solid and liquid shear. These types of mechanical procedures of lysing do not involve adding chemicals or enzymes to the system [61]. However, the energies required when using these 'harsh' protocols can be high and destroy the very proteins being extracted [61]. The cell membrane destruction is influenced by exposing the cells to the following:

- shear through liquid flow;
- exploding through pressure differences between the inside and outside of the cell;

- collision forces through the effects of beads or paddles; or
- a combination of these forces.

All these energies should be optimized properly to expose the cell to the optimum level of energy [61].

During solid shear, frozen (−20 °C) microbial paste is placed in a cylindrical hole (0.1–1 mm in diameter) in a metal block. Then a tight fitting plunger is inserted to introduce 1000–4000 atmospheric pressure. This level of pressure is applied from the top of this plunger. The majority of the cells are ruptured by this method. In liquid shear, the microbial suspension is permitted to pass through a narrow orifice at pressure up to 40 000 psi. Occasionally a French press is also used for this purpose. Cells experience disruption owing to the extreme level of shear during passage from the orifice. Nearly 90% of cell breakage was reported with baker's yeast after a single passage at 20 000 psi.

Concussion. During concussion, microbial cells can be disrupted by bombardment with hard particles such as glass beads. Numerous types of mills are used for this purpose, such as agitator bead mills, ball mills, colloidal mills, etc [62].

2.3.5.3 Aqueous and solvent extraction

The growing interest in industrial enzymes emphasizes the need for the development of new downstream approaches to make best use of enzyme recovery. Considerable efforts have been focused on the development of newly adapted technologies to purify enzymes in their catalytically active form. Recently, an aqueous two-phase system was developed as a promising tool for effective extraction and purification of enzymes due to the versatility, lower cost, process integration capability and easy scale-up of this system [63]. Three-phase partitioning has also been championed for enzyme enrichment as a promising technique for efficiently integrated bioseparation [63]. Currently, CLEAs technology and organic–inorganic nanoflower preparation are also utilized as novel approaches for simultaneous extraction, purification and immobilization of enzymes [63]. Microbial cells lysis does not necessarily result in breakdown of the molecular complexes of other cell components, e.g. lipids, nucleic acids and carbohydrates. The liquid extraction of the enzyme from insoluble particles can offer a technique for fractionation, in which extractants of increasing eluting power are employed. Amid *et al* reported a novel liquid–liquid extraction process composed of surfactant and acetonitrile for purification of the enzyme polygalacturonase from *D. zibethinus.* Glyk *et al* reported polyethylene glycol (PEG)–salt aqueous two-phase systems as a promising, efficient liquid–liquid extraction technology for the downstream processing of various biomolecules, such as proteins and enzymes [28, 64]. There are two general procedures for extraction of enzymes from broken cells:

- Using salt solution as a solvent (in which most of the enzymes are stable), extract all possible materials under mild conditions.
- Selective extraction of enzymes utilizing the different solubility of enzymes in different solvents. In this procedure the initial extraction is achieved by using a solvent in which only a few enzymes are soluble and then repeating the same

> process with other solvents in which other enzymes are soluble. In stirred jacketed vessels, microbial cells are extracted batchwise. In this procedure, particle size governs not only the extent of extraction, but also the amount of extract which gets adsorbed on the particle surface. With a known quantity of extracting fluid, the use of many fractions of the liquid results in a more nearly complete removal of the desired solute than does the use of the entire liquid in a single extraction. Further improvements in extraction efficiency may be obtained through arranging the staged extraction in a counter-current continuous flow. After extraction of enzymes, the spent solids are removed by filtration, centrifugation or sedimentation.

Aqueous two-phase systems (ATPSs) are one of the most common tools for the separation of proteins. They involve mixing a polymer (usually polyethylene glycol, PEG) and a salt (e.g. phosphate, sulfate or citrate), or two polymers and water, to successfully separate and purify the proteins [65]. The surface properties of the proteins and the properties of the two-phase system determine the partitioning between both phases. The complex mechanism of partitioning is somewhat dependent on the level of protein hydrophobicity. Hydrophobicity is the main factor in the partitioning of proteins and can be determined in many different ways. The procedures that are more advantageous, depending on the ATPS used, are those that consider the three-dimensional structure and the degree of hydrophobicity of amino acids on the surface and that based on precipitation with ammonium sulfate [65]. The influence of charge has a comparatively small effect on the partitioning of proteins in PEG/salt systems, but is more important in PEG/dextran systems. Protein concentration plays an important role in the partitioning of proteins in ATPSs [65], where it produced higher levels of solubility of the protein in both phases, and thus the partitioning reported at low protein concentrations can produce very different results to that reported at high concentrations. This protein precipitate is in equilibrium with the protein solubilized in each of the phases. The practial application of ATPSs has been shown in numerous cases, including a number of industrial applications with excellent levels of purity and yield [65].

2.3.6 Purification of enzymes

Batchwise adsorption and elution from ion-exchange celluloses is now often used and has largely replaced traditional practices such as precipitation techniques for large-scale purification [66]. Procedures such as concentration, dilution and reconcentration with the use of hollow-fiber ultrafiltration equipment has replaced dialysis in the effective purification of enzymes [66]. Additionally, antiphonally direct scaling up of column chromatographic procedures can also be utilized for purification purposes [66]. Alterations to column geometry to enhance flow rates are often desirable, however, the purification factors and recovery are comparable to those derived at the laboratory scale and can be achieved comparatively easily. Conventional affinity chromatographic tools have not been considered for large-scale purification, primarily because of their cost and the rather short life of the matrices. However, quasi-affinity chromatography performed using triazine dye conjugates has proved to be of great benefit. The materials are cheap to prepare [66]. The coupling methods are both easy and quick and do not contain the use of poisonous chemicals such as cyanogen bromide [66]. In addition, the triazine linkage is more stable under different conditions than the isourea formed in cyanogen bromide coupling [66].

2.3.6.1 Lipid removal

Lipid removal is usually done as early as possible as lipids obstruct in the separation of proteins. The traditional procedure of lipid removal is to make an acetone powder of the ground cells. In this process, the ground cells are mixed with cold acetone (−10 °C). This is repeated with acetone at 0 °C and finally with acetone at 20 °C. The method predominantly eliminates water and some lipid. The lipid is removed later with petroleum ether or ether at room temperature.

Triton X-100 (using a nickel column) is frequently used to aid lysis and solubilize lipids and membranes [67]. Removing lipids from membrane proteins can be involved, but most protein purifications remove lipids as a matter of course. Hydrophobic interaction chromatography can remove even minute quantities of lipopolysaccharides and lipids, and BioBeads can be used in spin preparations [67]. Separation is again dependent on factors such as the structural configuration of the protein, its solubility and whether it is free or membrane bound. Simply washing inclusion bodies with levels of detergent and/or urea can also be done until the sample is lipid free and quite pure. 1 M urea and 1% Triton X-100 are regularly used, although both concentrations should be optimized to prevent protein solubilization [67]. Different enzymes and their respective solvents for extraction are listed in table 2.5.

Additional methods of lipid removal are the separation of lipids from solutions of enzymes in 20%–50% v/v n-butanol at 0 °C, and lipid extraction using different gases under supercritical conditions. In the latter procedure, liquid CO_2 is most frequently used for the removal of lipids from biological materials.

2.3.6.2 Nucleic acid removal

Several methods have been developed to remove nucleic acid contaminants, given the general concern of accidentally introducing recombinant genes into humans. Due to this concern, FDA has recommended an upper limit for nucleic acid of

Table 2.5. Various enzymes and their respective solvent for extraction.

Enzyme	Source	Solvent
Cholesterol esterase	Pancreas	Dilute H_2SO_4, in the presence of protease inhibitor
Fungal lipase	Fungi	Water
Glycerol phosphate dehydrogenase (GPDH)	Rabbit muscle	1 mM disodium EDTA containing 2 mM 2-mercaptoethanol

10 pg/dose [68]. A number of methods are available for removing nucleic acid contaminants during protein isolation, e.g. treatment with cation exchangers or precipitation by salts (e.g. MnCl, NaCl), acids (e.g. acetic, trifluoroacetic), streptomycin sulfate, polycations (e.g. protamine, clupeine, polyethyleneimine), and heat [68]. The selection of the method to be used in any specific protein purification scheme depends mainly on the nature of the protein of interest, for example strongly basic protein products can form ionic complexes with nucleic acids leading to co-purification of nucleic acid contaminants with the product [68].

Purification of intracellular enzymes is a challenge as most of the intracellular enzyme preparations contain nucleic acids which can increase the viscosity, which may further interfere with enzyme purification procedures, in particular ultra-filtration. This type of purification is complicated by the presence of nucleic acid. Nucleic acid can be precipitated by high molecular weight polyvalent cations such as protamine sulfate, cetyl triethyl ammonium bromide, streptomycin sulfate and polyethyleneimine [68]. These polyvalent cations form a complex between negatively charged phosphate residues of the nucleic acid molecules and positively charged groups of precipitants. The resulting complex is then separated by centrifugation [68]. Several microorganisms contain satisfactory nuclease enzyme to circumvent this problem, however, the nucleic acids must be eliminated by precipitation or degraded by the supplementation of exogenous nucleases. Ammonium sulfate precipitation can be very effective in eliminating nucleic acids but also eliminates some protein at the same time. Many positively charged material precipitants such as polyethyleneimine, cetyltrimethyl ammonium bromide, streptomycin sulfate and protamine sulfate have been used. Generally, these can easily form complexes with the negatively charged phosphate residues of the nucleic acids. All of these precipitants are expensive and sometimes toxic (mainly streptomycin sulfate). Moreover, they form complexes with certain enzymes.

2.3.6.3 Purification by precipitation and differential solubility

Differential protein precipitation is a rapid and less expensive stage in protein purification and is based on using the inherent physio-chemical properties of the polypeptide [69]. Precipitation of proteins, lysed from the host cell, is generally used to concentrate the protein of choice before further refining procedures with more selective purification columns (e.g. His-tag, size exclusion, etc) [69]. Proteins can also precipitate naturally as inclusion bodies owing to various influences during over-expression in the host cell. While this phenomenon allows convenient initial separation from native proteins, these inclusion bodies must be carefully differentially solubilised so as to achieve functional, correctly folded proteins. Solubilization is the most frequently used method for enzyme purification. It is based on precipitation of the active enzyme or other proteins and soluble substances [69].

2.3.6.3.1 Salting-out

The solubility of globular proteins increases upon addition of salt (<0.15 M), which is called salting-in [70]. At higher salt concentrations protein solubility usually declines, resulting in the precipitation of protein, which is called salting-out [70].

A salt that decreases the solubility of proteins also tends to increase the stability of the native conformation. In comparison, salting-in ions are usually denaturants. The salting-out mechanism is based on superior solvation due to elimination of the cosolvent (salt) from the layer of water closely associated with the surface of the protein (the hydration layer) [70]. The hydration layer, typically 0.3–0.4 g water per gram protein, plays a significant role in conserving solubility and the correctly folded native conformation. During this procedure, the precipitation of proteins is achieved by a high concentration of neutral salts. The most often used salts are ammonium sulfate and sodium sulfate. Ammonium sulfate is inexpensive and is highly soluble ($767\ g\ l^{-1}$) which permits salting-out of practically all proteins [70].

2.3.6.3.2 Temperature and pH

Biological macromolecules have been developed to execute their function in a particular cellular environment (subcellular compartments or tissues); thus, they should be adjusted to the biophysical features of the corresponding environment. Several macromolecular features are pH-dependent, e.g. activity and stability [71]. However, only activity is biologically significant, while stability may not be essential for the corresponding reaction [71]. Most proteins exhibit increased solubility with temperature elevation [71]. At high temperatures, the differential stability of enzymes is quite significant and selective heat denaturation is frequently used at the industrial scale. Thus, inert protein materials may be denatured by controlled heating of extracts. This process is used in the purification of α-amylase, ribonuclease, adenyl kinase, cholesterol esterase and glutamate dehydrogenase [71]. Alteration of pH is also used as a method of fractional precipitation. The different proportions of basic and acidic groups of different enzymes lead to a wide range of pH values at which enzymes exhibit isoelectric zero net charge characteristics. The principal difficulty in using differential pH precipitation is the pH stability of the desired enzymes, which is limited. Almost every biological process is pH-dependent, which indicates the significance of the local pH on all processes in the cell [71]. Therefore, various biologically relevant effects are significantly influenced by the pH of the water phase including:

- functional pH dependence;
- structural conformations associated with the function; and
- subcellular translocation.

Additionally, the role of the concentration of H^+ ions on protein stability is confirmed by acidic/basic unfolding and protein pH-dependent stability. Variation in pH is proven to activate the development of amyloid fibers and aggregation.

2.3.6.3.3 Organic solvents

Organic solvents have not been commonly used for the separation of enzymes, as they denature proteins at room temperature. During World War II, an ethanol precipitation method was developed. At low temperatures and low ionic strengths, various protein fractions were isolated from blood plasma. Ethanol fractionation has several benefits over the salting-out method. At low ionic strengths, the interaction between proteins and salts depends on specific features of protein molecules, e.g. the distribution of electric charges [72]. Small differences in dielectric constant and ionic strength will produce large and specific changes in the solubility of proteins. As discussed above, organic solvents are frequently used in fractional precipitation of proteins based on their dielectric constants [72]. Once an organic solvent is mixed with the aqueous solution of an enzyme, the dielectric constant of the solution is decreased, thus the solubility of the enzyme is reduced, however, enzymes should retain their internal hydrophobic amino acid residues and remain comparatively loosely folded [72]. Sometumes adding an organic solvent causes the molecule to refold into a new and inactive form with the hydrophobic residues exposed on the surface. The risk of refolding and subsequently denaturation is larger as temperature increases. This results in a requirement for low temperature, often below 0 °C, and fractionation with organic precipitants. Some organic solvents used in protein purification are methanol, ethanol, isopropyl alcohol and acetone [72]. Ethanol is the most frequently and extensively used organic solvent owing to its suitability for use in the food and pharmaceutical industry [72].

2.3.6.3.4 Nonionic polymers and multiphase systems

Biological macromolecules with high molecular weight polymers, e.g. dextrans and polyethylene glycols (PEG), have been used extensively in the isolation of biological material in three main ways:

- For the concentration of biological components including viruses by dialysis and by liquid–liquid extraction in aqueous two-phase mixtures.
- As a stabilizer on a particular component in a solution.
- As a precipitant which causes the formation of a solid protein phase.

Two-phase systems can be used to separate enzymes from cell homogenates and at the same time achieve a certain degree of purification. Dextran–PEG two-phase systems have been used in the production of commercial intracellular food enzymes. Based on a report from 1981, PEG helps in the precipitation of various proteins ranging in size between 14 000 and 670 000 daltons (Da). This was analyzed by excluded volume [73–75].

The nondenaturing, water-soluble, high molecular weight polymer referred to as PEG can precipitate protein from aqueous solutions, which can be qualitatively examined in terms of an excluded volume mechanism. The increase in PEG amount required to decrease solubility is distinctive for a given protein–polymer pair. This distinctiveness is not sensitive to solution conditions and is mainly reliant on the size of the protein and polymer [74]. The solubility of specific proteins can be selectively manipulated by controlling their state of association or ligand environment. PEGs for protein precipitation are typically classified by molecular weight. The higher molecular weight PEGs can efficiently precipitate but this may result in higher viscosity [76]. It has now been realized that the hydrodynamic radius of the PEG plays an important role in selecting suitable PEG precipitants. Moreover, it also offers more insight into understanding precipitation mechanisms [76].

2.3.6.3.5 Crystallization

Crystallization is compulsory to derive the three-dimensional structure of proteins and nucleic acids; it frequently signifies the bottleneck in structure determination [76, 77]. The crystallization of biological macromolecules (proteins, nucleic acids and viruses), depends on the formation of a solution that is supersaturated in the macromolecule, but also displays conditions that do not considerably perturb its natural state [80, 81]. Supersaturation is produced by the supplementation of mild precipitating agents, e.g. neutral salts or polymers, and by the manipulation of different parameters, which include temperature, ionic strength and pH. Factors that can disturb the structural state of the macromolecule, such as metal ions, inhibitors, co-factors or other conventional small molecules, play an important role in the crystallization process [76, 77]. A number of approaches have been established that combine a range of factors that affect and promote crystallization. Among the most extensively used are vapor diffusion, dialysis, batch and liquid–liquid diffusion. Crystallization is often performed after extraction and purification of the enzyme. The first crystals of the enzyme may contain a number of other proteins. Crystallization and recrystallization are effective procedures in enzyme purification. The most extensively used procedure of crystallization is via ammonium sulfate solutions. In this procedure the salt is supplemented to a concentrated enzyme solution until a slight turbidity appears. It is then permitted to stand, however, the salt concentration is enhanced by:

- Supplementing a strong solution of the salt dropwise at long intervals.
- Through a fine capillary.
- Through a dialysis membrane.
- The solution may simply be permitted to evaporate slowly.

Crystallization may be introduced by altering pH or temperature at a constant salt concentration. Glycerol phosphate dehydrogenase, pyruvate kinase, lactate dehydrogenase, urease and glutamate dehydrogenase are the most prominent examples of enzymes that have been purified using crystallization procedures [76, 77].

2.3.6.4 Protein purification using chromatographic methods

To attain a high level of purity in the purification of recombinant proteins for therapeutic or analytical applications, it is essential to use numerous chromatographic steps [78], which are based on the differential migration of enzyme. A variety of techniques are available, e.g. adsorption, anion and cation exchange (which can be performed at different pHs), hydrophobic interaction chromatography, gel filtration and affinity chromatography [78].

2.3.6.4.1 Adsorption chromatography

Adsorption in stable expanded beds allows proteins to be recovered directly from particulate-containing feedstocks, e.g. fermentation broths and preparations of disrupted cells, without the requirement for prior elimination of the suspended solids, which would usually lead to the blockage of packed beds [79]. The implementation of this method significantly reduces the complexity of downstream processing by removing certain filtration, centrifugation and concentration steps [79]. Aspects that are vital for the success of the procedure include the right choice of adsorbent, together with careful design of the apparatus in which the separation is performed. The design, optimization and scale-up of appropriate operating protocols for expanded-bed procedures are very similar to those used for the operation of packed beds [79].

The first chromatographic purifications were performed using inorganic compounds that were adsorbed by the biochemicals via van der Waal's forces and steric interaction [79]. The most extensively used adsorbent in enzyme purification is calcium phosphate gel, in particular its crystalline form hydroxyapatite (HA). The calcium and phosphate ions on the surface of HA crystals form bonds with charged groups of proteins. Acidic and neutral proteins form bonds with the calcium sites on the HA. The elution of acidic and neutral proteins is usually achieved with low concentrations of phosphate buffers of pH 6.8. Basic proteins associate and form bonds with the phosphate group on the HA crystals. Bacteria-derived alkaline phosphatase was purified using HA. *E. coli* derived amino transferases have also been purified, with a six-fold increase in specific activity.

2.3.6.4.2 Ion-exchange chromatography

The principle of ion-exchange chromatography is based on the separation of proteins, and hence has numerous applications in protein science, such as the discovery of proteins, high-resolution purification and the industrial production of proteins. Ion-exchange chromatography includes the separation of ionizable molecules based on their total charge, often used for the separation and purification of biomolecules such as proteins, polypeptides and nucleic acids [80–82]. Virtually all enzymes are polar in nature and can be charged. Ion-exchange chromatography is usually used for enzyme purification. Separation is achieved with the help of derivatives of cellulose, agarose, dextrans or resins. Agarose is the most commonly used cross-linked matrix for the purification of bioactive enzymes and pharmaceuticals because of the following properties:

- stable bed volume;
- high capacity;
- high flow rate and resolving power;
- good chemical stability between pH 3 and 10; and
- good thermal stability up to 70 °C, which makes it suitable for autoclaving.

The anion exchangers most frequently used are diethylaminoethyl cellulose, triethylamino cellulose and triethanolamine coupled to cellulose through glycerol and polyglycerol chain mixed groups (ECTEOLA cellulose) [80–82]. Carboxymethyl cellulose, phospho cellulose, sulfoethyl cellulose, acrylic acid resins are used as cation exchangers. Ion-exchange chromatography based enzyme fractionation can be achieved in a column or by a batch method. Enzymes, whose isoelectric points are well removed from neutral pH, are preferably separated by ion-exchange chromatography. For l-asparaginase (with an isoelectric point of 6.8) a 100-fold purification is possible using a carboxymethyl cellulose batch column. The batch method is also beneficial in eliminating nucleic acids from enzymes [80–82].

2.3.6.4.3 Gel filtration chromatography

Gel filtration (GF) chromatography is termed as separation of proteins exclusively on the basis of molecular size. This is done by using a porous matrix to which the molecules, for steric reasons, have different degrees of access, i.e., smaller molecules have greater access and larger molecules are excluded from the matrix. Therefore, proteins are eluted from the gel filtration column in decreasing order of size [82]. The sample is applied on the surface of a column of appropriate porous beads of hydrated gel and solvent is percolated through the column [82]. The molecules that are too large in size to penetrate porous structure of the beads are excluded and allowed to pass through in the void volume of the column. Molecules which are smaller in size can enter porous beads and move more slowly via the column, as they spend a proportion of their time in the beads, thus molecules are eluted in order of decreasing molecular size. This technique is also known as permeation, molecular sieve, molecular exclusion, restricted diffusional or steric chromatography. For enzyme purification there are three available gel filtration media:

- Partially cross-linked dextrans with a fractionation range up to 250 000 Da. Dextran is a polysaccharide made up of glucose residues. Dextran gels (Sephadex) are the first for which a close association between molecular size and elution behavior was established.
- Cross-linked granulated polyacrylamide gels with a fractionation range up to 400 000 Da. Cross-linked polyacrylamides form gels with water, which are used in various biochemical separations.
- Granulated agarose gel (Sepharose) with a fractionation range up to 50 000–40 000 000 Da.

Allyl dextran cross-linked with *N,N*-methylene bis acrylamide (Sepharoyl) is preferred for large-scale production. By using a 25 × 80 cm column of Ultrogel Ac and Sepharcyl S-200, two enzymes, alkaline phosphatase and restriction endonucleases, have been purified.

2.3.6.4.4 Affinity chromatography

Affinity chromatography is among the best chromatographic methods for the purification of a specific molecule or group of molecules from complex mixtures [88]. The principle is based on highly specific biological interactions between two molecules, such as interactions between an enzyme and substrate, receptor and ligand, or antibody and antigen [83]. These reversible interactions are used for purification by placing one of the interacting molecules, called the affinity ligand, onto a solid matrix to form a stationary phase, whereas the target molecule is in the mobile phase. Effective affinity purification needs a certain degree of knowledge of the nature of interactions between the target molecule and the ligand to help determine the selection of an appropriate affinity ligand and purification procedure [83]. Recently, matrices with distinctive features which bypass the limitations of more traditional materials have been established. Affinity purification can offer significant time savings and higher purification, however, the effectiveness of this method depends on the type of procedure used [83]. Therefore, it is important to optimize the purification protocol to attain efficient capture and maximum recovery of the target.

The entire procedure depends upon exact interaction between the analyte and the opposite group which is covalently bound to the column packing. A column comprising an insoluble polymer or gel to which a specific competitive inhibitor or other ligand has been covalently bound is used for this purpose. The solution containing macromolecules to be purified is allowed to pass through this column. Those proteins that have high affinity with the ligand will be retained, whereas those with less affinity will pass unretarded through the column. Using certain procedures, such as washing the ligand–protein complex with a solution of displacing agent such as an inhibitor, or by changing the pH or ionic strength of the elution solvent to favor dissociation, exactly retained proteins can then be eluted. Various insoluble supports are used for enzyme purification by affinity chromatography, such as hydrophilic cellulose derivatives, polystyrene gels, cross-linked dextrans, beaded agarose, glass beads and polyacrylamide gels. Some chemical derivatives of agarose and polyacrylamide have also been used for enzyme purification. The affinity matrices used for enzyme purification can be divided into two categories:

- Those which are specific for the desired enzyme by the specificity of the ligand such as the substrate, substrate analogs, inhibitors or antibody of the enzyme.
- Those which will interact with a related group of enzymes because of an immobilized general ligand such as a co-factor (5′-AMP, 2′,5′-ADP, NAD′ and others), which is specific for a class of enzymes and hydrocarbon ligands or dyes. This will interact with a large number of different enzymes.

The total expense of enzyme isolation can be minimized by the incorporation of an affinity step. One of the most common examples is purification of tissue plasminogen activator (t-PA) from cultures of human kidney cells, which is purified using α-benzylsulfonyl-p-amino-Sepharose [84].

2.3.6.4.5 Electrophoresis and ultracentrifugation

During electrophoresis, a molecule with an overall charge will move in an electric field. Electrophoresis offers a potential means of separating proteins and other macromolecules, such as DNA and RNA. The velocity of migration (v) of a protein (or any molecule) in an electric field depends on the electric field strength (E), the net charge on the protein (z) and the frictional coefficient (f). Considering all these, one can see that electrophoretic purification is based on the movement of proteins when placed in an electrical field. This process is capable of the highest resolution of enzymes employing physico-chemical separation. This procedure is now mainly used as a technique for separation of isoenzymes and other enzymes linked for diagnostic purposes. The procedures often used at the laboratory scale for enzyme purification and characterization are: free-boundary electrophoresis; zone electrophoresis with the help of supports such as paper, starch, and cellulose powder; electrophoresis in agarose and acrylamide gels; and isoelectric focusing. Recently, a continuous electrophoretic separator has been developed for large-scale separation of proteins. The separator can draw as many as 29 separate fractions. This application can be utilized for the isolation and purification of high value pharmaceutical enzymes and other proteins.

Electrophoresis-based separations are always performed in gels as the gel assists as a molecular sieve that enhances separation. Molecules that are small in comparison with the pores in the gel easily move from the gel, while molecules with a larger size than the pores are almost immobile. Intermediate-sized molecules move from the gel with different degrees of ease. Electrophoresis is performed in a thin, vertical slab of polyacrylamide and the direction of flow is from top to bottom [85]. One of the most suitable supporting media for electrophoresis is polyacrylamide gels, formed by the polymerization of acrylamide and cross-linked by methylenebisacrylamide, as they are chemically inert and are readily formed. Electrophoresis is the reverse of gel filtration, in that all of the molecules, irrespective of size, are forced to move through the same matrix [85]. In a solution, proteins have the tendency to sediment at high centrifugal force, so it is tricky to separate a protein from a mixture by centrifugation. Enhanced separation of proteins has been accomplished by density gradient centrifugation. In this process, sucrose or glycerol is used as density gradient [85]. With more sophisticated continuous flow ultracentrifugation, whole cells, viruses and subcellular components can be separated. With ultracentrifugation, we can determine parameters such as mass and density, study something about the shape of a molecule and examine the interactions between molecules [85].

2.3.7 Finishing operations

Its well-known that all enzymes are antigenic. After issues occurred in the late 1960s when workers manufacturing enzymes suffered from severe allergic responses after breathing enzyme dusts, methods have now been applied to reduce dust formation [3]. These include delivering enzymes as liquids wherever possible, or enhancing the particle size of dry powders from 10 μm to 200–500 μm by either prilling (mixing the enzyme with polyethylene glycol and preparing small spheres by atomization) or marumerizing (mixing the enzyme with a binder and water, extruding long filaments, converting them into spheres in a marumerizer, drying them and covering them with a waxy coating) [3]. Finishing operations such as enzyme desalting, concentration, purity control and storage are of greater importance [3].

2.3.7.1 Desalting

Ammonium sulfate (AS) fractionation is frequently used in protein and enzyme purification; however, the final protein pellets have a high salt content and desalting by dialysis is required prior to subsequent analysis [86, 87]. Unnecessary amounts of inorganic salts must be eliminated from enzyme preparations. The salts existing in one enzyme are perhaps inhibitory to other enzymes present in clinical diagnostic reagents. Also, desalting may be crucial at intermediate stages of enzyme isolation, e.g. before ion-exchange adsorption. The simplest and oldest method of salt removal is dialysis [86, 87]. The main function of dialysis is to eliminate small molecules such as salts from larger ones, in particular the enzymes to be purified. Mixed bed ion exchange, the conventional method of removing small ions, has been applied to some of the more robust enzymes. Mixed bed cation and anion exchange resins are used to eliminate both positive and negative ions. Wang *et al* developed a phenol-based method for rapid desalting and concentration of proteins after ammonium sulfate fractionation of complex olive leaf protein extract [86, 87]. After re-dissolving, ammonium sulfate precipitates were desalted with phenol extraction and a lot of β-glucosidase was observed in each fraction using a specific antibody [86, 87].

2.3.7.2 Concentration of enzymes

Once extraction is performed, both intracellular and extracellular enzymes are received as a dilute solution and must be further concentrated prior to further use. On the pilot scale, precipitation and adsorption are employed to concentrate the enzymes. On the large scale ultrafiltration has been used.

2.3.7.2.1 Ultrafiltration

A semi-permeable membrane allows the separation of solvent molecules from larger enzyme molecules, as only the smaller molecules can enter the membrane when the osmotic pressure is exceeded. Ultrafiltration is performed to separate macromolecules and colloidal particles by means of a membrane. Hydraulic pressure is employed as the active force for the solvent molecules to pass through the membrane, whereas the microporous membrane does not allow the passage of large solute molecules. Membranes with exclusion limits of 2000–300 000 Da are available for ultrafiltration. Ultrafiltration has a tendency to remove small molecules. The enzyme solution is fed into a cell fitted with a membrane which retains the selected protein while being permeable to the solvent and small molecules. Negative pressure is applied to the collecting chamber and positive pressure to the solution, which acts as the driving force that causes the flow of solvent and small solute molecules across the membrane. Large volumes can be reduced to a few milliliters in only one or two hours. Diafiltration is a very useful procedure for eliminating salts and other low molecular weight substances in the form of contaminants from dilute enzyme solution [88]. During this procedure the water is fed to the ultrafilter cell so that molecules other than water are successfully eliminated from the system. Cellulose acetate and organic polymers, e.g. polysulfone, have proven to be useful as membrane materials. With the exception of cellulose acetate, these membranes can easily be cleaned with alkali or acid and stream sterilized [88].

2.3.7.2.2 Drying

Drying procedures have long been established for food and pharmaceuticals and have now been applied successfully to enzymes. The extracellular enzymes in the food industry are often used as dried free-flowing powders. The drying of enzymes mainly depends upon the thermal stability of enzymes. The drying of enzymes has commonly been carried out by spray-drying and freeze-drying [32]. Spray-drying is a common method for producing powder from a liquid, whereas lyophilization, or freeze-drying, is a procedure for preserving food and biological materials (enzymes, proteins, vitamins, etc), floral products, drugs and whole animals. Robust enzymes may be vacuum dried or spray-dried, while the delicate ones are freeze-dried or spray-dried. Spray-drying is extensively used for extracellular bacterial enzymes, while most intracellular enzymes are dried using freeze-drying processes [32].

2.3.7.2.3 Vacuum evaporation

Enzymes are labile molecules, so evaporation must be conducted under rather high vacuum conditions to prevent denaturation. During the production of extracellular enzymes, the diluted enzyme solution is reduced under vacuum pressure at temperatures below 40 °C. At the industrial scale, enzymes are concentrated in a similar manner, with the same equipment as is used for the concentration of fruit juices at a reduced temperature [89]. In a characteristic application, an enzyme solution was reduced in two stages from 8% or 12% to 35% solids, then to 65% solids. Vacuum-based evaporation of enzymatic solution is always achieved by the addition of sugar alcohol such as sorbitol or sugars such as lactose in higher concentrations [89].

2.3.7.3 Storage

Good storage conditions are of paramount importance in the industrial production of enzymes. One of the major concerns is that the loss of activity during storage will result in the loss of product in its purest and most expensive form. Most enzymes have a restricted shelf-life owing to inherent active-conformation liability in the minority of molecules present in high energy states, at any temperature at any particular time. This loss can be suspended by cross-linking, immobilization or by using enzyme stabilizers, e.g. sugars, certain ions and co-factors. Most enzyme products are marketed as dry powders; a few enzymes are available in a liquid or suspension form. These products usually contain compounds which decrease the loss of enzyme activity during storage and check microbial growth, i.e., enzyme stabilizers and co-factors. Proteins (in particular enzymes) must be stored at in a suitable temperature and pH range and frequently in the presence of concentrated (approximately 1 M) glycerol, sucrose, or a similar substance, for the proteins to retain activity and prevent aggregation [90]. The compounds generally used for these purposes are glycols, propylene glycol, ethylene glycol, sorbitol, mannitol, thiol, reducing agents, sodium chloride, salts of organic hydroxy acids and other salts of buffers, sodium benzoate, and esters of parahydroxy benzoic acid. Recently, compounds such as gelatin, dextrans, partially hydrolyzed collagen, gum arabic, albumin, polyamines, poly-l-lysine and glycerol monoethers have been used as stabilizers. Enzyme containers should be kept sealed to prevent the escape of the stabilizing atmosphere and also to maintain the low moisture content (below 50%) of the solid product. The storage temperature should be low but not freezing, as freezing may cause denaturation of certain enzymes [90].

2.4 Recombinant proteins from algae

As photosynthetic organisms, microalgae can efficiently convert solar energy into biomass. Microalgae are currently used as an important source of valuable natural biologically active molecules, such as carotenoids, chlorophyll, long-chain polyunsaturated fatty acids, phycobiliproteins, carotenoids and enzymes. Significant

Table 2.6. Recombinant proteins from algae.

Algae name	Products	Expression location
Amphidinium sp.	β-Glucoronidase	Nucleus
C. reinhardtii	Anti-HSV glycoprotein D lsc, Anti-CD22-gelonin sc, Anti-CD22-ETA sc, VP1-CTB, 14FN3, Metallothionein-2, TRAIL, Allophycocyanin, Anti-PA 83 anthrax IgG1, E7GGG, VEGF, HMGB1	Chloroplast
C. reinhardtii	GBSS-PfMSP$_{1-19}$ GBSS-PbAMA$_{1\text{-}C}$	Nucleus

advances have been achieved in microalgae biotechnology over the last decade, and the use of microalgae as bioreactors for expressing recombinant proteins is receiving increased interest. Compared with the bioreactor systems that are currently in use, microalgae may be an attractive alternative for the production of pharmaceuticals, recombinant proteins and other valuable products (table 2.6) Products synthesized via the genetic engineering of microalgae include vaccines, antibodies, enzymes, blood-clotting factors, immune regulators, growth factors, hormones, and other valuable products, such as the anticancer agent Taxol. Here, we briefly compare the currently used bioreactor systems, summarize the progress in genetic engineering of microalgae, and discuss the potential for microalgae as bioreactors to produce pharmaceuticals.

2.5 Enzyme immobilization techniques

The process of immobilizing enzymes for usage in biotechnology requires the essential step of affixing soluble enzymes onto a solid substrate or matrix. This step is necessary since immobilization cannot occur without it. There are several benefits to using this technique, including improved enzymatic activity and stability, versatility, and a straightforward separation procedure (table 2.7).

2.5.1 Advantages and applications of enzyme immobilization

Compared to the usage of set-free soluble enzymes, the process of immobilizing enzymes, which is a common approach in biotechnology, possesses many benefits that, depending on the specifics of the situation, make it an additionally advantageous choice [91]. The immobilization of enzymes onto solid substrates or matrices has enhanced their stability, reuse ability, and activity as catalysts. This objective may be accomplished because they are restricted to a rigid surface. The immobilization of enzymes is currently used in many production methods, including conventional and innovative biotechnological techniques [92]. This section presents a complete overview of the benefits linked with immobilizing enzymes [93].

Table 2.7. A comparative analysis of widely utilized techniques for enzyme immobilization.

Method	Principle	Advantages	Examples
Entrapment	Isolation inside a gel or porous matrix	Simple to put together; keeps the action going	Glucose isomerase is used to manufacture high-fructose corn syrup; Lactase is used in the dairy sector to hydrolyse lactose.
Covalent bonding	Establishment of permanent enzyme-support chemical bonds	Strong ties, permanent solidity	Pharmaceutical companies rely on penicillin G acylase in the production of antibiotics.
Adsorption	Weakly interacting connection to a supporting surface	Easy to set up, flexible	Choline oxidase for choline sensing biosensor study and creation
Encapsulation	Getting stuck inside a capsule or membrane that lets some light through	Enzyme prevention and sustained activity	Enzymes that have been immobilized for use in enzyme microcapsules for timed-release
Cross-linking	Enzyme-enzyme or enzyme-support-enzyme covalent link formation	Improvements in stability and resistance to enzyme leaching	Binding enzyme with glutaraldehyde for better stability

2.5.1.1 Advantages of enzyme immobilization

The immobilization of an enzyme enhances resilience against several factors, such as fluctuations in temperature or pH. Additionally, this technique facilitates enzymes' immobilization, enhancing their ease of separation and reusability. Immobilized enzymes have a more extended period during which they may catalyze reactions, contributing to their increased catalytic efficiency [94]. Immobilizing an enzyme allows it to be retrieved and used several times, which is one of the most significant benefits of this technique [95]. In contrast to loosened enzymes, which may get denatured or destroyed during reactions, immobilized enzymes can be removed from the reaction mixture, regenerated, and reintroduced into subsequent processes with little loss of activity. This reusability factor affects the efficiency and longevity of biocatalytic processes [96]. Immobilized enzymes may be readily extracted from the reaction mixture using simple procedures like filtration or centrifugation. The ease of product recovery and further processing upstream means that elaborate purification techniques may be avoided [97]. Multiple enzymes may be attached to a single support via various immobilization methods, allowing for the co-immobilization of enzyme cascades or multi-enzyme systems. Synergistic enzymatic reactions result from this approach, expanding the scope of possible uses and boosting the efficiency of the process overall [98]. Immobilization simplifies the construction of continuous flow reactors, in which the immobilized enzyme remains stationary inside the reactor

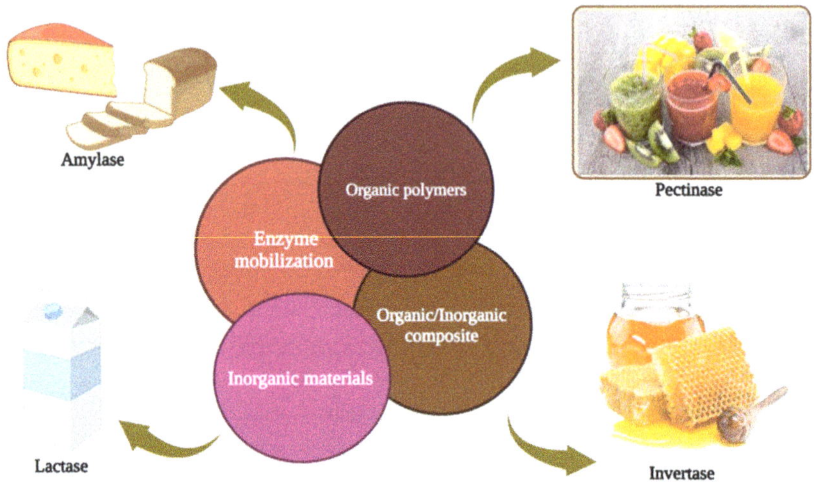

Figure 2.6. Applications of enzymatic reactions in food and beverage industries, highlighting the use of amylase, lactase, pectinase, lipase, and invertase.

Table 2.8. The utilization of enzyme immobilization in several industrial sectors.

Industry	Enzyme	Application
Food stuff and drinks	Invertase	The manufacture of speciality sugars, such as inverted sugar, is a topic of interest in food science and technology
	Lactase	Making dairy products that do not include lactose
	Penicillin G Acylase	Antibiotic making
Pharmacological	Chymotrypsin	Peptide creation
Bioremediation	Urease	The breakdown of urea in water treatment plants
The manufacturing of biodiesel	Lipases	Making biodiesel from vegetable oils using transesterification.
Biosensors	Glucose oxidase	Medical gadget glucose monitoring

while the reaction substrates pass over it. The advantages of this design include better reaction control, less enzyme loss, and enhanced enzymatic process stability [99]. Several enzymatic reactions in food and beverages used in industries are mentioned in figure 2.6 (table 2.8).

2.5.2 Methods of enzyme immobilization

Enzymes are turned into immobilized forms by using the central biotechnology technique of enzyme immobilization, in which they are attached to a stable substrate or matrix. Improved stability, reusability, and ease of separation from reaction mixtures make this technique essential for biocatalysts, figure 2.7.

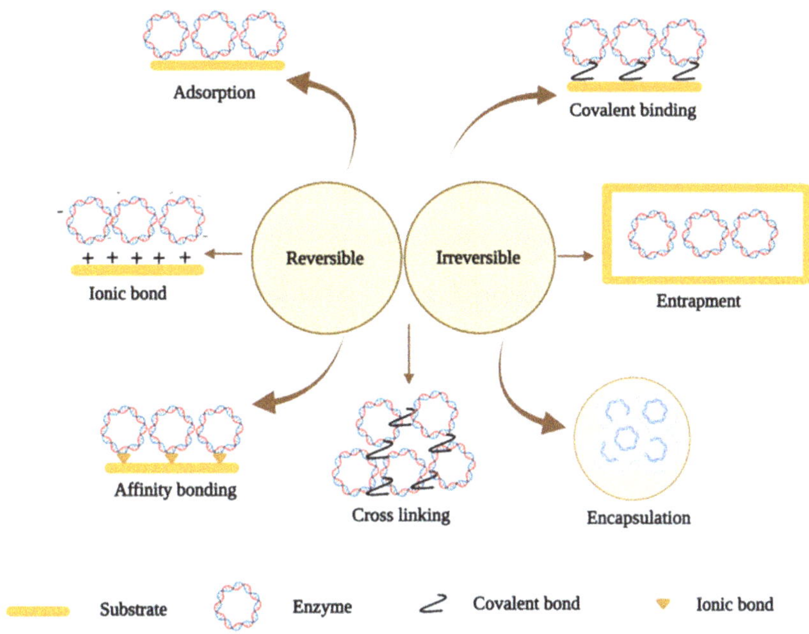

Figure 2.7. Comparison of reversible and irreversible enzyme immobilization methods such as adsorption, ionic binding, and encapsulation.

Table 2.9. Examples of enzymes immobilized by entrapment and their applications.

Enzyme	Application
Glucose isomerase	Making corn syrup sweetened with high fructose
Lactase	Hydrolysis of lactose for the dairy sector and urea for wastewater treatment
Urease	The creation of a choline-detecting biosensor
Choline oxidase	The making of biodiesel
Lipases	Making corn syrup sweetened with high fructose

2.5.2.1 Entrapment

One non-covalent method of immobilizing enzymes is physically confining them within a porous matrix or gel. The gel formation process isolates the enzyme in a protective matrix, allowing substrate and product transfer. Matrixes for trapping are commonplace, including agar gel, polyacrylamide, and calcium alginate. Immobilized glucose isomerase produces high-fructose corn syrup [100], while immobilized lactase is used for lactose hydrolysis in the dairy industry. Table 2.9 provides some other instances of how enzymes that have been captured and immobilized might be put to use.

2.5.2.2 Covalent bonding

When an enzyme is covalently immobilized, strong chemical linkages are formed between the enzyme and the support matrix. The approach's high adherence ensures the immobilized enzymes' long-term stability and reusability. Bifunctional reagents or linkers are often used to promote covalent bonding. Covalent immobilization has been used in the pharmaceutical industry to immobilize penicillin G acylase and chymotrypsin to produce antibiotics and peptides [99]. Table 2.10 displays some more examples of covalently immobilized enzymes and their respective applications.

2.5.2.3 Adsorption

Adsorption is a simple and widely used method in which enzymes are bound to the surface of a solid support material through weak contacts such as hydrophobic interactions, van der Waals forces, and hydrogen bonds. Common adsorption support materials include silica gel, activated carbon, and ion exchange resins. Adsorption has been employed in a wide variety of biotechnological contexts. Choline oxidase, for instance, may be detected in some diagnostic tools thanks to its adsorption onto support materials for biosensor development. In addition, lipases have been absorbed into activated carbon for use in biodiesel production [101] (table 2.11).

2.5.2.4 Encapsulation

During encapsulation, enzymes are enclosed in semi-permeable membranes or capsules. The encapsulating medium allows substrates and products to circulate, preventing enzyme leakage and protecting sensitive enzymes. This method is suitable when working with enzymes that must be shielded from harsh reaction conditions. The regulated release of enzymes has led to their encapsulation into

Table 2.10. Examples of enzymes immobilized by covalent bonding and their applications.

Enzyme	Application
Penicillin G acylase	Biosynthesis of antibiotics
Chymotrypsin	Manufacturing of peptides
Catalase	Breakdown of hydrogen peroxide
Glucose oxidase	Glucose sensing biosensor study and creation
Urease	Biological waste treatment

Table 2.11. Examples of enzymes immobilized by adsorption and their applications.

Enzyme	Application
Choline oxidase	The creation of a choline-detecting biosensor
Lipases	The making of biodiesel
Glucose oxidase	Biomedical gadget glucose monitoring
Invertase	Manufacturing of inverted sugar and other specialized sugars
Catalase	Catalysis in a natural setting

Table 2.12. Examples of enzymes immobilized by encapsulation and their applications.

Enzyme	Application
Various enzymes	Methods of medication administration with controlled release
Glucose isomerase	Making syrup from corn sweetened with high fructose
Urease	Wastewater treatment by urea hydrolysis
Lipases	Biological catalytic membranes' carefully regulated enzyme secretion
Catalase	Biological waste treatment

Table 2.13. Examples of enzymes immobilized by cross-linking and their applications.

Enzyme	Application
Various enzymes	Pharmaceutical and specialized chemical manufacturing
Glucose isomerase	Making corn syrup sweetened with high fructose
Lipases	Pharmaceutical intermediate synthesis
Invertase	Manufacturing of inverted sugar and other specialized sugars
Urease	Wastewater treatment by urea hydrolysis

microcapsules. Microencapsulated enzymes that have been immobilized offer a highly accurate and prolonged enzymatic response inside formulations that allow for regulated release. Encapsulation research has also focused on developing biocatalytic membranes for utilization in diverse biotechnology and environmental remediation applications [102] (table 2.12).

2.5.2.5 Cross-linking

Chemical agents are utilized in cross-linking to facilitate covalent connections between enzymes and the support matrix. This method generates enzymes with immobilization that demonstrate endurance and lifespan due to increased stabilization of enzymes and the avoidance of enzyme leach. The use of glutaraldehyde as a cross-linker in the enzymatic immobilization process is widely employed. An instance of a method used in biocatalysts to augment the activity and stability of enzymes is the application of glutaraldehyde bridging. Several commercial uses, such as the manufacture of speciality chemicals and pharmaceutical intermediates, have been found to use cross-linked enzymes [103] (table 2.13).

2.6 Enzyme engineering for enhanced stability and activity

Enzyme manufacturing is significant to biotechnology, given its capacity to improve the stability and function of enzymes, which may boost their economic and therapeutic usefulness [104]. This phenomenon may be attributed to the limited number of approaches capable of achieving this objective. Researchers may engage in structural and property alterations to improve the functioning of an enzyme under certain environmental circumstances to improve its catalytic stability and effectiveness. This section will look at the various techniques used in enzymatic engineering [105].

2.6.1 Protein engineering strategies

The study of protein engineering is a multidisciplinary field that aims to increase the functioning of proteins and enzymes by improving their balance, procedure, and substrate selection *via* a holistic strategy. Protein engineering uses a broad number of strategies to accomplish these objectives. This study will examine various methodologies frequently employed in protein engineering [106]. In rational protein design, one of the most critical steps is the alteration of the amino acid sequence of an enzyme on purpose. This modification must be based on previous knowledge of the connection between the structure of the enzyme and its function. The combined application of computational analysis and molecular modelling approaches enables the identification of specific amino acids that might be modified to enhance the stability, attachment of substrates, and catalytic effectiveness of an enzyme [107]. Enzymes with thermophilic properties may be produced in a controlled laboratory setting. Scientists have effectively created thermophilic enzymes, which are characterized by high levels of catalytic effectiveness and stability. This phenomenon may be linked to their capacity to operate at heightened temperatures with optimum efficiency. Thermophilic DNA polymerases have shown benefits for polymerase chain reaction (PCR) and other molecular biology techniques, owing to their increased resilience against denaturation at high temperatures [108] (table 2.14).

2.6.1.1 Directed evolution

The method of continually changing the enzyme *via* regulated mutagenesis and choosing mutants with desired features is directed evolution. Mutants with improved stability, substrate selectivity, or activity may be generated by subjecting the enzyme to different selection pressures. Temperature stability of evolved enzymes, enzyme thermostability, has been successfully enhanced by researchers using directed

Table 2.14. Examples of rational protein design for enhanced stability and activity.

Enzyme	Modification	Impact on stability/activity
DNA polymerase	Mutations that are heat-resistant are introduced	A more stable and active state at elevated temperatures
α-Amylase	Creating mutations at specific sites to enhance the binding of substrates	Increased catalytic activity
Proteases	Designed protection from proteolytic breakdown	Sustained steadiness under pressure
Lipases	Durability in organic solvents is much improved	Enhanced behaviour in non-aqueous settings
Chimeric enzymes	Combining the work of multiple enzymes into one	Increased substrate and catalytic diversity

Table 2.15. Examples of directed evolution for enhanced stability and activity.

Enzyme	Mutation technique	Impact on stability/activity
Lipases	PCR errors, DNA jiggery-pokery, and site-specific mutagenesis	Heat regulation and reactivity are both improved
Cellulases	Development on a cellulose-based substrate via guided development	Enhancement of substrate binding and catalytic activity
Proteases	Saturation mutagenesis iteratively	Modified stability and substrate specificity
Peroxidases	Hydrogen peroxide-mediated laboratory evolution	Peroxide reduction catalysis is accelerated

Table 2.16. Examples of immobilization-assisted enzyme engineering.

Enzyme	Immobilization strategy	Impact on stability/activity
Lipases	High-throughput screening by immobilization on solid frameworks	Finding more effective variations for catalysis in organic solvents
Glucose oxidase	Adherence to biosensor surfaces	Improved glucose detection stability and sensitivity
Proteases	Capture on chromatographic resins	Proteolytic processes with enhanced substrate selectivity and stability
Cytochrome P450s	Investigations of drug metabolism via immobilization in microreactors	Streamlined variant screening for medical uses

evolution. Guided evolution has resulted in more robust lipases to higher temperatures, allowing them to function in high-temperature industrial settings [109] (table 2.15).

2.6.1.2 Immobilization-assisted enzyme engineering

Enzyme immobilization has the potential to serve as a convenient platform for testing mutant libraries for enhanced stability and activity in enzyme engineering. Screening immobilized enzymes using high-throughput technologies might expedite the development of superior variants. For enzyme immobilization at high throughput in a lipase engineering study, immobilization facilitated a rapid screening of mutant libraries for improved catalytic efficiency and substrate selectivity. This technique was used to identify variations of lipase with enhanced activity in organic solvents. These are helpful for commercial uses that do not include water [110] (table 2.16).

2.6.1.3 Site-directed mutagenesis

The protein-coding gene is targeted for precise modification in site-directed mutagenesis. Amino acid substitutions brought on by these mutations alter the protein's

Table 2.17. Examples of site-directed mutagenesis for enhanced protein properties.

Protein	Mutation(s)	Impact on protein properties
HIV protease	Sub-stratum-binding residues	improved catalytic activity and substrate selectivity
Green fluorescent protein (GFP)	Fluorescence-altering amino acid substitutions	Fluorescence emission tuning for various uses
Serine protease	Mutations that are thermostable are introduced	Enhanced stability and activity in the presence of heat
α-Amylase	Substrate-specific amino acid substitutions	Increased catalytic activity on some substrates
Peroxidase	Substrate specificity modification by site-directed mutagenesis	Peroxide reduction now works in a broader variety of substrates.

amino acid sequence and, by extension, its structure and function. Researchers may study an enzyme's stability and activity after introducing different amino acids to tailor an enzyme to a particular task. Enhanced thermostability of DNA polymerase site-directed mutagenesis has been used to introduce thermostable mutations into DNA polymerases for use in PCR. These modifications have increased the enzyme's stability against denaturation in PCR processes at high temperatures [111] (table 2.17).

2.6.1.4 Circular permutation

Protein engineering techniques like circular permutation allow for modifying a protein's amino acid sequence. In this technique, the peptide backbone is cleaved in a specific spot and then rejoined to create a circularized variant. This procedure results in the creation of novel N- and C-termini for the protein, which may drastically change its structure and function [112]. Circular permutation may be used to study unexplored protein conformations, tune protein stability, and alter ligand-binding properties. The presence of a circular mutation in the green fluorescent protein (cpGFP) One prominent illustration of this phenomenon is the circular permutation of green fluorescent protein (cpGFP). In the cpGFP variant, the N- and C-termini of the native GFP molecule are connected, resulting in the formation of novel termini. GFP's potential reorganization could impact its folding and fluorescence characteristics, diminishing its utility as a research tool for investigating protein folding and biological processes [113] (table 2.18).

2.6.1.5 Domain swapping

The approach of domain swapping in protein engineering enables the assembly of oligomeric structures by the exchange of domains among protein subunits, irrespective of their structural resemblance [114]. Domain flipping can lead to the formation of novel, more complicated protein structures in certain circumstances [115]. Antibodies are Y-shaped proteins with two heavy chains and two light chains that are similar to one another. Light and heavy chain variable domains combine to

Table 2.18. In protein properties caused by circular permutations.

Protein	Strategy based on iterative permutations	Effects on protein features
Green fluorescent protein (GFP)	Changing the order of the ends to make a circle	Changed fluorescence characteristics and protein folding
β-Lactamase	Rearrangement of the active site's loop in a circle	Elevated beta-lactam antibiotic resistance
Lipases	Rotation in a circle of the eyelid	Activation at the interface and altered substrate specificity
Protein kinases	The kinase domain undergoes a circular permutation	Substrate recognition and kinase activity are altered
Eukaryotic initiation factors	The RNA-binding domain undergoes a circular permutation	Shifts in the control of RNA binding and translation

Table 2.19. This study examines instances of domain swapping in proteins and investigates the effects on protein properties.

Protein	Domain name swap technique	Effects on protein features
Immunoglobulins (antibodies)	Antibody fragments swapping variable domains	Adaptations in antigen binding and immunological responses
α-Amylase	Interchange of domains between monomeric components	The stability was improved, and the substrate specificity was changed
Serpins	Inter-serpin family reactive centre loop exchange	Changes in substrate specificity and protease inhibition
Tissue plasminogen activator (tPA)	Kringle domains allow for domain shifting	Modified plasminogen ligand binding and interactions
Hemagglutinin protein (influenza virus)	Flu hemagglutinin domain swapping	Variations in viral entry characteristics and receptor binding

form the antigen-binding site. Domain swapping occurs in immunoglobulins, wherein dimeric or higher-order complexes are formed from the interchangeable domains of different antibody subunits. Immune reactions and antigen-binding properties may be affected by this technique [116] (table 2.19).

2.6.2 Improving enzyme thermostability

Enzymes' capacity to withstand heat is crucial for their use in various industrial procedures. Enzymes may be more robust and efficient catalysts if protein engineering techniques are used to increase their stability at high temperatures. Enzyme

Table 2.20. Modifications that increase the thermal stability of enzymes.

Enzyme	Method for increasing thermal stability	Thermodynamic effect
DNA	polymerases	Extremophiles' thermostable mutations are incorporated into the population.
Enhanced high-	temperature stability and activity	
Lipases	Improved thermal stability through guided evolution	High-temperature organic synthesis with enhanced performance
Amylases	Disulfide linkages and salt bridges that make sense	Increased resistance to heat and denaturation
Cellulases	The addition of disulfide bonds and tweaks to the loop structure	Increased resistance to deterioration from high temperatures in biomass
Proteases	Substitution of residues in deformable domains	Increased catalytic activity and thermal stability

thermostability may be improved in several ways, including rational protein design, controlled evolution, and the incorporation of thermostable patterns seen in extremophilic species [117]. The development of thermostable DNA polymerases like Taq polymerase has dramatically impacted the field of molecular biology by making PCR possible at higher temperatures. The thermostability of DNA polymerases has been significantly enhanced by protein engineering. PCR amplification has become more efficient and reliable by extending the half-life of DNA polymerases, as shown in thermostable mutations in extremophilic bacteria [118] (table 2.20).

2.6.3 Enhancing enzyme substrate specificity

Substrate specificity is a crucial characteristic of an enzyme that determines its ability to recognize and bind specific substrates, leading to efficient catalysis. Protein engineering to improve enzyme substrate specificity might expand the range of substrates that enzymes can process [119]. To do so, we must use rational design or controlled evolution to alter the enzyme's active site or binding pockets. The substrate specificity of chymotrypsin was altered. Chymotrypsin is a protease that cleaves peptide bonds in specific spots within proteins. Using directed evolution, scientists have developed variations of chymotrypsin with altered substrate specificities. Since these improved forms can now break peptide bonds at a wider variety of amino acid residues, they are of greater use in proteolytic processes and peptide synthesis [120] (table 2.21).

2.7 Upstream process intensification

In bioprocessing, upstream process intensification refers to improving the efficiency and output of the first steps in producing industrial and biopharmaceutical enzymes. Increased yields, shorter production cycles, and reduced production costs may be

Table 2.21. Improving the substrate's specificity of enzymes: a few case studies.

Enzyme	Method for improving substrate selectivity	Substrate specificity effects
Chymotrypsin	Substrate recognition evolution with a purpose	Enhancements to peptide synthesis and the number of sites for cleavage
Lipases	Designing residues in the active site	Increased generality in enantioselective reactions
Cytochrome P450s	Changes to the substrate-binding residues	Accelerated reaction on selected substrates
β-lactamase	Mutations introduced into the active site	The hydrolysis substrate range of beta-lactam antibiotics has been expanded.
Glycosidases	Evolutionary manipulation of substrate-binding sites	A shift in the glycosylation reaction's specificity

Table 2.22. The benefits of high cell-density fermentation are numerous.

Advantages	Explanation
Increased productivity	Increased cell densities lead to elevated product concentration levels and enhanced overall production efficiency.
Reduced production time	Reduced fermentation cycles result in accelerated manufacturing, facilitating increased frequency of product batches.
Lower production costs	Increased crop productivity and decreased fermentation duration lead to decreased utilization of resources and reduced expenses.
Decreased risk of contamination	Increasing cell densities can mitigate the potential for contamination, enhancing the output's overall quality.
Simplified downstream processing	Increased concentrations of the product result in enhanced efficiency and cost-effectiveness of downstream purifying procedures.

achieved by enhancing and optimizing the fermentation, cell culture, and enzyme manufacturing processes. Process intensification aims to enhance efficiency by maximizing output while decreasing inputs [121].

2.7.1 High cell density fermentation

High cell density fermentation is a method of upstream process intensification that includes cultivating microorganisms at densities far higher than those employed in conventional fermentation. This is achieved via the use of upgraded bioreactor designs, medium formulation improvement, and cutting-edge control methods. High cell-density fermentation can boost yields, decrease fermentation periods, and cut production costs [122] (table 2.22).

2.7.2 Solid-state fermentation

Solid-state fermentation (SSF) is a technique used in bioprocessing in which microorganisms are cultured in the absence or minimal presence of free-flowing water on solid substrates. It is an alternative to conventional submerged fermentation that is just as efficient at making bioproducts, including enzymes, organic acids, bioactive compounds, and more [123]. The solid substrate provides food and structural support for the microbes in solid-state fermentation. Solid-state fermentation has been widely used in the production of several enzymes. One such instance is the evolution of amylases, enzymes that catalyze the breakdown of starch into more straightforward carbohydrates. *Aspergillus oryzae* and *Rhizopus* species are two common filamentous fungi used in SSF-based amylase production. SSF is a valuable and cost-effective method of enzyme production since the fungus can grow and release amylases directly onto solid substrates like wheat bran or rice husk [124] (table 2.23).

2.7.3 Continuous fermentation

The fermented broth is constantly drained from the bioreactor and replaced with fresh nutrient-rich medium in the bioprocessing method known as continuous fermentation [125]. In contrast to batch fermentation, which occurs in a sealed vessel with a finite capacity, continuous fermentation permits continuous growth and is, therefore, well-suited for long-term and enormous bioproduct synthesis. The production of biofuels like ethanol relies heavily on continuous fermentation. In a bioreactor, sugar-containing feedstock such as sugarcane juice or molasses is continuously added, and the fermented broth containing the ethanol is continuously removed to produce ethanol in a continuous process. This setup ensures a steady substrate supply and a consistent condition, boosting productivity and efficiency in the process [126] (table 2.24).

Table 2.23. The benefits of solid-state fermentation.

Advantages	Explanation
Lower water requirements	The utilization of SSF results in reduced water consumption and subsequent expenditures due to its minimal water requirements.
Cost-effectiveness	The utilization of solid substrates is typically more cost-effective than liquid media, leading to cost reduction.
Enhanced enzyme stability	Enzymes generated using SSF frequently demonstrate enhanced stability, rendering them well-suited for various applications.
Higher product concentrations	The absence of diluting effects in SSF can increase product concentrations.
Simplicity of scale-up	The method of scaling up SSF is very uncomplicated due to its little requirement for liquid handling procedures.

Table 2.24. Benefits of constant fermentation.

Advantages	Explanation
Steady-state operation	Constant substrate addition and product removal are possible during continuous fermentation.
Increased process productivity	A more extended fermentation period is achieved through continuous operation, increasing product yields.
Reduced labor and downtime	There is less downtime due to interruptions and less need for manual intervention when fermentation is continuous.
Enhanced process control	Continuous fermentation allows for fine-tuned regulation of critical process parameters thanks to its steady-state character.
Scalability	Manufacturing bioproducts on a massive scale is well suited to continuous fermentation because of its scalability.

Table 2.25. Benefits of enzyme production by microbial consortia.

Advantages	Explanation
Enhanced enzyme production	Microbial consortiums exploit synergistic interactions to increase enzyme production and productivity.
Efficient substrate utilization	The various microorganisms in the consortium each have their area of expertise, allowing for more efficient substrate use.
Process robustness and stability	When a wide variety of microorganisms are present, the process becomes more stable and resistant to external changes.
Expanded substrate range	Multi-enzyme synthesis is made possible by microbial consortia' increased substrate versatility.
Lower production costs	Increases in efficiency and output lower the price per unit of enzyme produced.

2.7.4 Microbial consortia for enzyme production

Groups of microorganisms called consortia work together to accomplish complex tasks like enzyme synthesis. Microbial consortia have gained popularity in the bioprocessing industry due to their increased efficiency in enzyme synthesis, substrate use, and product diversity. These consortia use the synergistic interactions between several microbial species to boost enzyme output and enhance bioprocess conditions [127]. Plant biomass contains cellulose, a complex polymer that is difficult to break down. However, bacterial and fungal cellulolytic microbial consortia can now break cellulose into simpler sugars, making it more digestible. The fungi in these groups secrete enzymes called cellulases that degrade cellulose into soluble sugars that the bacteria may then consume. The microorganisms' collaborative activity results in higher cellulase yields and more efficient biomass conversion than with individual cultures alone [128] (table 2.25).

Table 2.26. There are benefits to using *in situ* product removal methods.

Advantages	Explanation
Shift in reaction equilibrium	Constant removal of the product prevents the buildup of the product and drives the reaction to completion.
Increased enzyme productivity	Enzyme output and overall reaction efficiency are improved due to less product inhibition.
Enhanced reaction yield	Keeping a positive concentration gradient via constant product removal allows for increased yields.
Prolonged enzyme lifespan	Enzyme inactivation is a possible side effect of product inhibition. Enzyme stability is improved through ISPR methods.
Efficient scale-up	ISPR methods are easily reproducible, opening the door to industrial-scale bioprocessing and enzyme manufacturing.

2.7.5 *In situ* product removal strategies

In situ, product removal (ISPR) removes product molecules from the reaction mixture in real time during bioprocessing. ISPR methods boost enzyme output by rebalancing the reaction in favour of product formation rather than product inhibition, hence shifting the equilibrium of the process [129]. Physical separation techniques such as adsorption, extraction, or membrane filtering may be used regularly or continuously to remove the product from the reaction fluid. The process of lactose hydrolysis is essential in producing lactose-free dairy products. Glucose and galactose are produced when lactase digests lactose. Keeping the reaction mixture free of by-products and maximizing lactose hydrolysis efficiency calls for a membrane filtration system that continuously removes glucose and galactose [130] (table 2.26).

2.8 Enzyme production from extreme environments

Enzymes produced by organisms that can survive in extreme conditions are of great interest in biotechnology and industry. Heat (thermophiles), cold (psychrophiles), acid, alkali, pressure, and salt (halophiles) are all examples of extreme environments in which certain organisms may thrive. High stability, activity, and selectivity under extreme conditions characterize extremophile enzymes, making them promising biocatalysts for various industrial applications [131]. Extremophiles that thrive in warm environments include thermophilic bacteria like *Thermus aquaticus*. Many biotechnological procedures, such as PCR, need thermostable enzymes produced by these microbes (PCR). *Thermus aquaticus* (Taq) polymerase is one of the most well-known thermostable enzymes in PCRs. Due to its stability up to 95 °C, it is ideal for PCR applications (figure 2.8) (table 2.27) [132].

2.8.1 Psychrophiles (cold-loving)

Psychrophiles are a subset of extremophiles that may thrive at temperatures as low as 20 °C. To overcome the challenges given by the cold, these bacteria have evolved

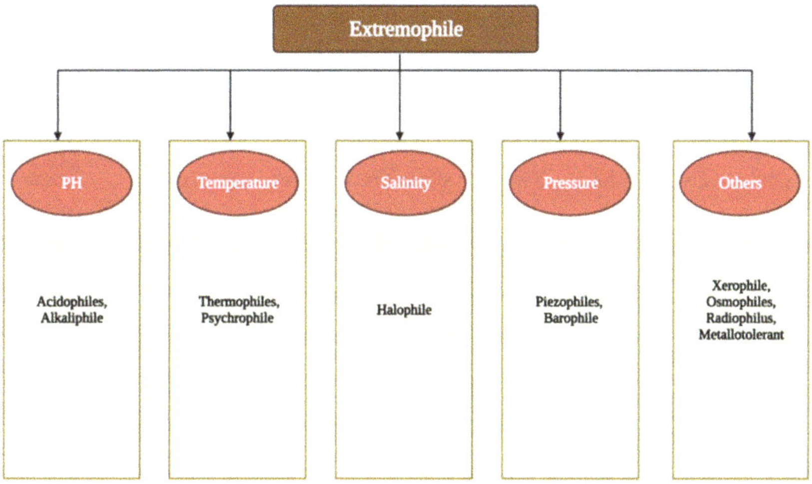

Figure 2.8. Classification of extremophiles based on environmental conditions, including pH, temperature, salinity, pressure, and other extreme factors.

Table 2.27. Extremophile enzymes are used as examples.

Enzyme	Source (extremophile)	Use of polymerase chain reaction in organic synthesis at low temperature	Dangerous situation
Taq polymerase	Aquatic thermophilus	Manufacturing of cleaning products and food	Thermophilic (loving heat)
Cold-adapted lipases psychrophile)	Psychotic-loving microbes	Fabric softeners and leather cleaners	Cold-loving (or
Acid proteases	Fungi with a low pH	The food and textile industries	Low pH (Acid lover).
Alkaline proteases	Alkali-loving microorganisms	Use of polymerase chain reaction in organic synthesis at low temperature	Low acidity (Basophile)
Halophilic α-amylase	Archaea that thrive in salty environments	Manufacturing of cleaning products and food	Halophilic (high salt)

enzymes with specific properties adapted for functioning well in such environments. Because of their high catalytic activity and versatility at low temperatures, psychrophilic enzymes play a significant role in various applications as biocatalysts. Lipases are enzymes that catalyze the breakdown of lipids, and it is known that psychrophilic bacteria may create cold-adapted lipases. These lipases are essential for the synthesis of organic molecules at mild temperatures. In producing fine chemicals and medications, for instance, cold-adapted lipases have been shown to

Table 2.28. Psychrophilic enzymes have these distinctive features.

Enzyme	Source (psychrophile)	Applications	Cold temperature range
Cold-adapted lipases	Psychrophilic bacteria	Organic synthesis, speciality compounds, and medicinal drugs	Below 20 °C
Psychrophilic proteases	Psychrophilic fungi	Industrial kitchens, detergent creation, and frigid cleaning agents	Below 15 °C
Cold-active amylases	Psychrophilic archaea	Baking resistant to low temperatures and starch hydrolysis	Below ten °C

Table 2.29. Characteristics of thermophilic enzymes.

Enzyme	Source (thermophile)	Applications	Temperature range
Thermostable DNA polymerases	*Thermus aquatics*	Industrial applications of PCR in the food and pharmaceutical sectors	50 °C–95 °C
Thermophilic proteases	Thermophilic bacteria	Baking and hydrolysis of starch	60 °C–80 °C
Heat-resistant amylases	Thermophilic fungi	Industrial applications of PCR in the food and pharmaceutical sectors	70 °C–90 °C

catalyze esterification and transesterification processes well, even at refrigerator temperatures [133] (table 2.28).

2.8.2 Thermophiles (heat-loving)

Thermophiles are a kind of extremophile that can survive at hot temperatures (over 50 °C). These creatures have adapted in unique ways to live in such extreme heat. Because of their remarkable durability and activity at high temperatures, thermophilic enzymes are an excellent choice for industrial applications that call for high heat. PCR requires thermostable DNA polymerases, which are generated by thermophilic bacteria like *Thermus aquaticus* (PCR). PCR is a vital tool in molecular biology since it allows for the amplification of DNA sequences. DNA polymerases from thermophiles may continue to operate and keep their catalytic efficiency even at the high temperatures required for DNA denaturation during the PCR process [134] (table 2.29).

2.8.3 Acidophiles (acid-loving)

Acidophiles are extremophiles that thrive in environments with a pH level of 3 or below. To thrive in these harsh conditions, these bacteria have evolved remarkably

Table 2.30. Characteristics of acidophilic enzymes.

Enzyme	Source (acidophile)	Applications	pH range
Acid proteases	*Aspergillus niger*	Manufacturing of cleaning products and food	pH < 3
Acid cellulases	Acidophilic bacteria	Hydrolysis of cellulose for use in making biofuels	pH < 4
Acidophilic amylases	Acidophilic archaea	Low-pH starch hydrolysis	pH < 4

stable enzymes and are active at low pH levels. Food processing and detergent manufacturing are only two examples of industries that benefit from using acidophilic enzymes. Fungi that thrive in acidic environments, such as *Aspergillus niger*, produce acid proteases, which are most active and stable at acidic pH values. In the food industry, these acid proteases play a vital role in cheesemaking, meat tenderization, and protein breakdown. Their high acidic activity facilitates protein hydrolysis and modification in several food processing contexts [135] (table 2.30).

2.8.4 Alkaliphiles (alkaline-loving)

Alkaliphiles are extremophiles that thrive in environments with a pH greater than 9. Because of the challenges of high alkalinity levels, these microorganisms have evolved to produce alkaliphilic enzymes. The capacity of alkaliphilic enzymes to function normally and remain stable in an alkaline environment sets them apart. Since many manufacturing procedures need an environment with a high pH, they have attracted much attention in biotechnology [136]. Bacillus species, which are alkaliphilic bacteria, produce alkaline proteases, an enzyme. Due to their stability and activity at high pH levels, these enzymes find widespread application in laundry detergents. Stains on clothes, such as those caused by food and blood, maybe more easily removed with the help of alkaline proteases, which are enzymes that break down proteins. Alkaline protease detergents allow for more eco-friendly, lower-temperature washing without sacrificing fabric quality [137] (table 2.31).

2.8.5 Halophiles (salt-loving)

Some organisms, called halophiles, can tolerate far higher salt concentrations than is typical, and hence, they thrive in environments like salt flats and salty lakes. These microorganisms produce halophilic enzymes to help them survive in salty conditions. Because of their stability and activity in high salt concentrations, halophilic enzymes play a significant role in various industrial applications. Halophilic archaea generate halophilic-amylases, enzymes that hydrolyze starch efficiently in high-salt environments. Enzymes like this are helpful in both the food and textile industries. In the textile industry, halophilic-amylases are used to break down starch-based

Table 2.31. Characteristics of alkaliphilic enzymes.

Enzyme	Source (alkaliphile)	Applications	pH Range
Alkaline proteases	Bacillus species	Cleaning agents, leather tanning	pH > 9
Alkaliphilic lipases	Alkaliphilic bacteria	Cleaning product creation and organic synthesis	pH > 9
Alkaline amylases	Alkaliphilic fungi	Detergent production and the hydrolysis of starch	pH > 9

Table 2.32. Characteristics of halophilic enzymes.

Enzyme	Source (halophile)	Applications	Salt concentration
Halophilic α-amylases	Halophilic archaea	Food processing and the de-sizing of textiles	High-salt environments
Halophilic proteases	Halophilic bacteria	Protein breakdown and bioprocessing	High-salt environments
Halophilic lipases	Halophilic fungi	Synthetic organic compounds and the creation of detergents	High-salt environments

sizing agents during the designing process. These enzymes aid in the starch hydrolysis process, improving processed foods' texture and quality [138] (table 2.32).

2.8.6 Applications of extremozymes in biotechnology

Extremozymes, enzymes produced by extremophiles, have several uses in biotechnological processes because of their unique properties and adaptability to extreme conditions. Several industries, including biofuels, food processing, detergents, and medications, have been revolutionized by these enzymes' increased efficiency and selectivity [139] (table 2.33).

2.9 Downstream process intensification

The enzyme synthesis processing steps in the bioprocessing pipeline may be made more efficient and productive using a novel approach known as downstream process intensification. The purification, separation, and recovery of enzymes must be accelerated and improved by incorporating and using state-of-the-art procedures as part of this process optimization. Researchers in biotechnology may be able to increase production output, lower costs, and develop greener production processes by concentrating on the process that follows [140].

Table 2.33. Applications of extremozymes in biotechnology.

Enzyme	Application
Cold-adapted lipases	Synthetic organic chemistry and detergent development
Thermostable DNA polymerases	Reverse transcription-PCR
Acid proteases	Manufacturing of cleaning agents and foods
Alkaline proteases	Cleaning agents, leather tanning
Alkaliphilic lipases	Cleaning product creation and organic synthesis
Alkaline amylases	Detergent production and the hydrolysis of starch
Halophilic α-amylases	De-sizing in the textile industry, industrial cooking
Halophilic proteases	Protein breakdown in bioprocessing
Halophilic lipases	Cleaning product creation and organic synthesis

2.9.1 Continuous chromatography

Ongoing chromatography has some benefits over batch chromatography, and is a cutting-edge method for improving downstream processes. Continuous chromatography was developed in the 1970s. It is a technique that facilitates the uninterrupted purification and segregation of enzymes in a way that allows for a continuous flow, resulting in increased efficiency and decreased processing duration [141]. Continuous chromatography, also sometimes called Simulated Moving Bed (SMB) chromatography, can be used to clean enzymes. SMB chromatography is a constant procedure whereby feed, adsorption, and eluent are continuously transported through a series of static columns. As a result, a counter-current flow pattern is noticed, leading to an improvement in the yield of the chromatographic splitting phase. SMB chromatography in industrial-scale enzyme manufacturing is beneficial since it needs a much lower amount of solvent, which lowers costs and enhances output rates [142]. Some advantages of continuous chromatography are:

- method of purification and isolation that occurs continuously;
- continuous tracking and regulation;
- decreased use of reducing agents;
- improvements in output and productivity;
- lower infrastructure requirements.

2.9.2 Process integration and optimization

Process integration and optimization include the systematic examination and improvement of various bioprocessing procedures to create a workflow that is both more efficient in terms of productivity and more economical in terms of cost. This technique utilizes several unit operations, state-of-the-art analytical techniques, and process modelling to improve enzyme synthesis and subsequent processing. The production of enzymes may be optimized with the use of computer-aided process design and cutting-edge software tools and algorithms. Biotechnologists may enhance process yields and decrease production costs by simulating different process settings and parameters to find the optimal operating conditions. Computer-aided process design (CAPD) is advantageous when dealing with complex multistage processes since it allows the exploration of various scenarios without extensive testing [143]. Benefits of process integration and optimization are:

- enhanced performance and output;
- reduced enzyme production costs Rapid prototyping and scaling;
- improved steady operation and stability;
- methods that do not harm the environment.

2.9.3 Advanced filtration techniques

One of the most critical ways cutting-edge filtering techniques contribute to ramping up downstream processes is by improving enzyme separation and purification. These strategies boost filtration output and efficiency using modern membrane materials, cutting-edge mediums, and specialized equipment.

2.9.3.1 Tangential flow filtration (TFF)

TFF is a more efficient filtering technology often used in the enzyme purification). It employs a semi-permeable membrane to size-separate enzymes from the other components of the feed solution. Compared to traditional dead-end filtration, TFF's cross-flow mode reduces the likelihood of filter clogging while increasing filtration efficiency. TFF may be used to concentrate and purify large volumes of fermentation broth, hence boosting the efficiency of the process [144]. Advantages of advanced filtration techniques are:

- enzyme purification and isolation at high yields;
- filter fouling is reduced, increasing filter life and decreasing processing times;
- production of enzymes on a massive scale is feasible;
- reduced loss of enzyme activity during filtering;
- enzyme purification and isolation at high yields.

2.9.3.2 Depth filtration

Depth filtration is often used in the enzyme industry for purification and downstream process intensification. This technique involves filtering the enzyme solution through a porous matrix, such as a fibre depth filter, which traps particles and impurities while letting the enzymes pass through. Depth filtering is a straightforward and cheap method for clarifying and partially purifying enzyme solutions. Clarifying the fermentation broth often involves depth filtration as part of the enzyme production process. Most of the time, the fermentation broth has foreign substances like microbial cells or cell debris. During a depth filtering step, the bulk of the solid particles in the broth are removed, leaving a somewhat clarified enzyme solution. This partial purification facilitates further downstream processing steps, including chromatography and ultrafiltration [145]. Advantages of depth filtration are:

- method of inexpensive purification;
- strong ability to trap particles;
- enzyme breakdown is kept to a minimum during filtration, making it feasible for industrial enzyme manufacturing;

- easy to understand and implement procedure;
- method of inexpensive purification.

2.9.3.3 Crossflow filtration

Crossflow filtration is a sophisticated downstream process intensification strategy for the concentration and purification of enzymes. In contrast to traditional dead-end filtration, in which the feed is constantly passed through the filter, cross-flow filtration employs a tangential flow that decreases filter clogging. This technique isolates and concentrates enzymes by permitting continuous feed circulation across the filter surface. Enzyme production using ultrafiltration often employs cross-flow filtration. Ultrafiltration concentrates enzymes by rejecting molecules too small to pass through the ultrafiltration membrane. This approach is ideal when dealing with enzymes that are easily damaged by heat since it may be used at milder temperatures. Ultrafiltration's ability to recover concentrated enzyme solutions aids in subsequent purification steps [146]. Advantages of cross-flow filtration are:

- effective and continuous separation method;
- reduced filter clogging and increased filter longevity;
- heat-sensitive enzymes can function at a low temperature;
- effective factor concentration at a high level;
- production of enzymes in large quantities.

2.9.4 Automation and robotics in downstream processing

Automation and robotics have made downstream processing more efficient, precise, and repeatable. Complex tasks, including sample management, liquid handling, chromatography, and filtration, may be performed by automated systems with little or no human intervention [147]. Adopting this technology allows scientists to increase enzyme output while decreasing processing times and improving efficiency. Automation and robotics have enabled high-throughput screening of enzyme variants to discover mutants with enhanced stability, activity, or substrate selectivity. Scientists can rapidly screen hundreds of mutant enzymes thanks to automated liquid handling systems' ability to produce and analyze various enzyme variants. These speed up enzyme engineering, allowing for the development of more valuable enzymes [148]. Advantages of automation and robotics in downstream processing are:

- increased effectiveness and output in all processes;
- prevention of mistakes made by humans;
- the engineering of enzymes sped up;
- improved ability to replicate studies;
- ability to expand manufacturing capacity.

References

[1] Payen A and Persoz J-F 1833 Mémoire sur la diastase, les principaux produits de ses réactions, et leurs applications aux arts industriels *Ann. Chim. Phys.* **53** 73–92

[2] Garg S K and Johri B N 1994 Rennet: current trends and future research *Food Rev. Int.* **10** 313–55

[3] Robinson P K 2015 Enzymes: principles and biotechnological applications *Essays Biochem.* **59** 1

[4] Gurung N *et al* 2013 A broader view: microbial enzymes and their relevance in industries, medicine, and beyond *BioMed Res. Int.* **2013** 329121

[5] Haitjema C H *et al* 2017 A parts list for fungal cellulosomes revealed by comparative genomics *Nat. Microbiol.* **2** 1–8

[6] Eckhard U *et al* 2017 Discovery of a proteolytic flagellin family in diverse bacterial phyla that assembles enzymatically active flagella *Nat. Commun.* **8** 521

[7] Mugabo Y *et al* 2016 Identification of a mammalian glycerol-3-phosphate phosphatase: role in metabolism and signaling in pancreatic β-cells and hepatocytes *Proc. Natl Acad. Sci.* **113** E430–9

[8] Jacobs A L and Schär P 2012 DNA glycosylases: in DNA repair and beyond *Chromosoma* **121** 1–20

[9] Aleku G A *et al* 2017 A reductive aminase from Aspergillus oryzae *Nat. Chem.* **9** 961–9

[10] Anbu P, Gopinath S C B, Chaulagain B P and Lakshmipriya T 2016 Microbial enzymes and their applications in industries and medicine *Biomed. Res. Int.* **2017** 2195808

[11] Murdoch B M and Murdoch G K 2015 Genetics of prion disease in cattle *Bioinf. Biol. Insights* **9** BBI. S29678

[12] Lieberman I and Ove P 1958 Enzyme activity levels in mammalian cell cultures *J. Biol. Chem.* **233** 634–6

[13] Djekrif-Dakhmouche S *et al* 2006 Application of a statistical design to the optimization of culture medium for α-amylase production by *Aspergillus niger* ATCC 16404 grown on orange waste powder *J. Food Eng.* **73** 190–7

[14] Amann R I, Ludwig W and Schleifer K-H 1995 Phylogenetic identification and *in situ* detection of individual microbial cells without cultivation *Microbiol. Rev.* **59** 143–69

[15] Ferrer M *et al* 2016 Estimating the success of enzyme bioprospecting through metagenomics: current status and future trends *Microb. Biotechnol.* **9** 22–34

[16] Narayanasamy S *et al* 2015 Integrated omics for the identification of key functionalities in biological wastewater treatment microbial communities *Microb. Biotechnol.* **8** 363–8

[17] Ghildyal N *et al* 1985 Economics of submerged and solid state fermentations for the production of amyloglucosidase *J. Food Sci. Technol.* **22** 171–6

[18] Hui L *et al* 2010 Direct microbial conversion of wheat straw into lipid by a cellulolytic fungus of *Aspergillus oryzae* A-4 in solid-state fermentation *Bioresour. Technol.* **101** 7556–62

[19] Souza P M d *et al* 2015 A biotechnology perspective of fungal proteases *Braz. J. Microbiol.* **46** 337–46

[20] Liu H F *et al* 2010 Recovery and purification process development for monoclonal antibody production *MAbs* (London: Taylor and Francis)

[21] Liang J *et al* 2009 Effective elimination of nucleic acids from bacterial protein samples for optimized blue native polyacrylamide gel electrophoresis *Electrophoresis* **30** 2454–9

[22] Coligan J E 2001 *Current Protocols in Protein Science* (Wiley)

[23] Wingren C and Hansson U-B 1996 Enzyme conformational alterations detected by partition column chromatography *J. Chromatogr. B: Biomed. Sci. Appl.* **680** 113–22

[24] Johansson G and Kopperschläger G 1987 Effects of organic solvents on the partitioning of enzymes in aqueous two-phase systems *J. Chromatogr.* A **388** 295–305

[25] Albertsson P-Å 1986 *Partition of Cell Particles and Macromolecules* (Wiley)

[26] Grimonprez B and Johansson G 1996 Liquid–liquid partitioning of some enzymes, especially phosphofuctokinase, from *Saccharomyces cerevisiae* at subzero temperature *J. Chromatogr. B: Biomed. Sci. Appl.* **680** 55–63
[27] Hatti-Kaul R 2001 Aqueous two-phase systems: a general overview *Mol. Biotechnol.* **19** 269–77
[28] Amid M *et al* 2015 A novel liquid/liquid extraction process composed of surfactant and acetonitrile for purification of polygalacturonase enzyme from *Durio zibethinus* *J. Chromatogr.* B **993** 1–8
[29] Yamadera K and DiMagno E P 1994 Separation of canine pancreatic juice proteins by hydrophobic interaction chromatography preserves enzyme activity *Pancreas* **9** 32–6
[30] Tomme P *et al* 1988 Chromatographic separation of cellulolytic enzymes *Methods in Enzymology* (Amsterdam: Elsevier) pp 187–93
[31] Alves N J *et al* 2016 Protecting enzymatic function through directed packaging into bacterial outer membrane vesicles *Sci. Rep.* **6** 24866
[32] De Jesus S and Maciel Filho R 2014 Drying of α-amylase by spray drying and freeze-drying-a comparative study *Braz. J. Chem. Eng.* **31** 625–31
[33] Roskoski R 2007 Modulation of enzyme activity *In xPharm: The Comprehensive Pharmacology Reference* ed S J Enna and D B Bylund (New York: Elsevier)
[34] Cirz R T *et al* 2005 Inhibition of mutation and combating the evolution of antibiotic resistance *PLoS Biol.* **3** e176
[35] Fijalkowska I J, Dunn R and Schaaper R 1993 Mutants of *Escherichia coli* with increased fidelity of DNA replication *Genetics* **134** 1023–30
[36] Mitchell J L, Choe C-y and Judd G G 1996 Feedback repression of ornithine decarboxylase synthesis mediated by antizyme *Biochem.* J **320** 755–60
[37] Sanchez S and Demain A 2008 Metabolic regulation and overproduction of primary metabolites *Microb. Biotechnol.* **1** 283–319
[38] Fujita Y 2009 Carbon catabolite control of the metabolic network in *Bacillus subtilis Biosci. Biotechnol. Biochem.* **73** 245–59
[39] Stülke J and Hillen W 2000 Regulation of carbon catabolism in *Bacillus* species *Annu. Rev. Microbiol.* **54** 849–80
[40] Kleijn R J *et al* 2010 Metabolic fluxes during strong carbon catabolite repression by malate in *Bacillus subtilis J. Biol. Chem.* **285** 1587–96
[41] Iwakuma H *et al* 2016 Generation of a glucose de-repressed mutant of *Trichoderma reesei* using disparity mutagenesis *Biosci. Biotechnol. Biochem.* **80** 486–92
[42] ter Schure E G, van Riel N A and Verrips C T 2000 The role of ammonia metabolism in nitrogen catabolite repression in *Saccharomyces cerevisiae FEMS Microbiol. Rev.* **24** 67–83
[43] Vieille C and Zeikus G J 2001 Hyperthermophilic enzymes: sources, uses, and molecular mechanisms for thermostability *Microbiol. Mol. Biol. Rev.* **65** 1–43
[44] Renge V, Khedkar S and Nandurkar N R 2012 Enzyme synthesis by fermentation method: a review *Sci. Rev. Chem. Commun.* **2** 585–90
[45] Lizardi-Jiménez M and Hernández-Martínez R 2017 Solid state fermentation (SSF): diversity of applications to valorize waste and biomass *3 Biotech.* **7** 44
[46] De Haan A B 2015 *Process Technology: An Introduction* (Walter de Gruyter GmbH & Co KG)
[47] Owusu-Apenten R 2004 *Introduction to Food Chemistry* (Boca Raton, FL: CRC Press)

[48] Manen J-F *et al* 2005 A fully automatable enzymatic method for DNA extraction from plant tissues *BMC Plant Biol.* **5** 1–9
[49] Boland M 1992 Extraction and purification of proteins from animal tissue using aqueous phase systems *Australas. Biotechnol.* **2** 47–52
[50] Geciova J, Bury D and Jelen P 2002 Methods for disruption of microbial cells for potential use in the dairy industry—a review *Int. Dairy J.* **12** 541–53
[51] Chisti Y and Moo-Young M 1986 Disruption of microbial cells for intracellular products *Enzyme Microb. Technol.* **8** 194–204
[52] Crapisi A *et al* 1993 Enhanced microbial cell lysis by the use of lysozyme immobilized on different carriers *Process Biochem.* **28** 17–21
[53] Moo-Young M 2019 *Comprehensive Biotechnology* (Amsterdam: Elsevier)
[54] Middelberg A P 1995 Process-scale disruption of microorganisms *Biotechnol. Adv.* **13** 491–551
[55] Nossal N G and Heppel L A 1966 The release of enzymes by osmotic shock from *Escherichia coli* in exponential phase *J. Biol. Chem.* **241** 3055–62
[56] Chaiyarit S and Thongboonkerd V 2009 Comparative analyses of cell disruption methods for mitochondrial isolation in high-throughput proteomics study *Anal. Biochem.* **394** 249–58
[57] Stathopulos P B *et al* 2004 Sonication of proteins causes formation of aggregates that resemble amyloid *Protein Sci.* **13** 3017–27
[58] McGann L E, Yang H and Walterson M 1988 Manifestations of cell damage after freezing and thawing *Cryobiology* **25** 178–85
[59] Tansey W P 2006 Freeze–thaw lysis for extraction of proteins from mammalian cells *CSH Protocols* **2006** pdb.prot4614
[60] Qi X, Sun Y and Xiong S 2015 A single freeze-thawing cycle for highly efficient solubilization of inclusion body proteins and its refolding into bioactive form *Microb. Cell Fact.* **14** 12
[61] Goldberg S 2008 Mechanical/physical methods of cell disruption and tissue homogenization *Methods Mol. Biol.* **424** 3–22
[62] Giza C C and Hovda D A 2001 The neurometabolic cascade of concussion *J. Athl. Train.* **36** 228
[63] Nadar S S, Pawar R G and Rathod V K 2017 Recent advances in enzyme extraction strategies: a comprehensive review *Int. J. Biol. Macromol.* **101** 931–57
[64] Glyk A, Scheper T and Beutel S 2015 PEG–salt aqueous two-phase systems: an attractive and versatile liquid–liquid extraction technology for the downstream processing of proteins and enzymes *Appl. Microbiol. Biotechnol.* **99** 6599–616
[65] Asenjo J A and Andrews B A 2011 Aqueous two-phase systems for protein separation: a perspective *J. Chromatogr.* A **1218** 8826–35
[66] Bruton C 1983 Large-scale purification of enzymes *Philos. Trans. R. Soc. Lond. B Biol. Sci.* **300** 249–61
[67] Palmer I and Wingfield P T 2012 Preparation and extraction of insoluble (inclusion-body) proteins from *Escherichia coli Curr. Protoc. Protein Sci.* **70** 6.3.1–20
[68] Zabriskie D and DiPaolo M 1988 Removal of nucleic acid contaminants using nuclease enzymes during protein isolation *Biotechnol. Bioeng.* **32** 100–4
[69] Ryan B J 2011 Differential precipitation and solubilization of proteins *Methods Mol. Biol.* **681** 203–13

[70] Duong-Ly K C and Gabelli S B 2014 Salting out of proteins using ammonium sulfate precipitation *Methods in Enzymology* (Amsterdam: Elsevier) pp 85–94
[71] Talley K and Alexov E 2010 On the pH-optimum of activity and stability of proteins *Proteins Struct. Funct. Bioinf.* **78** 2699–706
[72] Askonas B A 1951 The use of organic solvents at low temperature for the separation of enzymes. Application to aqueous rabbit muscle extract *Biochem.* J **48** 42
[73] Mahadevan H and Hall C K 1990 Statistical-mechanical model of protein precipitation by nonionic polymer *AIChE J.* **36** 1517–28
[74] Ingham K C 1984 Protein precipitation with polyethylene glycol *Methods in Enzymology* (Amsterdam: Elsevier) pp 351–6
[75] Atha D H and Ingham K C 1981 Mechanism of precipitation of proteins by polyethylene glycols. Analysis in terms of excluded volume *J. Biol. Chem.* **256** 12108–17
[76] Sim S-L *et al* 2012 Protein precipitation by polyethylene glycol: a generalized model based on hydrodynamic radius *J. Biotechnol.* **157** 315–9
[77] McPherson A and Gavira J A 2014 Introduction to protein crystallization *Acta Crystallogr. F: Struct. Biol. Commun.* **70** 2–20
[78] Asenjo J and Andrews B 2009 Protein purification using chromatography: selection of type, modelling and optimization of operating conditions *J. Mol. Recognit.: Interdiscip. J.* **22** 65–76
[79] Chase H A 1994 Purification of proteins by adsorption chromatography in expanded beds *Trends Biotechnol.* **12** 296–303
[80] Yigzaw Y *et al* 2009 Ion exchange chromatography of proteins and clearance of aggregates *Curr. Pharm. Biotechnol.* **10** 421–6
[81] Jungbauer A and Hahn R 2009 Ion-exchange chromatography *Methods Enzymol.* **463** 349–71
[82] Rahimzadeh M *et al* 2016 Purification, characterization and comparison between two new L-asparaginases from *Bacillus* PG03 and *Bacillus* PG04 *Open Biochem. J.* **10** 35
[83] Urh M, Simpson D and Zhao K 2009 Affinity chromatography: general methods *Methods Enzymol.* **463** 417–38
[84] Bernik M B and Kwaan H C 1969 Plasminogen activator activity in cultures from human tissues. An immunological and histochemical study *J. Clin. Investig.* **48** 1740–53
[85] Berg J M, Tymoczko J L and Stryer L 2002 Lectins are specific carbohydrate-binding proteins *Biochemistry* (Macmillan) pp 333–5
[86] Smárason S V and Smith A V 2005 Method for desalting nucleic acids *Google Patents*
[87] Wang W, Liu Q J and Cui H 2007 Rapid desalting and protein recovery with phenol after ammonium sulfate fractionation *Electrophoresis* **28** 2358–60
[88] Aehle W 2007 *Enzymes in Industry: Production and Applications* (New York: Wiley)
[89] Fazaeli M, Hojjatpanah G and Emam-Djomeh Z 2013 Effects of heating method and conditions on the evaporation rate and quality attributes of black mulberry (*Morus nigra*) juice concentrate *J. Food Sci. Technol.* **50** 35–43
[90] Simpson R J 2010 Stabilization of proteins for storage *Cold Spring Harb. Protoc.* **2010** pdb. top79
[91] Miletić N, Nastasović A and Loos K 2012 Immobilization of biocatalysts for enzymatic polymerizations: possibilities, advantages, applications *Bioresour. Technol.* **115** 126–35
[92] Homaei A A *et al* 2013 Enzyme immobilization: an update *J. Chem. Biol.* **6** 185–205

[93] Nisha S, Karthick S A and Gobi N 2012 A review on methods, application and properties of immobilized enzyme *Chem. Sci. Rev. Lett.* **1** 148–55
[94] Bashir N, Sood M and Bandral J D 2020 Enzyme immobilization and its applications in food processing: a review *Int. J. Chem. Stud* **8** 254–61
[95] Chapman J, Ismail A E and Dinu C Z 2018 Industrial applications of enzymes: recent advances, techniques, and outlooks *Catalysts* **8** 238
[96] Krajewska B 2004 Application of chitin-and chitosan-based materials for enzyme immobilizations: a review *Enzyme Microb. Technol.* **35** 126–39
[97] Brentjens R J *et al* 2013 CD19-targeted T cells rapidly induce molecular remissions in adults with chemotherapy-refractory acute lymphoblastic leukemia *Sci. Transl. Med.* **5** 177ra38–18
[98] Singh A *et al* 2018 Methods of enzyme immobilization and its applications in food industry *Enzymes in Food Technology: Improvements and Innovations* (Springer) pp 103–24
[99] Brena B, González-Pombo P and Batista-Viera F 2013 Immobilization of enzymes: a literature survey *Immobilization of Enzymes and Cells* (Springer) (Methods in Biotechnology vol 22)3rd edn pp 15–31
[100] Zhu Y *et al* 2020 Microfluidic immobilized enzyme reactors for continuous biocatalysis *React. Chem. Eng.* **5** 9–32
[101] Jesionowski T, Zdarta J and Krajewska B 2014 Enzyme immobilization by adsorption: a review *Adsorption* **20** 801–21
[102] Betancor L and Luckarift H R 2008 Bioinspired enzyme encapsulation for biocatalysis *Trends Biotechnol.* **26** 566–72
[103] Sheldon R, Schoevaart R and Van Langen L 2005 Cross-linked enzyme aggregates (CLEAs): a novel and versatile method for enzyme immobilization (a review) *Biocatal. Biotransform.* **23** 141–7
[104] Cummings C *et al* 2013 Tailoring enzyme activity and stability using polymer-based protein engineering *Biomaterials* **34** 7437–43
[105] Murata H *et al* 2013 Polymer-based protein engineering can rationally tune enzyme activity, pH-dependence, and stability *Biomacromolecules* **14** 1919–26
[106] Carlsson A-C C *et al* 2018 Increasing enzyme stability and activity through hydrogen bond-enhanced halogen bonds *Biochemistry* **57** 4135–47
[107] Bornscheuer U T and Pohl M 2001 Improved biocatalysts by directed evolution and rational protein design *Curr. Opin. Chem. Biol.* **5** 137–43
[108] Wollert T *et al* 2007 Extending the host range of *Listeria monocytogenes* by rational protein design *Cell* **129** 891–902
[109] Buchholz K, Kasche V and Bornscheuer U T 2012 *Biocatalysts and Enzyme Technology* (New York: Wiley)
[110] Tatsumi Y 2006 High-Mg andesites in the Setouchi volcanic belt, southwestern Japan: analogy to Archean magmatism and continental crust formation? *Annu. Rev. Earth. Planet. Sci.* **34** 467–99
[111] Acharyya S *et al* 2004 Cancer cachexia is regulated by selective targeting of skeletal muscle gene products *J. Clin. Investig.* **114** 370–8
[112] Yu Y and Lutz S 2011 Circular permutation: a different way to engineer enzyme structure and function *Trends Biotechnol.* **29** 18–25
[113] Qian Z and Lutz S 2005 Improving the catalytic activity of *Candida antarctica* lipase B by circular permutation *J. Am. Chem. Soc.* **127** 13466–7

[114] Ostermeier M and Benkovic S J 2001 Evolution of protein function by domain swapping *Adv. Protein Chem.* **55** 29–77
[115] Gronenborn A M 2009 Protein acrobatics in pairs—dimerization via domain swapping *Curr. Opin. Struct. Biol.* **19** 39–49
[116] Lutz S and Benkovic S J 2000 Homology-independent protein engineering *Curr. Opin. Biotechnol.* **11** 319–24
[117] Yu H *et al* 2017 Two strategies to engineer flexible loops for improved enzyme thermostability *Sci. Rep.* **7** 41212
[118] Moraïs S *et al* 2016 Enhancement of cellulosome-mediated deconstruction of cellulose by improving enzyme thermostability *Biotechnol. Biofuels* **9** 1–12
[119] Hu J *et al* 2013 The synergistic action of accessory enzymes enhances the hydrolytic potential of a 'cellulase mixture' but is highly substrate specific *Biotechnol. Biofuels* **6** 1–12
[120] Cho C M-H, Mulchandani A and Chen W 2004 Altering the substrate specificity of organophosphorus hydrolase for enhanced hydrolysis of chlorpyrifos *Appl. Environ. Microbiol.* **70** 4681–5
[121] Douglas K T 1992 Alteration of enzyme specificity and catalysis *Curr. Opin. Biotechnol.* **3** 370–7
[122] Stratton J, Chiruvolu V and Meagher M 1998 High cell-density fermentation *Methods Mol. Biol.* **103** 107–20
[123] Pandey A 2003 Solid-state fermentation *Biochem. Eng. J.* **13** 81–4
[124] Krishna C 2005 Solid-state fermentation systems—an overview *Crit. Rev. Biotechnol.* **25** 1–30
[125] Raghavarao K, Ranganathan T and Karanth N 2003 Some engineering aspects of solid-state fermentation *Biochem. Eng. J.* **13** 127–35
[126] Maxon W D 1955 Continuous fermentation: a discussion of its principles and applications *Appl. Microbiol.* **3** 110–22
[127] Zhang S *et al* 2018 Interkingdom microbial consortia mechanisms to guide biotechnological applications *Microb. Biotechnol.* **11** 833–47
[128] Qian X *et al* 2020 Biotechnological potential and applications of microbial consortia *Biotechnol. Adv.* **40** 107500
[129] Freeman A, Woodley J M and Lilly M D 1993 *In situ* product removal as a tool for bioprocessing *Biotechnology* **11** 1007–12
[130] Baez A, Cho K-M and Liao J C 2011 High-flux isobutanol production using engineered *Escherichia coli*: a bioreactor study with *in situ* product removal *Appl. Microbiol. Biotechnol.* **90** 1681–90
[131] Littlechild J A 2015 Enzymes from extreme environments and their industrial applications *Front. Bioeng. Biotechnol.* **3** 161
[132] Cabrera M Á and Blamey J M 2018 Biotechnological applications of archaeal enzymes from extreme environments *Biol. Res.* **51**
[133] Magan N 2007 Fungi in extreme environments *Mycota* **4** 85–103
[134] Rothschild L J and Mancinelli R L 2001 Life in extreme environments *Nature* **409** 1092–101
[135] Kendall A 1910 Observations on aciduric (acidophilic) bacteria *J. Med. Res.* **22** 153
[136] Wiegel J and Kevbrin V 2004 *Alkalithermophiles* (Portland Press Ltd)
[137] Banciu H L and Sorokin D Y 2013 Adaptation in haloalkaliphiles and natronophilic bacteria *Polyextremophiles: Life Under Multiple Forms of Stress* (Berlin: Springer) pp 121–78
[138] DasSarma S and Arora P 2001 Halophiles *Encyclopedia of Life Sciences* (Wiley-Blackwell)

[139] Raddadi N *et al* 2015 Biotechnological applications of extremophiles, extremozymes and extremolytes *Appl. Microbiol. Biotechnol.* **99** 7907–13
[140] Mesbah N M 2022 Industrial biotechnology based on enzymes from extreme environments *Front. Bioeng. Biotechnol.* **10** 870083
[141] Mahajan E, George A and Wolk B 2012 Improving affinity chromatography resin efficiency using semi-continuous chromatography *J. Chromatogr.* A **1227** 154–62
[142] Bechtold M *et al* 2006 Integrated operation of continuous chromatography and biotransformations for the generic high yield production of fine chemicals *J. Biotechnol.* **124** 146–62
[143] Zhang K *et al* 2018 Microplastic pollution in China's inland water systems: a review of findings, methods, characteristics, effects, and management *Sci. Total Environ.* **630** 1641–53
[144] Van Reis R *et al* 1997 High performance tangential flow filtration *Biotechnol. Bioeng.* **56** 71–82
[145] Cushing R S and Lawler D F 1998 Depth filtration: fundamental investigation through three-dimensional trajectory analysis *Environ. Sci. Technol.* **32** 3793–801
[146] Song L and Elimelech M 1995 Theory of concentration polarization in crossflow filtration *J. Chem. Soc., Faraday Trans.* **91** 3389–98
[147] Bensch M, Selbach B and Hubbuch J 2007 High throughput screening techniques in downstream processing: preparation, characterization and optimization of aqueous two-phase systems *Chem. Eng. Sci.* **62** 2011–21
[148] Singh N and Herzer S 2018 Downstream processing technologies/capturing and final purification: opportunities for innovation, change, and improvement. A review of downstream processing developments in protein purification *Adv. Biochem. Eng. Biotecnol.* **165** 115–78

IOP Publishing

Introduction to Pharmaceutical Biotechnology, Volume 2 (Second Edition)

Enzymes, proteins and bioinformatics

Ahmed Al-Harrasi, Saurabh Bhatia and Ajmal Khan

Chapter 3

Industrial enzymes and their applications

3.1 Industrial enzymes

Microbial enzyme production is an essential industrial process, owing to the extraordinary performance and multitude of applications of enzymes from various microbes. These microbes are active under a varied range of physical and chemical conditions [1]. Microbial enzymes are a potential source of replacement in the absence or deficiency of human enzymes. In addition, microbial enzymes are the favored source of industrial enzymes as they can be produced in large quantities in a short time. Microbes have short generation times, and genetic manipulation can be performed more easily on bacterial cells to enhance enzyme production. The industry is still seeking novel microbial strains to furnish different enzymes to meet requirements [1]. Of the 3000 enzymes reported to date, only a few are industrially used, such as hydrolytic enzymes which degrade naturally occurring polymers such as starch, proteins, pectins and cellulose. Progress in biochemistry leading to the isolation and characterization of many enzymes made it essential to standardize the enzyme nomenclature. Based on the type of reaction catalyzed, enzymes are classified into six main classes, as listed in table 3.1.

Broad applications of enzymes in different bioprocesses can be employed to deliver a range of products in different industries. Table 3.2 summarizes a number of applications used to deliver a range of products. The industrial production of microbial enzymes is presented in figure 3.1.

3.2 Bacterial α-amylases

Amylases are one of the key enzymes used in industry. These enzymes breakdown starch molecules into polymers composed of glucose units [2, 3]. Amylases have wide applications at the industrial level, e.g. in the food, fermentation and pharmaceutical industries. Based on the source, α-amylases are classified into various categories

doi:10.1088/978-0-7503-5387-8ch3

Table 3.1. Enzyme classification.

S. no.	Enzymes	Class	Reactions
1	Dehydrogenases, oxidases, oxygenases, peroxidases	Oxidoreductases	Transfer of hydrogen or oxygen or electrons between molecules.
2	Fructosyltransferases, transketolases, acyltransferases, transaminases	Transferases	Transfer of groups of atoms from one molecule to another.
3	Isomerases, epimerases, racemases	Isomerases	Transfer of a group from one position to another within one molecule.
4	Pectate lyases, hydratases, dehydratases, decarboxylases, fumarase, argino succinase	Lyases	Non-hydrolytic cleavage by elimination or addition reactions.
5	Proteases, amylases, acylases, lipases, phosphatases, cutinases	Hydrolases	Hydrolytic cleavage of bonds.
6	Synthetases, ligases	Ligases	Covalent joining of two molecules coupled with the hydrolysis of an energy rich bond in ATP or similar triphosphates.

Table 3.2. Enzymes and their applications.

Enzyme	Microorganism(s)	Function
Acid proteinase	*Aspergillus* spp.	Milk coagulation
Acyltransferase	*Bacillus* sp. APB-6	Synthesis of hydroxamic acids
Alkaline protease	*Alcaligenes faecalis*	Dehairing, bating
Amidase	*Rhodococcus erythropolis*	Degradation of nitriles containing wastes
Aminopeptidase	*Lactobacillus* spp.	Faster cheese ripening
Aminopeptidases	*Lactobacillus brevis*, *Lactobacillus plantarum*	Protein breakdown during mashing
Amylase	*Aspergillus* spp., *Bacillus* spp.	Flour adjustment, bread softness
Amylase	*Bacillus licheniformis*	De-inking, drainage improvement
Amylase	*Aspergillus* spp., *Bacillus subtilis*	Carbohydrate stain removal
Amylase	*Aspergillus* spp., *B. subtilis*	Fiber splitting
Amylase	*B. licheniformis*, *Aspergillus* spp.	Bioremediation of vegetable waste
Amyloglucosidase	*Aspergillus niger*	Starch hydrolysis for bioremediation
Catalase	*A. niger*	Cheese processing
Cellulase	*A. niger*, *Trichoderma atroviride*	Fruit liquefaction
Cellulase	*Bacillus* spp., *A. niger*	De-inking, drainage improvement
Cellulase	*A. niger*, *Bacillus* spp.	Color clarification

Cutinase	*Fusarium solani f. pisi*	Triglyceride removal
Cutinase	*F. solani f. pisi*	Degradation of plastics, polycaprolactone
Endoglycosidase	*Mucor hiemalis*	Teeth and gum tissue care
Glucose isomerase	*Corynebacterium* spp., *Streptomyces murinus*	Production of high-fructose corn syrup
Glucose oxidase	*A. niger*, *Penicillium chrysogenum*	Dough strengthening
Glucose oxidase	*A. niger*	Oxygen removal from beer
Glucose oxidase	*A. niger*, *P. chrysogenum*	Polymerization of anilines
Glycosyl tranferase	*Bacillus* spp.	Synthesis of oligosaccharides
Laccase	*B. subtilis*	Non-chlorine bleaching, delignification
Laccase	*Trametes hirsute*	Polymerization of bisphenol A
Laccase	*B. subtilis*, *Trametes versicolor*	Hair dye
Laccase	*T. versicolor*, *B. subtilis*	Production of textile dyes, cosmetic pigments, flavor agents and pesticides
Laccase	*T. versicolor*	Degradation of waste containing olefin unit, polyurethane and phenolic compounds
Lactase (β-galactosidase)	*Escherichia coli*, *Kluyveromyces* spp.	Lactose reduced milk and whey products
Lignin peroxidase	*Phanerochaete chrysosporium*, *Coprinus cinereus*	Degradation of phenolic compounds
Limoninase	*A. niger*, *Aspergillus oryzae*	Debittering
Lipase	*A. niger*, *A. oryzae*	Faster cheese ripening, flavor customized cheese
Lipase	*A. niger*	Dough stability and conditioning
Lipase	*Candida antarctica*	Pitch control
Lipase	*C. antarctica*	Polycondensation, ring-opening polymerization of lactones, carbonates
Lipase	*A. oryzae*, *Aspergillus flavus*	Fat stain elimination
Lipase	*A. oryzae*, *A. flavus*,	Degreasing
Lipase	*A. oryzae*, *A. flavus*	Skin care
Lipase	*A. oryzae*, *A. flavus*	Synthesis of pharmaceuticals, polymers, biodiesels, biosurfactants
Lipase	*A. oryzae*, *Candida tropicalis*	Degradation of crude oil hydrocarbons
Maltogenic α-amylase	*Bacillus stearothermophilus*	Enhancing the shelf life of breads
Manganese peroxidase	*P. chrysosporium*, *C. cinereus*	Degradation of phenolic compounds
Mannanase	*Bacillus* spp.	Mannan spot removal
Naringinase	*A. niger*	Debittering
Neutral protease	*A. niger*, *A. flavus*, *B. subtilis*	Dehairing, soaking

(*Continued*)

Table 3.2. (*Continued*)

Enzyme	Microorganism(s)	Function
Neutral proteinase	*B. subtilis*, *A. oryzae*	Faster cheese ripening, debittering
Nitrile hydratase	*Rhodococcus rhodochrous* PA-34, *Bacillus* spp. APB-6	Synthesis of acrylamide, butyramide and nicotinamide
Nitrile hydratase	*Rhodococcus* spp.	Degradation of nitriles containing wastes
Oxygenase	*Pseudomonas* spp., *Rhodococcus* spp.	Degradation of halogenated contaminants
Pectinase	*A. oryzae*, *Penicillium funiculosum*	Depectinization
Phytase	*A. niger*	Hydrolyze phytic acid to release phosphorous
Protease	*A. niger*	Restrict haze formation
Protease	*B. subtilis*	Biofilm removal
Protease	*A. oryzae*, *B. subtilis*	Protein stain removal
Protease	*A. niger*, *A. flavus*, *B. subtilis*	Removal of dead skin
Protease	*Chrysosporium keratinophilum*	Bioremediation of keratinic wastes
Pullulanase	*Bacillus* spp., *Klebsiella* spp.	Starch saccharification
Superoxide dismutase	*Corynebacterium glutamicum*, *Lactobacillus plantarum*	Free radical scavenging, skin care
Transglutaminase	*Streptomyces* spp.	Protein crosslinking
Transglutaminase	*Streptoverticillium* spp., *Streptomyces* spp.	Laminated dough strength
Transglutaminase	*Streptomyces mobaraensis*	Protein crosslinking
Tyrosinase	*Trichoderma reesei*	Polymerization of lignin and chitosan
Xylanase	*A. niger*	Dough conditioning
Xylanase	*Aspergillus* spp., *Bacillus* spp.	Enhanced digestibility of starch
Xylanase	*Trichoderma reesei*, *Thermomyces lanuginosus*, *Aureobasidium pullulans*	Bleach boosting
α-amylase	*Bacillus* spp., *Aspergillus* spp.	Starch hydrolysis
β-amylase	*Bacillus* spp., *Streptomyces* spp., *Rhizopus* spp.	Starch hydrolysis
β-glucanase	*B. subtilis*, *Aspergillus* spp.	Restrict haze formation
β-glucanase	*A. niger*	Digestive aid

such as α-amylases from bacteria, fungi, plants, animals and microorganisms, whereas enzymes from fungal and bacterial sources have a considerable number of applications in industry. α-Amylase production is necessary for the conversion of starches into oligosaccharides. Starch, a major storage product of many economically important crops, is a vital constituent of the human diet. Starch-converting enzymes are used in the production of maltodextrin, modified starches, and glucose and fructose

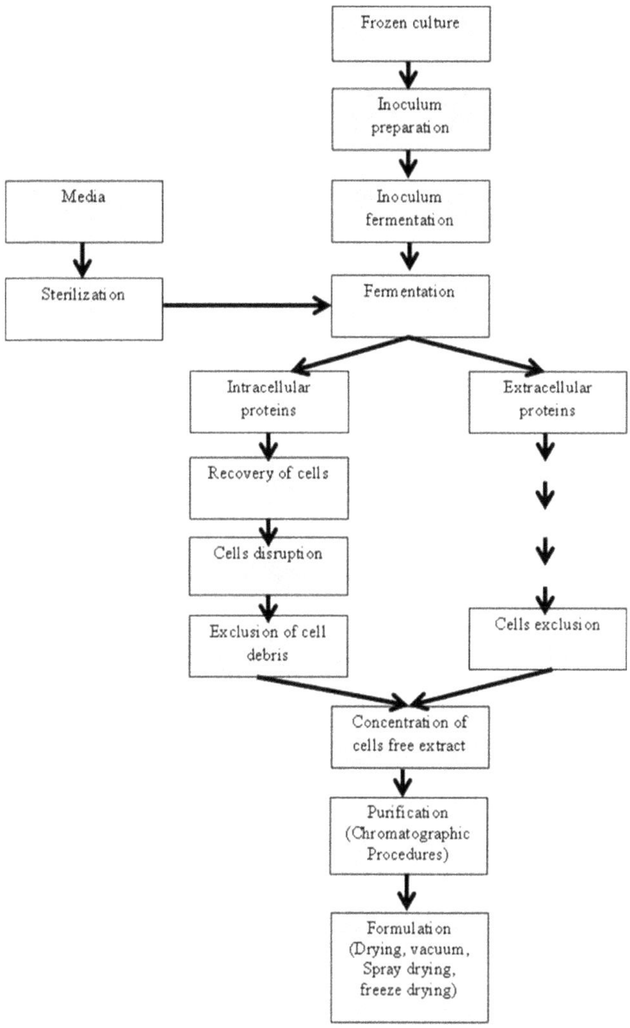

Figure 3.1. Basic outline of industrial production of enzymes.

syrups. A large number of microbial α-amylases have applications in different industrial sectors such as the food, textiles, paper and detergent industries [2, 3]. α-Amylase production is usually performed using submerged fermentation, although solid-substrate fermentation systems also provide reliable technology. The thermostability, pH profile, pH stability, Ca independence and other properties of each α-amylase play an important role in the development of fermentation processes [2, 3].

α-Amylases (both bacterial and fungal) are enzymes which have been produced industrially on a large scale. The general procedure for amylase production is depicted in figure 3.2. The bacterial α-amylase endoenzyme breaks down α-1,4 bonds in amylose and amylopectin, resulting in a sudden fall in the viscosity of gelatinized starch solutions (endohydrolysis of starch, also known as starch

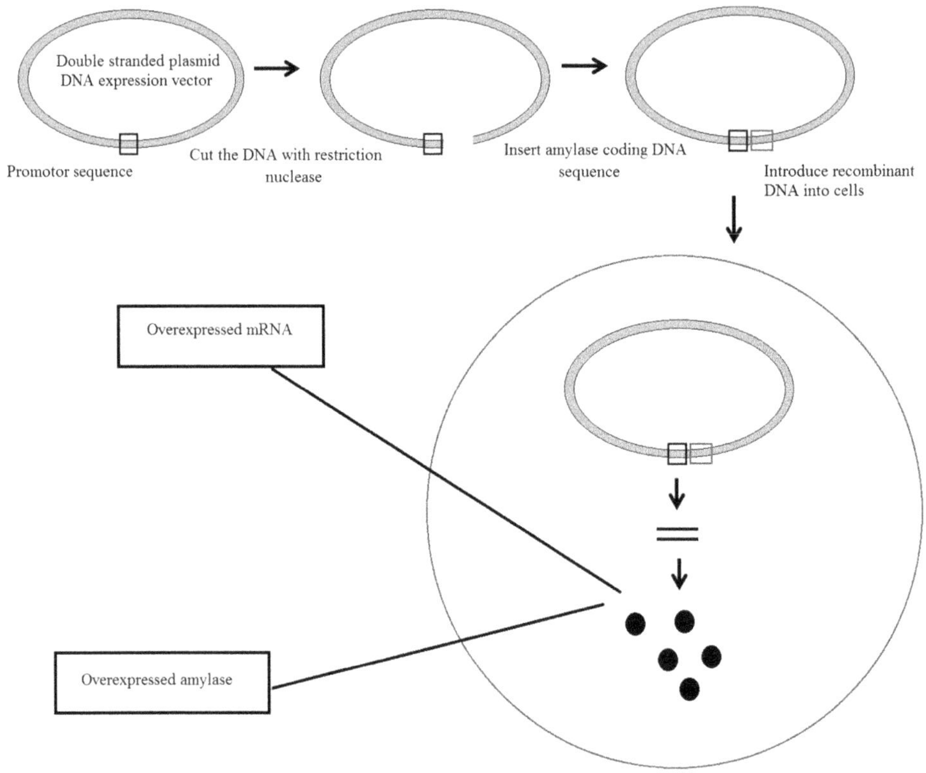

Figure 3.2. Amylase production using rDNA technology.

liquefaction) [2, 3]. After the action of α-amylase, the final product recovered is dextrans, together with small quantities of glucose and maltose. Before treatment with amylases, the native starch is exposed to hydration (gelatinization of starch). According to the literature, α-amylase derived from *Bacillus amyloliquefaciens* is active up to 90 °C and this high temperature stability (for gelatinization purpose) has been used at the industrial scale. Another strain belonging to the same genus, *Bacillus licheniformis*, has also been used industrially for the production of α-amylases. α-Amylases are metallo-proteins, containing at least one mol of calcium ions (they are stabilized by Ca^{2+} and inhibited by chelate forming agents) [2, 3]. The activity and stability of α-amylase obtained from *B. licheniformis* is not dependent on the calcium content of the solution, in contrast to α-amylase from *B. amylolequefaciens.* pH 6.5–7 is the optimum range of pH, at which these enzymes show maximum activity. At neutral pH and temperature (30 °C–40 °C), fermentation of bacterial amylases is performed in submerged culture. Cereal meal and starch rich medium are usually used along with an organic source of nitrogen. After an interval of 10–20 h, α-amylase formation starts and lasts for another 100 h [3]. The pH of the medium must be less than 6 during fermentation to avoid the denaturation of α-amylase. The α-amylase is accompanied by other extracellular enzymes.

B. licheniformis synthesizes a serine protease, whereas *B. amyloliquefaciens* synthesizes a neutral protease along with hemicellulase and β-glucanase. Starch liquefaction using α-amylase is performed in a continuous or batch reactor. The degree of anticipated starch hydrolysis is determined by the intended later use. The manufacture of coating compounds, surface sizing of paper and paints requires a colloidal starch solution with a final viscosity [3]. Incomplete degradation of starch is brought about by α-amylase to attain a specific viscosity. During the production of glucose syrup, α-amylase is used in the first step of enzymatic degradation resulting in a mixture of glucose and fructose with high-fructose content. During the production of dextrans, the degradation of starch required is as high as 10 dextrose equivalents. The increasing production of alcohol as a fuel from starch-containing raw material is opening greater prospects for the utilization of α-amylases and glucoamylases at large scales [3].

3.3 Fungal α-amylases

Fungal amylases have been extensively used in large-scale industrial production owing to their many merits, for example, their cost-effectiveness, consistency, smaller temporal and spatial requirements, and ease of process modification and optimization [4]. These enzymes account for around 30% of the world's enzyme production [3]. Amylases belong to a class of starch degrading enzymes that catalyze the breakdown of internal glycosidic bonds in polysaccharides with the retention of the anomeric configuration in the products. As mentioned above, most amylases are metalloenzymes, which require calcium ions (Ca^{2+}) for their activity, structural integrity and stability [5]. Endo-amylases, exo-amylases, debranching enzymes and glycosyltransferases are further examples of the starch degrading class of enzymes [6]. In the starch processing industry, enzymatic hydrolysis is favored over acid hydrolysis, owing to the specificity of the reaction, stability of the synthesized products, lower energy requirements and exclusion of neutralization steps [7]. Due to the high demand for these enzymes at large scales, there is great interest in developing enzymes with better properties, e.g. raw starch degrading amylases suitable for industrial applications and cost-effective production techniques. Most amylases have been synthesized from soil fungi, e.g. *Aspergillus, Penicillium* and *Rhizopus* [7]. Only little evidence is available on amylases from endophytic fungi, which are primarily explored for beneficial secondary metabolites with different bioactivity [8]. Fungal α-amylases are mainly derived from the *Aspergillus* genus (*Aspergillus niger*, *Aspergillus oryzae*). Because of their low deactivation temperature, low optimum pH (pH 4–5) and high saccharifying action, they significantly differ from the bacterial amylases [3–8]. They are less fit for the liquefaction of starch than bacterial α-amylases. The synthesis of fungal α-amylase is accomplished in solid-substrate culture and occasionally in submerged culture for specific strains of *Aspergillus*. The fermentation medium used remains the same as for bacterial α-amylases, but the concentration of glucose hinders the formation of amylase, thus the concentration of glucose in the fermentation medium must be measured and kept low [3–8]. Other fungal enzymes are produced in solid-substrate culture. The protease content is found to be higher when produced by solid-substrate culture in comparison to α-amylase produced by submerged culture [3–8]. The glucoamylase level is low in both methods. Fungal α-amylases are employed in the manufacturing of baked goods, where this enzyme is added to amylase-poor flour to reduce and standardize the proving time of dough. In addition, they are also used in the production of maltose-rich syrups and various other areas of the food industry [3–8].

3.4 Bacterial proteases

Microbial proteases are among the most important hydrolytic enzymes and have been studied widely. Proteases derived from microorganisms have gained great attention in the last decade because of their biotechnological applications in various industrial processes, e.g. detergent, textile, leather, dairy and pharmaceutical preparations. Proteolytic enzymes derived from microorganisms are preferred in industrial applications of enzymes owing to their technical and economic advantages [9]. The category of microbial proteases signifies one of the largest groups of industrial enzymes and accounts for approximately 60% of total enzyme sales in the world [9]. The majority of bacterial proteases are produced from *B. licheniformis*. The bacterium is cultured in a fermentation medium supplemented by protein and protein hydrolysate. The medium's pH is adjusted to neutral and the temperature is kept between 30 °C–40 °C. Supplementation of carbohydrates *in situ* enhances the productivity of enzymes. Production begins when the culture passes into the stationary phase (after 10–20 h) and takes place at an almost constant rate for several hours, providing that the protein is still present in the medium. Starch hydrolysates are degraded and assimilated by *B. licheniformis*, however, at the end of the fermentation serine protease is virtually the only protein in the culture suspension. Proteases can also be synthesized by fermentation of *B. amyloquefaciens*, but the final yield of protease is higher in the case of *B. licheniformis* (at least 10% more protein added to the medium). In the case of *B. amyloliquefaciens*, the culture supernatant contains other enzymes, in particular, a large amount of α-amylase. Alkaline proteases derived from *B. amyloliquefaciens* and *B. licheniformis* represent the lead molecules for subtilisin. Serine proteases have been derived from species of *Bacillus*. These proteases have better pH stability (up to pH 12) compared to subtilisins (pH 8–11). The bulk of alkaline proteases are used as additives to detergents in the form of granulates, prills or marumerizer pellets. Proteases enhance the cleansing power of a detergent and, in addition, this allows the elimination of protein-containing soils, e.g. blood, egg yolk and chocolate, and enhances the detachment of soil from the fibers. The stability of subtilisins is independent of metal ions, hence complexing additives in detergents, e.g. EDTA or tripolyphosphates, do not significantly interfere. Currently, almost 80% of the detergents on the market contain enzymes in concentrations of about 0.015%–0.025%. The high alkali resistance of alkaline proteases makes them suitable for the leather industry, for the dehairing (nuding) of skins and to reduce softening times. They exhibit much better stability in detergents when the complexing agent EDTA or tripolyphosphate is substituted by citrate or gluconate.

3.5 Fungal proteases

Fungal proteases have attracted the attention of researchers as fungi can grow on low-cost substrates and secrete large quantities of enzymes into the culture medium, which could ease downstream processing [10]. Fungal proteases can be employed for hydrolyzing protein and other components of soybeans and wheat in soy sauce production. Proteases can be synthesized in large amounts in a short time by established methods of fermentation [10]. Parameters such as the C/N ratio and the presence of some sugars, in addition to several other physical factors, are significant in the development of the fermentation process. Fungus-derived proteases can be produced cost effectively, and also have the advantages of fast production, ease of enzymes modification and the easy removal of mycelium by filtration. Protease production has mainly been achieved by using submerged fermentation, however, the conditions in solid-subtrate fermentation result in several potential merits for the production of fungal enzymes [10].

Fungal proteases are synthesized from the genus *Aspergillus*, in particular the two species *A. oryzae* and *A. niger* [11, 12]. When cultured on a solid substrate, large quantities of proteases are produced by these species. The yield can be further improved by the addition of inorganic nitrogen. Other than proteases, reasonable amounts of α-amylase, glucoamylase, cellulases and pectinases are also produced. As far as applications are concerned, *Aspergillus* proteases are employed for hydrolysis of soybean protein in the production of soya sauce, as a component of enzymatic preparations for the treatment of digestive disturbances and in the baking industry. The supplementation of protease into flour incompletely hydrolyzes the gluten, reduces the viscosity of dough and thus reduces the kneading time. Fungal proteases are deactivated at 50 °C, so a quick denaturation takes place in the beginning of the baking process and circumvents the complete hydrolysis of proteins. Acid proteases can be derived from *Mucor* strains, in particular from the species *Mucor pusillus* and *Mucor michei*. During the fermentation of *Mucor* strains, esterases and lipases are also formed, which are mainly used in the manufacture of cheese [13].

3.6 Glucose isomerase (d-xylose ketol-isomerase; EC. 5.3.1.5)

Glucose isomerase is the first intracellular enzyme used on a large scale. It catalyzes the reversible isomerization of d-glucose and d-xylose to d-fructose and d-xylulose, respectively [14]. This enzyme has the largest market in the food industry because of its application in the production of high-fructose corn syrup (HFCS) [14]. This mixture contains 42% fructose, 50% glucose and 8% other mono- and disaccharides used as liquid sugar in the food industry. The entire process is based on starch hydrolysis by α-amylase and glucoamylase, and then isomerization to a mixture of glucose and fructose. Fructose has a better sweetening power than sucrose and glucose. HFCS, an equilibrium mixture of glucose and fructose, is 1.3 times sweeter than sucrose and serves as a sweetener for use by diabetics [14]. Interconversion of xylose to xylulose by glucose isomerase acts as a nutritional requirement in saprophytic bacteria and has a potential application in the bioconversion of hemicellulose to ethanol. The enzyme is generally found in prokaryotes. The microbial strain development accomplished by utilizing xylan-containing raw materials for the development of or screening for constitutive mutants of glucose isomerase is expected to result in discontinuation of the use of xylose as an inducer for the production of the enzyme [14]. Removal of Co^{2+} from the fermentation medium is necessary to prevent health issues arising from human consumption of HFCS. Glucose isomerase is synthesized by submerged cultivation of the various organisms listed in table 3.3 in the pH range 6.5–8.5 at 30 °C. Enzyme isolation is typically omitted and whole or disintegrated cells are immobilized. Glucose isomerase immobilization requires adsorption or heat treatment together with cross linkage [14]. Glucose isomerase offers an efficient means for its easy recovery and reuse, and lowers the cost. X-ray crystallographic and genetic engineering reports support a hydride shift mechanism for the action of glucose isomerase. Glucose isomerase cloning in homologous as well as heterologous hosts has been performed, with the main aim of overproducing the enzyme and interpreting the genetic makeup of individual genes (xylA, xylB and xylR) in the xyl operon of different microorganisms [14]. Using a low-cost inducer in the fermentation medium devoid of Co^{2+} and redesigning a tailor-made glucose isomerase with improved thermostability, greater affinity for glucose and lower optimum pH will contribute considerably to the growth of an economically viable industrial process for enzymatic isomerization of glucose to fructose [14]. Various glucose isomerase sources and immobilization techniques are listed in table 3.3.

Different varieties of reactor have been compared and it has been reported that continuous fixed-bed reactors are the most suitable [14]. The isomerization is in a pH range of 7.0–8.5 at 60 °C–65 °C. The substrate solution contains 40%–50% glucose and oligosaccharide and has a viscosity of 0.8–3 mPa s. A magnesium salt concentration 0.5–5 mM l^{-1} is supplemented to activate and stabilize the enzyme. Alkali-catalyzed transformation of fructose into mannose and psicose can be averted by decreasing the pH of the product solution. The purification of fructose syrup is achived by treatment with activated charcoal and using ion exchangers. The fructose syrup is concentrated to 71% dry matter. The procedure for the production of fructose syrup is represented in figure 3.3.

Table 3.3. Glucose isomerase sources and immobilization techniques.

Name of organism	Immobilization technique	Final form
Streptomyces olivaceus	Whole cell; cross-linked with glutaraldehyde	Granules
Streptomyces olivochromogenes	Aluminum oxide support	Powder
Arthrobacter	Immobilized in the cells with a flocculating agent	Cylindrical particles
Actinoplanes missouriensis	Mycelium encapsulated in gelatin cross-linked with glutaraldehyde	Microspheres

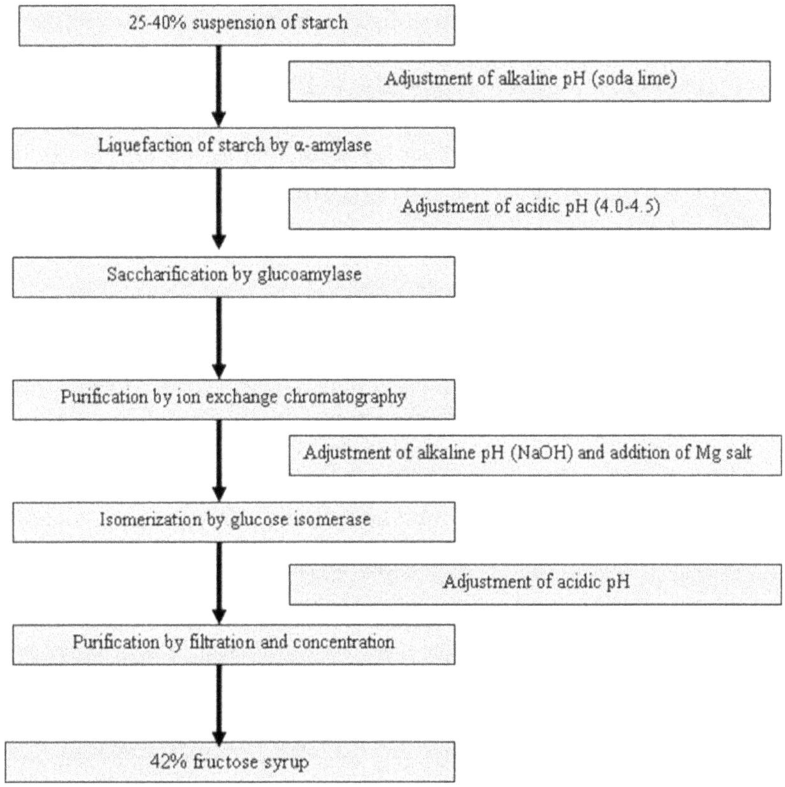

Figure 3.3. Flow diagram for the production of fructose syrup.

3.7 Penicillinase

Penicillinases are produced on the inner surface of the bacterial cell membrane and perhaps pass through the membrane to the external surface while they are being synthesized [14]. Generally, a gram-positive bacterium produces an ample amount of penicillinase and the majority is released into the surrounding medium. This is called exopencillinase. On the other hand, gram-negative bacteria synthesize β-lactamase in smaller amounts. The production and processing of penicillinase by the gram-positive organism *B. licheniformis* has been investigated. When the bacterium is exposed to inducers (e.g. penicillin), there is a sudden rise in penicinillase production [15]. This process is accompanied by the development of many vesicles with high enzymatic activity. There are considerable differences in the way that β-lactamases protect gram-positive and gram-negative bacteria from the β-lactam antibiotic. Generally, β-lactamase production in a gram-positive organism is inducible and a large quantity of penicillinase is released into the surrounding medium [15].

Because of its inactivation property against penicillin and certain cephalosporins, penicillinase (a bacterial enzyme) has gained wide attention. Several other hydrolytic enzymes which are also capable of inactivating penicillin have been explored, and a number of penicillinase producing pathogenic bacteria have been explored, e.g. staphylococcus species and some gram-negative bacteria of intestinal origin. This was first reported when some species showed resistance against penicillin. In particular, it was evidenced among patients infected by *Staphylococcus aureus*. Many common genera of fungi, such as *Penicillium*, *Aspergillus* and *Mucor*, synthesize the enzyme *Penicillin amidase* [16–18]. Based on their activity penicillinase can be divided into two major classes:

- p-lactamase or penicillinase, and
- *Penicillin amidase* or *Penicillin acylase*.

Penicillinase reverses the therapeutic potential of penicillins. The activity of the enzyme penicillin amidase is based on a specific attack on the acyl group attached to the basic nucleus, i.e., 6-aminopenicillanic acid [16–18], therefore, it is also called penicillin acylase. Penicillin acylase specifically acts on the enzyme which is more specific to penicillin V and K. p-Lactamase acts specifically on the basic nucleus itself, i.e., by cleaving the β-lactam bond and finally generating penicilloic acid. p-Lactamase is more specific against penicillin G and X, and to a lesser extent against penicillin V [16–18].

As discussed earlier, certain bacteria have the capability to synthesize penicillinase in constitutents, whereas in others it may be inducible. The final effects can be established with the following case. If the antibiotic concentration is found to be non-lethal in a penicillin-treated patient, at that point, it can encourage the formation of penicillinase after which the bacteria becomes resistant to the antibiotic. A similar example is also reported when the penicillinase synthesizing bacteria are greater in number in comparison to the amount of antibiotic present in a certain time period. Under these conditions, although the bacteria lesser numbers are vulnerable to penicillin, they are resistant when present in greater numbers, as the concentration of penicillinase released by each bacterium adds up to an amount which can inactivate the antibiotic. In several clinically resistant strains of bacterium, the synthesis of β-lactamase is regulated by extra-chromosomal genetic elements. There are a number of notable differences between the enzymes synthesized by gram-positive and gram-negative bacteria. Considering molecular weight as a factor of comparison, gram-negative bacterium enzymes are generally small in molecular weight (22 000 Da), whereas gram-positive bacterium enzymes are large in molecular weight (28 000 Da) [19]. The concentration of β-lactamase synthesized by gram-positive bacteria is greater and, since the antibiotic is more specific against gram-positive bacteria than gram-negative bacteria, the enzyme β-lactamase is more sensitive against penicillin when synthesized by gram-positive bacteria. This is because the concentration of enzyme synthesized by gram-negative bacteria is far less and they do not secrete the enzyme into the external environment. This can also be linked in an alternative way, i.e., as there is no β-lactamase secreted into the external environment, there is no dilution (loss) of β-lactamase in gram-negative bacteria, and therefore the need for production of β-lactamase by the cells is quenched.

3.8 Chloramphenicol acetyltransferase

Chloramphenicol has been widely used to treat typhoid fever since 1948 and is the drug of choice in the treatment of typhoid fever and certain infections caused by organisms such as *Haemophilus influenza* [20]. A major typhoid epidemic was first countered by chloramphenicol in Mexico [21]. During this period certain strains of the gram-negative bacterium *Salmonella typhi* came to light. It was later reported that the chloramphenicol resistance facilitated by R-factors in gram-negative bacteria and by transducible plasmids in *S. aureus* is due to the occurrence of the enzyme chloramphenicol acetyltransferase (CAT), which acetylates the hydroxyl groups of the side chain of the chloramphenicol (see figure 3.4) [22].

The product derived from the two-stage inactivation process involving chloramphenicol acetyltransferase is 1,3-dicetoxychloramphenicol (which is inactive) [23]. Chloramphenicol acetyltransferase production in gram-positive bacteria is stimulated by chloramphenicol. Chloramphenicol acts as a protein synthesis inhibitor, thus producing an initial lag period in which the antibiotic prevents protein synthesis with simultaneous induction of chloramphenicol acetyltransferase. Therefore, an initial low amount of chloramphenicol acetyltransferase does not affect the antibiotic, however, at a later phase, it brings down the inhibitory level, i.e., when the amount of chloramphenicol acetyltransferase is high enough to break the drug moiety. As mentioned earlier for penicillinase, there exists a difference between enzymes released by gram-positive bacteria and gram-negative bacteria. However, in this case there is no such substantial difference. The molecular weight of chloramphenicol acetyltransferase produced by both gram-positive and -negative cells is almost the same (80 000 Da).

3.9 Aminoglycoside antibiotic inactivating enzymes

Aminoglycoside antibiotics are also susceptible to inactivation. Different strains of *Streptomyces* have aminoglycoside-modifying enzymes. *Streptomyces kanamyceticus* synthesizes an enzyme that acetylates the 6′-amino group of kanamycin A and B, gentamicin C(1a) and neomycin. *Streptomyces spectabilis* synthesizes an enzyme that acetylates the 2′-amino group of the hexose ring of gentamicin C(1a). These

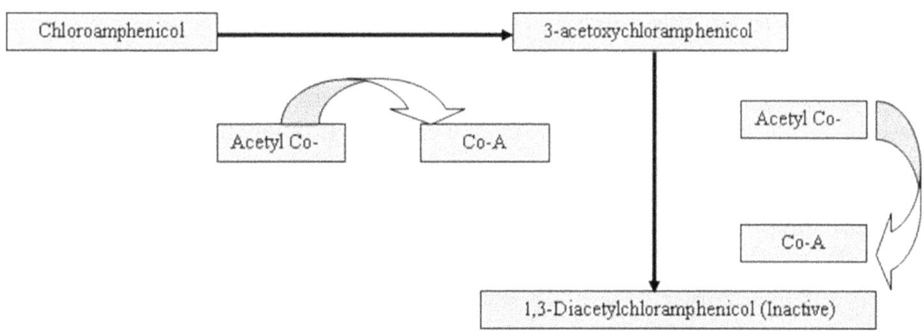

Figure 3.4. The two-stage chloramphenicol inactivation reaction involving chloramphenicol acetyltransferase.

Table 3.4. Different aminoglycoside antibiotic inactivating enzymes.

Enzymes	Substrates (aminoglycoside antibiotics)
Streptomycin/spectinomycin adenyltransferases	Streptomycin, spectinomycin
Streptomycin phosphotransferase	Streptomycin
Lividomycin phosphotransferase	Neomycin, paromomycin
Kanamycin/neomycin phosphotransferases I and II	Kanamycins, neomycins, gentamicin A
Kanamycin acetyltransferase	Kanamycin A and B, neomycin, gentamicin
Gentamicin adenyltransferace	Kanamycins, gentamicins
Gentamicin acetyltransferases I and II	Gentamicin

enzymes catalyze reactions similar to those catalyzed by enzymes present in gram-negative bacteria having R(antibiotic resistance)-factors. The breakthrough of these enzymes proposes the likelihood of an evolutionary relationship between the aminoglycoside inactivating enzymes (synthesized by resistance determinants) in bacteria containing R-factors and similar enzymes found in the actinomycetes [24].

Despite the range of enzymes presenting full or partial resistance to antibiotics, there are only three types of inactivation reactions:

- N-acetylation of susceptible amino groups.
- Adenylation of hydroxyl groups. Phosphorylation of hydroxyl groups. Table 3.4 shows different enzymes that are accountable for the inactivation of aminoglycoside antibiotics.

Acetylation of the drug is performed by the co-factor, acetyl-CoA which serves as the source of the acetyl group, while the source of the phosphoryl and adenyl groups is adenosine triphosphate (ATP). Inactivation occurs in the periplasmic space (periplasm) or on the external surface of the cytoplasmic membrane. Intracellular accumulation of active aminoglycosides is determined by the induction of an energy-dependent process. The modified aminoglycoside is unable to stimulate intracellular accumulation after inactivation of the aminoglycosides by the enzymes. If somehow they succeed in entering a cell, they are incapable of restricting ribosomal function [25].

3.10 Fibrinolytic enzymes

Conversion of fibrinogen to fibrin inside blood vessels leads to thrombosis, resulting in myocardial infarction and other cardiovascular diseases. Generally, there are four therapy options: surgical operation or the intake of antiplatelets, anticoagulants or fibrinolytic enzymes [15]. Microbe-derived fibrinolytic enzymes have been gaining much attention compared to traditional thrombolytic agents because the latter are expensive and have side effects. Fibrinolytic enzymes have been successively derived from various microorganisms, the most significant among which is the genus *Bacillus* [15]. Microbial fibrinolytic enzymes, particularly those from food-grade microorganisms, have the capability to be established as functional food additives and drugs to avert or cure thrombosis and other associated diseases. There are numerous assay methods for these enzymes; this might be due to the insolubility of the substrate, fibrin. Current assay approaches can be categorized into three main groups:

- The first group involves the assay of fibrinolytic activity with natural proteins as substrates, such as fibrin plate methods.
- The second and third groups of assays are appropriate for kinetic investigations and are based on the determination of hydrolysis of synthetic peptide esters.

The fibrinolytic enzyme dissolves intravascular clots due to the action of plasmin (enzyme that digests fibrin) [15]. Plasminogen (the inactive precursor) is converted to plasmin by breakdown of a single peptide bond. For this reason, infusion of two types of enzymes can be considered, those with direct and general proteolytic activity, such as plasmin or trypsin, and those such as the plasminogen activators which increase the level of native plasmin [15]. In this respect, lyokinase plasminogen activators, such as streptokinase urokinase, and tissue plasminogen activators (t-PA) have gained more attention.

3.10.1 Streptokinase

Streptokinase is a proteolytic enzyme (47-kDa protein) derived from the culture of β-hemolytic streptococci of Lancefield group C. It is a potent activator of the fibrinolytic enzyme system in humans [26]. The protein molecule has molecular weight 47 600 Da and an isoelectric point of pH 4.7. The thrombolytic capability of this enzyme catalyzes the transformation of human plasminogen to plasmin by hydrolytic cleavage of the Arg–Val bond. The enzymatic action of streptokinase is based upon a 1:1 noncovalent complex with a zymogen from which the active plasmin is released [26]. This protein complex can be dissociated into two parts, one with plasmin activity and the other with plasminogen activity. Figure 3.5 depicts a positive feedback mechanism, in which complexation first occurs between streptokinase and the plasmin contaminant of plasminogen. This complex is later free to convert a second plasminogen molecule [26].

As mentioned above, streptokinase can be utilized in the management of thromboembolic occlusive vascular disease. The major reasons behind acute arterial occlusion are embolism, thrombosis and trauma. The objective of thrombolytic treatment is to restore blood flow and to preserve life and limb. Antithrombotic therapy during chronic disease is considered to avoid the progression and development of thrombotic occlusion, and also to avoid thrombotic problems after vascular reconstructions. During acute arterial occlusion in the form of embolism or thrombosis, active anticoagulant treatment will avoid the spread of thrombi and also avoid re-occlusion after surgical or interventional procedures to re-establish flow; or, in the case of embolism, may prevent recurrence. In this thrombolytic treatment of occlusive vascular disease, both circulating and intrinsic thrombus plasminogen are activated. This is usually done by forming an activator complex (plasmin, as well as plasminogen, can form an activator complex with streptokinase)

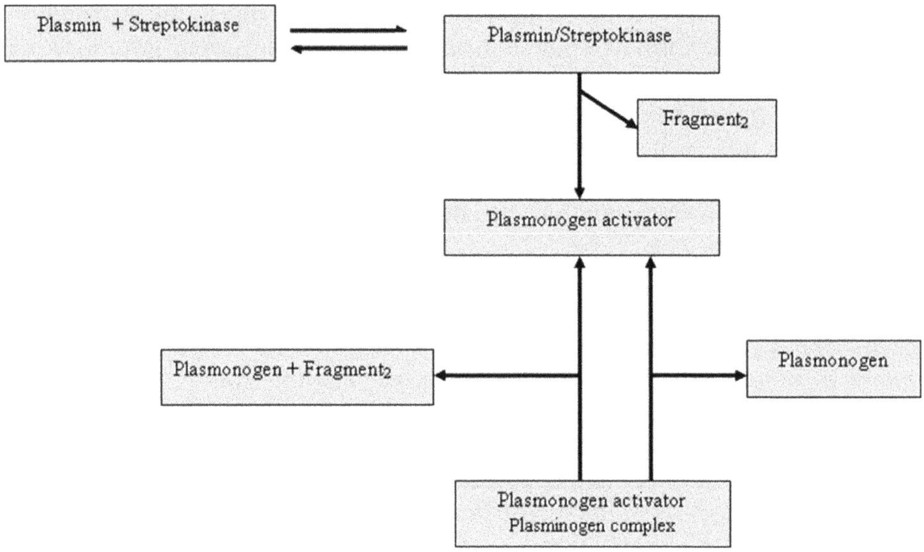

Figure 3.5. Proposed feedback mechanism attributed to streptokinase.

with the plasminogen molecule itself. Simultaneously, streptokinase can also encourage coagulation defects (depending on the dosage used) due to the induction of a hyperplasminaemic state [26]. So far the role of streptokinase therapy in the management of occlusive vascular disease is not clear. However, as per a recent report, streptokinase-based treatment can be utilized in acute massive or major pulmonary embolism, arterial occlusion and in deep-vein thrombosis (iliofemoral) and peripheral venous segments [26]. Based on a recent report it was suggested that zinc chelation (Ca-EDTA) can improve the efficacy of streptokinase in thrombolysis. Thus zinc reduced streptokinase-induced thrombolysis and zinc chelation can promote the effects of streptokinase-induced thrombolysis [27]. It was also observed that PEGylation of truncated streptokinase resulted in a formulation with increased *in vivo* half-life, reduced immune-reactivity and clot-specificity [28]. Additionally, streptokinase has also been employed in the management of chronic arterial occlusions and acute myocardial infarction. Streptokinase can also be utilized in the management of several other diseases associated with thromboembolic occurrences, however, more supporting research is essential before these conditions become definite indications for streptokinase treatment. Streptokinase-based thrombolytic treatment differs significantly with certain conditions. It has been observed that newly formed thrombi can be more easily broken down than old ones. Similarly, venous thrombi can be more easily broken down than arterial thrombi. The action of streptokinase is also dependent on the degree of occlusion and the amount of blood supply in that particular region. Similarly to other thrombolytic agents, streptokinase also faces problems related to bleeding from sites of vascular puncture [26]. Another challenge is the development of antibodies after foreign protein (streptokinase) administration, which limits the course of treatment to 3–5 days. There should be two years between repeated administrations of streptokinase.

Reports have also confirmed its cross reaction with anti-streptococcal antibodies. This may result in the development of resistance against therapy. However, this can be overcome by the administration of booster doses.

Streptokinase is superior in artificially dissolving induced coronary thrombi and pulmonary embolisms. The power of streptokinase over heparin in decreasing mortality in myocardial infection has also been well recognized. A streptokinase–plasminogen complex (antistreplase) in which lys-plasminogen is acylated at its catalytic site, serine is also used for coronary thrombolysis. Under *in vivo* conditions, the acyl group is allowing complex to bind to fibrin before activation, and this change confers some specificity towards clots during the fibrinolytic process. Owing to its bacterial origin, streptokinase is antigenic and may bind to antibodies and nonspecific inhibitors. The immune response presented by streptokinase affects the modification of urokinase.

3.10.2 Urokinase

Urokinase (molecular weight 54 500 Da) is a serine protease comprising 411 amino acid residues, synthesized and isolated from cultured human kidney cells [27]. This enzyme is single polypeptide and very stable against temperatures and extremes of pH [27]. Urokinase efficiently digests blood clots. Human urokinases often act as plasminogen activators by specifically binding to cleave peptide bonds adjacent to lysine and arginine side chains. As it is derived from humans, it is non-immunogenic and its action is very similar to that of trypsin, catalyzing the activation of plasminogen in a first order reaction with cleavage of the Arg–Val bond [27]. The current focus on the management of mortality due to thrombovascular disorders is providing openings for various cardiovascular agents, particularly plasminogen activators, to avoid strokes and heart attacks [27]. Therefore, urokinase, one of the most potent plasminogen activators, is gaining a great deal of attention. Progress in cell lines and bioprocessing technique has made it conceivable to synthesize urokinase from *in vitro* cell cultures. Efforts are now underway to increase urokinase synthesis from cell culture through medium optimization, bioreactor cultivation and advanced purification methods [27].

3.10.3 Tissue plasminogen activator (t-PA)

t-PA (527 amino acid residues) is a protein involved in the breakdown of blood clots. This enzyme belongs to the serine protease class and binds to fibrin via lysine binding sites at its amino terminus, and further activates bound plasminogens several hundred fold more quickly than it activates plasminogen in circulation. In the absence of fibrin it acts as a poor plasminogen activator. Under biological conditions (5–10 ng ml^{-1}), the specificity of t-PA for fibrin restricts the systemic development of plasmin and the introduction of a systemic lytic state. It can successfully break down thrombi during treatment of acute myocardial infarction. t-PA is produced by recombinant DNA technology. Currently it is recommended for coronary thrombolysis. The major side effect is severe hemorrhage. The cost of t-PA is high, several times more than streptokinase per therapeutic dose.

The production of this drug in plants such as cucumber, one of the more common vegetables in the world, could reduce its production costs. In a study it was concluded that the presence of three expressions of regulatory factors (CaMV 35S, Kozak, NOS) and the KDEL signal in the construct caused the increase of t-PA gene expression in cucumber plants [28]. In another study a protease-deficient strain of *Aspergillus niger* was used as a host for the production of human tissue plasminogen activator (t-PA). Production was increased (up to 1.9 mg t-PA (g biomass)(−1)) by the addition of soy peptone to the defined medium [29]. However, the total t-PA (detected by enzyme-linked immunoassay) also eventually disappeared from culture supernatants, confirming significant extracellular proteolytic activity, even though the host strain was protease-deficient [29].

3.11 Biotechnological applications of enzymes

3.11.1 Algae and plant research

As mentioned above, there are various applications of enzymes in different disciplines, however, some of the applications are restricted to plant discipline. Recently, interest related with plant enzymes has augmented considerably. Plants are considered as the main source for secondary metabolites. Plant-based enzymes such as peroxidases are extensively used in medicine as diagnostic tools and in the bioremediation and biobleaching industries, among others. Earlier these enzymes were derived from a natural source, a process that is sometimes difficult and influenced by environmental conditions and low yields. To prevent this obstacle, some inputs have been made to develop plant cell cultures *in vitro* to use the system as a continuous source of plant enzymes.

3.11.2 Immobilization

Different types of carriers and procedures have been implemented in the recent past to improve traditional enzyme immobilization targeted to increase enzyme loading, activity and stability to reduce the enzyme biocatalyst cost at large scale. These include:

- recently nanoparticle-based immobilization of enzymes;
- microwave-assisted immobilization;
- mesoporous supports;
- cross-linked enzyme aggregates;
- click chemistry technology.

In nanotechnology method, mixture of the specific physical, chemical, optical and electrical properties of nanoparticles, especially catalytic properties of biomolecules, has resulted in the appearance of countless novel biotechnological applications. Nanoparticles offer high surface-to-volume ratio resulting in an increase in the concentration of the immobilized entity that is considerably higher than that afforded by experimental protocols based on immobilization on planar 2D surfaces. Enzymes immobilized on nanoparticles presented a broader working pH and temperature range and higher thermal stability than the native enzymes. In contrast with traditional procedures, nanoparticle-based immobilization served three important features:

- nano-enzyme particles are easy to synthesize in high solid content without using surfactants and toxic reagents;
- homogeneous and well-defined core–shell nanoparticles with a thick enzyme shell can be obtained;
- particle size can be conveniently changed within utility limits. Moreover, with the growing attention paid to cascade enzymatic reaction and *in vitro* synthetic biology, it is possible that co-immobilization of multi-enzymes could be achieved on these nanoparticles.

3.12 Industrial enzymes

3.12.1 Glucoamylase

Theoretically, glucoamylase (GA) can convert 100% of the starch in your diet into glucose. As the chain length of the dextrin substrate gets shorter, the reaction rate drops. To produce mostly maltose and isomaltose, GA can catalyze a reversal of the typical hydrolysis reaction [30]. High quantities of sugars (up to 40%) can occur in industrial processes, and these conditions favor some maltose production. The saccharification of starch, brewing, and distilling are just a few examples of how GA is used in the food and fermentation sectors. The production of glucose, fructose syrups, and other sweeteners relies heavily on fungal GA [31]. It is common practice in the food business to use an enzymatic technique to create high-glucose syrups, and glucose may also play a crucial role as a substrate in fermentative processes that generate by-products like ethanol, amino acids, and organic acids. Bread's texture and appearance can be enhanced by using GA because of its decrease in the dough's viscosity. In addition, researchers discovered use in manufacturing pharmaceutically active gastrointestinal supplements [32]. The glucoamylase catalytic domain (CD) of *A. niger* is shown in figure 3.6.

3.12.1.1 Classification of GA

When it comes to converting starch and pertaining to dextrin's into glucose, Fleming in 1968 classified GA into two groups: those that turn 80% of the starches and 40% of the restrict dextrin's into glucose, and those that convert just 80% of the starch. However, both classes can convert panose and α-limit dextrins to glucose without intermediate products. The rate of hydrolysis by the GA is determined by the substrate's molecular size, structure, bond position, and bond type. Substrate pretreatment increases the hydrolysis rate and enhances product recovery. Amylopectin, starch, amylose, maltodextrins, dextrin, malt sugar, isomaltose, dextrin, panosian, oligo, di, and polysaccharides, etc, are all substrates for the enzyme [33].

3.12.1.2 Sources

All living things, from plants to mammals, bacteria, fungi, and yeasts, produce GA. The fungi *Aspergillus*, *Rhizopus*, and *Endomyces* species are responsible for most GA

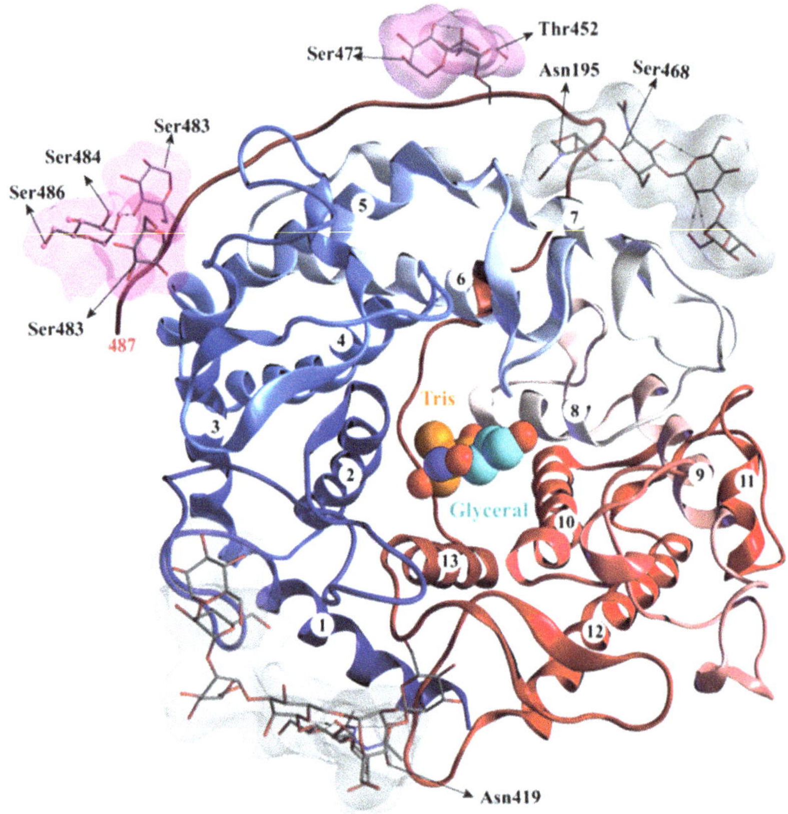

Figure 3.6. Structure of glucoamylase. The catalytic domain (CD) of *Aspergillus niger* GA (blue) to 487 (red) residues. 13 α-helices, indicated as cartoon, are counted from N-terminus. The active-site-bound Tris (orange) and glycerol (cyan) are highlighted.

production, this process is typically extracellular, and the enzyme could be retrieved from culturing remains [34]. GA derived from *Aspergillus awamori* or *A. niger* is widely used in manufacturing. In addition to *Rhizopus*, *R. oryzae*, *R. niveus*, *R. Delmar*, and *R. javanicus*, several other *Rhizopus* species, are significant GA producers. Some *Penicillium* species are also known to generate GA. In addition to pigment, *Monascus* species can also generate GA. *T. viride* and a few other *Trichoderma* species have also been reported to produce GA. GA has also been traced back to several thermophilic fungi [35]. *Thermomyces lanuginosus*, *Scytalidium thermophilum*, and Thermomucor 05 °C for 5–10 min, followed by 95 °C for 2 h. GA then sacrifice starch at a pH of 6.0 and 60 °C. If maltose is desired as a by-product, only then will amylase be utilized in the saccharification process. To increase the ratio of dextrose to maltose, pullulanase must be used. The benefits of amylases have led to their replacement of acid hydrolysis of starch. *Stamfordii*, *Humicola grisea*, *Talaromyces flavus*, and *Streptosporangium* spp. [30, 36], *Flavobacterium* species, *Bacillus stearothermophillus*, *Halobacterium sodamense*, *Sclerotinia sclerotiorum*, *Lactobacillus-amylovorus*, and *Sclerotium-rolfsii* are some of the aerobic bacteria that are known to create GA. Other known producers of GA include *Sclerotinia sclerotiorum. Clostridium thermosaccharolyticum* and *Clostridium thermohydrosulfuricum*, two anaerobic bacteria, have also been implicated as GA producers [30]. GA has been traced back to various yeast species, including *Candida antarctica, Saccharomyces's fibuligera, Pichia sub-pelliculosa*, and *Saccharomyces diasticus* [37].

3.12.1.3 Production of GA

Submerged fermentation (SmF) has been the standard industrial method for producing GA for many years; however, solid-state fermentation (SSF) has recently been seen as a viable alternative. By-products encompass several substances such as wheat bran, rice bran, rice husk, gram flour, flour, tea waste, wheat, corn flour, and copra waste, among others [38]. Fragment size, humidity content, and liquid endeavor of the substrate are significant determinants in enzyme synthesis in SSF. Due to the significance of the plane zone on hydrolysis/growing rates, the substrate's atom dimension significantly impacts the development rate and enzyme-generating action of the organisms [39]. The ability of oxygen to fill empty space is influenced by the dimension of the particles. For substrates like wheat bran particles between 425 and 500 μm in size, dissolution improves with decreasing particle size because smaller particles give greater surface area. [40]. GA activity was minimized on surfaces with particles between 1.4 and 180 μm in size. Therefore, a trade-off must be made when deciding on an appropriate particle size to improve mass transfer. The efficient transport of both water and solutes along the cellular membrane is highly contingent upon water-related activity present in the surrounding environment. Greater GA yields were seen at higher initial substrate water activity values [41]. The moisture content of the substrate used in SSF for GA production varies from about 50%–70% for starchy substrates (based on the chemical makeup of the substrate for carbohydrates, cellulose, and so forth) to higher values (depending on the temperature used in the process). Adding a carbon source (easily accessible source) to the substrates can sometimes boost culture activity [42]. It could be polymeric polymers like starch or simple sugars like glucose, maltose, sucrose, etc. For instance, adding com starch to a wheat bran medium usually results in increased GA synthesis by fungal culture. Similarly, increasing GA yields in SSF has been achieved through the successful application of substrate supplementation with exogenous nitrogen sources (of either organic or inorganic form). A wide array of biological compounds, spanning from basic ammonia or nitrates salt to the urea as well as intricate substances such as steep liquid, can be employed as a source of nitrogen. The latter method has been extensively employed in sustainable seafood farming for genetic improvement and increased production of genetically advanced individuals [30]. *Aspergillus* sp. and *A. niger* produce more GA in SSF when the substrate, such as wheat bran, is supplemented with fructose, ammonium sulfate, urea, and yeast extract. Using urea instead of ammonium sulfate resulted in a 100% increase in GA production by *A. awamori*, however, using C/P ratios between 5.1 and 28.7 did not affect GA production. The efficiency and impact of bioreactor construction on the SSF processing of GA has been evaluated using the laboratory large-scale biological reactors such as Erlenmeyer flasks, Erlenmeyer trays, roux bottles, and the glass columns. [43]. The *A. niger* enzyme synthesis was shown to be quicker in trays (36 h) than in flasks (96 h). As was previously indicated, SmF has historically been employed in GA manufacturing. The nutritional needs of SmF are typically more nuanced than those of SSF. The formation of GA is profoundly affected by the nature of the media used. The fermentation process requires a continual supply of oxygen and a pH of –4.5, with starch as the carbon source [44]. High concentrations of GA were generated by *Rhizopus* sp. A-11 in a liquor medium with added zinc and calcium. The type of nitrogen and carbon sources, as well as the pH of the medium and salts like K2HPO4 and KH2PO4, had a significant impact on GA synthesis by *Thermomyces lanuginosus*. Cultures of *Streptosporangium* sp. on starch-czapek medium yielded a thermostable glucoamylase. pH 4.5 and 70 °C were optimal for glucoamylase activity. To distinguish between the definite growing rate and the GA production rate, Ricci Queiroz investigated GA making through A [45] Awamori to develop the rheological parameter uniformity index (*K*) from the Power law. The presence of oxygen is crucial during the synthesis of GA. The kinetic properties of a fungal culture play a vital role in formulating a fermentation medium for the industrial-scale synthesis of GA. The environmental conditions, including temperature, oxygen levels, pH, and other factors, can significantly influence the kinetic parameters of a fungal growth. The GA indicator and feed rate control were derived from the specific glucose consumption rate. A feeding regimen for the cultivation was devised utilizing the statistical regression model. The organism's growth rate exhibited a 34% increase when compared to the outcomes achieved under conditions of a consistent feeding rate [46].

3.12.1.4 Genetic engineering of GA

Using recombinant DNA technology and genetic engineering has significantly enhanced the production of innovative gene products. Now, gene modification is the predominant approach utilized to produce microbial enzymes with notable commercial importance [47]. Various genetic engineering strategies have been utilized to enhance the production of the GA-generating strain, attain thermodynamic stability of GA, and enhance selectivity in glucose production, among other aims. Considerable research has been undertaken about the methodology of site-directed mutagenesis, which involves the intentional modification of specific amino acid residues [48]. The combination of beneficial genetic changes has led to a notable decrease, around 50%, in the enzyme's ability to produce isomaltose. Isomaltose is a key secondary product in the glucose production process facilitated by the enzyme GA. Furthermore, incorporating these mutations has significantly augmented the enzyme's thermodynamic stability, resulting in a remarkable increase of several orders of magnitude [49]. Moreover, there has been a significant increase of 15% in enzyme activity. In addition, investigations using mutational analyses have improved the catalytic efficiencies of the hydrolysis of maltose compared to the hydrolysis of isomaltose. Reilly conducted a study on the improvements in genetic algorithms achieved through protein engineering, focusing on the role of heterologous gene expression in these advancements [50]. The complementary DNA (cDNA) of *R. oryzae* GA was inserted into the area downstream of the alcohol oxidase (AOD 1) promoter obtained from *Candida boidinii*. The transformant *C. boidinii*'s gibberellic acid was purified and analyzed next to the enzyme made by *S. cerevisiae*. It was discovered that the enzyme that *C. boidinii* generated had a larger molecular size than the enzyme produced by *S. cerevisiae*. The reason for this change in molecular weight was that the proteins that were made had different N-linked glycosylated sugar structures [51]. The study also showed how a hybrid yeast strain was created that can make both GA and isoamylase enzymes. The achievement of this conclusion was realized by the effective integration of the (*Pseudomonas amylodermosa*) gene into a chromosome of the integrant G23-8. The recombinant yeast reached a utilization rate of 95% for soluble starch. The employment of both growth rate independent and dependent promoters can exemplify the phenomenon of boosting the production of recombinant proteins is carried out in fed-batch growing platforms. [52]. The point was successfully shown by using *Fusarium venanatin* JeRS 325, a strain exhibiting transgenic GA expression according to the control of an expansion rate distinct promoter. The strain was transformed by utilizing a plasmid that carried the *A. niger* GA gene. This gene's expression was controlled by its promoter, which was linked to the strain's growth rate [53]. When grown in fed-batch cultures, the double transformant produced an amount of GA comparable to that produced by the JeRS 325 strain. Recombinant yeast, namely *S. cerevisiae* SR93, was bred and tested for its ability to produce GA. The over-expression of the GA gene can be traced back to the disruption of the MAT locus, which caused a repressor protein to be produced [54]. As a result, there was a 1.6-fold spike in GA activity per cellular concentration. The specific growth rate and rate of GA synthesis were found to be significantly greater in comparison to *S. cerevisiae* SR93. The gene responsible for producing a thermally stable GA (glycosyl hydrolase) derived from *Talaromyces emersonii* was successfully cloned and then expressed heterologously in the organism *A. niger* [55]. The gene under investigation in this study encodes a protein consisting of six to eight amino acids, resulting in a predicted molecular weight of 62 827 Da. *T. emersonii* GA is classified within the glucoside hydrolase family 15, with a sequence similarity of around 60% to the GA enzyme found in *A. niger* [56]. The enzyme under investigation exhibits significant specificity towards maltose, isomaltose, and maltoheptaose, with a kcat value that is 3–6 times higher than that of the GA enzyme derived from *A. niger*. The thermosensitivity of *T. emersonii* GA was greatly enhanced, exhibiting a half-life of 48 h at 65 °C in a 30% (w/v) glucose solution [57]. In comparison, GA derived from *A. niger* had a half-life of just 10 h under the same conditions. The expression of the catalytical domain (GAc) of *A. awamori* GA was reported in *Pichia pastoris*, resulting in the production of GAc at a concentration of 0.4 g per liter of medium. In an independent inquiry, the investigators analyzed the consequences of upregulating and releasing a comparable prototype glycoprotein, GA the 'GAM-1' [58]. This study investigates glycosylation patterns in *A. niger*, comparing a wild-type parent strain with a single gene copy to transformants with numerous gene copies. The strain of *A. niger* that was overexpressed exhibited an increased number of copies

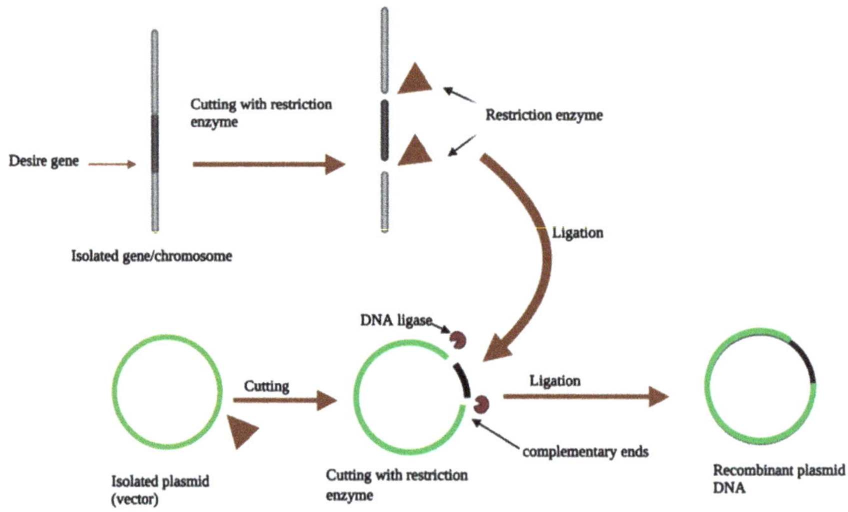

Figure 3.7. Overview of recombinant DNA technology: restriction enzyme-mediated gene splicing and plasmid vector insertion.

(20 and 80) of the glaA (GAM-1) gene, resulting in the secretion of a protein at levels 5–10 times higher than the normal strain [59] (figure 3.7).

3.12.2 Cellulases

The yearly production of biomass in terrestrial and marine ecosystems on Earth is estimated to be around 1.9×11^{13} tons. Approximately 60% of the biomass consists of lignocellulose, the primary structural component of plant cell walls. Approximately 30%–60% of the composition of lignocellulose consists of cellulose. Lignocellulose, specifically cellulose, represents a consistent and renewable reservoir of power and feed stocks for many chemicals [60]. Cellulose is a structured arrangement of lined ~-1,4-D glucan chain up, while hemicelluloses encompass a diverse range of substances, including xylenes, xyloglucans, arabinoxylans, and mannans. These compounds form complicated branching structures with various substituents near their backbone, such as acetyl ester. Hemicelluloses primarily establish hydrogen bonds with cellulose and other hemicelluloses, stabilizing the cell wall matrix and providing the cell wall with insolubility in aqueous conditions [61]. Hemicelluloses are found in plants. Cellulose comprises elongated, non-branching glucose polymers that are densely arranged in a manner that gives rise to exceedingly insoluble crystalline structures. Cellulolytic organisms with high enzymatic activity, such as *Trichoderma*, can produce intricate combinations of essential enzymes for effectively breaking down the substrate. The enzyme Endo and Exo glucanase and cellobiohydrolases (CBH) are the main components of *T. reesei*'s extrinsic enzyme framework, which also includes β-glucosidases and cellob [62]. Endoglucanases exhibit specificity in hydrolyzing the internal 1,4-glycosidic linkages in celluloses that are amorphous, swollen, and substituted. This enzymatic activity results in the liberation of glucose, cellobiose, and cello-oligosaccharides. Endoglucanases facilitate the generation of additional chain ends for CBH by inducing random cleavage inside the central region of long cellulose chains. In contrast to CBH, endoglucanases possess the ability to hydrolyze substituted celluloses, including carboxymethylcellulose (CMC) and hydroxyethyl cellulose (HEC). The exoglycanases, also known as CBH, are enzymes that catalyze the cleavage of cellobiose units from the terminals of polysaccharide chains. These enzymes are known to possess significant activity on crystalline cellulose. On the other hand, glucosidases are responsible for cleaving cellobiose and other soluble oligosaccharides into glucose [63]. This step is crucial as cellobiose has been observed to hinder the effectiveness of various cellulase components. In natural environments, organic matter containing lignocellulose undergoes various physio-chemical and biological degradation processes, producing simpler molecules. In animals, this lignocellulosic material is metabolized as a primary nutrient in symbiotic relationships with microorganisms, such as those seen in ruminants and termites. The lignocellulolytic enzyme complex serves as the agent for this bioconversion process. The primary constituents of the lignocellulolytic enzyme complexes consist of cellulases, hemicelluloses, pectinases, and other enzymes involved in lignin degradation [64]. These enzymes engage in a symbiotic connection during plant cell wall disintegration. Cellulases, a category of enzymes that catalyze the hydrolysis of cellulose, have significant industrial importance. Considerable focus has been directed towards the production and characteristics of cellulases due to the significant role of cellulose as a primary structural element in textiles, paper, and building materials, as well as its importance as a primary food for ruminant animals. The degradation of cotton textiles utilized by the US Army during tropical warfare in World War II was a significant catalyst for advancing cellulase research. During the period spanning from 1950 to 2000, extensive research efforts were dedicated to the description and characterization of the cellulase system [65]. The most efficient microorganisms with high production capabilities have been identified and subjected to genetic enhancements. The industrial-scale generation of cellulase by SmF has been successfully achieved. Currently, cellulase preparations are mostly targeted towards specialized markets characterized by low volume and high value. These industries include food administration, fabric management, and washing cleaners, which can accommodate the recent elevated cost of cellulase enzymes. Cellulases find application in the food industry to extract and/or clarify fruit and vegetable juices, treat wines, extract oils, and enhance the quality of baked products. Cellulase is employed within the textile industry for bio-stoning and/or fading denim, as well as for the polishing of cellulosic fabric. Cellulases have the potential to be utilized in the recycling of wastepaper within the pulp and paper sector [66]. The increasing demand for sources of renewable energy and the imperative for responsible resource management has prompted a significant emphasis on cellulase development and manufacturing within the realm of agricultural and biotechnological usage. This research primarily aims to convert lingo-cellulose into solvable sugar, which can be further treated as biofuel or other biological and chemical products. The primary objective of the industrial processing strategy for lignocellulose is the process through which cellulose, hemicellulose, and pectin are converted into reducing sugars by bioconversion. The aforementioned procedure might potentially provide lignin as an additional item or need the improving delignification of the feed stock prior to biological conversion. Consequently, the key enzymes implicated in the process of bioconversion encompass cellulases, hemicelluloses, and pectinases. Cellulase stands out as the most prominent enzyme among the group of enzymes [67].

Cellulases and related enzymes have significant agro-biotechnological implications, particularly in the context of animal feed supplements. These enzymes play a crucial role in enhancing the digestibility of lignocellulosic feed materials. The use of agro-biotechnological applications necessitates the availability of more precise, focused, specific targets that are more cost-effective than the enzymes presently accessible [68]. Cellulases, hemicelluloses, and pectinases collectively constitute around 20% of the global enzyme market. The phenomenon is expected to exhibit substantial growth because of the heightened utilization of agrobiotechnology solutions. Extensive reviews have been conducted in the past on cellular research and production. This chapter focuses on current endeavors in economic cellulase production, particularly evaluating submerged and solid-substrate fermentation technologies. Additionally, the chapter explores the latest developments in developing highly efficient microbial strains for specific applications [69].

3.12.2.1 Sources

Numerous species, both marine and terrestrial, produce cellulases in their native habitats. Commercial cellulase production relies primarily on filamentous fungi found in various habitats, including soil, plants, and the ocean. Some microorganisms can potentially act as important sources for the production of cellulase on a large scale [70]. Biochemical and enzyme studies of cellulases have historically focused primarily on aerobic mesophilic fungi. Included in this group of molds were *Trichoderma viride*, *Sporotrichum pulverulentum*, *Trichoderma reesei*, *Penicillium pinophilum*, *Trichoderma koningii*, *Fusarium solani*, *Penicillium funiculosum*, and *Aspergillus niger* [71].

Over the last 20 years, there has been an increasing acknowledgment of diverse microorganisms that can synthesize cellulase and hemicellulase enzymes. The microorganisms in question include thermophilic fungi, including *Humicola insolens*, *Chaetomium thermophilum*, *Talaromyces emersonii*, *Sporotrichum thermophile*, and *Thermoascus aurantiacus*. Furthermore, it has been observed that certain types of anaerobic fungi, specifically *N. patriciarum*, *Orpinomyces* sp., *Neocallimastix frontalis*, and *Sphaeromonas communis*, as well as aerobic bacteria of both mesophilic and thermophilic nature, such as *Bacillus* spp., *Cellulomonas fimi*, *Cellvibrio* sp., and *Pseudomonas fluorescens* subsp. cellulosa exhibit the presence of these enzymatic systems [72]. Furthermore, mesophilic and thermophilic anaerobic bacteria, including *Fibrobacter succinogenes*, *R. flavefaciens* Bacteroides cellulosomes, *Clostridium thermocellum*, *Ruminococcus albus*, and *Clostridium stercorarium*, have been identified as cellulase and hemicellulase producers. Lastly, actinomycetes such as *Microbispora bispora*, *Streptomyces flavogriseus*, and *Thermomonospora fusca* have also been observed to exhibit highly active cellulase and hemicellulase systems. Furthermore, it is worth noting that hyperthermophilic microbes, like *T. neapolitana*, *Thermotoga maritema*, *Pyrococcus furiosus*, and *Anaerocellum thermophilum* microbial organisms that exhibit optimal growth within the temperature range of 85 °C to 110 °C can synthesize cellulases and hemicelluloses with improved stability [73]. Typically, cellulases demonstrate comparatively reduced specific activity, frequently exhibiting a minimum of a 100-fold decrease compared to amylases. The goal of the research study was to find wild types that are more productive. After that, strain mutation was used to boost the specific activity of enzymes and speed up the catalytic cycle rate at the active site. The first modification program was done at the US Army Natick Laboratories using the wild strain *Trichoderma reesei*. In the early 1970s, the mutant QM 9414 was effectively isolated [74]. A research study was undertaken to isolate indigenous strains that exhibit enhanced productivity. Following this, the introduction of strain mutation has been employed to enhance the activity of enzymes and elevate the catalytic turnover rate at the active site. The mutation experiment was carried out at the US Army Natick Laboratory Services via the natural strain of *Trichoderma reesei* 'QM 6a,' formerly known as *T. viride* QM 6a. During this study, a mutant designated as QM 9414 was successfully identified in the early 1970s. The use of UV light and nitrosoguanidine resulted in mutagenesis [75]. Numerous *T. reesei* mutants, such as Rut NG-14, that can produce cellulase despite considerable catabolite suppression, have been identified and isolated using this method. The cellulolytic enzyme activity of the mutant strain NG-14 was about three times greater than that of the wild-type strain *T. reesei* QM 6a. After exposure to ultraviolet (UV) radiation, the strain *T. reesei* Rut NG-14 was isolated, leading to the discovery of a new strain known as *T. reesei* Rut C30. The cellulase production level of the mutant strain Rut C30 exhibited a significant increase, about 4–5 times greater, compared to the wild-type parent strain QM 6a. Several other labs, including Cetus Corporation, VTT in Finland, and a French laboratory, used the same procedures to identify other highly cellulolytic *T. reesei* mutants [71]. The plate clearance technique has since been successfully employed in isolating cellulase-producing mutants from *Penicillium pinophilum*, *P. occitanis*, and *P. purpurogenum*. While the mutant strains of *T. reesei* have shown an enhancement in the quantity of released protein, the relative distribution of cellulase components has exhibited no variation compared to the original strains [76]. Therefore, screening several mutant colonies on plates has shown to be impractical for developing customized enzyme mixes for diverse biotechnological applications. Genetically engineered *T. reesei* strains, capable of producing modified combinations of cellulases, have been developed since the late 1980s. Novel strains have been developed by employing cloned *T. reesei* genes and their corresponding promoters, resulting in cellulase profiles that differ significantly from the original strains [77]. These modified strains exhibit the absence of one or more cellulase components. Additionally, the expression of fungal cellulase genes can be regulated by the *T. reesei* promoter. These strategies facilitate the large-scale manufacture of a certain cellulase component, often endoglucanase, while minimizing the presence of other components with substantial activity. Mono-component enzymes exhibit a higher degree of selectivity in their actions, making them particularly suitable for application in specialized domains such as bio-stoning and fading of denim fabric (often found in blue jeans) and laundry detergents [78]. Current endeavors are being made to acquire cellulase-generating mutants and/or recombinants that exhibit enhanced efficiency. To achieve these objectives, the United States Department of Energy (DOE) has provided money to two prominent manufacturers specializing in enzymes. In the year 2000, Genencor International received a grant of USD 17.1 million from the National Renewable Energy Laboratory, located in Golden, Colorado, and operated by the DOE. The purpose of this funding was to support Genesco International's efforts in developing cost-effective cellulases and other enzymes that can be utilized to synthesize ethanol from biomass [79]. The aim of this study is to investigate and create enzyme systems that have the potential to significantly improve the cost-effectiveness of decomposing cellulosic material and other complex carbohydrates into fermentable sugars, with a target enhancement of tenfold. The DOE has provided money for USD 14.8 million to Novozymes Inc. over three years from 2001 to 2003. This financial support was allocated to facilitate the development of cellulase enzymes that are more economically viable for manufacturing bioethanol. Currently, the expenditure associated with the enzyme totals USD 0.50 for every gallon of ethanol generated [80].

3.12.2.2 Production

Multiple businesses industrially manufacture cellulases using SmF methodology. The selection of production technology is contingent upon the intended application of the cellulase preparation [81]. In specific applications within the textile industry, pulp and paper industry, and specific sectors of the food business, there is a requirement for cellulases that have been partially or extensively purified or particular components of the cellulase enzyme complex. A crude enzyme complex comprising cellulases, hemicelluloses, and pectinases may be deemed appropriate for agro-biotechnological purposes. Ongoing endeavors are being made to decrease production costs due to the comparatively elevated expenses associated with cellulases. The existing hyper-cellulolytic fungal mutants utilized for cellulase production through SmF exhibit much lower yields than antibiotics or other high-quality biochemical compounds [82]. The exorbitant cost associated with commercial cellulases poses a significant barrier for the majority of agrobiotechnology applications, hence rendering them commercially unviable. The potential reduction in application costs can be achieved by implementing on-site or *in situ* production methods. The aforementioned techniques encompass the inclusion of substrate residue in the enzymatic production process, wherein it is utilized in the synthesis of end products like feed additives or the saccharification of pretreated lignocellulose for the purpose of bio-alcohol production. [83].

3.13 The role of enzymes in the synthesis of functional foods

Considerable investigation has examined the utilization of enzymes in bioprocessing to produce components and functional foods. The phenomenon can be principally ascribed to the enzymes' capacity to augment the occurrence of bioactive chemicals in food, promote solubility and stability, and mitigate specific unfavorable

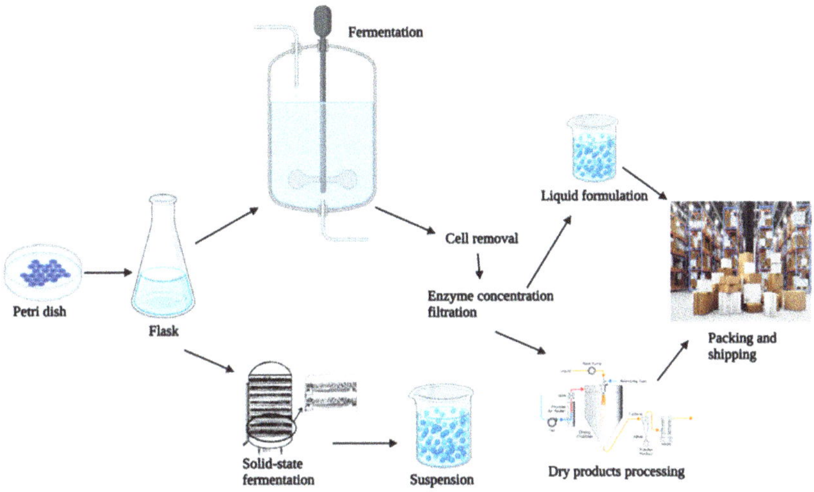

Figure 3.8. Biotechnological production pipeline: from culture initiation to fermentation and final product formulation.

nutritional characteristics in food items [84]. Using commercial enzymes from various sources, scientists have created procedures for microbial fermentation and enzymatic breakdown or conversion to create functional foods. A fermentation pipeline was described in figure 3.8. These functional foods provide one or more beneficial benefits to one's health. Enzymes, including the peptidases tannases, lipases, L-asparaginase, carbohydrate modifying enzymes, and phytases, are vital components in producing functional meals [85].

3.13.1 Lipases

Hydrolases, of which lipases are members, catalyze the hydrolysis of triacylglycerols (TAGs) into glycerol and fatty acids (FAs). Lipases are a class of enzyme catalysts that play crucial roles in the biochemical process of lipid metabolism [86]. Triacylglycerol (TAG) hydrolases are a class of enzymes that can catalyze the hydrolysis of triacylglycerol molecules. Biocatalysts, like enzymes, have been used increasingly in the last few decades to help make esters, polyunsaturated fatty acids (PUFAs), and long-chain FAs. In these processes, enzymes are used more often because they can be used in many ways. The functional classification of meals formulated from lipases is attributed to the diverse qualities of oils and fats because of their enzymatic action. The sources of this enzyme exhibit significant variability, encompassing a wide range of species such as plants, animals, fungi, and bacteria [87]. Microbial-derived lipases are favored due to their cost-effectiveness in procurement, genetic manipulability, straightforward isolation and production processes, and various biochemical functionalities. In contrast, previous studies have demonstrated that enzymes produced from plants and animals have comparatively lower stability when compared to their counterparts. This proposal introduces a possible replacement approach and has been utilized for the production of enzymes using biologic procedures that are financially and energy viable [88]. Nevertheless, a significant hurdle that persists is the disparity in the number and quality of molecules that can be extracted compared to alternative technologies. Lipases are frequently employed in food processing to enhance and formulate various dairy products and derivatives, including cheeses. They are also utilized in bakery products, the processing of fats and oils to produce modified acylglycerols, and in the fruit juice business. Lipase is employed in the dairy industry to alter the lengths of FA chains, augmenting the flavor of cheeses by the hydrolysis of milk fat. Furthermore, this technique can be utilized to expedite the aging process of cheese and impart distinct flavors primarily to varieties of soft cheeses. The functional characteristics of lipases have contributed to their widespread use in various industrial applications, particularly in the food industry, as well as in the creation of pharmaceuticals and cosmetics, among other commercial products. The multifunctionality and potential applications of these enzymes constitute compelling reasons to advance further cutting-edge technologies that facilitate the generation and utilization of lipases as a valuable resource for ingredient sourcing and the development of functional food products [89].

3.13.2 Proteases

Proteases are a diverse group of enzymes that are capable of the ability to catalyze the hydrolysis of bonds made up of peptides. The categorization of enzymes is contingent upon several variables, encompassing the characteristics and chemical qualities of the active site, the specific process in which the molecule functions as a catalyst, and the development of a protease shape along with its associated relationships [90]. An alternative and captivating classification may be derived by analyzing the active site of the molecule, resulting in the categorization of several types, such as cysteine, serine, aspartic, asparagine peptide lyases, threonine, glutamic, and metalloproteases. Proteases can be derived from several sources, including plants, animals, and microbes, and exhibit considerable potential in functional food manufacturing. Proteases have been employed in food to facilitate protein modification, enhance flavor profiles, extend the shelf life of protein sources, optimize digestibility, and reduce allergenic potential [91]. Protease is employed in several food production processes, such as manufacturing cheese, bread goods, hydrolyzed soybeans, and meat tenderization. The generation of proteases by microbes and their application in the food industry have been extensively studied. One instance that exemplifies this phenomenon is the Flavoenzyme enzyme, which is synthesized by specifically chosen strains of *Aspergillus oryzae*. The utilization of this enzyme, in conjunction with Protamex, serves the purpose of transforming meat by-products into a broth imbued with flesh-like flavor [92]. This broth is subsequently incorporated into meat processing procedures, diminishing the salt required in the ultimate products. Neutrase is employed in the context of drinks to ensure consistent yeast proliferation, leading to enhanced beer performance and quality. However, it is crucial to do a safety evaluation of the generating strain when considering enzymes derived from microbes. In addition to meeting safety requirements for consumer health, the microbe resulting from the enzyme must be the intended product. The Joint FAO/WHO Experts Committee on Food Additives (JECFA) is recognized as one of the entities within the regulatory framework that offers certification. Certain plant-derived enzymes, such as papain, have acquired significant commercial significance due to their exceptional performance under diverse operational circumstances. Furthermore, these enzymes have demonstrated noteworthy proteolytic activity against various protein substrates [93]. One illustration of this phenomenon is the utilization of papain as a substitute in the process of cheese production since it has demonstrated efficacy in developing semisoft and creamy cheese varieties. Nevertheless, it is crucial to consider that the coagulation rate of this enzyme exhibits variability when employed with various milk variants [94].

3.13.3 Carbohydrate-modifying enzyme

Carbohydrates refer to a class of enzymes that play a crucial role in catalyzing the breakdown of carbohydrates. Enzymes, including amylases, indulines, galactosidases, glucosidases, pectinases, glucosyltransferases, and fructosyltransferases, play a significant role in the food industry by producing advantageous biological substances that contribute to the development or enhancement of functional foods [95]. Extensive research has been conducted on lactic acid bacteria due to its advantageous characteristics in promoting human health. One illustrative instance is the b-galactosidase enzyme, which is notable for its utilization in the dairy sector due to its ability to enhance the breakdown of lactose, thereby ameliorating the manifestations seen by lactose-intolerant individuals. The utilization of b-galactosidase has been employed in the manufacturing and retrieval of galacto-oligosaccharides (GOSs). The intake of GOS has been associated with immunomodulatory effects because of its direct interaction with immune cells, enhancing the abundance of beneficial bacteria. The utilization of microorganisms as a source for enzymes with carbohydrate activity offers a cost-effective alternative and a more sustainable technique from an environmental standpoint [96]. The utilization of *Lactobacillus paracasei* BGP1 in the fermentation process of GOS derived from diverse plant species has demonstrated promise as a viable substitute for generating valuable prebiotic components in the formulation of functional food products. An illustration of functional foods can be observed in developing beverage prototypes fortified with GOS and possessing antibacterial qualities. These prototypes are created through fermentation involving lactic acid bacteria and apple by-products. The findings indicate a favorable level of acceptability in the end product and the proposition of novel beverage prototypes that possess prebiotic and antibacterial properties. The utilization of sustainable materials in the development of food packaging, which serves the dual purpose of preserving food and minimizing environmental impact, has garnered significant attention and widespread adoption. This study focused on investigating the production of edible prebiotic films using whey protein that was enhanced with GOS and XOSs. The objective was to develop semipermeable packaging materials that could be used for coating fresh fruits and vegetables and bakery foods. This hypothesis elucidates the extensive research that pertains to the development and enhancement of functional foods through the utilization of enzymes derived from various biotechnological sources. Glycosaminoglycans (GAGs) and xyloglucans (XGs) constitute a significant proportion of the oligosaccharides that are widely present [97]. Cross-linked oligosaccharides (XOSs) hold significant importance in commercial oligosaccharide development. The enzymatic synthesis of these compounds is exceptionally viable as it effectively reduces the occurrence of undesired reactions and the formation of secondary products during enzymatic hydrolysis. *Xylo oligosaccharides* (XOSs) can be found in various natural sources, including fruit, vegetables, honey, and milk. Furthermore, many agro-industrial by-products, such as wheat oat bran, rice straw, wheat, and maize, have the potential to serve as abundant sources for the synthesis of *X. oligosaccharides* (XOSs). Utilizing *X. oligosaccharides* in the improvement of efficient foods enhances the presence of functional and nutritional components within traditional food products. One instance of this phenomenon can be observed using symbiotic soy milk supplemented with *X. oligosaccharides* and an inoculum of *Weissella cibaria* FB069. This specific formulation has been developed to investigate its impact on the spread of malignant cells within the colon in comparison to alternative agitated soybean stuffs [98].

3.13.4 Tannase

Like other enzymes, tannase exhibits a broad distribution across several ecosystems, encompassing plants, animals, and microbes. The mechanism by which it operates involves the cleavage of ester and depside linkages present in hydrolyzable tannins, resulting in the liberation of glucose and gallic acid. Consequently, tannase significantly contributes to the production of gallic acid [99]. Within the realm of the food business, this substance finds application in the manufacturing process of instant tea and serves as an enhancer for the overall quality of various beverages, including fruit juices, beer, and wine. The utilization of microorganisms to manufacture tannase is a highly prevalent and extensively researched approach due to its widespread availability. Fungal species, including *Aspergillus fumigatus*, *Aspergillus* sp., and *Aspergillus versicolor*, as well as bacterial strains such as *Lactobacillus para Plantarum*, *Lactobacillus plantarum*, and *Klebsiella pneumoniae*, *Pseudomonas aeruginosa*, have demonstrated promising capabilities in the production of this enzyme to a satisfactory extent. The utilization of tannase derived from microorganisms in food production has been documented. This pertains specifically to the enzymatic extraction of tannase from green tea, employing tannase sourced from *A. niger* [100].

3.13.5 Asparaginase

L-asparaginase, an enzyme, is ubiquitous in many organisms, including algae, plants, microorganisms (such as bacteria and fungi), and certain animal species. Extensive research has been conducted to investigate its efficacy as a potent anticancer agent. Several microbes have been reported to produce L-asparaginase, including *Erwinia aroideae*, *P. aeruginosa*, *Aspergillus tamari*, *Vibro succinogenes*,

Aspergillus terreus, *Pseudomonas stutzeri*, and *Staphylococcus* sp. In food science, this method is notable for its efficacy in the mitigation or diminishment of acrylamide, a chemical molecule found in carbohydrate-rich foods that have undergone high-temperature cooking processes. This compound is known to potentially exhibit carcinogenic properties when consumed by individuals [101].

3.13.6 The phytases

Phytase functions as an enzymatic catalyst in the hydrolysis of phytate, a compound indigestible by the human body. It is predominantly present in non-plant-based meals in higher concentrations. Fortifying food items with phytase can enhance components' and functional foods' performance and nutritional quality. Like other enzymes, phytase can be found in various organisms such as herbs, mammals, fungus, bacteria, and yeast. The categorization of enzymes is contingent upon several variables, encompassing the characteristics and chemical qualities of the active site, the specific process in which the molecule functions as a catalyst, and the development of a protease shape along with its associated relationships. The enzyme in question plays a crucial part in the digestive process by mitigating the antinutritional effects of phytates and phytic acid [102]. Furthermore, it facilitates the improved absorption of minerals and proteins, contributing to better health. Phytase has been employed in several applications within the food sector, such as bread preparation, which enhances plant-based products' nutritional composition. Additionally, it is utilized in cereal bran fractionation, grain wet milling, and the isolation of plant proteins [103].

3.14 Enzymes used as additives to food

Food manufacturing enzymes are subjected to the same regulations as other food additives because of their role in food production. According to projections, the global market for food enzymes is anticipated to reach US$ 3.23 billion by 2023 [104]. Enzymes are presently employed as food additives in various food applications. The applications that garner the highest level of popularity are observed in the bakery field, wherein they modify the rheology of dough, enhance crumb softness, and improve gas retention. Similarly, these applications find extensive use in brewing and winemaking processes, effectively mitigating the Influence of long-chained molecules such as pectins and enhancing fermentation. Furthermore, these applications are also employed in producing fruit. Enzymes intended for utilization in food applications must satisfy the following criteria [105].

3.14.1 The enzymatic synthesis of dietary antioxidants

The use of antioxidants helps keep the food fresh and extends its shelf life. The food and edible oil industries have widely adopted synthetic antioxidants such as butylated hydroxytoluene (BHT) and butylated hydroxy anisole. However, concerns have arisen regarding their potential toxicity or the formation of carcinogenic components during their degradation [106]. As a result, manufacturers have started to focus on natural antioxidants as an alternative. Their inadequate solubility hinders the efficacy of most natural antioxidants in lipid-based dietary products. To address this issue, many enzymatic approaches have been devised to enhance the solubility characteristics of these compounds through the attachment of FAs, hence augmenting their hydrophobic nature [107].

3.14.2 The use of ascorbyl esters

Vitamin C ascorbyl esters are a popular form of this vitamin because they are fat-soluble and may effectively fight free radicals due to their improved solubility and ability to mix with other substances. These lipophilic derivatives exhibit exceptional antioxidant properties and are commonly employed to inhibit the process of lipid peroxidation [108]. According to Pohanka *et al* [109], the utilization of ascorbyl stearate (E305) and ascorbyl palmitate (E304) as antioxidants is authorized in accordance with the food additives regulations established by the European Union. Enzymatic methods are often favored over chemical production methods due to their ability to avoid the generation of by-products, their operation under mild experimental settings, and their capacity to generate 6-O-ascorbyl esterLipases derived from *Thermomyces lanuginosus*, *Rhizomucor miehei* and *Candida antarctica*, that are extensively employed in the production of ascorbyl esters [110]. The enzymes have the ability to facilitate esterification that results in transesterification processes that involve ascorbic acid and various acyl donors. These acyl donors encompass free FAs, such as oleic, stearic, palmitic, and omega-3 FAs, as well as triacylglycerol, including olive oil, palm oil, and soybean oil, and FA esters, such as methyl, ethyl, and vinyl esters. In order to mitigate the substantial expenses associated with enzymatic procedures, it is possible to immobilise enzymes for the purpose of repeated utilization. Multiple investigations have demonstrated that the immobilization of lipases enhances their catalytic performance and significantly increases the production yield of ascorbyl esters, reaching up to 80% within a time frame of less than 24 h. The antioxidant effects of ascorbyl oleate and ascorbyl palmitate, synthesized by the utilization of immobilized lipases derived from *C. antarctica* and *T. lanuginosus*, utilizing olive oil and triolein as substrates, were found to be highly effective in soybean oil [111]. The researchers discovered that the application of ascorbyl esters had a notable inhibitory effect on the formation of peroxides in soybean oil. Ascorbyl esters have also been employed for the purpose of oxidative inhibition in lipid-based food products, such as mayonnaise, salad dressing, milk, and dairy derivatives. A prior investigation similarly discovered that the inclusion of ascorbic palmitate effectively inhibited primary oxidation and hexanal generation in the process and preservation of cookies containing chocolate cream and milk.

3.14.3 Polyphenolic esters

Polyphenols encompass a diverse group of naturally occurring organic chemicals originating from plants, exhibiting notable antioxidant properties, and conferring various health advantages. Dietary sources rich in these substances are prevalent and renowned for their capacity to mitigate the onset of degenerative ailments, including cancer and cardiovascular disorders [112]. Polyphenols may be classified into many categories, including hydroxybenzoic acid, hydroxycinnamic acids, flavonoids, which contain acid chlorogenic, stilbenes, and the lignans. The utilization of polyphenols as food additives in the food industry is a common practice. However, their application in lipid-based food products presents a significant challenge due to their extremely limited solubility in oil. One effective strategy for addressing this challenge involves enhancing hydrophobicity through the enzymatic esterification step catalyzed by lipase, wherein an FA is attached [113]. The utilization of lipases has been employed in the synthesis of several lipophilic esters derived from polyphenols. The synthesis of acyl esters of quercetin-3-O-glucoside was conducted with immobilized lipase B from *Candida antarctica* (Cal B). The chemicals show the ability to impede the initial oxidation process in both fish oil and fish oil emulsion. It has been shown that lipase is responsible for the esterification process that occurs during the production of esters between epigallocatechin gallate 'EGCG' and polyunsaturated FAs, more especially eicosatetraenoic acid (EPA) and docosahexaenoic acid 'DHA'. The antioxidant activity of these EGCG esters was observed to be greater in comparison to that of EGCG alone. Furthermore, the integration of EPA and DHA into the EGCG molecule has the potential to provide supplementary health advantages, hence making them suitable for utilization in food and natural health commodities. A series of lipophilic esters of hydroxy-tyrosyl were synthesized utilizing the enzyme Cal B [114]. The research revealed that the EPA ester of hydroxy-tyrosyl had superior antioxidant properties compared to BHT and α-tocopherol in various forms of fish oil, including bulk fish oil, fish-oil-in-water emulsion, and microencapsulated fish oil. The stability of the substance was seen to persist for a duration of one year when subjected to storage conditions of −20 °C. Additionally, a separate study discovered that the process of esterification of tyrosyl resulted in an increased antioxidant efficacy when applied to infant formula. Previous studies have documented the existence of lipophilic esters of polyphenols generated by lipase, which possess food-grade properties.

3.14.4 Synthesis of sugars esters surfactants by enzymes

Glucose esters of FAs are non-ionic surfactants that are widely used in the dietary supplement, pharmaceuticals, and cosmetics sectors due to their advantageous characteristics, including low toxicity, biodegradability, and sustainable sourcing from natural resources [115]. Sugar esters are used extensively in the food sector, and the most common types used are sucrose esters, alkyl polyglycolide esters, and sorbitan esters. The chemicals discussed in this context are synthesized by the esterification process, which involves the combination of sugar molecules with different FA chains. The synthesis of sugar esters with diverse lipophilic and hydrophilic properties may be achieved by the manipulation of both the sugar moiety and the length of the FA chain. The user's text is too short to be rewritten academically. In industrial settings, the production of sugar esters involves chemical synthesis utilizing homogenous acid or base catalyst systems. Nevertheless, there are certain limitations involved with these approaches, such as their substantial financial implications, the potential for soap creation, and the environmental implications that need to be considered [115]. The enzymatic synthesis of sugar esters has been extensively documented in literature. Sugar esters can be synthesized through two different methods: direct esterification of sucrose with an FA chain, or trans-esterification of sucrose with FA methyl esters using lipases. These techniques have resulted in the synthesis of sugar esters characterized by elevated levels of purity and reduced formation of by-products. The lipases derived from *C. antarctica*, *R. miehei*, and *Candida rugosa* are the most employed enzymes in the production of sugar esters. Sugar esters have been granted approval for utilization as food additives in numerous countries. Sucrose esters of FAs have received international approval and are authorized for use in several regions, including the European Union, the United Kingdom, and the United States. E473 is a food additive that finds applications in many food products such as ice cream, soup, and mayonnaise [116]. A prior investigation revealed that sugar esters generated by lipase, namely fructose laurate, exhibited inhibitory effects on the proliferation of *Streptococcus mutans*, a pathogenic bacterium commonly associated with food-borne illnesses. In a separate investigation, the application of a diluted solution containing sucrose Mon myristate and Mon palmitate at a concentration of 0.05% showed significant inhibitory properties against the proliferation of *S. aureus*, *Escherichia coli*, and *Salmonella enteritidis*. These findings indicate that sugar esters of FAs possess potential as antimicrobial agents in the context of food applications. Additional applications of sugar esters in the food sector encompass the facilitation of cheese maturation, enhancement of flavour profiles, and incorporation into the manufacturing processes of cakes, biscuits, sauces, sausages, wine, and dairy goods [117].

References

[1] Anbu P *et al* 2017 *Microbial Enzymes and their Applications in Industries and Medicine 2016* (London: Hindawi)

[2] Souza P M d 2010 Application of microbial α-amylase in industry—a review *Braz. J. Microbiol.* **41** 850–61

[3] Van Der Maarel M J *et al* 2002 Properties and applications of starch-converting enzymes of the α-amylase family *J. Biotechnol.* **94** 137–55

[4] Burhan A *et al* 2003 Enzymatic properties of a novel thermostable, thermophilic, alkaline and chelator resistant amylase from an alkaliphilic *Bacillus* sp. isolate ANT-6 *Process Biochem.* **38** 1397–403

[5] Bordbar A-K, Omidiyan K and Hosseinzadeh R 2005 Study on interaction of α-amylase from *Bacillus subtilis* with cetyl trimethylammonium bromide *Colloids Surf. B: Biointerfaces* **40** 67–71

[6] Khajeh K *et al* 2006 Acidic and proteolytic digestion of α-amylases from *Bacillus licheniformis* and *Bacillus amyloliquefaciens*: stability and flexibility analysis *Enzyme Microb. Technol.* **38** 422–8

[7] Pandey A *et al* 2000 Advances in microbial amylases *Biotechnol. Appl. Biochem.* **31** 135–52

[8] Pimentel M R *et al* 2011 The use of endophytes to obtain bioactive compounds and their application in biotransformation process *Biotechnol. Res. Int.* **2011** 576286

[9] Saran S, Isar J and Saxena R K 2007 A modified method for the detection of microbial proteases on agar plates using tannic acid *J. Biochem. Biophys. Methods* **70** 697–9
[10] Anitha T and Palanivelu P 2013 Purification and characterization of an extracellular keratinolytic protease from a new isolate of *Aspergillus parasiticus Protein Expr. Purif.* **88** 214–20
[11] Ogawa A *et al* 1995 Production of neutral protease by membrane-surface liquid culture of *Aspergillus oryzae* IAM2704 *J. Ferment. Bioeng.* **80** 35–40
[12] Vishwanatha K, Rao A A and Singh S A 2009 Characterisation of acid protease expressed from *Aspergillus oryzae* MTCC 5341 *Food Chem.* **114** 402–7
[13] Andrade V S *et al* 2002 Production of extracellular proteases by *Mucor circinelloides* using D-glucose as carbon source/substrate *Braz. J. Microbiol.* **33** 106–10
[14] Bhosale S H, Rao M B and Deshpande V V 1996 Molecular and industrial aspects of glucose isomerase *Microbiol. Rev.* **60** 280–300
[15] Fantin B *et al* 1996 Importance of penicillinase production for activity of penicillin alone or in combination with sulbactam in experimental endocarditis due to methicillin-resistant *Staphylococcus aureus Antimicrob. Agents Chemother.* **40** 1219–24
[16] Savidge T and Cole M 1975 [54b] Penicillin acylase (bacterial) *Methods in Enzymology* (Amsterdam: Elsevier) pp 705–21
[17] Cole M and Sutherland R 1966 The role of penicillin acylase in the resistance of gram-negative bacteria to penicillins *Microbiology* **42** 345–56
[18] Holt R and Stewart G 1964 Production of amidase and β-lactamase by Bacteria *Microbiology* **36** 203–13
[19] Silhavy T J, Kahne D and Walker S 2010 The bacterial cell envelope *Cold Spring Harb. Perspect. Biol.* **2** a000414
[20] De la Maza L, Miller S and Ferraro M 1990 Use of commercially available rapid chloramphenicol acetyltransferase test to detect resistance in *Salmonella* species *J. Clin. Microbiol.* **28** 1867–9
[21] Olarte J and Galindo E 1973 *Salmonella typhi* resistant to chloramphenicol, ampicillin, and other antimicrobial agents: strains isolated during an extensive typhoid fever epidemic in Mexico *Antimicrob. Agents Chemother.* **4** 597–601
[22] Shaw W, Bentley D and Sands L 1970 Mechanism of chloramphenicol resistance in *Staphylococcus epidermidis J. Bacteriol.* **104** 1095–105
[23] Derrick J *et al* 1992 Analysis of the binding of 1,3-diacetylchloramphenicol to chloramphenicol acetyltransferase by isotope-edited proton NMR and site-directed mutagenesis *Biochemistry* **31** 8191–5
[24] Benveniste R and Davies J 1973 Aminoglycoside antibiotic-inactivating enzymes in actinomycetes similar to those present in clinical isolates of antibiotic-resistant bacteria *Proc. Natl Acad. Sci.* **70** 2276–80
[25] Kotb E 2013 Activity assessment of microbial fibrinolytic enzymes *Appl. Microbiol. Biotechnol.* **97** 6647–65
[26] Brogden R, Speight T and Avery G 1973 Streptokinase: a review of its clinical pharmacology, mechanism of action and therapeutic uses *Drugs* **5** 357–445
[27] Bansal V and Roychoudhury P K 2006 Production and purification of urokinase: a comprehensive review *Protein Expr. Purif.* **45** 1–14
[28] Asgari M *et al* 2014 Production of human tissue plasminogen activator (tPA) in *Cucumis sativus Prep. Biochem. Biotechnol.* **44** 182–92

[29] Wiebe M G *et al* 2001 Production of tissue plasminogen activator (t-PA) in *Aspergillus niger Biotechnol. Bioeng.* **76** 164–74
[30] Pandey A 1995 Glucoamylase research: an overview *Starch-Stärke* **47** 439–45
[31] Sauer J *et al* 2000 Glucoamylase: structure/function relationships, and protein engineering *Biochim. Biophys. Acta Protein Struct. Mol. Enzymol.* **1543** 275–93
[32] Thivend P, Mercier C and Guilbot A 1972 Determination of starch with glucoamylase *General Carbohydrate Method* (Amsterdam: Elsevier) pp 100–5
[33] Kim K *et al* 1994 Cloning of a new allelic variant of a *Saccharomyces diastaticus* glucoamylase gene and its introduction into industrial yeasts *Appl. Biochem. Biotechnol.* **44** 161–85
[34] Norouzian D *et al* 2006 Fungal glucoamylases *Biotechnol. Adv.* **24** 80–5
[35] Karim K M R and Tasnim T 2018 Fungal glucoamylase production and characterization: a review *Biores. Commun. (BRC)* **4** 591–605
[36] Marín-Navarro J and Polaina J 2011 Glucoamylases: structural and biotechnological aspects *Appl. Microbiol. Biotechnol.* **89** 1267–73
[37] Lincoln L, More V S and More S S 2019 Isolation, screening and optimization of extracellular glucoamylase from *Paenibacillus amylolyticus* strain NEO03 *Biocatal. Agric. Biotechnol.* **18** 101054
[38] Kosugi A *et al* 2009 Production of ethanol from cassava pulp via fermentation with a surface-engineered yeast strain displaying glucoamylase *Renew. Energy* **34** 1354–8
[39] Hostinová E and Gašperík J 2010 Yeast glucoamylases: molecular-genetic and structural characterization *Biologia* **65** 559–68
[40] Li H *et al* 2007 Glucoamylase production by the marine yeast *Aureobasidium pullulans* N13d and hydrolysis of potato starch granules by the enzyme *Process Biochem.* **42** 462–5
[41] Shigechi H *et al* 2004 Energy-saving direct ethanol production from low-temperature-cooked corn starch using a cell-surface engineered yeast strain co-displaying glucoamylase and α-amylase *Biochem. Eng. J.* **18** 149–53
[42] De Moraes L, Astolfi-Filho S and Oliver S 1995 Development of yeast strains for the efficient utilisation of starch: evaluation of constructs that express α-amylase and glucoamylase separately or as bifunctional fusion proteins *Appl. Microbiol. Biotechnol.* **43** 1067–76
[43] Yamashita I and Fukui S 1984 Isolation of glucoamylase-non-producing mutants in the yeast *Saccharomyces diastaticus Agric. Biol. Chem.* **48** 131–5
[44] Soccol C R *et al* 2006 Glucoamylase *Enzyme Technology* (Springer) pp 221–37
[45] Ricci Queiroz M C, Facciotti M C R and Schmidell W 1997 Rheological changes of *Aspergillus awamori* broth during amyloglucosidase production *Biotechnol. Lett* **19** 167–70
[46] Saito S *et al* 1996 Breeding of a new type of baker's yeast by δ-integration for overproduction of glucoamylase using a homothallic yeast *J. Ferment. Bioeng.* **81** 98–103
[47] Gen M and Cheng R 1999 *Genetic Algorithms and Engineering Optimization* **vol 7** (New York: Wiley)
[48] Chipperfield A, Fleming P and Fonseca C 1994 Genetic algorithm tools for control systems engineering *Proc. Adaptive Computing in Engineering Design and Control*
[49] Chaudhry S and Luo W 2005 Application of genetic algorithms in production and operations management: a review *Int. J. Prod. Res.* **43** 4083–101
[50] Reilly P J 1999 Protein engineering of glucoamylase to improve industrial performance - a review *Starch-Stärke* **51** 269–74

[51] Reeves C and Rowe J E 2002 *Genetic Algorithms: Principles and Perspectives: A Guide to GA Theory* (Berlin: Springer Science & Business Media) vol 20
[52] Man K-F, Tang K S and Kwong S 2001 *Genetic Algorithms: Concepts and Designs* (Berlin: Springer Science & Business Media)
[53] Ribeiro Filho J L, Treleaven P C and Alippi C 1994 Genetic-algorithm programming environments *Computer* **27** 28–43
[54] Coit D W and Smith A E 1996 Reliability optimization of series-parallel systems using a genetic algorithm *IEEE Trans. Reliab.* **45** 254–60
[55] Oh I-S, Lee J-S and Moon B-R 2004 Hybrid genetic algorithms for feature selection *IEEE Trans. Pattern Anal. Mach. Intell.* **26** 1424–37
[56] Joines J A, Culbreth C T and King R E 1996 Manufacturing cell design: an integer programming model employing genetic algorithms *IIE Trans.* **28** 69–85
[57] Wang D, Yung K L and Ip W 2001 A heuristic genetic algorithm for subcontractor selection in a global manufacturing environment *IEEE Trans. Syst. Man, Cybern., Part C (Appl. Rev.)* **31** 189–98
[58] Leu Y Y, Matheson L A and Rees L P 1994 Assembly line balancing using genetic algorithms with heuristic-generated initial populations and multiple evaluation criteria *Decis. Sci.* **25** 581–605
[59] Chu P C and Beasley J E 1997 A genetic algorithm for the generalised assignment problem *Comput. Oper. Res.* **24** 17–23
[60] Tolan J S and Foody B 1999 Cellulase from submerged fermentation *Recent Progress in Bioconversion of Lignocellulosics* (Springer) pp 41–67
[61] Turner M B *et al* 2003 Ionic liquid salt-induced inactivation and unfolding of cellulase from *Trichoderma reesei Green Chem.* **5** 443–7
[62] Li X-h *et al* 2009 The most stirring technology in future: cellulase enzyme and biomass utilization *Afr. J. Biotechnol.* **8** 11
[63] Beckham G T *et al* 2012 Harnessing glycosylation to improve cellulase activity *Curr. Opin. Biotechnol.* **23** 338–45
[64] Gusakov A V and Sinitsyn A P 1992 A theoretical analysis of cellulase product inhibition: effect of cellulase binding constant, enzyme/substrate ratio, and β-glucosidase activity on the inhibition pattern *Biotechnol. Bioeng.* **40** 663–71
[65] Sajith S *et al* 2016 An overview on fungal cellulases with an industrial perspective *J. Nutr. Food Sci.* **6** 461
[66] Shirai T *et al* 2001 Crystal structure of alkaline cellulase K: insight into the alkaline adaptation of an industrial enzyme *J. Mol. Biol.* **310** 1079–87
[67] Kim M *et al* 1982 Surface deactivation of cellulase and its prevention *Enzyme Microb. Technol.* **4** 99–103
[68] Barati B *et al* 2015 Introduction of cellulase and its application *In Silico Engineering of Disulphide Bonds to Produce Stable Cellulase* (Springer) pp 1–5
[69] Subhedar P B and Gogate P R 2014 Enhancing the activity of cellulase enzyme using ultrasonic irradiations *J. Mol. Catal. B: Enzym.* **101** 108–14
[70] Zhang X Z and Zhang Y H P 2013 Cellulases: characteristics, sources, production, and applications *Bioprocessing Technologies in Biorefinery for Sustainable Production of Fuels, Chemicals, and Polymers* (Wiley) pp 131–46
[71] Bollok M and Reczey K 2000 Cellulase enzyme production by various fungal strains on different carbon sources *Acta Aliment.* **29** 154–68

[72] Feng Y, Jiang J-x and Zhu L-w 2009 Recent developments in activities, utilization and sources of cellulase *For. Stud. Chin.* **11** 202–7

[73] Juhasz T *et al* 2005 Characterization of cellulases and hemicellulases produced by *Trichoderma reesei* on various carbon sources *Process Biochem.* **40** 3519–25

[74] Chatterjee S *et al* 2015 Cellulase enzyme based biodegradation of cellulosic materials: an overview *Cellulose* **5** 271–82

[75] Sharada R *et al* 2013 Production of cellulase—a review *Int. J. Pharm. Chem. Biol. Sci.* **3** 4

[76] Jahangeer S *et al* 2005 Screening and characterization of fungal cellulases isolated from the native environmental source *Pak. J. Bot.* **37** 739

[77] Gado H *et al* 2007 Enzymatic treatments of sugarcane bagasse by different sources of cellulase enzymes *Egypt. J. Nutr. Feeds* **10** 607–20

[78] Vázquez-Montoya E L *et al* 2020 Moringa straw as cellulase production inducer and cellulolytic fungi source *Rev. Argent. Microbiol.* **52** 4–12

[79] Dashtban M, Buchkowski R and Qin W 2011 Effect of different carbon sources on cellulase production by *Hypocrea jecorina* (*Trichoderma reesei*) strains *Int. J. Biochem. Mol. Biol.* **2** 274

[80] Hideno A *et al* 2011 Production and characterization of cellulases and hemicellulases by *Acremonium cellulolyticus* using rice straw subjected to various pretreatments as the carbon source *Enzyme Microb. Technol.* **48** 162–8

[81] Milala M *et al* 2005 Studies on the use of agricultural wastes for cellulase enzyme production by *Aspergillus niger Res. J. Agric. Biol. Sci.* **1** 325–8

[82] Persson I, Tjerneld F and Hahn-Hägerdal B 1991 Fungal cellulolytic enzyme production: a review *Process Biochem.* **26** 65–74

[83] Acharya S and Chaudhary A 2012 Bioprospecting thermophiles for cellulase production: a review *Braz. J. Microbiol.* **43** 844–56

[84] Piironen V *et al* 2000 Plant sterols: biosynthesis, biological function and their importance to human nutrition *J. Sci. Food Agric.* **80** 939–66

[85] Havrlentová M *et al* 2011 β-Glucans and their significance for the preparation of functional foods-a review *Czech J. Food Sci.* **29** 1–14

[86] Alemzadeh I *et al* 2022 Enzymes in functional food development *Novel Food Grade Enzymes: Applications in Food Processing and Preservation Industries* (Berlin: Springer) pp 217–52

[87] Jideani V 2011 Functional properties of soybean food ingredients in food systems *Soybean-Biochemistry, Chemistry and Physiology* (IntechOpen) pp 345–66

[88] Xue N, Svensson B and Bai Y 2022 Structure, function and enzymatic synthesis of glucosaccharides assembled mainly by $\alpha 1 \rightarrow 6$ linkages—a review *Carbohydr. Polym.* **275** 118705

[89] Mirmiran P, Bahadoran Z and Azizi F 2014 Functional foods-based diet as a novel dietary approach for management of type 2 diabetes and its complications: a review *World J. Diabetes* **5** 267

[90] Van den Berg H *et al* 2000 The potential for the improvement of carotenoid levels in foods and the likely systemic effects *J. Sci. Food Agric.* **80** 880–912

[91] Shi Y and Cheng D 2009 Beyond triglyceride synthesis: the dynamic functional roles of MGAT and DGAT enzymes in energy metabolism *Am. J. Physiol. Endocrinol. Metab.* **297** E10–8

[92] Wells M L *et al* 2017 Algae as nutritional and functional food sources: revisiting our understanding *J. Appl. Phycol.* **29** 949–82
[93] Raigond P, Ezekiel R and Raigond B 2015 Resistant starch in food: a review *J. Sci. Food Agric.* **95** 1968–78
[94] Eskin N M and Shahidi F 2012 *Biochemistry of Foods* (Academic Press)
[95] Nimbkar S *et al* 2022 Medium chain triglycerides (MCT): state-of-the-art on chemistry, synthesis, health benefits and applications in food industry *Compr. Rev. Food Sci. Food Saf.* **21** 843–67
[96] Shvachko N A *et al* 2021 Bioactive components in oat and barley grain as a promising breeding trend for functional food production *Molecules* **26** 2260
[97] Méndez-Carmona J, Ascacio-Valdés J and Aguilar C N 2022 Enzyme technology for production of food ingredients and functional foods *Value-Addition in Food Products and Processing Through Enzyme Technology* (Amsterdam: Elsevier) pp 1–11
[98] Florowska A *et al* 2016 Prebiotics as functional food ingredients preventing diet-related diseases *Food Funct.* **7** 2147–55
[99] Yao J *et al* 2014 Production, characterization and applications of tannase *J. Mol. Catal. B: Enzym.* **101** 137–47
[100] van de Lagermaat J and Pyle D L 2006 Tannase *Enzyme Technology* (Springer) pp 381–97
[101] Batool T *et al* 2016 A comprehensive review on L-asparaginase and its applications *Appl. Biochem. Biotechnol.* **178** 900–23
[102] Castro D *et al* 2021 L-asparaginase production review: bioprocess design and biochemical characteristics *Appl. Microbiol. Biotechnol.* **105** 4515–34
[103] Muneer F *et al* 2020 Microbial L-asparaginase: purification, characterization and applications *Arch. Microbiol.* **202** 967–81
[104] Fraatz M A, Rühl M and Zorn H 2014 Food and feed enzymes *Adv. Biochem. Eng. Biotechnol.* **143** 229–56
[105] Pariza M and Foster E 1983 Determining the safety of enzymes used in food processing *J. Food Prot.* **46** 453–68
[106] Benzie I F 2003 Evolution of dietary antioxidants *Comp. Biochem. Physiol. Part A: Mol. Integr. Physiol.* **136** 113–26
[107] Andre C M, Larondelle Y and Evers D 2010 Dietary antioxidants and oxidative stress from a human and plant perspective: a review *Curr. Nutr. Food Sci.* **6** 2–12
[108] Burham H *et al* 2009 Enzymatic synthesis of palm-based ascorbyl esters *J. Mol. Catal. B: Enzym.* **58** 153–7
[109] Pohanka M, Pejchal J, Snopková S, Havlickova K, Z Karasova J, Bostik P and Pikula J 2012 Ascorbic acid: an old player with a broad impact on body physiology including oxidative stress suppression and immunomodulation: a review *Mini Rev. Med. Chem* **12** 35–43
[110] Viklund F, Alander J and Hult K 2003 Antioxidative properties and enzymatic synthesis of ascorbyl FA esters *J. Am. Oil Chem. Soc.* **80** 795–9
[111] Karmee S K 2009 Biocatalytic synthesis of ascorbyl esters and their biotechnological applications *Appl. Microbiol. Biotechnol.* **81** 1013–22
[112] Hsieh H J *et al* 2005 Synthesis of mixed esters of ascorbic acid using methyl esters of palm and soybean oils *Prep. Biochem. Biotechnol.* **35** 113–8
[113] Ćorović M *et al* 2020 Enzymatically derived oil-based L-ascorbyl esters: synthesis, antioxidant properties and controlled release from cosmetic formulations *Sustain. Chem. Pharm.* **15** 100231

[114] Stojanović M *et al* 2015 Influence of fatty acid on lipase-catalyzed synthesis of ascorbyl esters and their free radical scavenging capacity *Biotechnol. Appl. Biochem.* **62** 458–66
[115] Neta N S, Teixeira J A and Rodrigues L R 2015 Sugar ester surfactants: enzymatic synthesis and applications in food industry *Crit. Rev. Food Sci. Nutr.* **55** 595–610
[116] Maruyama T, Nagasawa S-i and Goto M 2002 Enzymatic synthesis of sugar amino acid esters in organic solvents *J. Biosci. Bioeng.* **94** 357–61
[117] Grüninger J, Delavault A and Ochsenreither K 2019 Enzymatic glycolipid surfactant synthesis from renewables *Process Biochem.* **87** 45–54

IOP Publishing

Introduction to Pharmaceutical Biotechnology, Volume 2
(Second Edition)
Enzymes, proteins and bioinformatics
Ahmed Al-Harrasi, Saurabh Bhatia and Ajmal Khan

Chapter 4

Immobilization of enzymes

4.1 Introduction

In modern science, biologically active natural compounds, mainly enzymes, have gained significant attention in medicine and various biotechnological processes where they are being employed commercially. At present a number of ailments related to lysosomal enzyme activities have been recognized. These diseases could ideally be cured by supplementation or replacement of defective or deficient enzyme. Additionally, enzymes with very specific activity are usually involved in the catalysis of several reactions. Enzymes have various significant clinical applications as bioreactors, biosensors and in other enzyme-based reactions, however, their use is restricted for a number of reasons, such as high cost, low availability and quick inactivation under physiological conditions followed by fast clearance, therefore there is the requirement for a greater amount of enzyme during the course of treatment. Moreover, possible antigenicity, inactivation by different endogenous natural inhibitors and, lastly, the challenge to achieving higher levels for therapeutic activity, are limitations on the practical clinical use of enzymes. Regardless of these limitations, enzymes have a vast range of possible applications covering therapeutic, analytical and industrial aims. The application potential of an enzyme is established by the distinctive enzyme properties of precise specificity for the substrate and reaction catalyzed. In order to be practically suitable, an enzyme must have excellent catalytic behavior, with specificity, stability and reusability. According to research, the majority of enzymes involved in particular reactions become comparatively less active during the last phase because of the accumulation and detrimental effect of the reaction product.

Immobilized enzymes are currently the subject of significant interest because of their benefits over soluble enzymes. In addition to their use in industrial processes, immobilization methods are the basis for making a number of biotechnology products with applications in diagnostics, bioaffinity chromatography and biosensors [1].

doi:10.1088/978-0-7503-5387-8ch4

Earlier, only single immobilized enzymes were employed, however, since the 1970s more complex systems including two-enzyme reactions with co-factor regeneration and living cells were explored. The enzymes can be attached to the support by interactions ranging from reversible physical adsorption and ionic linkages, to stable covalent bonds. Although the choice of the most suitable immobilization method depends on the nature of the enzyme and the carrier, in the last few years immobilization technology has gradually become a matter of rational design [1]. As a result of enzyme immobilization, some important features, such as catalytic activity or thermal stability, are changed. These properties have been demonstrated and exploited [1]. The concept of stabilization has been an important driving force for immobilizing enzymes. Furthermore, true stabilization at the molecular level has been established, e.g. proteins immobilized through multipoint covalent binding [1].

Enzymes exist as bioproteins and thus are environmentally sensitive to different pH and temperature. Therefore, stability remains a challenge for the effective cure of problems associated with enzymes and enzyme technology. The major focus of immobilization is characteristically the economic application of enzyme systems. Additional merits of the immobilized enzyme system are ease of control and uniformity of conversion. The solution to qualifying the economic concerns is the evaluation of the cost of the constituents of the immobilized system against the value of its performance. During immobilization, the enzyme utilizes the carrier phase for stealth, and safe homing. The immobilization matrix or support facilitates exchange, but remains separate from the bulk phase in which substrate, effect or inhibitor molecules are present and isolated. This entails limiting soluble protein catalysts or the individual buoyancy of cells in reactor systems, which can require constant changes of fresh solution. Usually the immobilized system is placed in an appropriate column through which the charge is allowed to pass constantly. The definition may be expanded to cover intact cells and biocatalysts under the category of guest. The process of immobilization, i.e., the restrictive localization of enzymes, may in the immediate future have great potential in the development of biosensors, bioelectronic sensors in fermentation technology and enzyme therapeutics [2]. The carrier phase, also known as the enzyme phase, is classically water insoluble but can be combined with as hydrophilic porous polymeric matrix, e.g. cellulose, agarose and acrylamide. In other words, immobilization is a general term that designates the retention of a biologically active catalyst within a reactor or analytical system with the help of a suitable carrier support. A unique procedure is planned by using immobilization techniques through which fluid can pass without any difficulty, converting the substrate into the product under controlled enzymatic reaction, and all together allowing the easy removal of the catalyst from the product as it leaves the reactor. The immobilization, also referred to as forced homing, of enzymes is achieved by covalent coupling using adsorption or physical entrapment of enzymes within the enzyme phase (polymeric matrix). The activity of immobilized enzymes is usually dependent on the type of matrix and enzyme phase. One of the most common immobilization matrices which utilizes anchoring on the surface of an insoluble polymeric matrix is cellulose or polyacrylamide via covalent bond formation. The enzyme phase is available in the form of fine particulate, membranous or monolithic spheres. The enzyme in turn may be bound to another enzyme via cross-linking. This may render the overall composite as an insoluble, but active, polymeric enzyme system. Once a support or carrier is employed for the purpose of enzyme immobilization, the stability of that carrier during its use is equally important. A carrier (membrane or matrix) that is not stable at a suitable pH, ionic strength or under the solvent conditions of the process, may be disrupted or dissolved releasing the enzyme component. This obviously suggests that it is not essential for a carrier to be insoluble and durable at all pHs, ionic strengths or solvent conditions. The different procedures most frequently employed for enzyme immobilization using solid supports can be categorized into two main classes on the basis of the approaches used to restrain biocatalysts: those with catalysts within the support and those which hold the biocatalyst on the surface of the support. Each class is further divided on the basis of their usage of covalent and noncovalent coupling procedures for surface immobilization, with cross-linking entrapment and encapsulation techniques for immobilization in or within a support. The different types of supports used in immobilization are shown in figure 4.1 and table 4.1.

4.2 Types of immobilization

On-surface immobilization involves [4]:

- Covalent coupling with polymers employing their functional group for anchoring, moreover, the groups must be non-functional or non-essential for biological activity [5].
- Adsorption on an inert support or ion-exchange resins.
- Complexation and chelation.

In the procedure of within-support immobilization, the enzyme is immobilized by cross-linking by multifunctional reagents, followed by entrapment within a structure of known/defined geometry. Entrapment can be achieved by:

- encapsulation in microcapsules, hollow fibers, liposomes, etc.
- occlusion within a cross-linked gel.

Immobilization frequently causes obvious changes in the apparent parameters of the enzyme related to the reaction it catalyzes. These parameters include the reaction rate, effect of the inhibitor (which may be lost completely in the case of an immobilized enzyme), Michaelis–Menten kinetics, and the optimum temperature and pH corresponding to maximum activity. The degree of variation among these parameters may not only be related to the technique of immobilization selected, but also to some extent to the enzyme reaction. Iso *et al* have demonstrated the microencapsulation of lipase (*Pseudomonas fluorescens*), carried out using a (W/O)/W two-phase emulsion technique [6].

4.2.1 Surface immobilization by covalent coupling

Immobilization of enzymes by covalent bonding to an insoluble polymer has the supposed benefit of irreversible binding of the enzyme to the support matrix. Many of the bonds usually employed are, however, not 100% stable in use. If insufficient

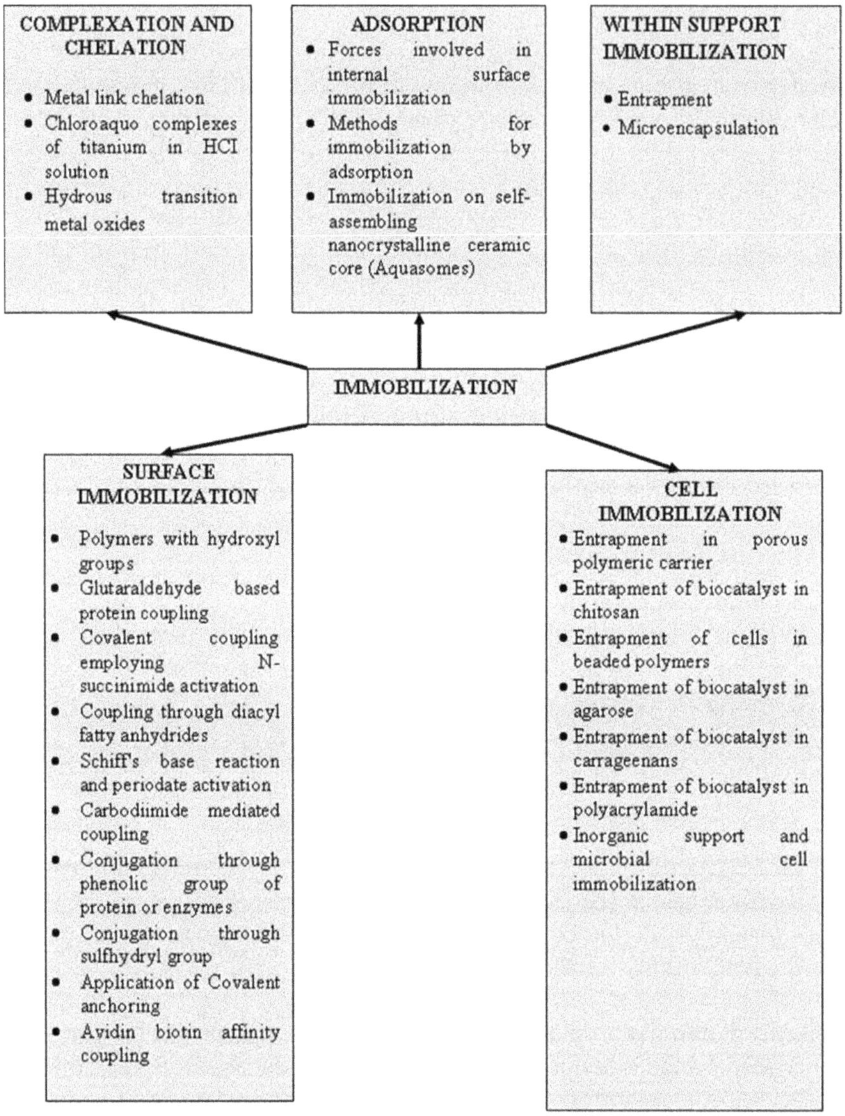

Figure 4.1. Schematic or immobilization techniques.

care is taken to confirm that the enzyme can survive the reaction conditions, considerable loss of enzyme activity will occur. Even under promising conditions, 60% loss of activity is not uncommon [7]. The covalent bond between a biocatalyst and a support matrix results in a complex which is significantly stable throughout the functional use of the enzyme. However, the process subjects the delicate three-dimensional structure of the biopolymer to strong disruptive physical and chemical forces or stresses. Thus, where the superior form and stability of an immobilized enzyme are more important than the irreversible loss of activity that is certainly associated with immobilization procesess, such enzymes are preferred over their

Table 4.1. Different types of supports used in immobilization [3].

Classification of supports
Organic
Natural polymers
• Polysaccharides: cellulose, dextrans, agar, agarose, chitin, alginate
• Proteins: collagen, albumin
• Carbon synthetic polymers
• Polystyrene
• Other polymers: polyacrylate polymethacrylates, polyacrylamide, polyamides, vinyl and allyl-polymers
Inorganic
Natural minerals Bentonite Silica processed materials: glass (nonporous and controlled pore) Metals Controlled pore metal oxides

soluble form. The functional groups fo und on enzyme proteins, by which a covalent bond with polymeric or other supports could be established, should be non-essential for enzymatic action. Moreover, the reactions which include comparatively mild conditions and principally utilize an aqueous medium are favored. This additionally requires broad information on the amino acids and their active groups involved in polymeric covalent bonding, the prospect of chemical amelioration or specific chemical modification on activity, the protection of active group(s) and the three-dimensional structure of the enzyme under consideration. The protein functional groups which could be employed in covalent coupling include:

- COOH: β and α of aspartic acid and glutamic acid, respectively.
- NH_2 lysine: N-terminal of polypeptide.
- OH: Phenol ring on tyrosine.
- SH: Group on cysteine.

The polymeric supports which have been considered as supports for covalent coupling based immobilization include [1]:

- Aldehyde and acetal groups of polymers.
- Amide group of polypeptides and polyamides (nylon).
- Amino and related groups of amino-ethyl coated polysaccharides and silica gel, poly(d-aminoglycine), etc.
- Carboxylic acid and related groups of poly(glutamic acid), maleic anhydride co-polymers, poly(acrylamide) and carboxymethyl cellulose.
- Hydroxyl groups of polysaccharides, PVA, polymethyl methacrylate (PMMA) and inorganic glasses.

The covalent coupling procedures usually employed for conjugation of enzymes with a solid/matrix support are cyanobromide, cyclic trans 2,3-carbonates and acid anhydrides. The approaches employed for covalent anchoring via support activation are: diazotization, Schiff's base formation, glutaraldehyde treatment, thiodisulfide and imido ester formation. With the help of these coupling agents and certain procedures, covalent bonds are developed between functional groups on enzymes and respective counter groups on polymeric support with a net result of an immobilized enzyme system formation.

4.2.2 Adsorption

Considering the functionality at the level of operation, adsorption appears to be a most economical and simple process, however, the forces involved are extremely complex. So far, practically no material has been reported which could be employed for adsorptive immobilization with its own surface contribution [1]. The nature of the carrier and the enzyme protein surface determines the bonds that exist between the enzyme protein and carrier, such as ionic, hydrogen, covalent, coordinated covalent or hydrophobic, or even a combination of any of these [1]. Immobilization can be achieved by coupling an enzyme to either the external or internal surface of a carrier. When an enzyme is immobilized externally, it is necessary that the particle size of the carrier must be small enough to offer a substantial surface for binding. These particles possibly have diameters ranging between 500 Å mm and 1 mm diameter [1]. The external surface binding employed during immobilization of the enzyme is beneficial as it does not include conditions such as pore diffusion. The drawbacks, however, include a comparatively small surface area for binding, exposure of enzymes against microbial attack, physical abrasion of the enzyme and inhibitory effects due to turbulence related to the bulk solution. Finally, the reduced particles cause a high pressure drop (gradient) in continuous packed-bed reactors [1]. While the internal surface participation of a porous carrier during enzyme immobilization has been a noticeable shortcoming, many adavatages can be gained from this approach. The main shortcoming of internal immobilization relates to pore diffusion. Therefore, the process calls for proper optimization of pore diameter, surface area, surface charges and other related parameters.

4.2.3 Complexation and chelation

Numerous techniques for the immobilization of enzymes have been developed. By choosing a suitable carrier material and coupling procedure, it is typically possible to obtain immobilized derivatives with good activity and stability [8]. However, the majority of these comprise irreversibly bonded enzymes, which means that the carrier cannot be regenerated and reused. This issue can be avoided by immobilization based on ion exchange, hydrophobic interaction or thiol disulfide interexchange [8].

4.2.3.1 Metal link chelation

This method provides an immediate coupling without chemical derivatization or activation of a support or matrix. The procedure is principally based on the chelation properties of transition metals, specifically titanium and zirconium, which are attractive due to their nontoxic nature [9]. A scheme based on titanium chloride–cellulose demonstrates the process of transition metal association–chelate formation.

Titanium metal has the feature of octahedral co-ordination with ionic molecules which function as ligands. In the majority of cases these ligands are water molecules or chloride ions. In the event where the chloride ion behaves as a ligand, its surplus electron density is employed in the development of a partial-covalent bond with the metal ion (Ti), thus the whole positive charge of titanium is minimized by a unit.

4.2.3.2 Chloroaquo complexes of titanium in HCI solution

These ligands may be substituted by other water-based ligands or other electron donating groups. The strength of association depends on the chemical nature of the ligand [10]. Hydroxyl ions are active ligands for transition metals; consequently they may well have the potential to create complexes with polysaccharides, where new ligating hydroxyl ions may be substituted for pre-existing ones if any are present [10]. Certain polysaccharides, e.g. cellulose, contain a vicinal diol group which is not involved in glycosidic linkage and is therefore accessible for free chelation by transition metals. The chelate is an outcome of the substitution of two ligands from the titanium ion by polysaccharide hydroxyl groups. For steric reasons the number of ligands which can be substituted by cellulose hydroxyl groups is limited [10].

4.2.3.3 Hydrous transition metal oxides

During this procedure hydrous metal oxides are used as the support for enzyme or cell immobilization [10]. The oxides can be prepared by precipitation after hydrolysis of the corresponding chloride. The method of immobilization is mainly based on chelation. Therefore the precipitation is achieved to obtain hydrous oxide in the presence of the enzyme, which may result in effective and efficient immobilization. However, all safety measures needed to account for potential detrimental conditions should be taken in to consideration [10]. The metal chlorides which may be employed for transformation to hydrous oxides include cobalt(ii), copper(ii), iron(ii), manganese(ii), tin(ii), zinc(ii), chromium(ii), vanadium(iii), tin(iv) and zirconium(iv). The complexes retain a considerable portion of the activity profile of the chelated immobilized enzyme. Due to the low operational stability of enzymes immobilized on metal hydrous oxide, a cross-linking step based on glutaraldehyde treatment has been recommended. This method of modification could avert protein loss into the solution during operation.

4.2.4 Within-support immobilization

The entrapment or encapsulation of enzymes can be achieved via their inclusion in a matrix that is based on highly cross-linked polymers, encapsulation in microcapsules or in distinct non-aqueous phases [11]. The characteristic feature of these procedures, mainly matrix inclusion and encapsulation, is that the enzyme is not attached to the matrix, thus any issues, such as the steric blockades related to covalent or electrostatic binding, are not encountered. The procedure offers scope for developing biocatalysts in various physical shapes and forms. While beads are most common, fibers, sheets, emulsions and gels have been used in bioreactors [11]. In conclusion, immobilization by means of entrapment methods is an attractive option where the difference in size of the catalyst and substrate should be characteristically large. Practically, membrane reactors are well adapted for enzymes which act on a low molecular weight substrate, whereas three-dimensional gel is favored for immobilizing cellular/particular biocatalysts and therefore is the scheme of choice for immobilization of live cells [11]. Usually entrapment is achieved by dissolving an enzyme in a solution that is required either for dissolution or for preparation of the enzyme phase (carrier), and then treating this solution so that a distinctive and discrete biphasic system is created in the form of dispersion.

4.2.5 Cell immobilization

Enzyme immobilization has now become a mature technology and a number of immobilization procedures have been developed. The groundbreaking attention has moved onto the development of immobilization of whole plant/animal cells, which offers another route to highly specific enzyme processes aimed at multistage processing and production of fine chemicals against first generation biocatalysts. In the last few decades, experience and expertise in the immobilization of microbial cells has improved such that a range of gentle procedures are now accessible to produce fine chemicals, fabrics and membranes incorporating a high number of viable cells. Hydrogels are being studied for mammalian cell immobilization. Their material features can be designed or structured for biocompatibility, selective permeability, mechanical and chemical stability, and other necessities as specified by the application, including uniform cell distribution and a given membrane thickness or mechanical strength [12]. These aqueous gels are a good choice for analytical and tissue engineering applications and can be employed for immobilization in therapies for various diseases as well as to generate bioartificial organs [12].

4.2.5.1 Distinctive features of plant and animal cells

In cell immobilization, currently most research is focused on using the prokaryotic bacterial cells as a subject [13]. The differences between prokaryotic and eukaryotic cells are clearly distinguishable and involve size, form and function. Prokaryotes lack of organelles, have a different cell wall composition and are typically one tenth the size or one thousandth the volume of plant and animal cells. Eukaryotic cells have different subcellular, membrane bound organelles such as nuclei, mitochondria, lysosomes, vacuoles and various other plastids. As a result of these major differences the metabolic functions of eukaryotes proceed more slowly than those of bacteria. Eukaryotic cells can express a superior amount of genetic information in a number of ways, to produce distinct, differentiated (i.e., specific) cells which frequently function co-operatively to develop tissues, organs or even whole organisms. As a result, they develop complex mechanisms for both intracellular and intercellular control and informative transfer, involving hormones, cell mediators and specific cell surface receptors. They are hence capable of more sophisticated responses than the basic survival-related reactions of bacteria. The whole complexity of their metabolism, affecting the gene expression in individual cells, presents problems in the maintenance and use of eukaryotes, even when successful immobilization has been achieved. However, these different levels of control could clearly offer valuable opportunities for the manipulation of cellular activity. Unfortunately, at present these mechanisms are so poorly understood at the molecular level, that bacteria continue to be considered for any applications where either cell type could be employed.

4.2.5.2 Products from eukaryotes

There is developing interest in the large-scale culture of plant and animal cells for the production of high value pharmaceuticals, flavors, hormones and immunological products, despite the difficulties associated with such cells. The complication of organization and regulation of biosynthetic pathways resulting in secondary products among eukaryotes is likely to be beyond the practical or economic limits, whereas the practical and economic limits of genetic manipulation of bacteria are yet to arise. In addition, certain operational and post-translational modifications, such as glycosylation, are unlikely to be accomplished by incorporating gene sequences into prokaryotes. It might also be claimed that the most satisfactory source of material for replacement therapy in the treatment of humans will be attained from genetically engineered human cell lines, and that the best way of synthesizing plant and animal cell products is by direct genetic manipulation of these cells and their use in an immobilized form.

4.2.5.3 Limitations of immobilization of eukaryotic cells

In contrast to enzymes, immobilized cells are less reactive to high substrate concentrations, surfactants, solvents and rapid changes in physical factors. Therefore, the process intensity and flexibility of response are likely to be lower. The substrate is the major nutrient of the cell and in a single-pass reactor, cells at the end of the process will either be exposed to nutrient starvation, or lower conversion must be accepted. The sensitivity of higher cells against environmental factors, e.g. osmotic shock, oxygen, shear, gas balance, pH, temperature and toxic chemicals, is a clear drawback to the procedures which might be employed for immobilization. Nevertheless, these issues are to some extent offset by the capacity of cells to regenerate after immobilization, if maintained under suitable conditions. The hormonal reactions of eukaryotes allow additional levels of control and flexibility compared to microorganisms, which often only respond to nutrient levels or gross environmental changes. To achieve the maximum merits of immobilization, cells must be reused and thus must be retained in a healthy condition. The rich nutrient media in which both plant and animal cells must be maintained are highly susceptible to microbial contamination and so all operations must be carried out in an aseptic environment. This further restricts immobilization methods and adds to the cost and complexity of the techniques. Moreover, stored medium can deteriorate and may become increasingly unreliable when continuous operation of a process is considered. It can be seen that some of these limitations are in fact related to the cells rather than the immobilization process. If synthesis by eukaryotic cells is selected, as discussed above, the advantages ensuing from immobilization can be very high, as long as satisfactory process control is available. However, it is obvious that the complexity involved in using cultured plant and animal cells will in general limit their application in the production of high value compounds.

4.2.6 Commercial production of enzymes

Enzyme production still requires attention in the modern biotechnology industry. The arrival of genetic engineering has allowed the industrial scale production of enzymes and other proteins which are synthesized naturally in only minute quantities [14]. This progress is mainly significant with regard to the synthesis of enzymes and other proteins of therapeutic importance, which are now accessible in clinically useful quantities [14]. The level of downstream processing to which any enzyme is exposed depends on its future application. The production of enzymes in bulk usually requires little downstream processing, and therefore these are comparatively crude preparations. Enzymes intended for therapeutic applications are subject to a far higher grade of downstream processing, frequently introducing three to four chromatographic steps. Although enzymology is one of the oldest recognized branches of the biochemical sciences, it continues to be an area of constant, active research. The repeated detection of new enzymes, and better knowledge of previously discovered enzymes and their functional implications, has suggested several novel applications for these catalytic activities [14].

4.3 Genetic engineering for microbial enzyme production

Enzymes are the large biomolecules that are obligatory for the many chemical interactions that sustain life. Enzymes produced from genetically modified microorganisms play an important role in food technology [15]. Enzymes accelerate all the metabolic developments in the body and each carries out a specific task. They are highly efficient, and can trigger reaction rates 100 million to 10 billion times quicker than any normal chemical reaction. Owing to developments in recombinant technology and protein engineering, enzymes have developed as vital molecules that have been extensively employed for different industrial and therapeutical purposes. Microbial enzymes are currently gaining much attention with fast expansion of enzyme technology [15]. Microbial enzymes are poplular due to their economic feasibility, high yields, consistency, ease of product modification and optimization, regular supply due to absence of seasonal fluctuations, rapid growth of microbes on inexpensive media, stability and greater catalytic activity [15]. Microbial enzymes play a significant role in the diagnosis, treatment, biochemical investigation and monitoring of various dreaded diseases. Amylase and lipase are two key enzymes that have been closely studied and have great significance in different manufacturing and therapeutic industries. The expression of a gene always results in the synthesis of a specific protein in the form of an enzyme, hormone, etc, for a specific function. We can say that the enzymes are functional proteins that are synthesized after the expression of specific sequences present in the gene that encode for that particular protein (enzyme) [15]. Currently genetic engineers are paying more attention to the production of these therapeutic proteins using rDNA technology. Due to their many advantages microbes are considered as an excellent source for the production of these therapeutic proteins. Recent developments in rDNA technology have allowed the efficient microbial production of commercial enzymes [15]. After the identification of an enzyme, especially those are with potential use in industry, multiple copies can be produced by cloning a suitable gene and introducing it into a suitable host.

4.3.1 Cloning methods

There are several cloning methods for the commercial production of enzymes, as mentioned in figure 4.2. cDNA templates are considered the best for the production of enzymes. cDNA, which can be synthesized from mRNA to establish a cDNA library, is required for the development of a suitable probe for a particular enzyme. The specific cDNA clones required can be identified on hybridization with oligonucleotide probes. This desired gene should be inserted into a suitable host such as *Aspergillus oryzae* for the expression of a desirable enzyme. This approach can be utilized to produce high quality industrial enzymes with better yield. There have been several reports based on enzyme synthesis using cloning methods:

- The fungal enzyme lipolase, present in *Humicola languinosa*, was recently shown to eliminate fat stains in fabrics [16]. However, commercial production of this fungal enzyme from this organism is not possible as it synthesizes in very low amounts. Thus the gene that encodes for this lipolase was initially

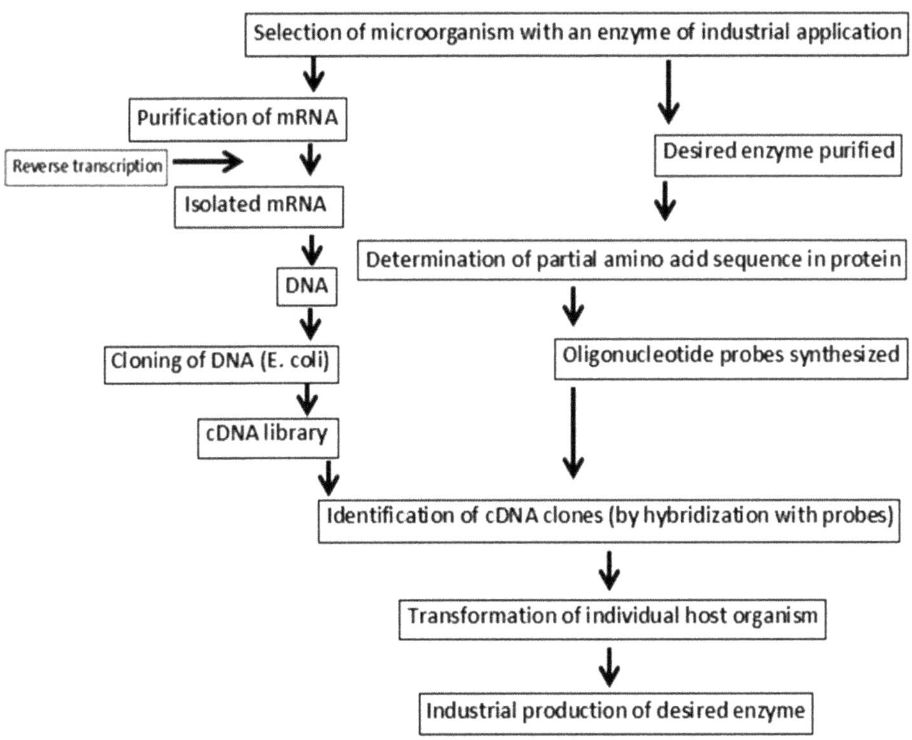

Figure 4.2. Cloning for the industrial production of enzymes.

identified and then separated, cloned and finally incorporated into *A. oryzae* to produce multiple copies [16]. By following this approach, commercial production of this enzyme can be positively attained. One of the most appreciated features of lipolase is its stability and resistance against degradation by the proteases that are usually employed in the detergent industry. These features make lipolase a good candidate for applications in the fabric and detergent industry.

- Rennet (major component is chymosin) is a milk clotting enzyme that can be isolated from different sources, in particular the stomach of a young calf. Generally, rennet is considered as combination of various enzymes, in particular chymosin, which is added to raw milk in the cheese industry to produce cheese. Usually this process involves curd cutting and fractional exclusion of the whey. Afterwards the prepared cubes are allowed to ripen in the whey until they change into slim blocks. Chymosin is extensively utilized commercially, in particular in cheese manufacturing [3]. Its commercial preparation also includes other proteases; bovine pepsin is usually present in varying concentrations. To meet the market requirements commercial production should be high. Unfortunately, using earlier or existing approaches it is not possible to produce the high amounts of rennet for the market demand. Therefore, using a cloning method, in particular by exploring the genes responsible for the production of chymosin, can be considered as a potential approach for its industrial production.

4.4 Protein studies for modification of commercial enzymes

By protein engineering and site-directed mutagenesis, it is now possible to modify the structure of a protein/enzyme. In enzyme research, most of the modifications in the enzymes are carried out to enhance enzyme stability, which can further improve its catalytic function. Modification also allows the development of degradation and oxidation resistant enzymes. Moreover, structural modification of enzymes can change their substrate preference and improve tolerance against alkali and organic solvents [15]. There are number of approaches available to achieve the aforementioned objective, one of the most common is site-directed mutagenesis. Enzymes can be redesigned by using site-directed mutagenesis. This requires the systematic alteration of protein structure by rDNA technology and chemical synthesis of DNA fragments to allow the superficial modification of proteins by site specific mutagenesis of their genes. Thus mutated genes can be utilized to produce enzymes with improve yield and novel properties. Kinetic investigation of mutant enzymes with high-resolution structural data from protein x-ray crystallography can be utilized to draw the relationships between structure and function [17]. In particular, the strength and nature of enzyme–substrate interactions and their roles in catalysis and specificity may be examined [17].

During mutagenesis a number of amino acids present in the target enzyme at a particular site are allowed to modify to produce an enzyme with desirable features, e.g. structural modification of phospholipase A2 by using fundamental knowledge of protein engineering to resist elevated concentrations of acid. This modification allows its efficient utilization as a food emulsifier. Commercial preparation of phospholipase A2 is mainly produced from the pancreas for the further production of lysolecithin. This allows its extensive utilization as an excellent emulsifier for the food, cosmetics and pharmaceutical industries. Most eukaryotic proteins are N-terminally altered by one or more processing enzymes. Enzymes acting on the very first amino acid of a polypeptide include different peptidases, transferases and ligases [18].

The tyrosyl–tRNA synthetase from *Bacillus stearothermophilus* is being scientifically examined by site-directed mutagenesis. A fine-structure inspection is revealing the subtle roles of hydrogen bonding in catalysis and specificity [17]. Alteration of the residues that hydrogen-bond with ATP and tyrosine display how the energetics must be examined in terms of an exchange reaction with solvent water. Based on this knowledge, and structural data, an enzyme of vastly improved enzyme–substrate affinity has been engineered [17].

4.5 Enzyme and cell immobilization

Usually, enzymes in free solutions (i.e., in soluble or free form) react with substrates to yield final products. This type of enzyme utilization is inefficient, mainly for large-scale production, as enzymes are not stable and they cannot be recovered for reuse.

Enzymes or cells immobilization emerged as a technique of confining/anchoring the enzymes or cells in or on an (inert) support for their stability and functional reuse. By means of this technique, the enzymes produced are more effective and economical for large-scale use. A number of researchers referred to immobilization as 'the goose that lays the golden egg' in enzyme technology. Immobilized enzymes retain their structural conformation necessary for catalysis. There are various benefits to immobilized enzymes:

- They are stable and more efficient in function.
- They can be reused repeatedly.
- Their products are enzyme-free.
- They are ideal for multi-enzyme reaction systems.
- The control of enzyme function is easy.
- They are appropriate for large-scale and therapeutic use.
- They reduce effluent disposal problems. There are, however, certain drawbacks related to immobilization:
- There is a possibility of loss of biological activity of an enzyme
- Immobilization is a costly process that frequently requires sophisticated equipment.

Immobilized enzymes are usually chosen over immobilized cells owing to their ability to produce the products in a pure form. However, there are numerous benefits to using immobilized multi-enzyme systems, e.g. organelles and whole cells, over immobilized enzymes.

4.6 Immobilization methods

The frequently used procedures for immobilization of enzymes are adsorption, entrapment, covalent binding and cross-linking.

4.6.1 Adsorption methods

Adsorption includes the physical binding of enzymes (or cells) on the surface of an inert support. The support materials may be inorganic (e.g. alumina, silica gel, calcium phosphate glass) or organic (starch, carboxymethyl cellulose, DEAE-cellulose, DEAE-sephadex). Adsorption of enzyme molecules on the inert support involves weak forces, e.g. van der Waals forces and hydrogen bonds (figure 4.3). Consequently, the adsorbed enzymes can be removed by minor changes in pH, ionic strength or temperature. This is a shortcoming for the large-scale utilization of enzymes.

4.6.2 Nonspecific adsorption

The immobilization procedure of nonspecific adsorption is generally based on physical adsorption or ionic binding [19, 20]. During physical adsorption the enzymes are attached to the matrix via hydrogen bonding, van der Waals forces, or hydrophobic interactions; while in ionic bonding the enzymes are bound via salt linkages. The types of forces present in noncovalent immobilization can be reversed by varying the conditions that affect the strength of the interaction (e.g. pH, ionic strength, temperature, or polarity of the solvent). Immobilization by adsorption is a gentle, easy to perform process, and generally conserves the catalytic activity of the enzyme. Such procedures are consequently economically attractive, but may suffer

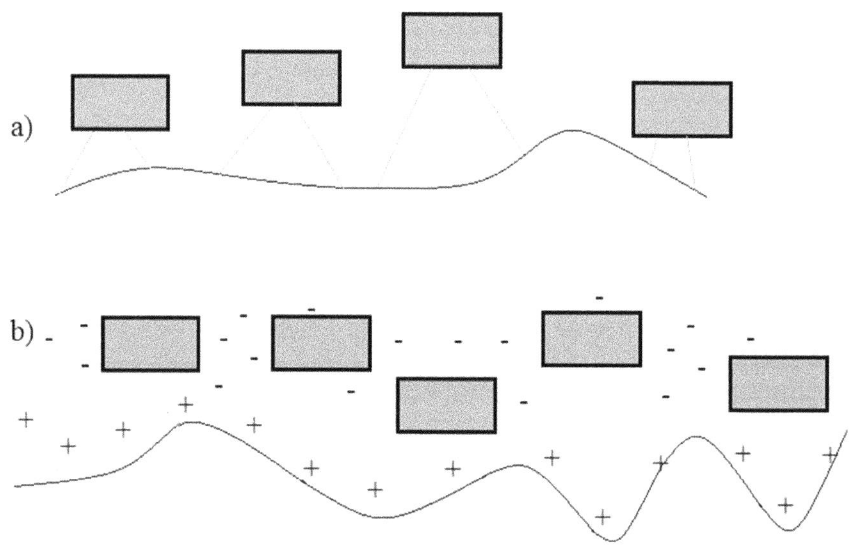

Figure 4.3. Immobilization of enzymes by absorption: (a) by van der Waals forces and (b) by hydrogen bonding.

from limitations, e.g. enzymes escape from matrix when the interactions are comparatively weak.

4.6.3 Ionic binding

One method for the reversible immobilization of enzymes is to use protein–ligand interactions based on the principles employed in chromatography. For instance, one of the first claims of chromatographic principles in the reversible immobilization of enzymes was the use of ion-exchangers [21, 22]. The procedure is simple and reversible, but it is generally challenging to discover conditions under which the enzyme remains both firmly bound and fully active. Currently, the use of immobilized polymeric-ionic ligands has permitted the modification of protein–matrix interactions and has thus enhanced the properties of the derivative. Some patents have been published on the use of polyethyleneimine to bind a rich variety of enzymes and whole cells [22]. However, issues may rise from the use of an extremely charged support when the substrates or products themselves are charged; the kinetics can be distorted resulting in partition or diffusion phenomena. Consequently, enzyme features, e.g. pH optimum or pH stability, may change [23, 24]. Although this could be a problem it could also be valuable to change the optimal conditions of a certain enzyme against more alkaline or acidic conditions, depending on the application [25].

4.6.4 Hydrophobic adsorption

Another approach is the use of hydrophobic interactions. During this procedure, it is not the development of chemical bonds but rather an entropically driven interaction that occurs. Hydrophobic adsorption has been employed as a chromatographic principle for more than three decades. It relies on well-known experimental variables such as pH, salt concentration and temperature [26]. The power of interaction relies on both the hydrophobicity of the adsorbent and the protein. The hydrophobicity of the adsorbent can be controlled by the degree of substitution of the support and by the size of the hydrophobic ligand molecule. The effective reversible immobilization of β-amylase and amyloglucosidase to hexyl-agarose carriers has been demonstrated [27, 28]. Several other examples of strong reversible binding to hydrophobic adsorbents have also been demonstrated [29, 30].

4.6.5 Affinity binding

The basis of affinity between complementary biomolecules has been applied to enzyme immobilization. The outstanding selectivity of the interaction is a key benefit of the procedure. However, the method often needs the covalent binding of a costly affinity ligand (e.g. antibody, or lectin) to the matrix [31, 32].

4.6.6 Entrapment method

By means of physical entrapment enzymes can be easily immobilized inside a polymer or a gel matrix. The size of the matrix pores is maintained in such a manner that the enzyme is retained, whereas the substrate and product molecules can easily pass through. During this procedure, also known as lattice entrapment, the enzyme (or cell) is not exposed against strong binding forces or structural distortions. During an immobilization process, the level of deactivation might be possible. This happens due to the fluctuations in pH or temperature or the addition of solvents. The matrices employed for entrapment of enzymes include polyacrylamide gel, collagen, gelatin, starch, cellulose, silicone and rubber. Enzymes can be entrapped in numerous ways. There are different approaches to entrapping enzymes such as gel [33] or fiber entrapping [34, 35] and microencapsulation [36, 37].

4.6.6.1 Enzyme inclusion in gels

This is achieved by enzyme entrapment inside gels (figure 4.4). The poly(vinyl alcohol) bearing styrylpyridinium groups (PVA-SbQ), a soluble pre-polymer bearing photo-cross-linkable group, has been used extensively to entrap enzymes, and numerous bioassays based on this immobilization matrix have been demonstrated [38, 39]. The sol–gel process was established on the capability to form solid metal or semi-metal oxides through the aqueous process of hydrolytically labile precursors. Enzymes can also be entrapped in an agarose gel [39]. In contrast to synthetic polymers, e.g. polyacrylamide, this matrix is biocompatible, nontoxic, provides a natural microenvironment to the enzyme and also offers adequate accessibility to electrons to shuttle between the enzyme and the electrode. The entrapment approaches are easy to perform, and allow the deposition of enzymes, mediators, and additives in the same sensing layer. Furthermore, the activity of the enzyme is conserved during the immobilization process, as the biological element is not altered [39]. Biosensors based on physically entrapped enzymes are frequently described by increased operational and storage stability.

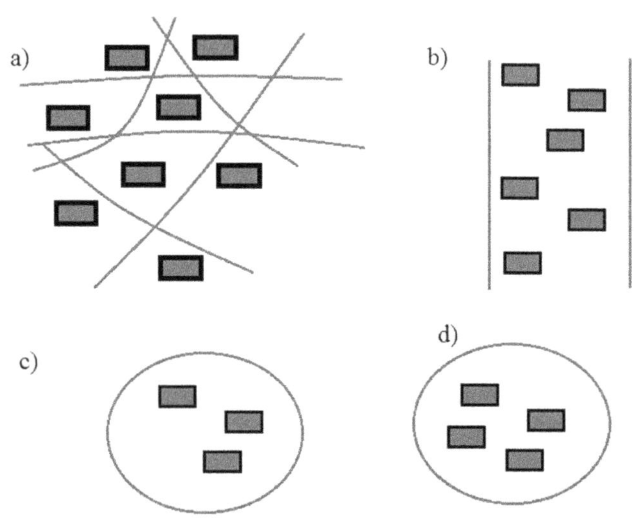

Figure 4.4. Immobilization of enzymes by entrapment. (a) Inclusion in gels. (b) Inclusion in fibers. (c) Inclusion in microcapsules.

4.6.6.2 Enzyme inclusion in fibers

Entrapment involves inclusion of an enzyme in a polymer network (gel lattice) such as an organic polymer, a silica sol–gel or a membrane device such as a hollow fiber or a microcapsule. Entrapment requires the synthesis of the polymeric network in the presence of the enzyme. The last step involves cross-linking of enzyme aggregates or crystals, using a bifunctional reagent, to prepare carrier-free macroparticles [40]. The enzymes are trapped in the fibers of the matrix.

4.6.6.3 Enzyme inclusion in microcapsules

During this procedure enzymes are trapped inside a microcapsule matrix (figure 4.4). The hydrophobic forms of the matrix polymerize to yield a microcapsule containing enzyme molecules [41]. The major limitation for entrapment of enzymes is the leakage from the matrix. Most of the researchers suggested utilizing this method of entrapment for immobilization of whole cells. Entrapped cells can be used in large-scale production of amino acids such as l-isoleucine, l-aspartic acid, l-malic acid and hydroquinone [41].

4.6.6.4 Micro-encapsulation

Micro-encapsulation is a kind of entrapment in which spherical particles in a liquid or suspension are enclosed in a semipermeable membrane [42]. The membrane may be polymeric, lipoidal, lipoprotein-based or non-ionic in nature. The three steps of microencapsulation are:

- Building superior membrane reactors.
- Formation of the emulsion.
- Stabilization of the emulsion to yield microcapsules [42].

Currently microencapsulation is employed for immobilization of enzymes and mammalian cells. For example, cultured pancreatic cells can be immobilized by microencapsulation; immobilized hybridoma cells have also been evidenced by this technique [43].

4.6.7 Covalent binding

Enzyme immobilization can be accomplished by formation of covalent bonds between the chemical groups of enzymes and the chemical groups of the support (figure 4.4). This procedure is extensively used. However, covalent binding is frequently linked with loss of some enzyme activity. Pretreatment (to form pre-activated support) of the inert support is typically required before it binds to an enzyme. The following are the common procedures of covalent binding. Immobilizations of proteins by procedures based on the formation of covalent bonds are among the most extensively used. A benefit of these procedures is that, because of the stable nature of the bonds developed between enzyme and the matrix, the enzyme is not released into the solution upon use. However, in order to attain high levels of bound activity, the amino acid residues vital for catalytic activity must not be involved in the covalent linkage to the support; this may prove a challenging condition to accomplish in some cases. A simple method that occasionally increases the activity yield is to perform the coupling reaction in the presence of substrate analogs [44]. Covalent methods for immobilization are used when there is a strict obligation for the absence of the enzyme in the product. An extensive range of reactions have been established depending on the functional groups accessible on the matrix [45]. Coupling procedures can generally be categorized in two main classes:

- Activation of the matrix by addition of a reactive function to a polymer.
- Alteration of the polymer backbone to synthesize an activated group.

The activation procedures are usually intended to make electrophilic groups on the support which, in the coupling step, react with the strong nucleophiles on the proteins. The basic principles governing the course of covalent coupling to the matrices are similar to those used for the chemical alteration of proteins. The most often used reactions include the following side chains of the amino acids: lysine (ε-amino group), cysteine (thiol group), and aspartic and glutamic acids (carboxylic group).

- *Cyanogen bromide activation:* The inert support materials such as cellulose, sepharose and sephadex enclosing glycol groups are activated by CNBr, which at that time binds to enzymes and immobilizes them (figure 4.5).
- *Diazotation:* A number of the support materials (aminobenzyl cellulose, amino derivatives of polystyrene, aminosilanized porous glass) are exposed to diazotation on treatment with $NaNO_2$ and HCI. They, in return, bind covalently to tyrosyl or histidyl groups of enzymes (figure 4.5).
- *Peptide bond formation*: Enzyme immobilization can also be achieved by the development of peptide bonds between the amino (or carboxyl) groups of the support and the carboxyl (or amino) groups of enzymes (figure 4.5). The support material is initially chemically treated to form active functional groups.
- *Activation by bi- or polyfunctional reagents*: A number of reagents, e.g. glutaraldehyde, can be used to build bonds between the amino groups of the enzymes and the amino groups of the support (such as aminoethylcellulose, albumin, amino alkylated porous glass). This is represented in figure 4.6.

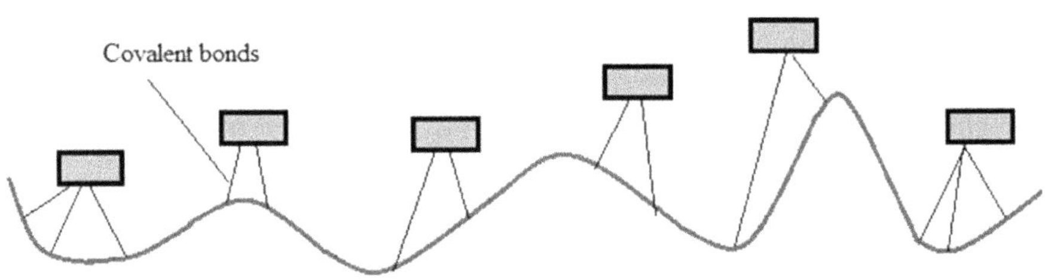

Figure 4.5. A general representation of the immobilization of enzymes by covalent binding.

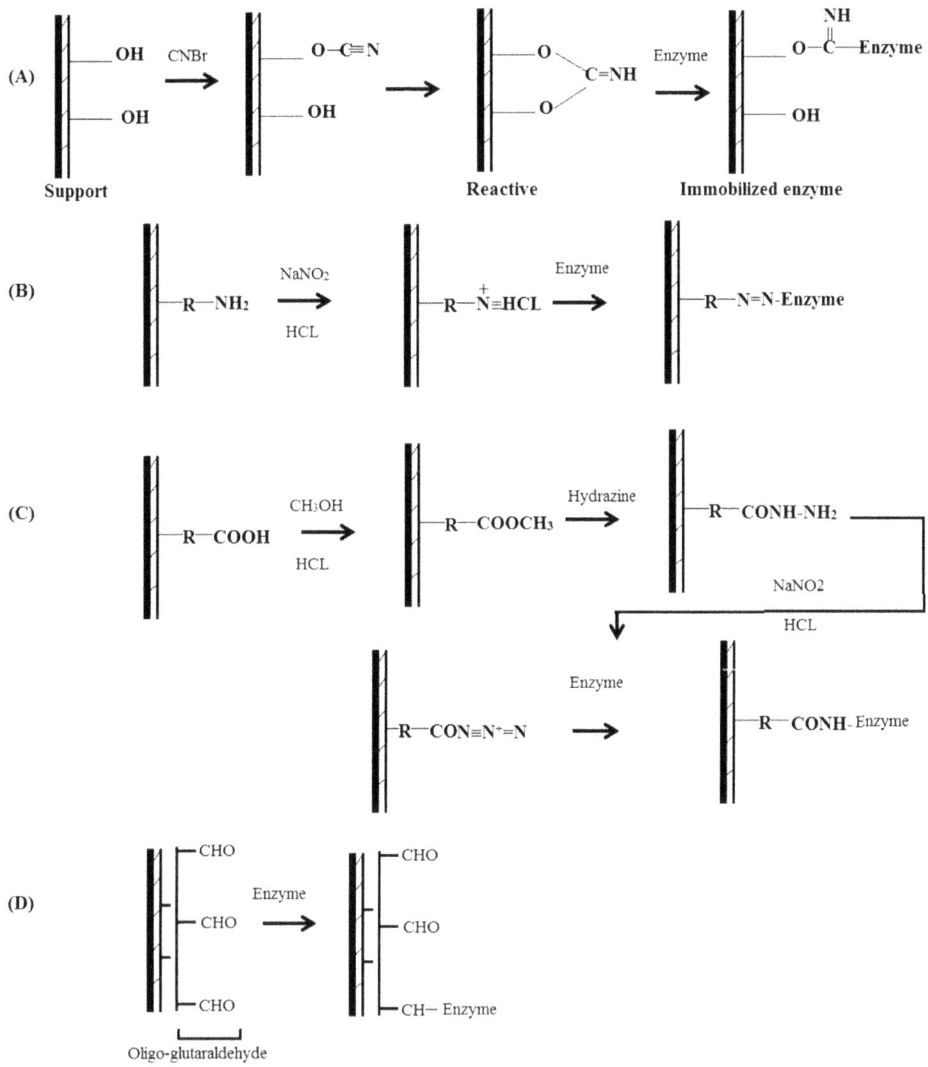

Figure 4.6. Immobilization of enzymes by covalent binding: (a) cyanogen bromide activation, (b) diazotation, (c) peptide bond formation and (d) activation by bifunctional agent.

4.6.8 Cross-linking

A characteristic feature of the immobilization of enzymes by cross-linking is the lack of a solid support. The enzyme molecules are immobilized by building cross-links between them, and by the participation of polyfunctional reagents. In fact, these reagents react with the enzyme and make bridges which further form the support to hold enzyme molecules (figure 4.7). There are a number of reagents used for cross-linking. These include glutaraldehyde, diazobenzidine, hexamethylene diisocyanate

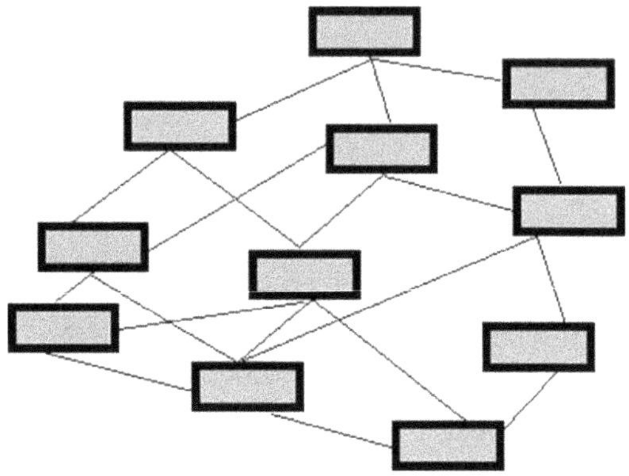

Figure 4.7. Immobilization of enzyme molecules by cross-linking.

and toluene di-isoth iocyanate. Glutaraldehyde is the most frequently used cross-linking reagent [38]. It successfully reacts with lysyl residues of the enzymes and finally yields a Schiff's base. The cross-links developed between the enzyme and glutaraldehyde are irreversible and can tolerate extreme pH and temperature. Glutaraldehyde cross-linking has been effectively utilized to immobilize a number of industrial enzymes such as glucose isomerase and penicillin amidase [38]. The method of cross-linking is very simple and cost-effective, but the drawback is that it includes the possibility of enzyme denaturation by the polyfunctional reagent.

4.7 Choice of immobilization technique

Selection of a particular procedure for immobilization of enzymes is based on a trial and error approach to select the perfect one. The enzyme catalytic activity, stability, regenerability and cost are the most important factors that decide a technique.

4.7.1 Immobilization of l-amino acid acylase

Japanese researchers [46] discovered the first enzyme immobilized on a matrix, known as l-amino acid acylase. Later, a number of immobilization procedures were attempted by these researchers, but only three showed promising results. These were:

- Covalent binding to iodoacetyl cellulose.
- Ionic binding to DEAE-sephadex.
- Entrapment with *n* polyacrylamide.

4.7.2 Stabilization of soluble enzymes

Enzyme stabilization is essential for any biomedical or industrial application of enzymes. In several applications, the objective is to deliver a prolonged active lifetime under normal environmental conditions with traditional substrates at low concentrations in buffered solutions [47]. However, as enzymes are being employed for more and more applications, there is a need to use them under extreme environmental conditions (i.e., high temperatures), in high substrate concentrations and in nontraditional solvent systems [47]. Certain enzymes cannot be immobilized as they should be used in soluble form, for example, enzymes used in liquid detergents, some diagnostic reagents and food additives. With the aid of a number of additives or by chemical modifications these enzymes can be stabilized. The stabilized enzymes have longer half-lives, although they cannot be recycled. Several significant procedures for enzyme stabilization are briefly described in the following [47]:

- *Solvent stabilization*: Some solvents at low concentrations stabilize the enzymes, whereas at high concentrations the enzymes become denatured, e.g. acetone (5%) ethanol (5%) can stabilize benzyl alcohol dehydrogenase.
- *Substrate stabilization*: By adding substrates the active site of an enzyme can be stabilized, e.g. starch stabilizes α-amylase; glucose stabilizes glucose isomerase.
- *Stabilization by polymers*: This type of stabilization can be achieved by the addition of polymers, such as gelatin, albumin and polyethylene, particularly at increased temperatures.
- *Stabilization by salts*: Metalloenzymes stability of can be attained by supplementing salts, e.g. Ca, Fe, Mn, Cu and Zn. Proteases are commonly stabilized by the addition of calcium.
- *Stabilization by chemical modifications*: During this procedure, enzymes can be stabilized by appropriate chemical modifications without loss of biological activity. There are different types of chemical modifications:– Addition of polyamino side chains, such as polytyrosine.
  - Acylation of enzymes by adding groups, e.g. acetyl, propionyl and succinyl.
- *Stabilization by rebuilding*: Ideally, enzyme stability is dependent on the hydrophobic interactions in the core of the enzyme. It was thus suggested that enzymes can be stabilized by increasing hydrophobic interactions. For this reason, the enzyme is initially unfolded and later rebuilt in one of the following ways (see figure 4.8):– The enzyme can be chemically treated (e.g. using urea and a disulfide) and then refolded.
  - The refolding can be done in the presence of low molecular weight ligands.
  - For certain enzymes, refolding at higher temperatures (around 50 °C) stabilizes them.
- *Stabilization by site-directed mutagenesis*: Site-directed mutagenesis has been fruitfully used to synthesize more stable and functionally more efficient enzymes such as subtilisin E.

4.8 Immobilization of cells

A single-step reaction procedure is suitable for the immobilization of an individual cell, but is not appropriate for multienzymes or for reactions demanding co-factors. During this procedure whole cells or cellular organelles can be immobilized, yielding a system which acts as a source for various enzymes, and hence is referred to as a multi-enzyme system. Furthermore, immobilized cells rather than enzymes are often favored even for single reactions, owing to the cost factor in isolating enzymes.

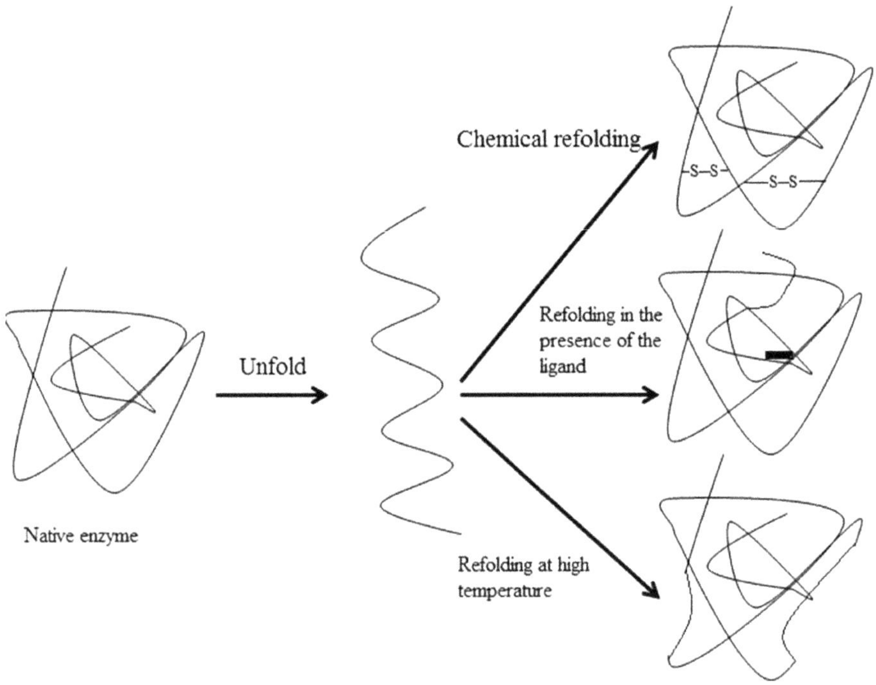

Figure 4.8. Stabilization of an enzyme by refolding.

For those enzymes which are dependent on the spacial arrangement of the membrane for their activity, cell immobilization is ideal. There are several significant applications of immobilized enzymes, for example, they are traditionally used for the treatment of sewage. The procedures used for the immobilization of cells are almost the same as those employed for the immobilization of enzymes, with appropriate modifications. Techniques such as entrapment and surface attachment are frequently used. Gels, and to some extent membranes, are also used.

4.8.1 Immobilization of viable cells

By means of gentle immobilization it is possible to preserve the viability of the cells. These immobilized cells are mainly useful for fermentation. Occasionally, mammalian cell cultures are made to function as immobilized viable cells.

4.8.2 Immobilized non-viable cells

In most cases, immobilized non-viable cells are considered over enzymes or even viable cells. This is primarily because of the expensive isolation and purification procedures. An excellent example is the immobilization of cells producing glucose isomerase for the large-scale production of high-fructose syrup.

4.8.3 Drawbacks of immobilizing eukaryotic cells

Prokaryotic cells (mainly bacterial) are generally used for immobilization. According to various reports it is also possible to immobilize eukaryotic plant and animal cells. Owing to the presence of cellular organelles, the metabolism of eukaryotic cells is slow. Consequently, for the large-scale production of biochemicals, prokaryotic cells are considered. However, for the synthesis of complex proteins (e.g. immuno-globulins) and for proteins that experienced post-translational modifications, eukaryotic cells may be used.

4.8.4 The effect of immobilization on enzyme properties

Cell immobilization is often linked to modifications in enzyme properties, particularly the kinetic properties of enzymes. Some of these are as follows:

- A considerable reduction in enzyme specificity. This may be because of conformational changes that take place when the enzyme becomes immobilized.
- The kinetic constants (K_m and V_{max}) of an immobilized enzyme differ from those of the innate enzyme. This is because of the conformational modifications of the enzyme which may further affect the affinity between the enzyme and substrate.

4.8.5 Immobilized enzyme reactors

Immobilized enzyme cells are exploited for large-scale production in the form of enzyme reactors [43]. They are generally of two types: batch reactors and continuous reactors. The frequently used enzyme reactors are depicted in figure 4.9.

Batch reactors. In these types of reactors, the immobilized enzymes and substrates are employed, and the reaction is allowed to start under constant stirring. As the reaction is finished, the product is isolated from the enzyme (typically by denaturation). Soluble enzymes are frequently used in batch reactors. It is somewhat challenging to isolate the soluble enzymes from the products, therefore, there is the drawback of their reuse. Special procedures have been developed for the recovery of soluble enzymes, which may occasionally result in loss of enzyme activity [48].

Stirred tank reactors. The most modest form of batch reactor is the stirred tank reactor (figure 4.9). It is composed of a reactor fixed with a stirrer that permits good mixing, and a suitable temperature and pH control. However, in this system there may be loss of some enzyme activity. The basket reactor is a modification of the stirred tank reactor. In this method, the enzyme is retained over the impeller blades. Both the stirred tank reactor and basket reactor have a well-mixed flow pattern [48].

Plug flow type reactors. These reactors are alternatives to flow pattern type reactors. The flow rate of fluids can be regulated by a plug system. Plug flow type reactors are available in the form of packed-bed or fluidized-bed reactors (figure 4.9). These reactors are mainly useful when flow type reactors furnish insufficient product formation. Moreover, plug flow reactors are also beneficial for obtaining kinetic data on the reaction systems [48].

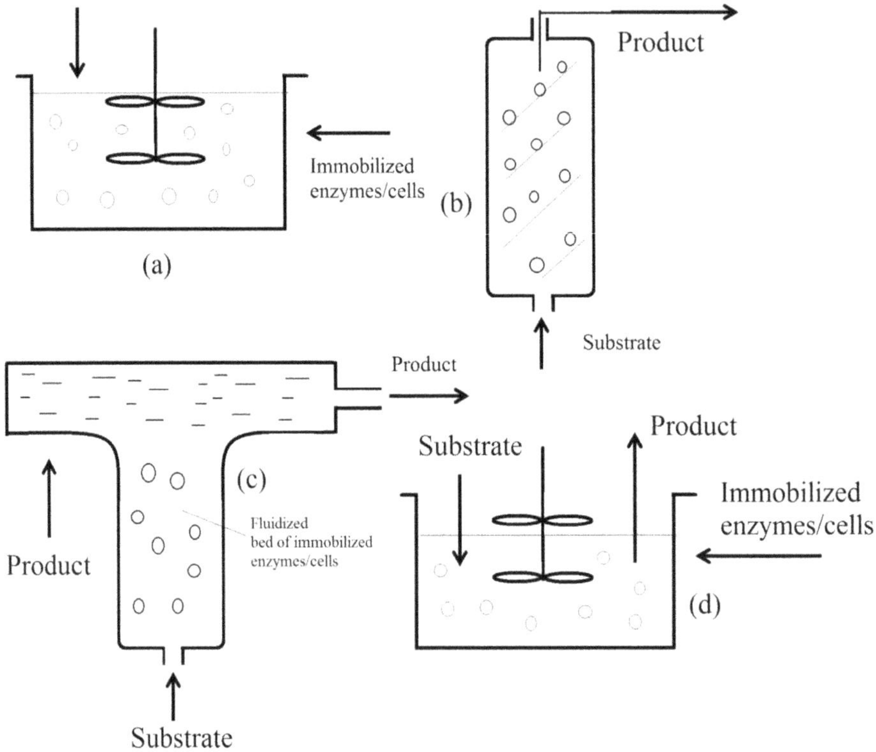

Figure 4.9. Immobilized enzyme/cell reactors: (a) batch stirred tank reactor, (b) packed-bed reactor, (c) fluidized-bed reactor and (d) continuous stirred tank reactor.

Continuous reactors. During this procedure the substrate is supplemented constantly, whereas the product is eliminated. Immobilized enzymes can also be employed for continuous operation. Continuous reactors have certain merits over batch reactors. These entail regulation over the product formation, suitable operation of the system and easy automation of the whole procedure. There are two main types of continuous reactors: the continuous stirred tank reactor (CSTR) and plug reactor (PR) [49]. A schematic depiction of CSTR is shown in figures 4.9 and 4.10. CSTR is suitable for good quality product formation.

Membrane reactors. A number of membranes with an array of chemical compositions can be used. Polysulfone, polyamide and cellulose acetate are the most often used materials for membranes. The biocatalysts (enzymes or cells) are usually retained on the membranes of the reactor. The substrate is added into reactor while the product passes out. Good mixing in the reactor can be attained using a stirrer (figure 4.10). In a continuous membrane reactor, the biocatalysts are held on membrane layers over which substrate molecules are passed (figure 4.10). In a recycle model membrane reactor, the contents, i.e., the solution containing enzymes, co-factors, and substrates, along with freshly released product, are recycled by using a pump (figure 4.10). The product passes out of the system and can be recovered [43–45].

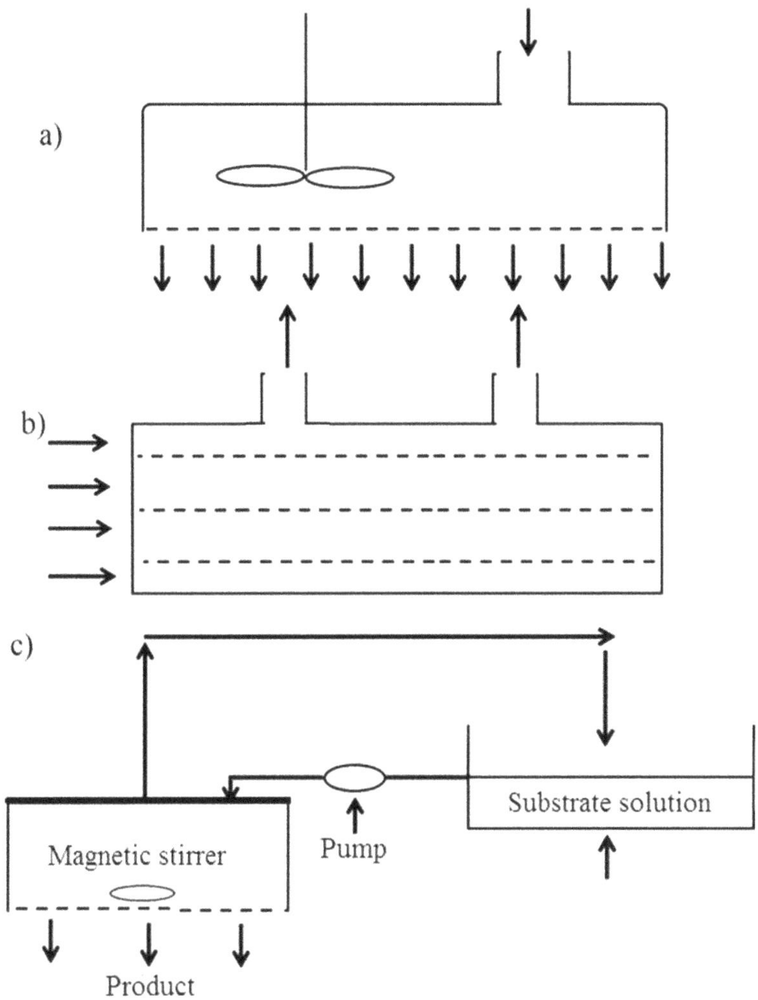

Figure 4.10. Membrane reactors: (a) batch membrane reactor, (b) continuous membrane reactor and (c) recycle membrane reactor (coloured lines indicate membranes).

4.8.6 Applications of immobilized enzymes and cells

Immobilized enzymes and cells are extensively utilized for industrial, analytical and therapeutic applications, including their utilization in food production and research in biochemistry, microbiology and other allied sciences [50]. A summary of industrial applications of immobilized cells is provided in table 4.2.

4.9 Manufacture of commercial products

A list of significant immobilized enzymes and their industrial applications is mentioned in table 4.2. Further details on the production of L-amino acids and high-fructose syrup are mentioned below.

Table 4.2. A selected list of important immobilized enzymes and their industrial applications.

Immobilized enzyme	Applications
β-Galactosidase	Splitting of lacrosse to glucose and galactose.
Ribonuclease	Synthesis of nucleotides from RNA.
Penicillin acylase	Commercial production of semi-synthetic penicillins.
Nitrilase	Production of acrylamide from acrylonitrile.
Invertase	Splitting of sucrose to glucose and fructose.
Histidine ammonia lyase	Production of urocanic acid from histidine.
Glucose isomerase	Production of high-fructose syrup from glucose (or starch).
Fumarase	Synthesis of malic acid from fumaric acid.
Aspartase	Production of aspartic acid from fumaric acid.
Amylase	Production of glucose from starch.
Aminocyclase	Production of l-amino acids from d, l-acyl amino acids.

4.9.1 Production of l-amino acids

l-Amino acids (and not d-amino acids) are very important for use in food and feed supplements and therapeutic applications [49, 51]. The chemical methods used for their production result in a racemic mixture of d- and l-amino acids. They can be acylated to yield d, l-acyl amino acids. The immobilized enzyme aminocyclase (frequently immobilized on DEAE-sephadex) can selectively hydrolyze d, l-acyl amino acids to produce l-amino acids.

$$\text{D, L-acyl amino acids} \longrightarrow \text{L-amino acids} + \text{D, L-acyl amino acids}$$

The free l-amino acids can be separated from the unhydrolysed d-acyl amino acids. The latter can be racemized to d, l-acyl amino acids and recycled via an enzyme reactor containing immobilized amnocyclase. Large amounts of l-methionine, l-phenylalanine, l-tryptophan and l-valine are produced worldwide using this method.

4.9.2 Production of high-fructose syrup

Among the monosacharaides, fructose is the sweetest, and has doubled the sweetening strength of sucrose. Glucose is about 75% as sweet as sucrose. Thus, glucose (the most abundant monosaccharide) cannot be a good replacement for sucrose for sweetening. Therefore, there is a great demand for fructose which is very sweet, but has a similar calorific value to that of glucose or sucrose. High-fructose syrup (HFS) contains about equivalent amounts of glucose and fructose. From the nutritional point of view high-fructose syrup is similar to sucrose [52]. High-fructose syrup is a good replacement for sugar in the manufacturing of soft drinks, processed foods and baking. High-fructose syrup can be manufactured from glucose by using an immobilized glucose isomerase. The starch-containing raw materials (wheat, potato, corn) are exposed to hydrolysis to produce glucose. Glucose isomerase then

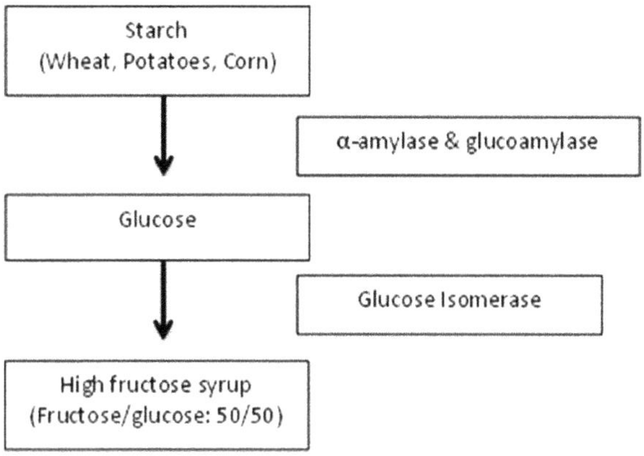

Figure 4.11. The production of high-fructose syrup from starch with glucose isomerase as the immobilized enzymes.

isomerises glucose to fructose (figure 4.11). The ultimate product formed is high-fructose syrup comprising 50% fructose.

4.9.2.1 Glucose isomerase

Glucose isomerase is an intracellular enzyme synthesized by several microorganisms. Species of *Arthrobacter*, *Bacillus* and *Streptomyces* are the preferred sources. As it is an intracellular enzyme, the separation of glucose isomerase without the loss of biological activity involves specialized and expensive methods. Often, whole or partly broken cells are immobilized and used [17].

4.9.3 Immobilized enzyme and cell analytical applications

4.9.3.1 In biochemical analysis

Immobilized enzymes (or cells) can be employed for the advancement of precise and specific analytical methods for the determination of several compounds. The main principle of analytical assays involves the action of the enzyme on the substrate. A decrease in the substrate concentration, an increase in the product or an alteration in the co-factor concentration can be used for the assay. Two types of detectors are commonly employed, thermistors and electrode devices.

Thermistors are heat measuring devices which can analyze the heat produced in an enzyme-calibrated reaction. Electrode devices are employed for determining potential differences in the reaction systems. In figure 4.12 an enzyme thermistor, enzyme electrode and a urease electrode are shown.

4.9.3.2 Affinity chromatography and purification

Proteins purification by traditional methods is often tedious and partial, and the yields are often low. Earlier isolation of enzyme is limited to certain concepts such as:

- its specific biological property;
- its reversible association capability with specific substrates;
- its reversible association capability with specific inhibitors.

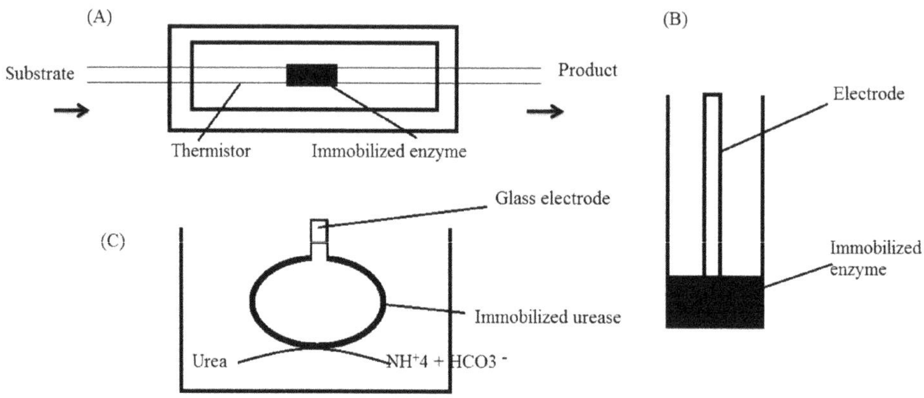

Figure 4.12. Immobilized enzymes or cells in analytical biochemistry. (a) Enzyme thermistor. (b) Enzyme electrode. (c) Urease electrode.

During affinity chromatography, the desired enzyme considered for the purification is allowed to pass through a column which usually contains a cross-linked polymer or gel. This specific competitive enzyme is covalently attached with polymer or gel present in the column. Enzymes without considerable affinity for the bound inhibitor present in the polymeric or gel matrix will pass directly or spontaneously through the column, whereas those that have substantial affinity, recognize the inhibitor and form in a complex way and are eventually retained by the matrix. Elution of complex or bound enzymes can be achieved by altering certain factors such as salt concentration or pH, or by addition of a competitive inhibitor in solution. Generally, the matrix is usually inert in nature, i.e., it shows minimal interaction with proteins, both before and after coupling to the specific binding group such as substrate or inhibitors. For affinity chromatography, the adsorbent must have a number of promising characteristics. A loose and porous matrix or gel allows easy entry and exit of macromolecules. Additionally, it also retains suitable flow properties during use. The chemical nature of the matrix must allow the suitable and extensive attachment of the particular ligand under mild conditions. This will only happen with chemical bonds that are stable to the conditions of adsorption and elution.

Affinity chromatography can be employed in several applications such as purification of nucleic acid and protein from cell free extracts and blood. Based on the property of affinity it is possible to purify several compounds e.g. antigens, antibodies and co-factors.

4.10 Immobilized enzymes for biomedical applications

The investigation of immobilized enzymes for biomedical purposes was initiated during the 1960s. The primary goal was to improve the stability of enzymes, lower their immunogenicity and toxicity, and increase their time in circulation in living organisms to be used clinically [53]. Since then, various approaches have been utilized in enzyme treatment. These methodologies have been employed for several objectives, encompassing the detection of bioactive compounds for disease diagnosis, and managing certain ailments. Fixing innate metabolic problems, heart problems, cancer, intestinal problems, and managing alcoholism are some examples of these kinds of conditions. There are two different ways that enzymes have been immobilized. The initial technique involves the immobilization of the enzyme through cross-linking or covalent attachment to a scaffold, commonly known as the process of immobility by attaching [54]. The second methodology is around the confinement of the enzyme within a matrix, commonly referred to as immobilization via inclusion. Polymer conjugation has emerged as a leading method for immobilization via binding, attracting a lot of attention in recent years. Enzyme immobilization is a process that could be accomplished with a wide variety of polymers. It is important to keep in mind, though, that the strict standards needed for a biological application make it very hard to test a lot of polymers. For the enzyme immobilization process, the polymers used should be completely biocompatible and biodegradable. They should also be very pure and have a regular distribution of molecular weights. Furthermore, it is crucial to consider that the covalent bonding of enzymes to polymers might result in alterations in molecular structure and a significant decrease in enzymatic functionality [55]. Polyethylene glycol (PEG) is currently a highly favored polymer for the purpose of modifying peptides and proteins that possess therapeutic promise PEG possesses several advantageous characteristics, including its cost-effectiveness, biocompatibility, non-toxicity, and existing approval by drug regulatory bodies. Pegylation can enhance the characteristics of enzymes without compromising their enzymatic performance, rendering them suitable for applications as protein-based pharmaceuticals or as catalysts in bioreactors. Currently, several enzyme/PEG conjugates are employed in clinical settings. Villard provides a comprehensive list of these conjugates in a recent review [56], which includes recombinant human tissue-plasminogen activator, adenosine deaminase, arginine deaminase, and asparaginase [57]. The methods of immobilization by inclusion offer several advantages compared to those employed for immobilization by binding. Firstly, there is no requirement for enzyme derivatization. A photobioreactor system powered by solar energy is depicted in figure 4.13.

Additionally, these systems afford a greater level of protection against enzymatic degradation and other detrimental factors. Furthermore, they enable higher drug loads to be accommodated. Finally, enzymes could be fixed in a more stable manner inside various systems, such as multi-enzyme networks, groups of enzymes, or the cells responsible for producing a particular enzyme [58].

Nevertheless, the implementation of inclusion methods is accompanied by certain drawbacks associated with the utilization of synthetic materials. However, these concerns can be addressed by employing biodegradable polymers, Examples of polymers and co-polymers that can be generated from lactic and glycolic acid, alginate, and chitosan are commonly utilized in many academic and scientific applications. In addition, the application of biodegradable anchoring transporters, like liposomes or red blood cells, presents an acceptable replacement method. Liposomes have been widely investigated as particle drug carriers and have been

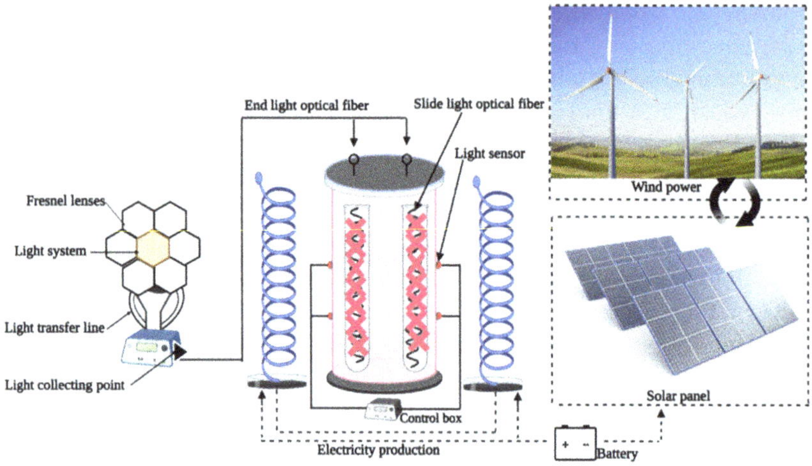

Figure 4.13. A diagram illustrating a photobioreactor system powered by solar energy. This system includes an internal light source, where optical fibers are excited by sunlight collected through a system, as well as a multi-LED light source powered by electricity generated from solar panels and a wind power generator.

found to possess highly favorable features for the encapsulation of polypeptides. Liposomes are nano-sized vesicles that consist of phospholipid bilayers resembling cell membranes, which enclose compartments filled with water-based solutions [59]. These substances exhibit biological inertness biocompatibility and induce little toxic or antigenic responses. Liposomal encapsulation of enzymes can increase their *in vivo* circulation through the bloodstream.

Additionally, liposomes can effectively conceal the antigen determinants of enzymes, hence mitigating the occurrence of undesirable immunological reactions. Controlled-release systems composed of biodegradable polymers, such as nanoparticles, present a viable alternative to liposomes [60]. Micro/nanoparticles refer to polymeric colloidal systems with sizes ranging from 10 nm to micrometers, wherein the drug is dissolved, entrapped, encapsulated, or adsorbed. Nanoparticles possess various desirable characteristics, including their ability to be formulated, sustained release capabilities, subcellular size, and compatibility with tissue and cells. These attributes make nanoparticles a potentially advantageous solution for immobilizing enzymes and protein medicines. Asparaginase, an enzyme that has garnered significant attention from researchers, has been immobilized on several supports. The enzyme L-asparaginase facilitates hydrolyzing L-asparagine, classified as an essential amino acid, into L-aspartic acid and ammonia. Leukemic cells that do not possess asparagine synthase cannot sustain their life [61]. L-asparaginase administration results in a fast reduction of extracellular asparagine, hence inducing targeted apoptosis of leukemic cells. Cells possessing the capacity to synthesize asparagine intracellularly exhibit heightened resistance to the cytotoxic effects of L-asparaginase.

In the treatment of leukemia, L-asparaginase therapy is often used. This treatment is generally administered with vincristine, daunomycin, methotrexate, or cyclophosphamide. The treatment effectively lowers the level in the blood of the amino acids, hence impeding the method of protein formation [62]. In normal use,

L-asparaginase is often created by *Escherichia coli* or *Erwinia chrysanthemums*. Asparaginase has shown promise in the therapy of lymphoblastic lymphoma and other lymphoid tumors in children, according to the results of many recent clinical studies. Despite its usage, L-asparaginase for treating acute lymphoblastic leukemia (ALL) is not as successful as other options [63]. Because of the short duration of its half-life *in vivo*, it must be administered by many injections before the desired therapeutic enzyme levels may be achieved. When L-asparaginase is administered, immunological adverse effects are a possibility as well. These can range from mild allergic responses to anaphylactic shock. These side effects happen because the enzyme is a foreign protein in people. This is especially true when given repeatedly to reach therapeutic enzyme levels. As a result, a significant amount of research has been undertaken in recent years to investigate alternative medicines or prospective substitutes for L-asparaginase. One of the ways investigated in clinical settings, which has demonstrated favorable outcomes in terms of reduced immunogenicity and extended half-life, involves the utilization of PEG for binding purposes. This technique has led to the developing of a novel molecule known as pegaspargase [64]. The technique has been approved by the US Food and Drug Administration (FDA) and is commercially available under the trade name Oncaspar. This alteration leads to a reduced delivery frequency and yields a less immunogenic response. However, several authors caution against the systematic replacement of L-asparaginase with pegaspargase due to a potential increase in pancreatitis linked to pegaspargase [65].

4.11 Detecting biomass with immobilized cells via bioluminescence and other biosensor uses

4.11.1 Bioluminescence

The incident of bioluminescence was initially documented over one hundred years ago, with its original observation being made in fireflies. The enzyme responsible for facilitating the oxidative reaction that produces light was subsequently identified and dubbed luciferase:

$$\text{Luciferin} + O_2 \xrightarrow{\text{luciferase}} \text{Oxyluciferin} + CO_2 + \text{AMP} + \text{light}$$

Subsequently, many more bioluminescent creatures were discovered, encompassing many taxa such as fish and microbes. The reaction 'luciferase', as depicted in the above equation, employs adenosine triphosphate (ATP) as a substrate for light production. However, in the case of marine luminous bacteria, reduced flavin is utilized instead of ATP [66]. Bioluminescent bacteria are naturally occurring microorganisms that inhabit many ecological niches, encompassing marine and terrestrial ecosystems. In addition to the utilization of naturally occurring microorganisms, genetically modified microbes are also employed in the development of bioluminescence-based biosensors. The process of mapping, isolating, and cloning the enzymes responsible for gene coding in bioluminescence was undertaken. Advancements in genetic technology have facilitated the transmission of bioluminescent properties to a diverse range of microbes. The utilization of genetically modified strains containing bioluminescent reporter plasmids is becoming significant in advancing microbial luminescent biosensors [67]. The initial documentation of the analytical utilization of bioluminescence emerged about a century ago, as Beijerinck elucidated the identification of oxygen produced during photosynthesis in leaf extract by employing luminescent bacteria. The utilization of bioluminescence as a basis for developing several biosensor approaches, both bioluminescent and chemiluminescent, has been seen. The practical uses of bioluminescence primarily lie in the advancement of instrumental approaches within the field.

1. The quantification of microbial and other cellular entities by assessing ATP levels [68].
2. The determination of active immobilized biomass, which encompasses the measurement of biologically active microorganisms attached to surfaces or within a matrix, critical for assessing the effectiveness of biofilm-based treatment systems
3. The primary focus of bioluminescence-based biosensors lies in their application within the field of environmental studies.

4.11.2 The measurement of biomass using bioluminescence-based techniques

The basis of bioluminescence has been expanded to encompass the detection of naturally nonluminescent species and fluorescent cells. The utilization of intracellular ATP, and perhaps other nucleotides, can facilitate luminescence production after introducing light-generating enzymes into the biological system. The initial studies focused on the quantification of biomass utilizing the principle of bioluminescence, and these investigations have been conducted for over three decades [69]. A comprehensive investigation examined the intracellular ATP levels in 19 distinct *E. coli* species. The results revealed a variation in ATP content, ranging from 0.29 to 8.7 × 11–10 μg of ATP per organism. Cell detection is often performed *in vitro*, relying on effectively extracting intracellular ATP while minimizing ATP hydrolysis. Following this, a light-generating system of luciferin and luciferase is introduced, and the resulting emitted light is quantified. Various substances have been examined for their efficacy in extracting ATP [70]. The range of substances includes solvents made from organic materials, inorganic acidic substances, and surfactants. Hence, examining ATP can be employed to identify microbial cells at exceedingly low concentration levels. The approach was modified to facilitate discerning various cellular classifications, encompassing bacterial constituents in liquids, microorganisms' mycobacteria, yeast cells, neoplastic cells, and other biological structures. The necessary components for the assay, namely luciferin and luciferase, can be readily obtained from commercial sources.

Additionally, commercial luminometers or other instruments capable of detecting light are also available for use in this context [71]. A recent study was undertaken to examine publicly accessible luminometers and imaging equipment specifically developed to conduct low-light level measurements. Other methods include using chromosome lux AB and GFP genes, which express bacterial luciferase and green fluorescent protein, accordingly, to observe cell number and metabolic performance directly. The relationship between bioluminescence output and cellular metabolic activity is attributed to the energy requirements of the metabolism [72].

4.11.3 Bioluminescence analysis for biomass captured in a microfluidic device

Estimating active immobilized biomass concentration using the luminometric approach is predicated on measuring ATP content within the cells. ATP functions as a vital chemical energy carrier within cells, wherein the energy is saved within the chemical bonds connecting the terminal phosphate groups. Following cellular demise, the quantity of ATP experiences a swift decline [73]. The ATP concentration relies on the quantity of active biomass, making it a reliable indication of cell viability. The determination of ATP concentration can be achieved by utilizing the bioluminescence method, as previously stated. The proper measurement necessitates the essential extraction of intracellular ATP. Various extraction procedures exist, and selecting an appropriate extractant is contingent upon the specific microbe under consideration [74]. The extraction protocol must effectively facilitate the complete release of nucleotides in a quantifiable manner while also ensuring the deactivation of any nucleotide changing enzymes that might be present within the halted cells. Ninety percent of the living cells that have been immobilized through entrapment within gel beads are concentrated within a 141 μm dense external layer of a 1.1 mm blob. Furthermore, it has been observed that these cells maintain over 91% of their activity following the immobilization process.

Consequently, the efficacy of ATP extraction from immobilized cells has been demonstrated [75]. While there is extensive literature on measuring free biomass using bioluminometry, a limited number of studies focus on estimating immobilized biomass with bioluminescence-based methods. The immobilized Benecken natriegens cells on silica particles were subjected to bioluminometry analysis to assess their content, which was then compared to the viability of the biomass in its free form. The determination of yeast biomass that has been immobilized in various ionotropic hydrogels has been documented in a published study. The experimental section comprehensively explains this specific procedure, serving as an informative scenario [76].

4.11.4 Biosensors relying on bioluminescence

The utilization of biosensor approaches that rely on bioluminescence and chemiluminescence has recently gained significant traction, mostly due to notable advancements in light sensing technology. The utilization of advanced photomultipliers and charge-coupled device (CCD) cameras enables highly efficient light detection. Furthermore, compared to other methodologies, contemporary instruments possess the advantageous characteristics of compactness, portability, and relative affordability. Luminometry has certain advantages compared to alternative optical techniques, namely its exceptional sensitivity and extensive dynamic range [77]. Luminometry exhibits a significantly higher level of sensitivity, reaching up to 105 times greater than absorption spectrometry. From a theoretical standpoint, detecting a single photon in a photomultiplier allows for potentially detecting a particular molecule of analyte or a separate cell. In practical applications, the efficiency of light detection may be limited.

Nevertheless, bioluminescent and chemiluminescent approaches have demonstrated the ability to detect minute quantities of analytes or organisms. The primary area of implementation for bioluminescence biosensors, which utilize immobilized intact cells, is the monitoring of the environment [78]. The detailed evaluation conducted by researchers focused on the applications of luminescence biosensors in environmental monitoring. Luminescence-based biosensor approaches have been widely employed in the surveillance of diverse organic and inorganic chemical pollutants. Numerous hazardous chemicals and environmental pollutants have the potential to disrupt energy metabolism and the electron transfer system in a general sense. The substances generate substrates that facilitate bioluminescence; hence, any disruption leads to observable consequences in the form of less luminescent activity [79]. The utilization of immobilized cells in luminescence biosensors has been the subject of recent publications. Given that bioluminescence relies on intracellular metabolism, it is reasonable to expect any alterations in bioluminescence to arise because of exposure to harmful substances that can enter the cell. The association between concentrations of active compounds is often unsatisfactory due to transport processes, and this correlation is typically highly particular to each system involving microorganisms and harmful compounds [80].

The immobilization procedures employed for bioluminescent cells are typically moderate approaches utilized in several other domains, which aim to maintain the vitality of the arrested cells. Another essential criterion is the optical characteristic of an immobilization substance, which should lead to a minimum reduction in bioluminescence intensity. Multiple immobilization materials and procedures were documented in the study, including alginate, agar, porous sol and gel glass, immobility on a gold surface, and various instances of immobilization on polyamide membranes. The utilization of bioluminescence biosensors holds significant promise in environmental monitoring due to its inherent simplicity and capacity to identify hazardous pollutants that pose risks to human health effectively. The bioluminescence approaches provide several key characteristics that render them highly appealing. The implementation is simple, and it can be used in portable field equipment. In contrast to other approaches, this one has an exceptionally high sensitivity and speed [81].

4.12 Bioluminescence-based microbial biosensors

Numerous methodologies have been devised in recent decades, establishing a foundation for the replacement of tissues and organs and the regulated and sustained delivery of therapeutic substances to the recipient. The process of encapsulating live cells refers to the technique of confining cells inside encapsulation systems that possess semipermeable properties [82]. These systems are fabricated using either naturally occurring or synthetic polymers and are specially designed to mitigate immune resistance. This biotechnology approach possesses two significant therapeutic potentials. Firstly, it involves the extended transplantation of bioactive compounds that can boost or revive normal tissue function. Secondly, it entails advancing and refining innovative drug delivery systems that enable the sustained release of therapeutic products over an extended period. Both approaches have a substantial influence in terms of therapy and economics. The utilization of a technologically optimized encapsulation system would effectively hinder the infiltration and subsequent destruction of encapsulated cells by antibodies and other immune cells [83]. Consequently, the continuous administration of immunosuppressant drugs could be minimized, leading to an improved quality of life for patients undergoing this therapeutic intervention. The first documented instances of cell transplantation within polymer matrices may be traced back to 1933, when Bisceglie conducted an experiment involving the introduction of tumor cells into a polymer framework, which was subsequently transplanted into a pig's abdominal cavity. During the 1960s, the term 'artificial cell' was used to describe the process of immuno-isolating cells and enzymes within microcapsules possessing semipermeable properties. Since that time, significant endeavors have been undertaken globally to enhance education in the fields of genetics, biology, science of polymers, and medicine [82]. Enhanced microcapsules with advanced technological features have been developed with the aim of enhancing the survivability and usefulness of encapsulated cells, while also improving their resistance to handling, transplantation, and stress within the host organism. Furthermore, a wide range of cell sources have been immobilized and evaluated as prospective drug-secreting entities. Based on the findings of many investigations, it has become evident that not all cells possess the necessary characteristics to be deemed acceptable for microencapsulation [82]. The proliferation of cells after encapsulation has the potential to completely occupy the capsular space, resulting in reduced effectiveness of therapeutic diffusion. This, in turn, may jeopardize the sustained viability of immobilized cells in the long run. In contrast, cell types that exhibit limited proliferation following encapsulation, such as myoblasts, possess the capacity to sustain the release of therapeutic agents over extended durations. It is worth noting that the application of the process of immobilizing transgenic cells from islets within alginate polylysine small capsules for the purpose of glucose control in diabetes has evolved beyond its initial implementation in the 1980s [84]. This biotechnological strategy has now been employed for various therapeutic purposes. Indeed, the efficacy of its medication delivery system and allogeneic transplantation has been effectively established in animal models for several diseases including cancer, haemophilia, and renal failure.

4.12.1 The microencapsulation process involves the utilization of polymers and cells

The effectiveness of the technology of cell microencapsulation relies heavily on the appropriate mix of its two primary components, namely cells and polymers. Numerous natural and synthetical polymers have been evaluated for their suitability as capsule matrices and outer membranes [85]. It is imperative that all these materials exhibit biocompatibility, ensuring that they do not disrupt the internal cellular balance or trigger an immune response from the host organism that could compromise the sustained effectiveness of the transplanted microcapsules. In addition, it is imperative that the microcapsules produced using these polymers have sufficient stability to withstand both mechanical stress and osmotic stress upon implantation [86]. Hence, it is imperative to meticulously choose the components that will comprise the ultimate composition of the immobilization apparatus.

Alginate, which consists of mannuronic and guluronic dimers, is widely used in scientific research due to its exceptional biocompatibility and biodegradability. Numerous investigations have been conducted to investigate the impact of alginate makeup, pureness, and concentration on encapsulated cells' viability and peptide synthesis. Typically, it is well accepted that the purification of alginates is of utmost importance to guarantee their biocompatibility [87]. However, there is ongoing discussion on the appropriateness of the monomer composition of the capsules. In recent times, there has been a notable advancement in the production of innovative materials, encompassing oligochitosans, cellulose sulfate, pectin, and various synthetic polymers. The application of a suitable semipermeable membrane to coat the produced capsule matrix is an area of research that is now gaining attention. The outer membrane will facilitate the bidirectional passage of nutrients, oxygen, and waste, while impeding the ingress of immune cells, antibodies, and other constituents of the immune response [88]. The membrane chemistry of Alginate-PLL complex has received much research attention, making it the most widely investigated. Nevertheless, alternate polycations such as polyethylene glycol, poly-vinyl alcohol, and poly-L-ornithine have also been examined in this situation. The selection of appropriate encapsulated cells plays a crucial role in determining the efficacy and viability of biological applications. Numerous cellular entities have been extensively investigated as prospective contenders for sustained release of medicinal substances. Once the appropriate polymers and therapeutic cells have been chosen, it becomes necessary to build technologically optimized microcapsules in order to achieve a functioning drug delivery system [89]. The selection of the microencapsulation technique and microencapsulation system will be contingent upon the chosen biomaterials. Consequently, distinct manufacturing techniques will be employed depending on whether natural or synthetical polymers are selected. In the first step, cells that produce therapeutic products are mixed with a solution of sodium alginate, typically at concentrations of 1.6% (w/v) or 3% (w/v). Using extrusion, the cell and gel suspension is introduced into a jellifying solution, such as $CaCl_2$ or $BaCl_2$. The interaction between sodium alginate, a part of the brown algae cell wall and the jellifying solution induces the polymerization of the matrix due to the ionic exchange, resulting in the formation of microbeads composed of calcium or barium alginate. After complete gelation, microbeads containing cells are chemically cross-linked with poly-L-lysine (PLL). Following a washing procedure, the beads undergo an additional coating with a layer of alginate. The latter is important in order to tackle the issue of immunological rejection, as the polycations employed in the creation of the semipermeable membrane have an affinity for inflammatory cells, hence triggering cells death of the captured cells. Once manufactured, microcapsules can be utilized in the therapeutic intervention of many medical conditions.

4.12.2 Microcapsule evaluation

A key focus within the domain of cell microencapsulation pertains to the endorsement and optimization of both the biomaterials and technology employed in constructing immobilization systems. Additionally, there is a need to develop and refine assays and techniques that facilitate the analysis and replication of these devices [90]. The proliferation of sophisticated procedures and assays in recent times has significantly expanded the possibilities for systematizing this therapeutic strategy. Extensive study is being conducted to investigate the purity and biocompatibility of various materials. Multiple procedures are being developed to facilitate the beneficiation of alginates. The methodologies used in this research include the utilization of chemical reagents and dialysis, the initiation of mortality in Jurka cells, and the evaluation of the growth of lymphocytes by assessment. The approach described above is a rapid and highly responsive methodology utilized to identify potential contaminants that can induce fibrosis in alginate samples [91]. Prior research has established heightened cytokine levels, such as tumor necrosis factor and human monocyte upon activation by alginates of diverse compositions. After the biomaterials have been characterized, their shape and *in vivo* biocompatibility as microcapsules must be evaluated. Several techniques are constantly refined and developed to help researchers get around these problems. Among them are photoelectron spectroscopy with x-rays (PES), atomic force microscopes (AFM), confocal laser scanning microscopy (CLSM), and enhanced nuclear magnetic resonance (NMR). These methods allow for a thorough study of the microcapsules and the parts that make them up. The CLSM method looks at how alginate and PLL are arranged in space within whole microcapsules [92]. Furthermore, NMR and AFM methods are used together to provide solid proof of the capsules' surface topography and the cross-linking properties between alginate and the gelling ion. Key parameters for producing biocompatible capsules are calculated using FT-IR and x-ray photoelectron spectroscopy, and the reactivity of the microcapsules is evaluated in the immediate post-transplant period. The comprehensive examination of histological and immunopathological aspects and *in vivo* antigenicity assessment significantly enhances the advantages of testing for biocompatibility for anchoring devices. Different studies have been designed to test their mechanical stability to make microcapsules stronger. A texture analyzer gadget can measure how resistant microcapsules are to compression [93]. An alternative approach to enhance comprehension of the mechanical characteristics of polymer systems involves subjecting the particles to destabilizing forces, such as exposure to swollen solution and application of shear stresses. An osmotic pressure test has been used to develop a new way to measure the strength of microcapsules. This test entails subjecting the microcapsules to a range of hypotonic solutions with varying concentrations and subsequently measuring the proportion of capsules that have ruptured as a percentage [94]. Another area of interest pertains to assessing the permeability characteristics of the semipermeable microcapsules, namely the entry and egress behavior. The viability of a membrane is contingent upon the extent to which control can be exercised over the selective exclusion of molecules based on size and the rate at which diffusion occurs. This control is crucial for regulating the survival and metabolic efficiency of the graft. The transport of species over a membrane, referred to as membrane permeability, is influenced by two key parameters: the equilibrium partition coefficient, which is a thermodynamic parameter, and the diffusion coefficient, which is a kinetic parameter. Several assays of immobilization devices have been optimized to assess the permeability characteristics, specifically the permeability to hemoglobin and immunoglobulin G (IgG) [95]. The tests used in this study involve the technique of mass refusal chromatography, which involves using dextran references with different molecular weights and calculating the coefficient of mass transfer ratio. The latest technique was successfully used in the first evaluation of microcapsules consisting of three different hurdle substances, including poly-L-ornithin, polymethylene hydrochloride, and PLL. The PLO small capsules had the highest level of success among each of the options. In future research, it is recommended that the optimization of encapsulated cells should include an evaluation of their mechanical stability, diffusion, and permeability qualities *in vivo*. The resolution of these challenges will have a substantial influence on the uniformity of immune isolation gadgets during the FDA phase [96].

4.12.3 Potential health benefits

The therapeutic applications of cell microencapsulation technology encompass a diverse array of areas, which can be categorized into five distinct groups. The categories mentioned above include the management of classical Mendelian disorders, therapeutic approaches for cancer, diseases affecting the central nervous system (CNS), the development of artificial tissues, and several other uses. Given the current severe scarcity of donor organs, researchers have explored the utilization of donor cells and tissues (both human and non-human) as potential therapeutic agents [97]. Xenografts have emerged as a significant source of apprehension because of the potential transmission of infectious organisms, including porcine endogenous retrovirus (PERV), from the donor to the recipient. Moreover, using genetically engineered cells has created novel opportunities for addressing conventional Mendelian illnesses, including cancer. Genes can serve as templates, while cells can function as reactors to produce and release the desired product. Additionally, capsules can be employed as immunoselection vehicles to deliver drugs within a living organism. Biosafety is a crucial factor to consider while employing genetically modified cells. Utilizing genetically modified cells necessitates a delicate equilibrium between ensuring the safety and stability of gene expression [98]. The scientific foundation for various clinical trials has been established by utilizing small and large animal models. These trials encompass a range of applications, such as the encapsulation of allogeneic islets to address diabetes, the encapsulation of cytochrome P450 enzyme-expressing cells to combat pancreatic cancer, and the immobilization of retinal pigmented epithelial (hRPE) cells on gelatin microcarriers for the treatment of advanced Parkinson's disease in patients [99].

4.12.4 Modern developments in cell encapsulation

Researchers are looking into the possibility of using settled cells that release the granulocyte macrophage-colony-stimulating factor (GM-CSF) as an immunomodulatory or adjuvant in the context of immunization for both humans and animals as a result of the rapid developments in cell biology, gene treatment, and chemical engineering and pharmaceutical technology. Live vaccines can potentially be used in cancer immunotherapy and the prevention of infectious illnesses [100]. Another potential use case is immobilizing genetically modified cells that produce therapeutic antibodies. Various cell types have been employed in this methodology, encompassing hybridomas, skin fibroblasts, keratinocytes, myogenic cells, and hepatocytes. Notably, in certain instances, antibodies generated through both *in vitro* and *in vivo* methods maintain the specificity and affinity of the original parenteral antibody without any observed idiotypic reaction in animals that create ectopic antibodies [101]. In a similar vein, the utilization of encapsulated cells that produce retroviral vectors has been examined to achieve sustained *in vivo* gene transfer, given the requirement for frequent vector administration to ensure effective delivery of the therapeutic gene. Significant endeavors are being undertaken by scientists in the advancement of a bioartificial pancreas by the process of immobilizing pancreatic islets within polymer microcapsules. Several research groups have focused their efforts on developing a neovascularized environment suitable for the implantation of encapsulated islets [102]. While not universally endorsed by all specialists, this methodology can enhance the interaction between the bloodstream and immobilized cells, potentially improving their long-term performance and functionality. This strategy can be readily implemented by employing the encapsulation technique of cells that secrete angiogenic factors or by utilizing gelatin microspheres impregnated with the administration of basic FGF or VEGF, which stands for vascular endothelial growth factor [103].

4.13 Immobilization of microalgae

The utilization of algae for commercial purposes has a substantial historical background, with numerous algae species employed as food, feed, and important chemical resources. Various kinds of macroalgae, such as *Iridaea*, *Porphyra*, *Gigartina*, *Caulerpa*, and *Ulva*, are commonly collected for human consumption or the extraction of hydrocolloids. The cultivation of *Porphyria*, commonly referred to as 'Nori' in Japan, is a significant sector within the aquaculture industry of Japan [104]. Furthermore, the industries manufacturing carrageenan, agar, and alginic acid from macroalgae have been firmly established. Certain microalgae, including specific *Nostoc* and *Aphanizomenon* species, are procured from natural habitats for human consumption. However, most microalgae utilized in commercial applications are cultivated. Several microalgae species are known for their potential to produce valuable compounds [105].

For instance, *Dunaliella* is recognized for synthesizing β-carotene, while *Chlorella* and *Spirulina* are commonly utilized for protein production. Spoehr and Milner (1949) proposed that the cultivation of microalgae on a large scale may address the issue of protein deficiencies worldwide. The rationale behind their positive outlook stemmed from algae having a crude protein content surpassing 50% and demonstrating a biomass production of approximately 25 tonnes per hectare per year. In addition, wastewater high in nitrogen and phosphorus is also considered a useful substrate for algae production. Cultivating algae in wastewater presents a dual benefit of treating the wastewater while generating algal biomass. Biomass has the potential to be used for a range of applications, such as the production of nutritional supplements and food additives for aquaculture, as well as for animal and human feed [106].

Additionally, it can be harnessed for energy production, such as biogas and fuels, and for applications in agriculture, such as fertilizers and soil conditioners. One of the primary obstacles in the utilization of microalgal biomass is in the process of harvesting or separating the algal biomass from the discharged water after treatment. Considerable attention has been dedicated to developing appropriate technology for the extraction of microalgae, encompassing several methods such as basic sand filtering and more energy-demanding centrifugation techniques. The practice of autoflocculation, which involves the self-aggregation of cyanobacteria by the cessation of aeration and subsequent decantation, has also been seen [107]. Experiments have also been conducted on the utilization of ultrasonic waves or ultrasound for the harvesting of microalgae. In this approach, the separating process relies on the gentle aggregation generated by acoustic forces, which is subsequently followed by an intensified sedimentation phase. In the present context, the immobilization of algal cells has been suggested as a potential solution to address the challenge of harvesting and to preserve the valuable algal biomass for subsequent processing [108].

4.13.1 Techniques for immobilization

Among the several techniques employed for immobilizing cells and enzymes, entrapment stands out as the predominant approach for algal immobilization. This specific application utilizes a range of natural polymers, including collagen, which is agar, agarose, or cellulose, and alginate, which and carrageenan, alongside synthetic polymers such as acrylamide, polyurethane, and polyvinyl [109]. In the algal immobilization process, it is important to acknowledge that the often-used natural gels contain alginate and carrageenan.

The gel is commonly converted into functioning biological catalysts pellets by the introduction of microalgae cells in solution to an aquatic solution that contains the gelling component. As mentioned above, the substance is subsequently transformed into small spherical particles by applying controlled droplet formation techniques, passing via a nozzle or orifice, and introduced into a solution containing interacting salts [110]. The droplets are later rendered stable through polymerization or other forms of cross-linking, resulting in biocatalyst beads containing the imprisoned organisms. As an illustration, alginate droplets have the potential to be rendered stable through the introduction of bivalent ions, such as calcium. Conversely, carrageenan beads are commonly subjected to cross-linking processes utilizing $K+$ ions. Monodisperse calcium alginate beads are generated within the size range of 0.2–1.0 mm through the laminar jet break-up, ensuring sterility and reproducibility. Implementing an *in situ* cleaning procedure for the nozzles is undertaken to ensure the completion of multiple batch process cycles and achieve a throughput level of up to $5.3\ l\ h^{-1}$ [111]. The beads were subjected to analysis, revealing that the relative disparity in the average diameter across several nozzles was below 0.3%. Recently, a study reported the comobilization of microalgae with the bacteria *Az spirillum Brasiliense*. This comobilization was observed to enhance the growth, pigment, and lipid contents, In addition to the cells and population density of the entangled algae. The results of this study indicate that the novel immobilized biocatalyst exhibited greater efficacy in the removal of nitrogen and phosphorus compared to the use of immobilized algae alone. Since 1990, half of the papers about immobilized microalgae have focused on their application in the removal of nitrogen and phosphorus from wastewater [112]. The remaining reports have explored the utilization of immobilized algae for the accumulation and removal of metals. Recently, there has been a notable development in the field of conductometric biosensors, namely in utilizing immobilized microalgae. Fiber optic biosensors are employed to detect environmentally hazardous substances, including heavy metals, herbicides, and other toxic compounds.

4.13.2 Use of cryopreserved algae

Research indicates that immobilization significantly affects the productivity of algal cells. Specifically, studies have shown a remarkable enhancement in hydrogen production from the filamentous alga *Anabaena*, with a threefold increase observed following immobilization. This demonstrates the profound impact that immobilization can have on algal cell function and output. Brouwers has demonstrated that immobilization notably enhances the production of ammonia and hydrocarbons in *Mastigocladus laminosus* [113]. The immobilization of '*Chlamydomonas reinhardtian*' cells in Ba-alginate offers a reliable and efficient approach for the photoproduction of ammonia. The study demonstrated that the generation of glycolate in cells entrapped in alginate was twice as high as in cells that were not entrapped and were free-living [114]. Leon and Galvan investigated glycerol production in *C. reinhardtian* cells fixed in Ca-alginate. The immobilized cells exhibited a production rate of 8 g l^{-1}, whereas their free-living counterparts achieved a invention rate of 4 g l^{-1}. The comparative competence of arrested cells and thylakoid vesicles of the microalga *C. reinhardtia* was assessed concerning their free-existing foils, specifically in hydrogen peroxide generation [28]. Hydrogen peroxide (H_2O_2) is a highly effective and environmentally friendly fuel in various applications such as rocket propulsion, motors, and heating systems. The molecule in question is generated through a catalytic cycle within the photosystems, wherein a redox mediator, namely Me viologen, undergoes reduction by the electrons derived from water [105]. The Ca-alginate-entrapped cells maintained a photoproduction rate of 33 μmol H_2O_2/mg Chl./h for several hours under ideal conditions, exhibiting an energy conversion efficiency of 0.25%.

On the other hand, the immobilized cyanobacteria, specifically *Anabaena variabilis* and *Anacystis nidulans*, demonstrated reduced catalase activity and attained productivities of 151 and 61 μmol hydrogen peroxide. A novel photobioreactor has been developed to enhance Maren nine production, as indicated by the findings of this study. In a recent study, the microalgae species *Butyraceous braunii* and *B. protuberans* were immobilized as entire cells within alginate beads during airlift batch culture. This immobilization technique led to a significant increase in rest phase development, during which both resting and hydrocarbon output are substantially enhanced [104].

4.13.3 Removal of nitrogen and phosphorous

Numerous publications have been dedicated to examining the application of immobilized microalgae to remove nitrogen and phosphorus from wastewater, specifically focusing on its potential as a tertiary treatment method. Typically, immobilized cells exhibit more efficiency in removing nitrogen and phosphorus than their free-living counterparts [115]. Furthermore, the removal of phosphate is shown to occur at a slower rate than that of nitrogen. Moreover, a progressive decrease in efficiency was also noted from the initial cycle to the succeeding ones. In 1986, Jeanfils and Thomas conducted a study involving alginate-immobilized *Scenedesmus obliquus*. Their findings indicated that the efficiency of nitrite uptake was not impacted by immobilization, except for a prolonged lag phase found in the immobilized cells compared to the free cells. The available research supports the notion that culture age has a negligible effect on nitrogen removal [116]. In contrast to those mentioned earlier, previous batch culture investigations on phosphate uptake by alginate-entrapped *Chlorella Emersonian* have demonstrated that the cells in the exponential growth phase exhibit a phosphate removal rate from the medium that is five times higher than that of cells in the late stationary phase. Significant variations in reactor performance can be observed when immobilized cells of varying ages are enclosed in Ca-alginate and placed within a small-scale packed-bed reactor. The rate of nitrogen intake in immobilized *S. obliquus* was significantly enhanced under conditions of nitrogen scarcity. Rai and Mallick (1992) observed a greater rate of uptake for nitrogen and phosphorus in immobilized *Chlorella* and *Anabaena* compared to their free-living counterparts [117]. In the following investigations, it was observed that immobilized algae with a cell density of 0.1 g dry weight per liter exhibited the highest efficacy in nutrient and metal removal within a pH range spanning from 6.0 to 8.0. Furthermore, using chitosan as a substrate for supporting algae has shown promise in enhancing the process of wastewater detoxification. The research done by Vilchez and Vega shows that using alginate-entrapped *C. reinhardtian* cells offers a dependable and efficient method for removing nitrogenous contaminants in wastewater [118]. To determine the most favorable operating parameters for the immobilized cells, many criteria were considered, such as the concentration of the matrix, the loading of cells, the temperature, and the pH. In the case of *C. reinhardtian* cells, using a 3% alginate concentration effectively addresses challenges related to substrate transport. This concentration level facilitates the attainment of the appropriate physical properties of the beads. This study aims to evaluate the efficacy of foam-immobilized devices in the removal of phosphate [119]. This study compared the performance of Phormium laminose in batch bioreactors to that of continuous flow bioreactors. Beds in funneled columns and beds housed in Erlenmeyer flasks were the first fluidized-bed designs to be invented. The bioreactors were treated to a continuous illumination employing cool white fluorescent lamps with 100 μmol photon m^2 s^{-1} irradiation. The bottom half of each bioreactor was immersed in a thermostatically controlled water bath to keep the temperature within at a constant 45 °C. Preboiled, cleaned, and dried foam cubes (now 5 mm in size) were mixed with algae suspension. The adsorption immobilization procedure was placed over two months. The foam cubes were put in the bioreactors once fully colonized [120]. Despite the excellent removal of nitrogen and phosphorus from the system by cyanobacteria immobilized on polymer foams, the utilization of fluidized-bed reactors led to the development of a heterogeneous system, rendering it unsuitable for laboratory standardization in most cases. However, numerous researchers have investigated the removal of nitrogen and phosphorus in packed-bed reactors. Limitations in the operation of these reactors include inadequate light penetration, lack of cell mixing, and the presence of gaseous fluxes. Kaya and Picard have successfully devised an innovative immobilized algal system for wastewater biotreatment. The present study involved the cultivation of *Scenedesmus bicellularis*, a green microalga obtained from a secondary decantation tank. The microalga was cultured in a synthetic medium for 12 days [121]. Following centrifugation, the harvested cells were immobilized on alginate screens. The screens were placed within a photochamber fully saturated with a relative humidity of 100%. The photochamber had a photoperiod of 16 h and was illuminated with an intensity of 150 μE m^2 s^{-1}. Following 48 h of nutrient deprivation, the immobilized cells were employed in the elimination of ammonium and orthophosphate from a synthetic secondary wastewater effluent within a flexiglass reactor. A second study additionally revealed that intermittent carbon dioxide (CO_2) enrichment expedites the process of tertiary wastewater treatment. Nevertheless, a significant issue associated with using gel materials pertains to the challenge of preserving the structural stability of alginate gels for an extended period, typically beyond a few weeks [121]. While agarose gel-based reactors have demonstrated greater stability compared to other types of reactors, it is important to note that these matrices, composed of polysaccharides, are very susceptible to microbial degradation when exposed to natural environments. In order to address these challenges, Robinson put out a novel design for a hollow-fiber reactor. A diverse range of sizes of hollow-fiber cartridges can be found in the commercial market. Robinson developed a hollow-fiber reactor consisting of 50 cylindrical tubes made of polysulfone. These tubes were bundled together and securely enclosed within a transparent cartridge measuring 20 cm long. Each fiber possessed an internal diameter (ID) of 1.1 mm, and the fiber wall exhibited many perforations in the form of pores. One potential method involves the use of algae cells contained within the fiber lumen of a cartridge. Nutrients can be introduced either through the shell space or in the reverse direction, depending on the specific requirements of the experimental setup. The initial findings indicate a rapid fall in the phosphate uptake rate within a short timeframe [122]. This decline is not attributed to decreased activity but to settling biomass within the reactor. Nevertheless, the settling rates of cells were seen to be considerably reduced when they were immersed in a solution containing 1% Na-alginate. The investigation focused on eliminating nitrate and phosphate from wastewater at 43 °C. This was achieved by providing a constant supply of a diluted growth medium for seven days, followed by introducing secondary-treated sewage for an additional 12 days [123]. Under identical conditions, the nitrogenous and phosphate ions eliminated from secondary-treated sewage were recorded as 0.25 and 0.12 mmol d^{-1} l^{-1}. The utilization of thermophilic cyanobacteria in a wastewater purification system offers distinct advantages due to their capacity to withstand elevated temperatures, hence minimizing the risk of contamination. The coimmobilization of *Azospirillum brasilense* within small alginate beads led to significant enhancements in the growth, pigment and lipid content, as well as the cell and population size of both *Chlorella* species. The simultaneous mobilisation of both microorganisms was found to be more efficient in the removal of nitrogen and phosphorus as compared to the use of just immobilized microalgae [124]. In a 6-day timeframe, this comobilization method removed up to 100% of ammonium, 15% of nitrate, and 36% of phosphorus, with some variation between wastewater types. Using microalgae alone, on the other hand, led to lower removal rates: 75% for ammonium, 6% for nitrate, and 19% for phosphorous.

4.13.4 Disposal of metals

Microalgae have garnered significant attention in the biotechnology field due to their potential applications in removing heavy metals and radionuclides from emissions and effluents. Furthermore, it is plausible to extract valuable elements such as gold, silver, and uranium alongside the detoxifying process by appropriately treating the algal biomass enriched with these metals. Numerous studies have been conducted on the sequestration of metals by microalgae-immobilized systems [125]. One particularly intriguing aspect is the development of 'AlgaSORB' at New Mexico State University. During this procedure, the algae are densely packed within a columnar structure composed of solid silica gel. The microorganisms are rendered non-viable by encapsulating the algae within a solid matrix. However, the cell walls of these organisms continue to serve as a rich source of binding sites that can effectively sequester heavy metal ions from the surrounding solution. The current work explored extracting mercury from an aqueous solution utilizing a packed-bed reactor (PBR) that included *Chlorella emersonii* immobilized inside alginate and agarose gels [126]. The process of microalgae cultivation using waste-water for biomass production was reported in figure 4.14.

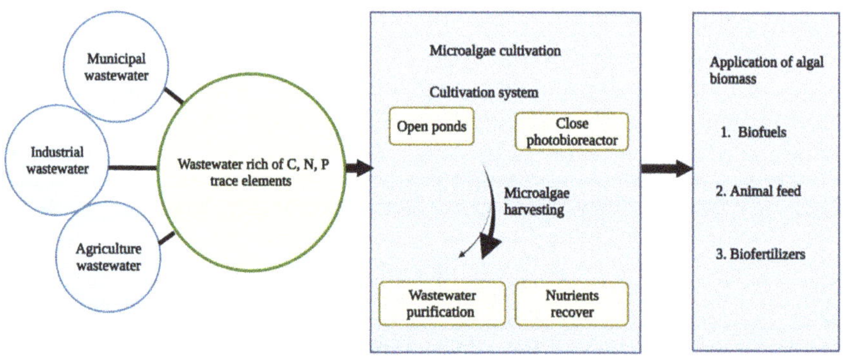

Figure 4.14. Integrated process of microalgae cultivation using wastewater for biomass production and its applications in biofuels, animal feed, and biofertilizers.

The reactors were made with chromatography columns filled with 200 gel particles between 4 and 6 mm across. The point of this study was to find out what happens to the mercury removal process when the cell packing density, the amount of mercury coming in, and the flow rate change. The investigation revealed that using agarose as an immobilizing matrix, as opposed to alginate, led to a reduction in the amounts of mercury volatilization. A laboratory-scale algal column reactor was created, utilizing *Chlorella vulgaris*, a species of green microalgae, with a combined volume of 75 ml of alginate-algal beads. The reactor was employed for the remediation of copper (Cu) and nickel (Ni) at a concentration of 30 mg l^{-1}, utilizing a hydraulic retention time (HRT) of 30 min. After the loading process of a 4 l metal solution was concluded, it was noted that a significant proportion of copper (Cu) and nickel (Ni), namely over 97% and 91%, respectively, were effectively extracted from the wastewater. It was discovered that up-flow is preferable to down-flow for keeping the flow rate stable. Gardea-Torresdey *et al* [127] immobilized *Synechococcus* sp. PCC7942 biomass in a silica-polymer matrix in their experiment. The ability of the immobilized biomass to bind metals was then studied under continuous flow conditions. The experimental findings demonstrated that the highest degree of adsorption was observed for lead (Pb), followed by cadmium (Cd), with copper (Cu) and nickel (Ni) exhibiting comparable levels of adsorption [128]. A concentration of 0.2 M hydrochloric acid was determined to be efficacious in the retrieval of the metals that had been adsorbed. A series of experiments were undertaken to ascertain the feasibility of many metal binding and stripping cycles by the immobilized biomass. The elements Cd, Cu, and Ni were shown to undergo sorption and desorption processes three times, whereas Pb exhibited as many as six sorption and desorption events. The study investigated the metallic elimination effectiveness of the *Scenedesmus acutus* and *Chlorella vulgaris*, immobilized in foam polyurethane and κ-carrageenan gel matrices. The effectiveness was evaluated in both fluidized-bed and packed-bed reactors. The tolerance of immobilized cells to heavy metals such as Cd, Cr, and Zn is greater than that of free cells, suggesting a significant potential for their application in wastewater treatment procedures. Singh and Prasad constructed a column named 'AlgaSORB' by combining silica, a polymer matrix (poly-N-xylene-N,N′-di cyclohexyl ethylenediamine dibromide), and a green microalga (Spirogyra) [129]. This column exhibited distinctive ion selectivity for copper (Cu) over other metal ions in the waste samples [130]. Standardizing factors such as flow rate, pH, and equilibrium time also impact the outcomes. The system's kinetics are advantageous, as it does not exhibit any issues related to clumping, clogging, or leaching of the stationary support. The present method possesses appealing characteristics that make it suitable for single-column ion chromatography due to its exceptional durability, straightforwardness, and cost-effectiveness. An experimental study was conducted to evaluate the effectiveness of a novel sorption system utilizing *Chlorella sorokiniana* immobilized on the biomatrix of *Luffa cylindrica*, commonly known as a vegetable sponge. The objective was to investigate the system's capability to remove Cd and Ni from a contaminated aqueous medium under continuous liquid flow conditions in a column setup, and the immobilized *Chlorella sorokiniana* exhibited notably superior efficiency compared to its free-living relatives. The metal desorption rate in the presence of a 0.1 M hydrochloric acid solution was shown to be 100%. Furthermore, the immobilized system, once desorbed, exhibited comparable efficiency throughout the subsequent cycle, indicating its potential for reusability. Microalga-luffasponge-immobilized-disks (MLIDs) have shown a remarkable ability to maintain around 93% of their original binding capacity for Ni throughout five consecutive reuse cycles [131]. Therefore, due to their notable efficiency, affordability, ease of preparation, and ability to be reused multiple times, MLIDs exhibit potential as a compelling biosorption technology for removing heavy metals. Nevertheless, the researchers employed a novel biosorbent material from the marine brown alga, *Ascophyllum nodosum*, within a packed-bed flow-through column. The study observed that removing Cd from an effluent with an initial concentration of 10 mg Cd/l achieved a 99.98% reduction. The metal removal efficacy of the bloom-forming cyanobacterium *Microcystis* was investigated. *Microcystis*, a cyanobacterium, is commonly found in eutrophic ponds and reservoirs in India and other tropical regions [132]. It is considered a nuisance due to its prolific presence. The immobilized state of this cyanobacterium results from a capsule or slime layer surrounding the cell in its natural habitat. The biosorption process was observed to be affected by variations in pH and temperature. It is worth noting that heat-killed, formaldehyde-treated, and metabolically inactive (DCMU-treated) *Microcystis* cells exhibited equivalent biosorption capability to metabolically active cells. This implies that deceased biomass may also possess comparable efficacy in the metal removal process. The present research team is actively investigating the viability of utilizing dried biomass for the widespread implementation of *Microcystis* as a 'AlgaSORB' for the purpose of removing metal build-up [133].

4.13.5 Biosensor development

The current scholarly attention in biotechnology is mostly directed toward using immobilized microalgae to develop biosensors that can effectively detect and identify potentially harmful substances, such as heavy metal and insecticides, within the natural environment [134]. This microalga was immobilized on a detachable membrane and positioned close to the point of an optical fibre bundle within a microcell constructed in-house. The identification of herbicides was predicated upon the assessment of chlorophyll fluorescence kinetics. A permanent culture system was established to generate algal cells under consistent circumstances for optimizing measurements. In heavy metal detection, a biosensor is developed utilizing the enzymatic activity of alkaline phosphatase (AP) located on the outer membrane of *Chlorella vulgaris*. The conductometric biosensors exhibited greater sensitivity compared to bioassays for detecting low concentrations of cadmium ions, with a detection limit of 1 ppb for Cd. One notable benefit of utilizing AP-based biosensors is their notable stability, which stems from their utilization of intact algal cells with APs on their cell walls, in contrast to enzymatic biosensors. The enzyme persists within its native habitat, which promotes prolonged stability and aligns with the mechanism of harmful inhibition, thereby rendering it of ecological significance (figure 4.15) [135].

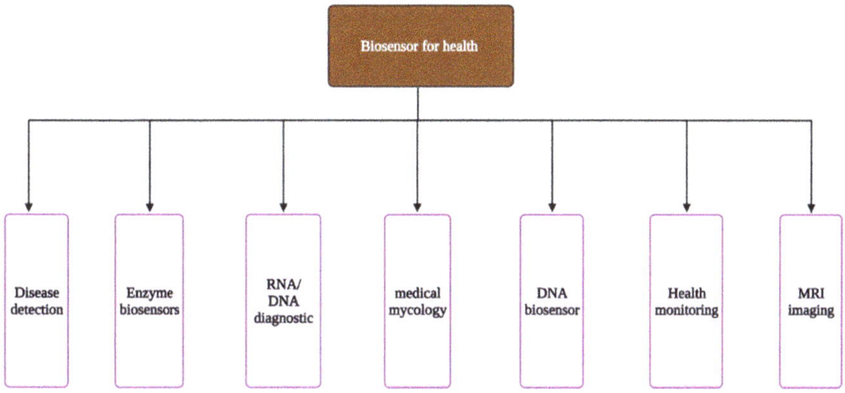

Figure 4.15. Applications of biosensors in healthcare: advancements from disease detection to diagnostic imaging and environmental monitoring.

References

[1] Brena B, González-Pombo P and Batista-Viera F 2013 Immobilization of enzymes: a literature survey *Immobilization of Enzymes and Cells: Methods in Molecular Biology* (Springer) 3rd edn1051 pp 15–31

[2] Mehrotra P 2016 Biosensors and their applications—a review *J. Oral Biol. Craniofac. Res.* **6** 153–9

[3] Fernandes P 2010 Enzymes in food processing: a condensed overview on strategies for better biocatalysts *Enzyme Res.* **2010** 862537

[4] Mohamad N R *et al* 2015 An overview of technologies for immobilization of enzymes and surface analysis techniques for immobilized enzymes *Biotechnol. Biotechnol. Equip.* **29** 205–20

[5] Kamra T *et al* 2016 Covalent immobilization of molecularly imprinted polymer nanoparticles on a gold surface using carbodiimide coupling for chemical sensing *J. Colloid Interface Sci.* **461** 1–8

[6] Iso M *et al* 1989 Immobilization of enzyme by microencapsulation and application of the encapsulated enzyme in the catalysis *J. Microencapsulation* **6** 165–76

[7] Trevan M 1988 Enzyme immobilization by covalent bonding *New Protein Techniques* (Springer) pp 495–510

[8] Coulet P, Carlsson J and Porath J 1981 Immobilization of enzymes on metal-chelate regenerable carriers *Biotechnol. Bioeng.* **23** 663–8

[9] Kennedy J F and Cabral J M 1986 Use of titanium etc species for the immobilization of bioactive compounds—enzymes *Transition Met. Chem.* **11** 41–66

[10] Kennedy J F *et al* 1997 Transition metal methods for immobilization of enzymes and cells *Immobilization of Enzymes and Cells: Methods in Molecular Biology* (Springer) pp 345–59

[11] Datta S, Christena L R and Rajaram Y R S 2013 Enzyme immobilization: an overview on techniques and support materials *3 Biotech.* **3** 1–9

[12] Jen A C, Wake M C and Mikos A G 1996 Hydrogels for cell immobilization *Biotechnol. Bioeng.* **50** 357–64

[13] Hall R, Holden M and Yeoman M 1988 Immobilization of higher plant cells *Medicinal and Aromatic Plants* I (Springer) vol 4 pp 136–56

[14] Headon D and Walsh G 1994 The industrial production of enzymes *Biotechnol. Adv.* **12** 635–46

[15] Gurung N *et al* 2013 A broader view: microbial enzymes and their relevance in industries, medicine, and beyond *BioMed. Res. Int.* **2013** 329121

[16] Hasan F *et al* 2010 Enzymes used in detergents: lipases *Afr. J. Biotechnol.* **9** 4836–44

[17] Fersht A and Winter G 1985 Redesigning enzymes by site-directed mutagenesis *Ciba Foundation Symposium 111-Enzymes in Organic Synthesis* (Wiley Online Library)

[18] Varland S, Osberg C and Arnesen T 2015 N-terminal modifications of cellular proteins: the enzymes involved, their substrate specificities and biological effects *Proteomics* **15** 2385–401

[19] Messing R A 1976 [11] Adsorption and inorganic bridge formations *Methods in Enzymology* (Amsterdam: Elsevier) pp 148–69

[20] Woodward J 1985 *Immobilised Cells and Enzymes: A Practical Approach* (IRL Press)

[21] Tosa T *et al* 1966 Studies on continuous enzyme reactions. I. Screening of carriers for preparation of water-insoluble aminoacylase *Enzymologia* **31** 214–24

[22] Sharp A, Kay G and Lilly M 1969 The kinetics of β-galactosidase attached to porous cellulose sheets *Biotechnol. Bioeng.* **11** 363–80

[23] Goldstein L 1972 Microenvironmental effects on enzyme catalysis. Kinetic study of polyanionic and polycationic derivatives of chymotrypsin *Biochemistry* **11** 4072–84

[24] Avineri-Goldman R *et al* 1968 Papain-collodion membranes. I. Preparation and properties *Biochemistry* **7** 486–500

[25] Guisan J M, Alvaro G, Rosell C M and Fernadez-Lafuente R 1994 Industrial design of enzymic processes catalysed by very active immobilized derivatives: utilization of diffusional limitations (gradients of pH) as a profitable tool in enzyme engineering *Biotechnol. Appl. Biochem.* **20** 357–69

[26] Porath J 1987 Salting-out adsorption techniques for protein purification *Biopolymers: Orig. Res. Biomolecules* **26** S193–204

[27] Caldwell K D *et al* 1976 Immobilization of enzymes based on hydrophobic interaction. I. Preparation and properties of a β-amylase adsorbate *Biotechnol. Bioeng.* **18** 1573–88

[28] Caldwell K D *et al* 1976 Immobilization of enzymes based on hydrophobic interaction. II. Preparation and properties of an amyloglucosidase adsorbate *Biotechnol. Bioeng.* **18** 1589–604

[29] Cashion P *et al* 1982 Enzyme immobilization on tritylagarose: reusability of both matrix and enzyme *Biotechnol. Bioeng.* **24** 1221–4

[30] Yon R J 1974 Enzyme purification by hydrophobic chromatography: an alternative approach illustrated in the purification of aspartate transcarbamoylase from wheat germ *Biochem.* J **137** 127

[31] Dixon J, Andrews P and Butler L G 1979 Hydrophobic esters of cellulose: properties and applications in biochemical technology *Biotechnol. Bioeng.* **21** 2113–23

[32] Solomon B *et al* 1987 Use of monoclonal antibodies for the preparation of highly active immobilized enzymes *Methods in Enzymology* (Amsterdam: Elsevier) ch 13 pp 160–70

[33] Bernfeld P and Wan J 1963 Antigens and enzymes made insoluble by entrapping them into lattices of synthetic polymers *Science* **142** 678–9

[34] Dinelli D, Marconi W and Morisi F 1976 Fiber-entrapped enzymes *Methods in Enzymology* (Amsterdam: Elsevier) ch 18 pp 227–43

[35] Wadiak D and Carbonell R 1975 Kinetic behavior of microencapsulated β-galactosidase *Biotechnol. Bioeng.* **17** 1157–81

[36] Mattiasson B and Kaul R 1991 Determination of coupling yields and handling of labile proteins in immobilization technology *Food Bioprocess Technol.* **14** 161–79

[37] Scouten W H 1987 A survey of enzyme coupling techniques *Methods in Enzymology* (Amsterdam: Elsevier) ch 2 pp 30–65

[38] López-Gallego F, Guisán J M and Betancor L 2013 Glutaraldehyde-mediated protein immobilization *Immobilization of Enzymes and Cells: Methods in Molecular Biology* (Springer) 3rd edn pp 33–41

[39] Sassolas A, Hayat A and Marty J-L 2013 Enzyme immobilization by entrapment within a gel network *Immobilization of Enzymes and Cells: Methods in Molecular Biology* (Springer) 3rd edn pp 229–39

[40] Cao L, van Langen L and Sheldon R A 2003 Immobilised enzymes: carrier-bound or carrier-free? *Curr. Opin. Biotechnol.* **14** 387–94

[41] Sheldon R A 2007 Enzyme immobilization: the quest for optimum performance *Adv. Synth. Catal.* **349** 1289–307

[42] Klibanov A M 1979 Enzyme stabilization by immobilization *Anal. Biochem.* **93** 1–25

[43] Sirkar K K, Shanbhag P V and Kovvali A S 1999 Membrane in a reactor: a functional perspective *Ind. Eng. Chem. Res.* **38** 3715–37

[44] Wöltinger J *et al* 2005 Membrane reactors at Degussa *Technology Transfer in Biotechnology: From Lab to Industry to Production* (Springer) pp 289–316

[45] Chang H N and Furusaki S 2005 Membrane bioreactors: present and prospects *Bioreactor Systems and Effects* (Springer) pp 27–64

[46] Tetsuya T *et al* 1969 Studies on continuous Enzyme reactions *Bull. Agr. Chem. Soc. Jpn.* **33** 1047–52

[47] Moehlenbrock M J and Minteer S D 2017 Introduction to the field of enzyme immobilization and stabilization *Enzyme Stabilization and Immobilization: Methods in Molecular Biology* (Springer) pp 1–7

[48] Roig M G *et al* 1987 Biotechnology and applied biology section applications of immobilized enzymes *Biochem. Educ.* **15** 198–208

[49] Lortie R 1994 Evaluation of the performance of immobilized enzyme reactors with Michaelis–Menten kinetics *J. Chem. Technol. Biotechnol.: Int. Res. Process, Environ. Clean Technol.* **60** 189–93

[50] Freed L *et al* 1993 Bioreactor based on suspended particles of immobilized enzyme *Ann. Biomed. Eng.* **21** 57–65

[51] Chibata I *et al* 1976 Production of l-amino acids by Aminoacylase adsorbed on DEAE-sephadex *Methods in Enzymology* (Amsterdam: Elsevier) ch 51 pp 746–59

[52] Jin L-Q *et al* 2017 Immobilization of recombinant glucose isomerase for efficient production of high fructose corn syrup *Appl. Biochem. Biotechnol.* **183** 293–306

[53] Esquisabel A *et al* 2006 Immobilized enzymes for biomedical applications *Immobilization of Enzymes and Cells: Methods in Biotechnology* (Springer) pp 283–93

[54] Liang J F, Li Y T and Yang V C 2000 Biomedical application of immobilized enzymes *J. Pharm. Sci.* **89** 979–90

[55] Costa S, Azevedo H S and Reis R L 2005 *Enzyme Immobilization in Biodegradable Polymers for Biomedical Applications* (CRC Press)

[56] Holz E, Darwish M, Tesar D B and Shatz-Binder W 2023 A Review of protein-and peptide-based chemical conjugates: past, present, and future *Pharmaceutics* **15** 600

[57] Lou-Franco J *et al* 2021 Gold nanozymes: from concept to biomedical applications *Nanomicro Lett.* **13** 36
[58] Rai M *et al* 2012 Biomedical applications of nanobiosensors: the state-of-the-art *J. Braz. Chem. Soc.* **23** 14–24
[59] Rocchitta G *et al* 2016 Enzyme biosensors for biomedical applications: strategies for safeguarding analytical performances in biological fluids *Sensors* **16** 780
[60] Guisan J M (ed) 2006 *Immobilization of Enzymes and Cells* **vol 22** (Berlin: Springer)
[61] Hage D S *et al* 2012 Pharmaceutical and biomedical applications of affinity chromatography: recent trends and developments *J. Pharm. Biomed. Anal.* **69** 93–105
[62] Liang D, Hsiao B S and Chu B 2007 Functional electrospun nanofibrous scaffolds for biomedical applications *Adv. Drug Delivery Rev.* **59** 1392–412
[63] Chang T M S 1975 Immobilized enzymes and their biomedical applications *Immobilized Enzymes, Antigens, Antibodies, and Peptides Preparation and Characterization* ed H H Weetall (New York: Marcel Dekker) pp 245–92
[64] Vunain E, Mishra A and Mamba B 2017 Fundamentals of chitosan for biomedical applications *Chitosan-Based Biomaterials* **vol 1** (Amsterdam: Elsevier) pp 3–30
[65] Peña-Parás L, Sánchez-Fernández J A and Vidaltamayo R 2018 Nanoclays for biomedical applications *Handbook of Ecomaterials* (Springer) vol 5 pp 3453–71
[66] Navrátil M, Švitel J and Gemeiner P 2006 Bioluminescence in immobilized cells for biomass detection and biosensor applications *Immobilization of Enzymes and Cells: Methods in Biotechnology* (Springer) pp 393–401
[67] Wong L S *et al* 2017 Bioluminescent microalgae-based biosensor for metal detection in water *IEEE Sens. J.* **18** 2091–6
[68] Reshetilov A, Iliasov P and Reshetilova T 2010 The microbial cell based biosensors *Intelligent and Biosensors* (IntechOpen) pp 289–322
[69] Weitz H J, Campbell C D and Killham K 2002 Development of a novel, bioluminescence-based, fungal bioassay for toxicity testing *Environ. Microbiol.* **4** 422–9
[70] Weinrich L A, Schneider O D and LeChevallier M W 2011 Bioluminescence-based method for measuring assimilable organic carbon in pretreatment water for reverse osmosis membrane desalination *Appl. Environ. Microbiol.* **77** 1148–50
[71] Jeong S *et al* 2013 A rapid bioluminescence-based test of assimilable organic carbon for seawater *Desalination* **317** 160–5
[72] Shama G and Malik D J 2013 The uses and abuses of rapid bioluminescence-based ATP assays *Int. J. Hyg. Environ. Health* **216** 115–25
[73] Fukuba T *et al* 2018 Adenosine triphosphate measurement in deep sea using a microfluidic device *Micromachines* **9** 370
[74] Efremenko E *et al* 2022 Luminescent analysis of ATP: modern objects and processes for sensing *Chemosensors* **10** 493
[75] Fukuba T *et al* 2011 A microfluidic *in situ* analyzer for ATP quantification in ocean environments *Lab Chip* **11** 3508–15
[76] Ristenpart W D, Wan J and Stone H A 2008 Enzymatic reactions in microfluidic devices: Michaelis–Menten kinetics *Anal. Chem.* **80** 3270–6
[77] Roda A *et al* 2011 A portable bioluminescence engineered cell-based biosensor for on-site applications *Biosens. Bioelectron.* **26** 3647–53
[78] Michelini E *et al* 2013 Field-deployable whole-cell bioluminescent biosensors: so near and yet so far *Anal. Bioanal. Chem.* **405** 6155–63

[79] Lopreside A *et al* 2021 Bioluminescence goes portable: recent advances in whole--cell and cell-free bioluminescence biosensors *Luminescence* **36** 278–93
[80] Michelini E *et al* 2006 Bioluminescent biosensors based on genetically engineered living cells in environmental and food analysis *Anal. Lett.* **39** 1503–15
[81] Syed A J and Anderson J C 2021 Applications of bioluminescence in biotechnology and beyond *Chem. Soc. Rev.* **50** 5668–705
[82] Christenson L, Dionne K E and Lysaght M J 1993 Biomedical applications of immobilized cells *Fundamentals of Animal cell Encapsulation and Immobilization* (CRC Press) pp 7–41
[83] Orive G *et al* 2006 Biomedical applications of immobilized cells *Immobilization of Enzymes and Cells: Methods in Biotechnology* (Springer) pp 427–37
[84] Seliktar D 2012 Designing cell-compatible hydrogels for biomedical applications *Science* **336** 1124–8
[85] Rathore S *et al* 2013 Microencapsulation of microbial cells *J. Food Eng.* **116** 369–81
[86] Murua A *et al* 2008 Cell microencapsulation technology: towards clinical application *J. Controlled Release* **132** 76–83
[87] Jyothi S S *et al* 2012 Microencapsulation: a review *Int. J. Pharm. Biol. Sci.* **3** 509–31
[88] Rabanel J M *et al* 2009 Progress technology in microencapsulation methods for cell therapy *Biotechnol. Progr.* **25** 946–63
[89] Tomaro-Duchesneau C *et al* 2013 Microencapsulation for the therapeutic delivery of drugs, live mammalian and bacterial cells, and other biopharmaceutics: current status and future directions *J. Pharm.* **2013** 103527
[90] Gasperini L, Mano J F and Reis R L 2014 Natural polymers for the microencapsulation of cells *J. R. Soc. Interface* **11** 20140817
[91] Hernández R M *et al* 2010 Microcapsules and microcarriers for *in situ* cell delivery *Adv. Drug Deliv. Rev.* **62** 711–30
[92] Orive G *et al* 2004 History, challenges and perspectives of cell microencapsulation *Trends Biotechnol.* **22** 87–92
[93] Opara E C 2017 Applications of cell microencapsulation *Cell Microencapsulation: Methods and Protocols* (Springer) pp 23–39
[94] Vandegaer J E 2012 *Microencapsulation: Processes and Applications* (Berlin: Springer Science & Business Media)
[95] Goh C H, Heng P W S and Chan L W 2012 Alginates as a useful natural polymer for microencapsulation and therapeutic applications *Carbohydr. Polym.* **88** 1–12
[96] Choudhury N, Meghwal M and Das K 2021 Microencapsulation: an overview on concepts, methods, properties and applications in foods *Food Front.* **2** 426–42
[97] de Vos P *et al* 2014 Polymers in cell encapsulation from an enveloped cell perspective *Adv. Drug Deliv. Rev.* **67** 15–34
[98] Onwulata C I 2013 Microencapsulation and functional bioactive foods *J. Food Process. Preserv.* **37** 510–32
[99] Lim F 1984 *Biomedical Applications of Microencapsulation* (Boca Raton, FL: CRC press)
[100] Mizrahi A 1986 Biologicals from animal cells in culture *Bio/Technol.* **4** 123–7
[101] Garg T, Singh S and Goyal A 2013 Stimuli-sensitive hydrogels: an excellent carrier for drug and cell delivery *Crit. Rev. Ther. Drug Carrier Syst.* **30** 369–409
[102] Hamidi M, Azadi A and Rafiei P 2008 Hydrogel nanoparticles in drug delivery *Adv. Drug Delivery Rev.* **60** 1638–49

[103] Sadoughi F, Mansournia M A and Mirhashemi S M 2020 The potential role of chitosan-based nanoparticles as drug delivery systems in pancreatic cancer *IUBMB Life* **72** 872–83
[104] Mallick N 2020 Immobilization of microalgae *Immobilization of Enzymes and Cells: Methods and Protocols* (Springer) pp 453–71
[105] Mallick N 2006 Immobilization of microalgae *Immobilization of Enzymes and Cells: Methods in Biotechnology* **vol 22** pp 373–91
[106] Moreno-Garrido I 2008 Microalgae immobilization: current techniques and uses *Bioresour. Technol.* **99** 3949–64
[107] Talukder M M R, Das P and Wu J C 2014 Immobilization of microalgae on exogenous fungal mycelium: a promising separation method to harvest both marine and freshwater microalgae *Biochem. Eng. J.* **91** 53–7
[108] Moreno-Garrido I *et al* 2005 Calcium alginate immobilized marine microalgae: experiments on growth and short-term heavy metal accumulation *Mar. Pollut. Bull.* **51** 823–9
[109] De-Bashan L E and Bashan Y 2010 Immobilized microalgae for removing pollutants: review of practical aspects *Bioresour. Technol.* **101** 1611–27
[110] Lebeau T and Robert J-M 2006 Biotechnology of immobilized micro algae: a culture technique for the future *Algal Cultures, Analogues of Blooms and Applications* (Enfield: Science Publishers) pp 801–37
[111] Vasilieva S *et al* 2016 Immobilized microalgae in biotechnology *Moscow Univ. Biol. Sci. Bull.* **71** 170–6
[112] Mallick N 2002 Biotechnological potential of immobilized algae for wastewater N, P and metal removal: a review *Biometals* **15** 377–90
[113] Brouwer P *et al* 2014 A zolla domestication towards a biobased economy? *New Phytol* **202** 1069–82
[114] Eroglu E, Smith S M and Raston C L 2015 Application of various immobilization techniques for algal bioprocesses *Biomass and Biofuels from Microalgae: Advances in Engineering and Biology* (Springer) pp 19–44
[115] Dai Y *et al* 2020 Utilization of biochar for the removal of nitrogen and phosphorus *J. Clean. Prod.* **257** 120573
[116] Brdjanovic D *et al* 2000 Modeling COD, N and P removal in a full-scale WWTP Haarlem Waarderpolder *Water Res.* **34** 846–58
[117] Rai L C and Mallick N 1992 Removal and assessment of toxicity of Cu and Fe to *Anabaena doliolum* and *Chlorella vulgaris* using free and immobilized cells *World J. Microbiol. Biotechnol.* **8** 110–4
[118] Vílchez C and Vega J M 1994 Nitrite uptake by *Chlamydomonas reinhardtii* cells immobilized in calcium alginate *Appl. Microbiol. Biotechnol.* **41** 137–41
[119] Busnardo M J *et al* 1992 Nitrogen and phosphorus removal by Wetland Mesocosms subjected to different hydroperiods *Ecol. Eng.* **1** 287–307
[120] Rasoul-Amini S *et al* 2014 Removal of nitrogen and phosphorus from wastewater using microalgae free cells in bath culture system *Biocatal. Agric. Biotechnol.* **3** 126–31
[121] Lau P, Tam N and Wong Y 1997 Wastewater nutrients (N and P) removal by carrageenan and alginate immobilized *Chlorella vulgaris Environ. Technol.* **18** 945–51
[122] Beuckels A, Smolders E and Muylaert K 2015 Nitrogen availability influences phosphorus removal in microalgae-based wastewater treatment *Water Res.* **77** 98–106

[123] Shi J, Podola B and Melkonian M 2014 Application of a prototype-scale twin-layer photobioreactor for effective N and P removal from different process stages of municipal wastewater by immobilized microalgae *Bioresour. Technol.* **154** 260–6
[124] Mennaa F Z, Arbib Z and Perales J A 2015 Urban wastewater treatment by seven species of microalgae and an algal bloom: biomass production, N and P removal kinetics and harvestability *Water Res.* **83** 42–51
[125] Liu Z and Tran K-Q 2021 A review on disposal and utilization of phytoremediation plants containing heavy metals *Ecotoxicol. Environ. Saf.* **226** 112821
[126] Marafi M and Stanislaus A 2008 Spent hydroprocessing catalyst management: a review: Part II. Advances in metal recovery and safe disposal methods *Resour. Conserv. Recycl.* **53** 1–26
[127] Gardea-Torresdey J L, Arenas J L, Francisco N M C, Tiemann K J and Webb R 1998 Ability of immobilized cyanobacteria to remove metal ions from solution and demonstration of the presence of metallothionein genes in various strains *J. Hazard. Substance Res* **1** 2
[128] Schell W R and Nevissi A 1977 Heavy metals from waste disposal in central puget sound *Environ. Sci. Technol.* **11** 887–93
[129] Singh R and Prasad B B 2000 Trace metal analysis: selective sample (copper II) enrichment on an AlgaSORB column *Proc. Biochem.* **35** 897–905
[130] Lester J, Sterritt R and Kirk P 1983 Significance and behaviour of heavy metals in waste water treatment processes II. Sludge treatment and disposal *Sci. Total Environ.* **30** 45–83
[131] Boutouchent-Guerfi N *et al* 2016 Disposal of metal fragments released during polycrystalline slicing by multi-wire saw *J. Cryst. Growth* **447** 27–30
[132] Dhir B and Srivastava S 2012 Disposal of metal treated Salvinia biomass in soil and its effect on growth and photosynthetic efficiency of wheat *Int. J. Phytorem.* **14** 24–34
[133] Vats M C and Singh S 2014 E-Waste characteristic and its disposal *Int. J. Ecol. Sci. Environ. Eng.* **1** 49–61
[134] Ziegler C and Göpel W 1998 Biosensor development *Curr. Opin. Chem. Biol.* **2** 585–91
[135] Berney H *et al* 2000 A DNA diagnostic biosensor: development, characterisation and performance *Sensors Actuators* B **68** 100–8

IOP Publishing

Introduction to Pharmaceutical Biotechnology, Volume 2 (Second Edition)
Enzymes, proteins and bioinformatics
Ahmed Al-Harrasi, Saurabh Bhatia and Ajmal Khan

Chapter 5

Biosensors

5.1 Introduction

The field of biosensors has developed hugely from the initial demonstration of the concept of biosensors by Leland C Clark Jr in 1962. Currently, the biosensor market is dominated by glucose biosensors, mass-produced enzyme electrodes for the quick self-diagnosis of blood-glucose levels by diabetes patients [1–3]. A biosensor is an analytical device containing an immobilized biological material (enzyme, antibody, nucleic acid, hormone, organelle or whole cell) which can specifically interact with an analyte and produce physical, chemical or electrical signals that can be measured. An analyte is a compound (e.g. glucose, urea, drug, pesticide) whose concentration needs to be measured [1–3]. Biosensors mainly consist of the quantitative analysis of different substances by altering their biological actions into quantifiable signals. The majority of biosensors have immobilized enzymes. The efficiency of biosensors is typically dependent on two important factors, the specificity and sensitivity of the biological reaction, in addition to the stability of the enzyme. The category of biosensors that utilizes enzymes as the recognition element is known as enzyme-based chemical biosensors. Their mechanism is based on biological recognition. Typically it is based on a mixture of a biocatalyst and a supporting material to transduce the biological signal, thus enzymes are allowed to participate in the biochemical reaction. During their participation and after completion of biochemical reaction, the enzyme should be stable under the normal functional conditions of the biosensor. Information about the target analyte always determines the structure of biosensors along with the type of matrix in which the analyte has to be introduced [1–3].

The two different components of a biosensor are (see figure 5.1):

- the biological component (enzyme, cell, etc); and
- the physical component (transducer, amplifier, etc).

doi:10.1088/978-0-7503-5387-8ch5

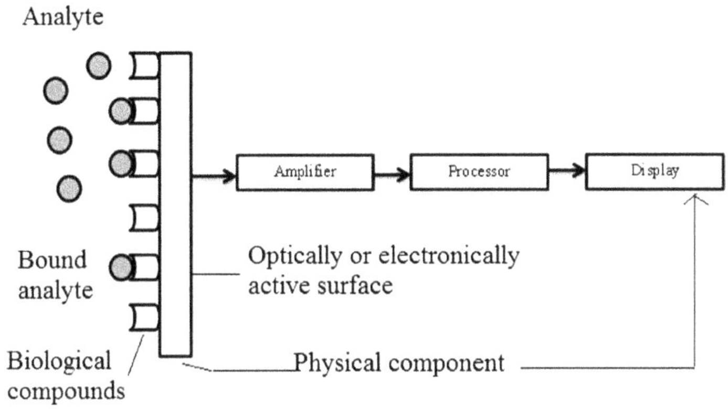

Figure 5.1. A schematic representation of a biosensor.

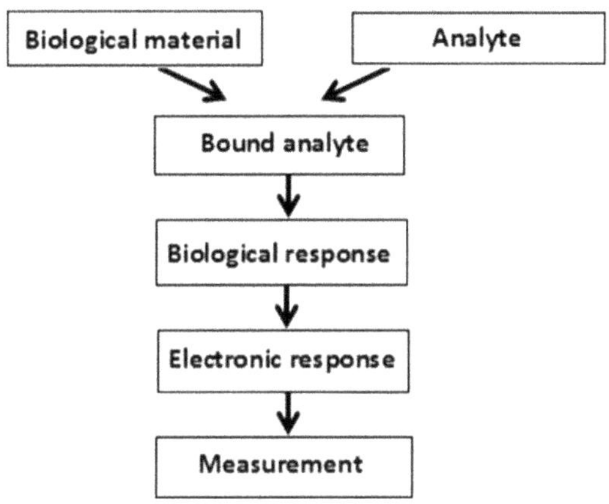

Figure 5.2. Principles of a biosensor.

The biological component identifies and interacts with the analyte to produce a physical change (a signal) that can be easily examined by the transducer. In practice, the biological material is properly immobilized on the transducer and the so prepared biosensors can be used several times (maybe about 10 000 times) for an extensive period (e.g. several months).

5.2 Principles of a biosensor

Biosensors are valuable analytical devices that can be assimilated with on-line process monitoring schemes [4]. The basic principle of a biosensor is dependent on the affinity between the biological material and analyte (figure 5.2) [4]. The selected biological material (usually a specific enzyme) is immobilized by conventional procedures (physical or membrane entrapment, non-covalent or covalent bonding). This immobilized biological material is in close interaction with the transducer.

The analyte binds to the biological material to form a bound analyte which in turn produces an electronic response that can be examined.

In a number of cases, the analyte is transformed into a product which may be related to the release of heat, gas (oxygen), electrons or hydrogen ions. The transducer can transform the product-associated changes into electrical signals which can be amplified and measured. The manufacture of biosensors, their resources, transducing devices and immobilization techniques entails multidisciplinary research in chemistry, biology and engineering. The resources used in biosensors are divided into three groups based on their mechanisms:

- the biocatalytic group comprising enzymes;
- the bioaffinity group including antibodies and nucleic acids; and
- the microbe-based group containing microorganisms.

A biosensor comprises three main parts:

- the biological recognition elements that differentiate the target molecules in the presence of various chemicals;
- a transducer that converts the biorecognition event into a measurable signal; and
- a signal processing system that converts the signal into a readable form [5–7].

The molecular recognition elements comprise receptors, enzymes, antibodies, nucleic acids, microorganisms and lectins [8, 9]. The five principal transducer classes are electrochemical, optical, thermometric, piezoelectric and magnetic [10]. Most currently available glucose biosensors are of the electrochemical type, due to their better sensitivity, reproducibility and easy maintenance, as well as their low cost. Electrochemical sensors may be further divided into potentiometric, amperometric or conductometric types [10–12]. Enzymatic amperometric glucose biosensors are the most common devices commercially available, and have been extensively investigated over the last few years. Amperometric sensors monitor currents generated when electrons are exchanged either directly or indirectly between a biological system and an electrode [13, 14].

5.3 Different types of biosensors

Biosensors were developed in the 1960s by the pioneers Clark and Lyons. Some types of biosensors currently in use are enzyme-based, tissue-based, immunosensors, DNA biosensors, thermal biosensors and piezoelectric biosensors. Enzyme biosensors have been developed based on immobilization procedures, i.e., adsorption of enzymes by van der Waals forces, ionic bonding or covalent bonding. The enzymes frequently employed for this function are oxidoreductases, polyphenol oxidases, peroxidases and aminooxidases [15–18]. The principal microbe-based or cell-based sensor was presented by Diviès. The tissues for tissue-based sensors are obtained from plant and animal sources. The analyte of interest can be an inhibitor or a substrate of these procedures. Rechnitz [19] established the first tissue-based sensor for the detection of the amino acid arginine. Organelle-based sensors were introduced, incorporating membranes, chloroplasts, mitochondria and microsomes. For this type of biosensor, stability is high, however, the recognition time is longer and the specificity is reduced. Immunosensors were based on the well-known fact that antibodies have high affinity towards their corresponding antigens, i.e., the antibodies exactly bind to pathogens or toxins, or interact with components of the host's immune system. DNA biosensors were developed based on the feature that a single-strand nucleic acid molecule is able to identify and bind to its opposite strand in a sample. This interaction is due to the development of stable hydrogen bonds between the two nucleic acid strands [20]. Magnetic biosensors and miniaturized biosensors distinguish magnetic micro- and nanoparticles in microfluidic channels by means of the magnetoresistance effect and have great efficiency in terms of sensitivity and size [21]. Thermal biosensors or calorimetric biosensors are devised by assimilating biosensor materials into a physical transducer. Piezoelectric biosensors are of two types: the quartz crystal microbalance and the surface acoustic wave devices. They are based on the extent of changes in the resonance frequency of a piezoelectric crystal because of mass changes in the crystal structure. Optical biosensors comprise a light source, as well as many optical components to produce a light beam with specific properties and to focus this light to a modulating agent, a modified sensing head along with a photodetector [22]. Green fluorescent protein and the subsequent autofluorescent protein (AFP) alternatives and the development of genetic fusion have supported the growth of genetically encoded biosensors [23–30]. This kind of biosensor is user-friendly, and easy to design, manipulate and transfer into cells. A single-chain Förster resonance energy transfer (FRET) biosensor is another example. They comprise a pair of AFPs, which are efficient in transferring fluorescence resonance energy between themselves when brought close together. Various procedures may be used to control variations in FRET signals based on the intensity, ratio or lifetime of the AFPs. Peptide and protein biosensors are simply fabricated via synthetic chemistry followed by enzymatic labeling with synthetic fluorophores. Owing to the individuality of the genetically encoded AFPs, they are easily employed to regulate target activity and constitute attractive alternatives to more traditional methods. They have an additional benefit of being able to improve the signal-to-noise ratio and the sensitivity of response via introduction of chemical quenchers and photoactivatable groups. Based on the sensor devices and the type of materials used, there are different types of biosensors. A number of them are discussed below.

5.3.1 Electrochemical biosensors

Electrochemical biosensors are simple devices based on electric current, ionic or conductance changes caused by bioelectrodes. Enzyme-based electrochemical biosensors are employed extensively in our day-to-day lives, such as in healthcare, food safety and environmental monitoring. Healthcare is a key area for biosensor applications, such as checking blood-glucose levels in diabetics using glucose biosensors. Moreover, the reliable determination of urea has potential applications for patients with renal disease, for use either at home or in the hospital. Large-scale applications for biosensors comprise observing fermentation broths or food processing events via monitoring amounts of glucose and other fermentative end products. The sensitive recognition of phenolic compounds is a significant topic for environmental research, as phenolic compounds are frequently present in the wastewaters of various industries, and can cause harm to our living environment, as many of them are very toxic [31].

5.3.1.1 Amperometric biosensors

Enzyme-based, amperometric electrochemical biosensing facilitates a highly selective and sensitive response in a complex environment. In comparison to other methods, such as microdialysis and nuclear magnetic resonance (NMR) spectroscopy, microsensors can rapidly and precisely measure extracellular low analyte concentrations within the tissue in near real time [15]. The principle of amperometric biosensors is based on the movement of electrons (i.e., determination of electric current) as a result of enzyme-catalyzed redox reactions (figure 5.3). Usually, a continuous voltage passes between the electrodes which can be easily measured. During an enzymatic reaction, the substrate or product can transfer an electron with the electrode surface to be oxidized or reduced. This results in an improved current flow that can be measured. The intensity of the current is proportional to the substrate concentration. The Clark oxygen electrode, which controls reduction of O_2, is one of the simplest forms of amperometric biosensor and glucose determination by glucose oxidase is a common example of this type of biosensor. There is a direct transfer of the electrons released to the electrode, which may pose some practical problems. After the first-generation amperometric biosensors, second-generation amperometric biosensors have been established wherein a mediator (e.g. ferrocenes) takes up the electrons and then transfers them to the electrode. These biosensors, however, are yet to become prevalent. One drawback of this sensor principle is the need for oxygen, which has inadequate solubility in aqueous fluids, only about 200 μM under physiological conditions. It is accessible only in lower concentrations within tissues due to the restricted supply by blood vessels and permanent cellular consumption [15, 32]. Thus when one is measuring higher analyte concentrations, the objective is to attain a diffusion-limited regime by restricting analyte diffusion using an additional membrane. Preferably, this membrane limits

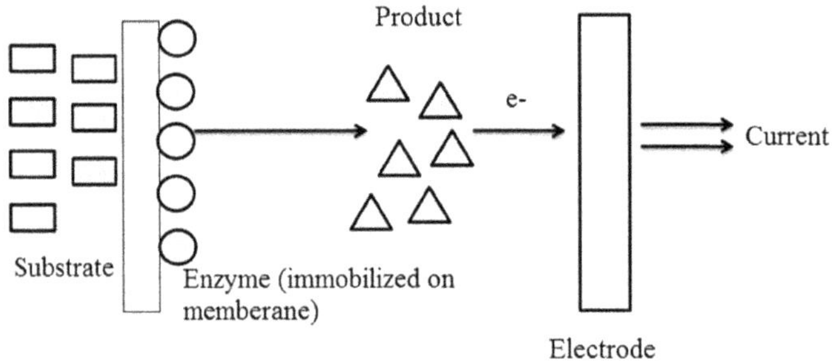

Figure 5.3. A schematic representation of an amperometric biosensor.

the transport of oxygen to a much lesser degree than analyte diffusion, and thus permits an unaltered enzymatic reaction even at high analyte concentrations. With the aim to eradicate oxygen dependence, second-generation reagentless biosensors use a surplus electron acceptor (mediator) as a replacement for oxygen [15, 32].

5.3.1.1.1 Blood-glucose biosensor

The blood-glucose biosensor is a good example of amperometric biosensors, and is extensively used all over the world by diabetic patients. The blood-glucose biosensor is a watch-like device and has a single-use disposable electrode. This electrode consist of a Ag/AgCl reference electrode and a carbon working electrode with glucose oxidase and ferrocene derivative (as a mediator). For uniform dispersal of a blood drop, the electrodes are covered with a hydrophilic mesh gauze. The disposable test strips, packed in aluminum foil, have a shelf-life of about 6 months.

Different types of amperometric biosensor can be used for measuring the freshness of fish. Compared to other nucleotides, the accumulation of inosine and hypoxanthine designate the freshness of fish, i.e., how long it has been dead and stored. For this purpose, a biosensor using immobilized nucleoside phosphorylase and xanthine oxidase over an electrode has been developed.

Usually, glucose measurements are based on interactions with one of three enzymes: hexokinase, glucose oxidase (GOx) or glucose-1-dehydrogenase (GDH) [32, 33]. The basic idea of the glucose biosensor is based on the fact that the immobilized GOx catalyzes the oxidation of β-d-glucose by molecular oxygen, generating gluconic acid and hydrogen peroxide [34]. To work as a catalyst, GOx requires a redox co-factor–flavin adenine dinucleotide (FAD). FAD works as the initial electron acceptor and is reduced to $FADH_2$:

$$\text{Glucose} + \text{GOx} - \text{FAD} + \rightarrow \text{Glucolactone} + \text{GOx} - \text{FADH}_2.$$

The co-factor is redeveloped by reacting with oxygen, resulting in the production of hydrogen peroxides:

$$\text{GOx} - \text{FADH}_2 + \text{O}_2 \rightarrow \text{GOx} - \text{FAD} + \text{H}_2\text{O}_2.$$

Hydrogen peroxide is oxidized at a catalytic, characteristically platinum (Pt) anode. The electrode easily identifies the number of electron transfers, and this electron flow is directly related to the number of glucose molecules present in the blood [35]:

$$\text{H}_2\text{O}_2 \rightarrow 2\text{H} + +\text{O}_2 + 2\text{e}.$$

Three overall strategies are employed for the electrochemical sensing of glucose: by determining oxygen consumption; by determining the concentration of hydrogen peroxide formed by the enzyme reaction; or by employing a diffusible or immobilized mediator to transfer the electrons from the GOx to the electrode. The number and types of GDH-based amperometric biosensors have been increasing. The GDH family includes GDH-pyrroquinolinequinone (PQQ) [36–38] and GDH-nicotinamide-adenine dinucleotide (NAD) [38–41]. The enzymatic reaction of GDH is independent of the dissolved oxygen. The quinoprotein GDH recognition element uses PQQ as a co-factor:

$$\text{Glucose} + \text{PQQ(ox)} \rightarrow \text{gluconolactone} + \text{PQQ(red)}.$$

This mechanism necessitates neither oxygen nor NAD^+. GDH–PQQ is a largely efficient enzyme system, with a rapid electron transfer rate, however, it is comparatively expensive.

GDH with NAD as a co-factor produces NADH rather than H_2O_2. NAD is a major electron acceptor in the oxidation of glucose, during which the nicotinamide ring of NAD^+ accepts a hydrogen ion and two electrons, equivalent to a hydride ion. The reduced form of this carrier generated in this reaction is called NADH, which can be electrochemically oxidized:

$$\text{Glucose} + NAD^+ \rightarrow \text{gluconolactone} + \text{NADHNADH} \rightarrow NAD^+ + H^+ + 2e.$$

5.3.1.2 Potentiometric biosensors

A potentiometric device determines the accumulation of a charge potential at the working electrode compared to the reference electrode in an electrochemical cell when zero or no considerable current flows between them [42–44]. In particular, potentiometry offers information about the ion activity in an electrochemical reaction [42–44]. The principle of this bioreactor is based on fluctuations in ionic concentrations which are determined using ion-selective electrodes (figure 5.4). The pH electrode is the most frequently used ion-selective electrode, as many enzymatic reactions include the release or absorption of hydrogen ions. Other significant electrodes are ammonia-selective and CO_2-selective electrodes. The potential difference found between the potentiometric electrode and the reference electrode can easily be determined. It is relative to the concentration of the substrate. One of the major limitations of potentiometric biosensors is the sensitivity of enzymes to ionic concentrations such as H^+ and NH^{4+}.

Potentiometry is also employed as a technique to electrically measure the point in a (bio)chemical reaction at which equal concentrations of opposing solutions reach a state of equilibrium (e.g. 0.1 mol HCl and 0.1 mol NaOH). This is called determining a titration end-point; the procedure is known as potentiometric

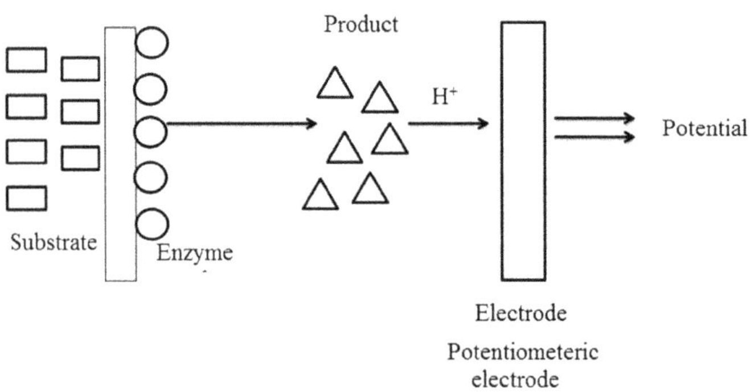

Figure 5.4. A schematic representation of a potentiometric biosensor.

titration. By carrying out a titration at constant or zero current, the end-point is recognized from the variations in electrode potential, which are produced by variations in solution concentration of the potential-determining ion. Numerous potentiometric devices are also based on many forms of field-effect transistor devices to determine pH variations, selective ion concentrations and the kinetics of biocatalytic reactions encompassing enzymes [45]. An additional example and novel optical/electrochemical hybrid method is called the light addressable potentiometric sensor [45–51]. This is a silicon-based detector that takes advantage of the photovoltaic effect to selectively detect the point of measurement. By scanning with a focused light source, it can measure the spatially resolved surface potential distribution along the interface of the sample and substrate surfaces [52].

5.3.1.3 Ion-selective field-effect transistors

For several years, much attention has been given to silicon-based biosensors in the area of bio-analytical applications owing to their promising features, which include sensitivity, speed, miniaturization and low cost [53–55]. This attention is obvious in the many investigations that have observed biological events, such as nucleic acid hybridization, protein–protein interaction, antigen–antibody binding and enzyme–substrate reactions, by means of these silicon-based biosensors. Among these, the ion-sensitive field-effect transistor (ISFET) is one of the most common electrical biosensors and was presented as the first miniaturized silicon-based chemical sensor [53–55]. The ISFET, usually known as a pH sensor, has been employed to determine ion concentration (H^+ or OH^-) in a solution through the effect of an interface potential on the gate insulator. The ISFET is a type of potentiometric device that functions similarly to a metal oxide semiconductor field-effect transistor. Consequently, so as to evaluate the performance of an ISFET, it makes sense to first recognize the overall principles behind the setup of the potentiometric sensor. ISFETs are the economic devices that can be employed for miniaturization (to manufacture ever smaller mechanical, optical and electronic products and devices) of potentiometric biosensors. An excellent example is the ISFET biosensor employed to monitor intramyocardial pH during bypass surgery [53–55].

5.3.1.4 Conductimetric biosensors

Conductometric biosensors were first introduced in 1961 to measure urea. The procedure is based on electrical conductivity variation. Formaldehyde, pesticides, insecticides and nitrate biosensors using conductometry were also established [56]. The urea biosensor was upgraded using a platinum electrode as a matrix for urease immobilization [56]. A conductimetric biosensor determines small variations in the conductivity of a solution by employing a conductimetric transducer, i.e., a conductivity meter. Conductivity determination is dependent on the biocatalytic reaction of the sample on an electrode. The reaction will generate ions which will result in the variation in conductivity [57]. The conductimetric transducer comprises two electrodes, a reference and a working electrode. Both electrodes are coated with a membrane referred to as the nata de coco membrane. The enzyme is immobilized on the working electrode, however, not on the reference electrode. Throughout the reaction, CO_2 is formed on the working electrode, which is soluble in water to form HCO_3^- and H_3O^+. Furthermore, no reaction takes place on the reference electrode, so the mobility of ions on the two electrodes is different and the conductivity is changed. There are a number of reactions in the biological systems that bring about changes in the ionic species. These ionic species change the electrical conductivity which can be determined. An outstanding example of conductimetric biosensor is the urea biosensor using immobilized urease. Urease catalyzes the following reaction:

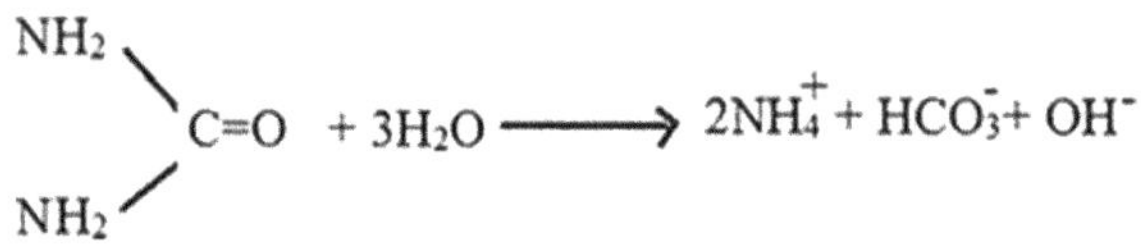

The above reaction is related to sudden modification in ionic concentration which can be used for monitoring urea concentration. Actually, urea biosensors are very fruitfully employed in dialysis and renal surgery.

5.3.2 Thermometric biosensors

Thermometric or calorimeteric biosensors utilize an essential property of biological reactions, i.e., absorption or emission of heat [57]. This is represented as a variation in the temperature within the reaction medium. In previous reports on calorimetry, the variation in heat was directly observed to measure the level of reaction (for catalysis) or structural dynamics of biomolecules in the dissolved state [58]. Its utilization in biosensors results in the development of thermometric devices [59]. These mainly determine the variation in temperature of the circulating fluid following the reaction of a appropriate substrate with the immobilized enzyme molecules. Thermometry basically means the determination of temperature. The most basic type of such a device is a thermometer, regularly used for determination of body or ambient temperature. However, simple mercury based-thermometers are restricted by their temperature sensitivity in addition to the toxicity of metallic mercury. Based on similar methods, in thermometric devices the heat is determined using sensitive thermistors [59]; such devices are generally called enzyme thermistors [60]. Calorimetric devices for regular use were restricted by the cost of the process and the comparatively long experimental processes. The creation of an enzyme thermistor based on flow injection examination in combination with an immobilized biocatalyst and heat-sensing element circumvented several of these limitations [61, 62]. A number of instruments were introduced in the past two decades that combined the principles of calorimetry, enzyme catalysis, immobilization on suitable matrices and flow injection analysis.

A schematic representation of a thermal biosensor is shown in figure 5.5. It includes a heat insulated box fitted with a heat exchanger (an aluminum cylinder). The reaction occurs in a small enzyme packed bed reactor. As the substrate comes into the bed, it is transformed into a product and heat is generated. The temperature

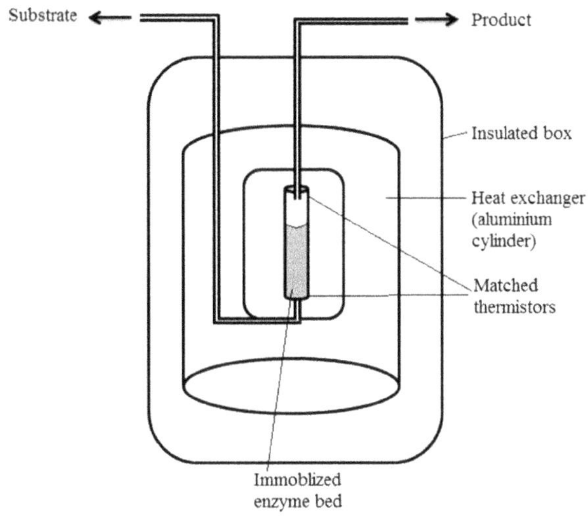

Figure 5.5. A schematic representation of a thermometric biosensor.

difference between the substrate and product is determined by thermistors. Even a small change in temperature can be measured by thermal biosensors. Thermometric biosensors are usually employed for the estimation of serum cholesterol. When cholesterol is oxidized by the enzyme cholesterol oxidase, heat is produced which can be determined. Similarly, measurements of glucose (enzyme glucose oxidase), urea (enzyme-urease), uric acid (enzyme-uricase) and penicillin G (enzyme β lactamase) can be achieved by these biosensors. Generally, however, their efficacy is limited. Thermometric biosensors can be employed as part of enzyme linked immunoassays (ELISA) and this technique is called thermometric ELISA.

5.3.3 Optical biosensors

The principle of this biosensor is based on optical measurements (absorbance, fluorescence, chemiluminescence, etc). Its utilization is based on the quality of the fiber optics and optoelectronic transducers used in fabricating these biosensors. The word optrode is used as a condensation of the words optical and electrode. Optical biosensors mainly involve enzymes and antibodies as the transducing elements. Optical biosensors facilitate safe non-electrical sensing of materials. An additional merit of optical biosensors is that these biosensors usually do not require reference sensors, as the comparative signal can be produced by means of the same source of light as the sampling sensor. Certain important optical biosensors are discussed below.

5.3.3.1 Fiber optic lactate biosensor

Figure 5.6 show a fiber optic lactate biosensor. Its functioning is based on the determination of changes in molecular O_2 concentrations by detecting the quenching effect of O_2 on a fluorescent dye. The subsequent reaction is catalyzed by the enzyme lactate mono-oxygenase.

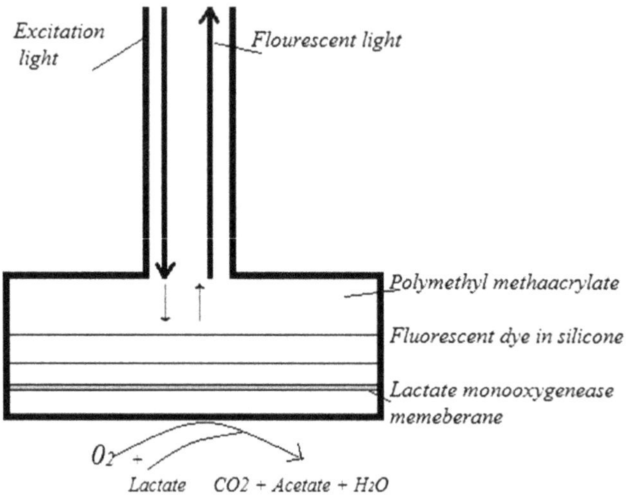

Figure 5.6. Schematic representation of a fiber optic lactate biosensor.

$$O_2 + \text{Lactate} \xrightarrow[\text{Lactate monooxygenase}]{} CO_2 + \text{ACETATE} + H_2O$$

The extent of fluorescence produced by the dyed film is dependent on O_2, because O_2 has a reducing effect on the fluorescence. As the concentration of lactate in the reaction mixture rises, O_2 is utilized, and as a result there is a proportionate decline in the quenching or reducing effect. Finally, there is an increase in fluorescent production which can be determined.

5.3.3.2 Optical biosensors for blood glucose

Optical biosensors exploit light and the selective nature of biological components to measure specific analytes [63–66]. Vast studies have been reported on optical biosensors [66], and great developments have been made [67] from the time when the first optical biosensor was introduced by Lübbers and Opitz [68]. The utilization of optical sensors can help circumvent many of the issues produced by electrochemical sensors [64, 69]. Unlike several other analytical approaches, such as electrochemical procedures, the light used is typically not damaging to the body or the system it is used in, and in theory the excitation and computing can be performed noninvasively from out the body [63]. Using fluorescence can be very sensitive [70] and the signal can travel great distances, making it possible to determine glucose concentrations in hard to reach places [5]. The device used is fairly cheap, convenient to use and is not disturbed by electrical or magnetic fields [69]. An additional advantage is that there are various procedures which can be utilized within the field of fluorescence; using a steady-state estimate by determination of the intensity differences, time-resolved fluorescence, Förster resonance energy transfer (FRET) and other procedures that can offer information about the microenvironment and structure of the molecules [63]. The first glucose biosensor was introduced in 1962 by Clark and Lyons [70] by means of glucose oxidase (GOx) entrapped over an oxygen electrode with a dialysis membrane. In 1975 the first available commercial glucose sensor was introduced by Yellow Spring Instruments Inc. [5]. A demonstration of *in vivo* glucose monitoring was presented in 1982 by Shichiri *et al* [71] and a wearable and noninvasive glucose sensor was created by Cygnus Inc. in 2000 [72]. In December 2011 Microsoft Research revealed that they were employed in making noninvasive glucose sensing contact lenses [73, 74]. After a couple of years Google started working on a similar project [75]. The fact that two multi-billion dollar companies like Microsoft and Google are investing time and money into noninvasive glucose sensors is evidence of how significant this field of research is, and that noninvasive sensors are the future.

Assessment of blood glucose is very significant for the monitoring of diabetes. This technique involves paper strips saturated with reagents. The strips contain glucose oxidase, horseradish peroxidase and a chromogen (e.g. toluidine). The following reactions occur:

$$\text{Glucose} \xrightarrow{\textit{Glucose oxidase}} \text{Gluconic acid} + H_2O_2$$

$$\text{Chromogen} + 2\,H_2O_2 \xrightarrow{\textit{Peroxidase}} \text{Colour dye} + 2H_2O$$

The intensity of the color (of the dye) can be determined by using a portable reflectance meter. Glucose strip production has now been commercialized worldwide. Colorimetric test strips of cellulose coated with suitable enzymes and reagents are also in use for the estimation of several blood and urine parameters.

5.3.3.3 Luminescent biosensors to detect urinary infections

Biosensors are being used widely in the medical field to detect infectious diseases. Various favorable biosensor technologies for urinary tract infection diagnosis along with pathogen identification and anti-microbial susceptibility are under development. The cause of urinary tract infections, i.e., the microorganisms in the urine, can be identified by employing luminescent biosensors. For this, an immobilized (or even free) enzyme called luciferase is used. The amount of light production can be determined by electronic devices. The principles of luminescent biosensors for detecting urinary infections are shown in figure 5.7. On lysis, the microorganisms release ATP.

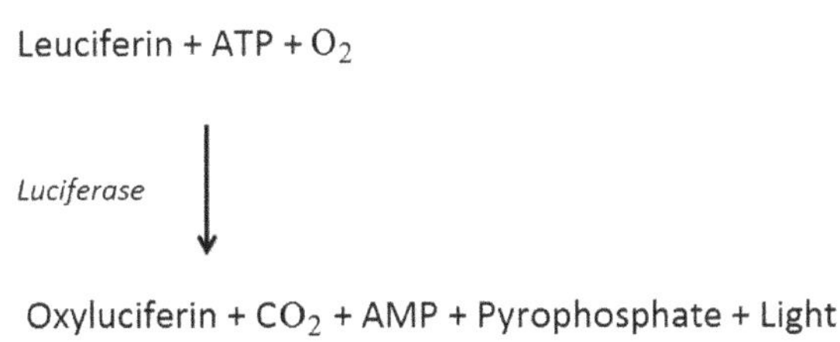

Figure 5.7. Principle of luminescent biosensors for detecting urinary infections.

5.3.3.4 Other optical biosensors

Optical fiber sensing devices are in use for determining pH, pCO_2 and pO_2 in critical care and surgical monitoring.

5.3.4 Piezoelectric biosensors

The piezoelectric effect is not an entirely new idea as it has been recognized since the nineteenth century with comprehensive scientific applications since the beginning of the twentieth century. The innovation of the piezoelectric effect is associated with the famous physicists Jacques Curie and Pierre Curie who documented the first anisotropic crystals, i.e., crystals without a center of symmetry that can produce an electric dipole when mechanically squeezed. The designated effect can work in the opposite way when an anisotropic crystal become distorted due to a voltage imposed on it [76]. This phenomenon is depicted figure 5.8.

The principle of piezoelectric biosensors is based on acoustics (sound vibrations), therefore, they are also known as acoustic biosensors. Piezoelectric crystals form the basis of these biosensors. These particles have characteristic frequencies and cystals with positive and negative charges vibrate with typical frequencies. Developed resonance frequencies are modified by the adsorption of certain molecules on the crystal surface. This resonance can be easily detected by electronic devices. Some

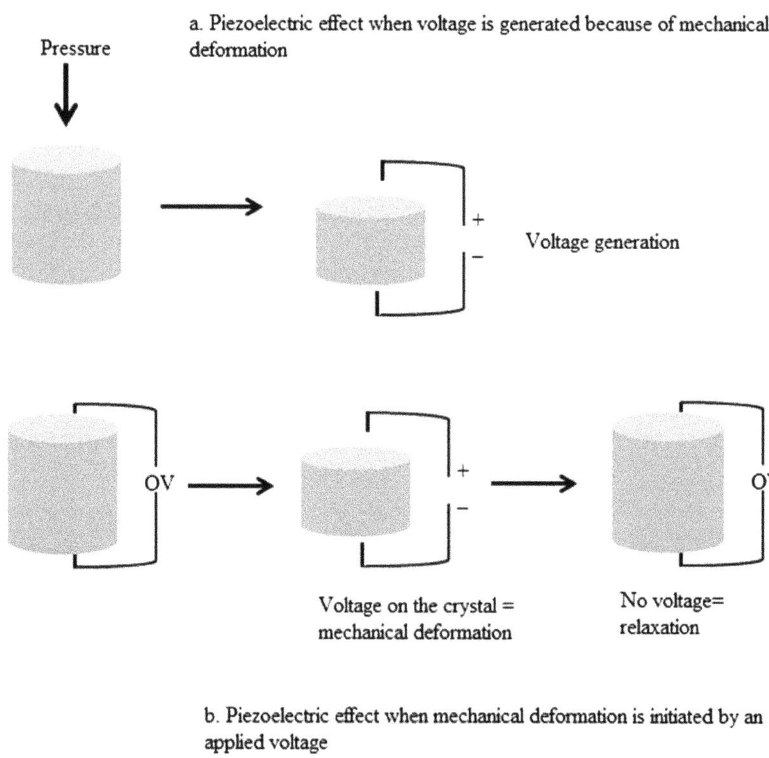

Figure 5.8. The principle of piezoelectric biosensors.

other biological compounds in different forms, such as enzymes with gaseous substrates or inhibitors, can also be attached to these crystals. By the introduction of acetylcholine esterase a piezoelectric biosensor for organophosphorus insecticide has been developed. Similarly, by introduction of formaldehyde dehydrogenase, a biosensor for formaldehyde has been created. Another example of a biosensor for cocaine (in the gas phase) has been developed by attaching cocaine antibodies to the surface of a piezoelectric crystal.

5.3.4.1 Drawbacks of piezoelectric biosensors

These biosensors cannot be utilized for the determination of substances in a solution. This is because the crystals may stop oscillating fully in viscous liquids.

5.3.5 Whole-cell biosensors

Whole-cell biosensors are mainly beneficial for multi-step or co-factor requiring reactions. These biosensors can be utilized for live or dead microbial cells. Certain examples of organisms along with the analytes and the types of biosensors used are listed in table 5.1.

Advantages of microbial cell biosensors. Microbial cells are economical as they have extended half-lives. Furthermore, in contrast to isolated enzymes, they are less sensitive to changes in pH and temperature.

Disadvantages of microbial cell biosensors. In general, whole cells entail extended periods of catalysis. Moreover, the specificity and sensitivity of whole-cell biosensors may be lower in comparison to that of enzymes.

5.3.6 Immunobiosensors

Immunosensors are compact analytical devices in which the development of antigen–antibody complexes is identified and converted, by means of a transducer, to an electrical signal, which can be processed, recorded and displayed [77]. Various transducing mechanisms are used in immunological biosensors, based on signal generation (such as an electrochemical or optical signal) or changes in properties (such as mass changes) following the formation of antigen–antibody complexes [77].

Table 5.1. A number of biosensor organisms along with the analytes and the types of biosensors.

Organism	Analyte	Type of biosensor
Sarcina flava	Glutamine	Potentiometric (NH_3)
Proteus morganii	Cysteine	Potentiometric (H_2S)
Nitrosomanas spp.	Ammonia	Amperometric (O_2)
Many organisms	Biological oxygen demand (BOD)	Amperometric (O_2)
Lactobacillus fermenti	Thiamine	Amperometric (mediated)
Lactobacillus arabinosus	Nicotinic acid	Potentiometric (H^+)
Escherichia coil	Glutamate	Potentiometric (CO_2)
Desulfovibrio desulfuricans	Sulfate	Potentiometric (SO_3)
Cyanobacteria	Herbicides	Amperometric (mediated)

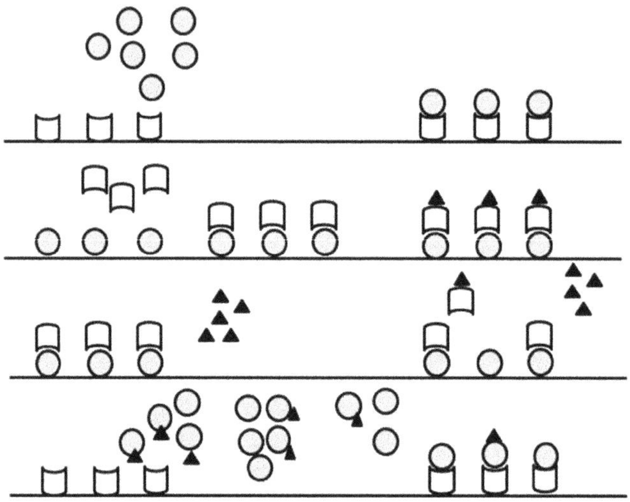

Figure 5.9. Diagrammatic representation of selected immunobiosensors. (a) Direct binding of an antigen to an immobilized antibody. (b) Antigen–antibody sandwiches (an immobilized antigen binds to an antibody and then to a second antigen). (c) An antibody binds to an immobilized antigen which is partially released by a competitive free antibody binding to a free antigen and an enzyme labeled antigen (in competition).

These are the biosensors which are based on the principle of immunological specificity, coupled with measurement (mostly) by amperometric or potentiometric biosensors. Immunobiosensors or immunochemical sensors have numerous possible configurations. Selected configurations are depicted in figure 5.9, and briefly explained in the following:

- It may contain an immobilized antibody to which the antigen can bind directly.
- It may also contain an immobilized antigen that binds to antibody which in turn can bind to a second, free antigen.

Enzyme immunosensors can be used for therapeutic applications. Some examples are as follows:

- Immobilized streptokinase and urokinase (on sephadex) can be employed for the treatment of thrombosis.
- Some success has been achieved in the management of congenital defects by employing immobilized enzymes, e.g. phenylalanine hydroxylase and lysosomal α-1,4-glucosidase to correct type II glycogen storage disease.
- Immobilized enzymes have been demonstrated in the treatment of congenital defects, e.g. phenylalanine in the treatment of phenylketonuria.

5.4 Applications of biosensors

Biosensors have become very popular in recent years. Due to their small size, easy handling, high specificity and sensitivity, and low cost, they are extensively used in various sectors. Certain important applications of biosensors are broadly described below.

5.4.1 Applications in medicine and health

Biosensors are effectively used for the quantitative assessment of several biologically vital substances in body fluids, e.g. glucose, cholesterol and urea. The glucose biosensor is of great benefit for diabetic patients for regular monitoring of blood glucose. Blood gas monitoring for pH, pCO_2 and pO_2 is performed during critical care and surgical monitoring of patients. The mutagenicity of numerous chemicals can be assessed by employing biosensors. Numerous toxic substances synthesized in the body can also be identified.

5.4.2 Applications in industry

Biosensors can also be employed for monitoring fermentation products and the assessment of various ions. Thus, biosensors assist in improving the fermentation conditions for superior yield. Currently, biosensors are used to detect the odor and freshness of foods. For example, the freshness of stored fish can be examined by ATPase. ATP is not found in spoiled fish and this can be examined by using ATPase. Some pharmaceutical companies have developed immobilized cholesterol oxidase system for the estimation of cholesterol concentration in foods (e.g. butter).

5.4.3 Applications in pollution control

Biosensors are very helpful in measuring environmental pollutants. Pesticides and biological oxygen demand can be measured by biosensors.

5.4.4 Applications in the military

Biosensors have been developed to detect toxic gases and other chemical agents used during war.

5.4.5 Immobilized enzymes and cell therapeutic applications

The industrial and analytical applications of immobilized enzymes are described in detail in an above section. There are several limitations on the direct utilization of enzymes for therapeutic purposes:

- Poor availability of the enzyme at the active site.
- Sensitivity to natural inhibitors.
- Interference by endogenous proteases.
- Immunogenicity of certain enzymes.

Further important therapeutic applications of immobilized enzymes and cells are briefly described in the following.

5.4.5.1 Improved drug delivery by using immobilized enzymes

Urea-urease modulated system. Drug delivery can be improved by using immobilized urease enzymes along with the substrate urea (figure 5.10). This procedure is dependent on the action of urease. Urease splits urea which may result in an increase in pH owing to the formation of ammonium hydroxide. Thus a therapeutic

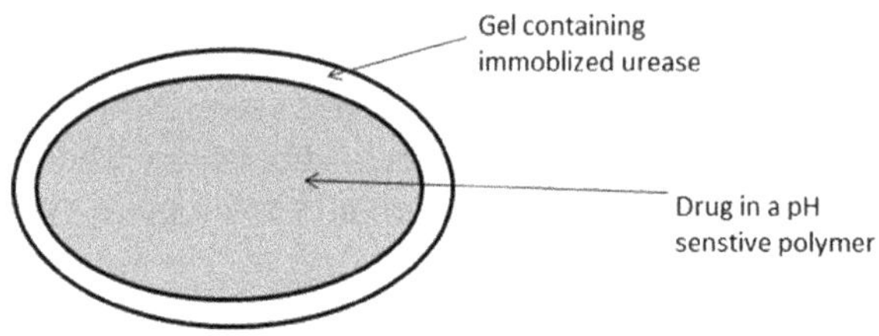

Figure 5.10. A schematic representation of immobilized urease for drug delivery.

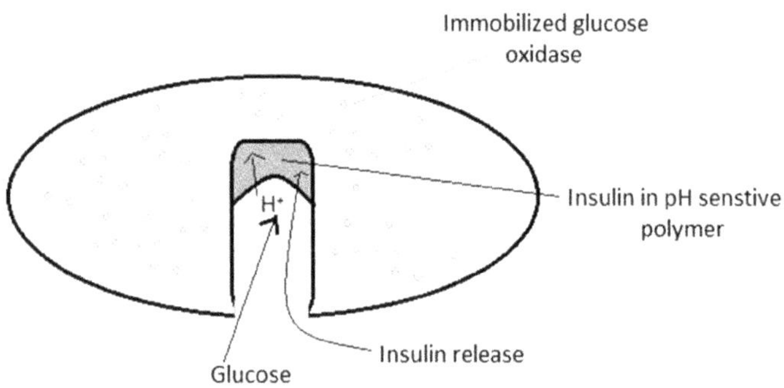

Figure 5.11. A schematic representation of immobilized glucose oxidase for insulin delivery.

drug present in a pH sensitive biodegradable polymer can be successfully released to perform its function (figure 5.11).

Glucose oxidase-glucose based system. A biodegradable polymeric system comprising insulin has been developed for efficient insulin delivery to the human body. By the help of immobilized glucose oxidase enzyme insulin delivery can be controlled (figure 5.11). After the action of glucose oxidase, gluconic acid is produced which can ultimately decrease the pH. The low pH, in turn, causes the release of insulin from the bio-erodible polymeric system.

5.4.5.2 Immobilization of artificial cells

An artificial cell mainly comprises a spherical semipermeable membrane with similar dimensions to a living cell. The biological materials, e.g. enzymes, enclosed within the artificial cells can be immobilized. The thus-immobilized compact artificial cells can function as artificial organs. Using this procedure, the most important artificial organs developed include artificial kidney, artificial liver, blood detoxifiers and immunosorbents. Their operation is, however, very restricted. Through multiple reactions, a multienzyme system can be immobilized in the form of artificial cells for the transformation of a substrate to a product.

5.5 Recent advancements in biosensor technology

A biosensor refers to an analytical instrument employed for the identification of a chemical compound, which integrates a biological element with a physicochemical detector. Notable advancements have been made in the advancement of precise and

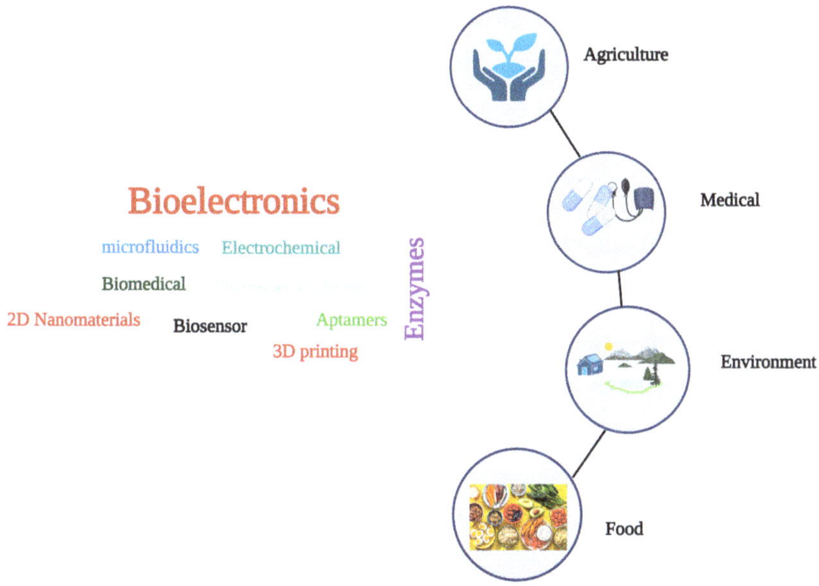

Figure 5.12. Subjects related to biosensing, including various subcategories and their potential applications as analytical tools.

resilient analytical techniques that include biological sensing elements, commonly known as biosensors [78]. Traditional to traditional methodologies, utilizing aptamers or nucleotides, affibodies, peptide arrays, and molecule imprinted polymers offers viable avenues for advancing innovative biosensors. The development of highly regenerative biosensors with precise and sensitive capabilities is greatly aided by integrated techniques. Biosensors made from bacteria, polymers, and nanomaterials all have the ability to be used in more situations. Biosensors with a wide array of applications necessitate the implementation of a variety of development methodologies [79]. Different subjects related to biosensors and their applications are shown in figure 5.12.

5.5.1 Electrochemical biosensors

The electrochemical aptamer-based (E-AB) biosensor has the capability to produce an electrochemical signal upon the binding of specified targets. The utilization of glucose biosensors is well recognized and valued within the medical field, among healthcare facilities and diagnostic centers. This is primarily attributed to its crucial function enabling routine blood glucose monitoring for diabetes patients. However, glucose biosensors may face some limitations due to unstable enzyme activity or lack of uniformity, requiring extra calibration procedures. The restrictions have led to the invention of several biomolecules that possess unique electrochemical properties [80]. This has subsequently enabled the investigation of glucose biosensors with enhanced effectiveness. In the present era, producing electrochemical biosensors often entails the surface alteration of metal and carbon electrodes by applying biomaterials, such as enzymes, antibodies, or DNA. The generation of the output signal in a biosensor is frequently facilitated by the occurrence of specific binding or catalytic reactions involving biomaterials on the surface of the electrode [81]. The necessity for the advancement of electrochemical sensors has become essential in the realm of clinical diagnostics, specifically in situations when the timely identification or surveillance of illnesses is considered crucial. Within this specific context, considering synthetic materials as viable alternatives to proteins is a common practice in developing non-enzymatic biosensors. It is important to note that various biomolecules display varying degrees of electrode stability and selectivity, hence playing a pivotal role in developing innovative electrochemical biosensors intended for a wide range of applications. Various electrochemical biosensors have been created to cater to various needs. As previously explicated, glucose biosensors have evolved quickly since their initial inception [82]. This research aims to examine the advancements made in using ferroceneboronic acid 'FcBA' and ferrocene modified boronic acids to create biosensors. These compounds have a significant potential because they have a binding site (in this case, a boronic acid moiety) and an electrochemically active component (in this case, an Fc residue). This combination gives them the ability to bind to a specific target. FcBA and its derivatives have a remarkable feature in which they preferentially bind to the 1,2- or 1,3-diol functional groups that are present in sugars. This results in the creation of cyclic boronate esters. As a result of the redox properties of the FcBA-sugar adduct exhibiting differences, electrochemical identification can be accomplished. This serves as a foundation for electrochemical identification. Furthermore, it is worth noting that boronic acids possess a notable affinity for attaching to Fe− ions. This characteristic presents an added advantage in developing non-conventional ion-selective electrodes targeting F− ions. The hydrocarbon chains found within the polypeptide structure of HbA1c can be quantified by utilizing FcBA-based electrochemical detection [83]. One significant constraint associated with this approach is the necessity to immobilize FcBA derivatives onto the electrodes' surface, given that these derivatives are introduced into the sample mixtures as components. The incorporation of polymers or silver electrodes, along with appropriate modifications of FcBA derivatives, have the potential to enhance the performance of FcBA electrochemical sensors in biomedical applications, particularly in the field of diabetes diagnosis, where the monitoring of glucose levels is of great importance [84].

Developing an electrochemical biosensor for evaluating antioxidant levels and reactive oxygen species in physiological systems is a notable contemporary innovation. One significant use in this field involves the identification of uric acid as the principal product of purine metabolism in bodily fluids. This serves as a diagnostic tool for a range of clinical abnormalities or diseases. Nevertheless, it is imperative to devise an economical and responsive approach. The utilization of an electrochemical-based methodology for the determination of uric acid oxidation and the quantification of glucose appears to be highly advantageous.

Nevertheless, the similarity between uric acid and ascorbic acid in terms of oxidation presents a significant challenge in developing a highly sensitive electrochemical biosensor [85]. To address this challenge, researchers have devised a biosensor utilizing amperometry sensing to quantify both reduction and oxidation potentials. Given the financial implications and the need for replicability in this process, it is crucial to immobilize or employ screen printing techniques to apply the enzyme onto nanomaterial-based electrodes. The latter option is particularly advantageous as it facilitates the creation of uric acid biosensors that are disposable, selective, cost-effective, and highly sensitive, making them suitable for routine analysis. Recent developments in 3D bioprinting have focused on creating biosensors incorporating living cells within 3D microenvironments [86]. A novel wireless mouth-guard biosensor has been created to enable real-time and continuous detection of salivary uric acid levels. This technology has the potential to be expanded to include wearable monitoring devices for a wide range of health and fitness applications. The utilization of electrochemical biosensors has proven to be effective in hormone measures. However, a comprehensive examination of its potential merits further investigation. One prospective domain of technological advancement in biosensors is specifically targeting nucleic acids. The scientific community widely recognizes the utilization of cellular miRNA expression as a biomarker for the identification of illness beginning and the enhancement of gene therapy efficacy for hereditary disorders. Typically, miRNAs are detected through techniques such as northern blotting, microarray analysis, and polymerase chain reaction (PCR). Contemporary technological advancements have facilitated the development of electrochemical biosensors that are very suitable for detecting miRNA [87]. These biosensors employ a label-free detection approach, wherein the detection process involves the oxidation of guanine following the formation of a hybrid between the miRNA and its capture probe, which is substituted with inosine. The advancements in biofortification techniques have played a significant role in developing electrochemical-based biosensor technologies in biomedicine.

Using biosensor technology is crucial for prompt detection of pesticide residues in environmental monitoring, as it plays a significant role in mitigating potential health risks [88]. Conventional techniques, including high-performance liquid chromatography, capillary electrophoresis, and mass spectrometry, have proven efficient in examining pesticides within the environment. However, these methods possess certain drawbacks, such as intricate procedures, time-intensive protocols, the need for sophisticated instrumentation, and operational constraints. Therefore, essential biosensors appear to offer significant benefits, yet developing a unified biosensor capable of evaluating several classes of pesticides is a complex task. To achieve this objective, researchers have created enzyme-based biosensors to assess the physiological consequences of pesticides on the environment and ensure food safety and quality management. Biosensors based on acetylcholinesterase inhibition (AChE) were developed to achieve this objective. There have been significant advancements in AChE inhibition-based biosensors in recent years, particularly in quick analysis [88]. These advancements have primarily focused on enhancing the approach through improvements in immobilization procedures and various fabrication strategies. Piezoelectric biosensors have been created to detect the environmental impact of organophosphate and carbamate pesticides. Organochlorine pesticides have been observed to significantly impact ecosystems, mainly when pesticides such

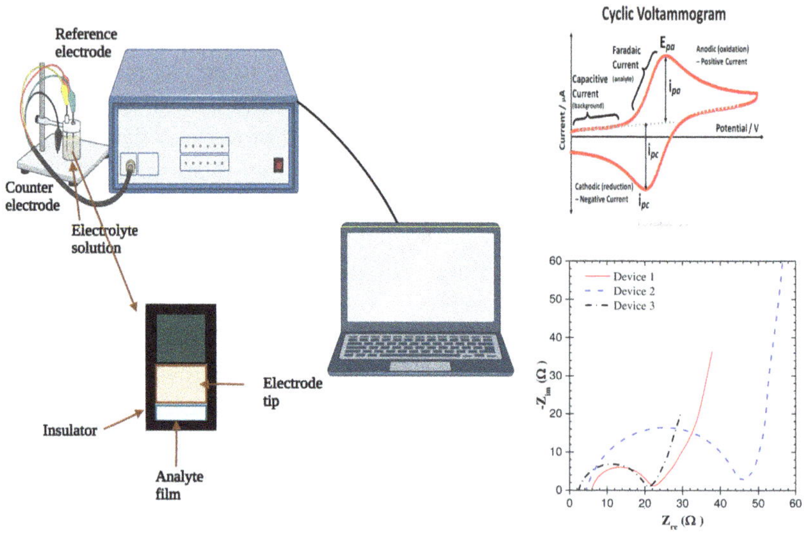

Figure 5.13. Diagram depicting an electrochemical biosensor.

as endosulfan are involved, leading to substantial ecological harm. Undoubtedly, the utilization of pesticides has distinct effects on the reproductive systems of male and female fish. Given these circumstances, the development of biosensors for assessing the aquatic ecosystem holds considerable importance, particularly considering the phenomenon of biomagnification [89]. In response to the increasing demand, the field of electrochemical biosensors has experienced a significant transformation characterized by notable advancements in the manufacturing and utilization of nanomaterials, quartz, and silica. Concerning biosensor implementations for food safeguarding, security of the environment, and surveillance, the choice of the receptor for biosensor advancement and the utilization of several different transduction mechanisms and efficient screening tactics have substantial importance. This is especially true when considering the issue of biosensor deployments in the safety of food. To facilitate this, the manufacture of biosensors appears to have significant importance, and the subsequent breakthroughs in this domain will be systematically elucidated in the following sections [90]. An electrochemical biosensor diagram is presented in figure 5.13.

5.5.2 Optical/visual biosensors

As previously elucidated, there is a growing need for the advancement of biosensors characterized by their simplicity, rapidity, and high sensitivity to meet the requirements of environmental and biological applications. This possibility can be realized using immobilizers, including a diverse range of materials such as gold substances made of carbon, quartz, silica, or glass. Integrating gold nanoparticles or quantum dots using microfabrication techniques presents a novel technological approach to advancing cytochrome P450 enzyme biosensors, offering enhanced sensitivity and portability for specific applications. Moreover, fiber-optic chemical sensors are essential in diverse domains, including drug innovation, biomedicine, and biosensing [91]. Recently, hydrogels have gained prominence as materials for restriction purposes in fiber-optic chemistry, particularly in the context of DNA-based sensors. In contrast to alternative materials, the process of immobilization within hydrogels takes place in a three-dimensional (3D) manner, hence enabling a substantial loading capacity for sensing molecules. Hydrogels, namely polyacrylamide, are polymers that have been cross-linked and have hydrophilic characteristics. These polymers can convert into several physical states, including thin films or nanoparticles, to enable immobilization [92]. Hydrogels' multiple benefits, including trapping, controlled release, analyte amplification, and DNA conservation, have made them a popular substrate for DNA immobilization. Hydrogels are substances that can help biomolecules stick to other molecules. They do this in a way that no other material can. Additionally, the helpful optical clarity that hydrogels exhibit makes them valuable visual evaluation tools. There is a consensus among scholars that the use of monolithic polyacrylamide gels and gel microparticles for immobilizing DNA biosensors signifies a notable advancement in biosensor technology. The DNA detection process has been used for the electrochemical oxidation of hydrazine. Using this technology, we can now track down specific DNA molecules [93].

5.5.3 Silica, quartz/crystal, and glass biosensors

Due to their distinctive characteristics, the utilization of silica, quartz, crystal, and glass materials has been prevalent in contemporary biosensor development. Silicon nanoparticles exhibit significant promise for driving technical advancements in biosensor applications, primarily attributable to their biocompatible nature, abundant availability, and notable electrical, optical, and mechanical capabilities. In addition, it is crucial for biomedical and biological applications that silicon nanoparticles exhibit no toxicity. Silicon nanoparticles have diverse applications encompassing bioimaging, biosensing, and cancer therapy [94]. Moreover, the utilization of fluorescent silicon nanoparticles exhibits significant potential for enduring applications in bioimaging. Notably, combining silicon nanowires with gold nanoparticles yields hybrids that serve as innovative silicon-based nano-reagents for efficacious cancer therapy. The covalent bonding of DNA oligomers modified with thiol groups onto silica or glass substrates offers the advantage of producing DNA films more suitable for UV spectroscopy and hybridization techniques. Despite the numerous advantages associated with the utilization of silicon nanoparticles, it is imperative to thoroughly assess prevailing problems, including the establishment of cost-effective, large-scale production techniques, as well as the evaluation of biocompatibility following biomolecular interaction [12]. Addressing these challenges will facilitate the integration of silicon nanoparticles as contemporary biosensor components. Quartz-crystal-microbalance biosensors, which do not need wires or electrodes, provide a new, more sensitive option for studying biomolecular interactions. The oscillatory oscillations of the quartz oscillator were initiated and seen using antennas, which enabled the wireless transmission of electromagnetic energies, obviating the need for mechanical cable connections. The potential to provide exact readings without the need for direct physical touch is essential for achieving ultrahigh sensitivity in detecting proteins in fluids utilizing gear constructed around quartz crystal biological sensors. Due to their unique properties, silica, quartz, and glass are used to develop cutting-edge biosensors. These biosensors use advanced technological advancements to enhance the efficacy of bio-instrumentation within the medical domain. However, it is crucial to address concerns about biological security and the associated financial implications [95].

5.5.4 Nanomaterials-based biosensors

A wide range of tiny materials, including silver, gold, silicon, and copper nanoparticles, in addition to materials made from carbon like graphite, graphene, and nanotubes made of carbon, are used in biosensor immobilization. In addition, the use of substances that involve nanoparticles has notable benefits in terms of increased specificity and sensitivity in the advancement of electrochemical and alternative biosensors. Because of their small size and resistance to oxidation, nanoparticles of gold are seen as a viable material for use in nanotechnology [96]. For example, silver nanoparticles may corrode and adversely affect intra-body operations like drug delivery. Utilizing nanomaterials in biosensors for biomedicine has significant obstacles that must be effectively addressed. In addition, it is crucial to consider the potential advantages and downsides of signal amplification systems based on nanoparticles. However, nanoparticles are widely regarded as crucial elements in bio-analytical instruments because they enhance sensitivity and improve detection limits for single-molecule analysis. It is pertinent to acknowledge the invention of platinum-based nanoparticles that were utilized for electrochemical amplification, which resulted in a solitary label response mechanism for detecting DNA at low concentrations. This information is pertinent because it is applicable to the current setting [97].

Similarly, the coupling of semiconductor quantum dots and iron oxide nanocrystals, which possess optical and magnetic characteristics, can be successfully achieved using tumor-targeted ligands. These ligands, including monoclonal antibodies, peptides, or small molecules, exhibit a strong affinity and specificity towards tumor antigens, hence facilitating precise targeting of tumors. The utilization of quantum dots technology holds the potential for comprehending the intricacies of the tumor microenvironment in the context of therapeutic interventions and facilitating the administration of nanomedicine. The assessment of beam size, which may be micro, milli and nano cantilever biosensors, is subject to severe examination owing to its prospective applications across diverse disciplines [98].

5.5.5 Fluorescent biosensors that are either genetically encoded or synthetic

The utilization of genetically encoded or synthetic fluorescence in creating tagged biosensors has facilitated the comprehension of biological processes, including a diverse range of biochemical pathways occurring inside the cellular environment. The development of fluorescent-tagged antibodies was first intended to visualize fixed cells. Utilizing natural amino acids, small-molecular interactions with substances, and additional messengers are unique approaches offered because of this approach, which has undoubtedly contributed to the development of sensors [99]. Recently, fluorescent biosensors have been developed that enable the analysis of motor proteins through single-molecule detection, which allows for the precise determination of analyte concentration. The technique that is used for probe identification and evaluation looks to present some difficulties, notwithstanding the benefits that have been discussed previously. The discovery of green fluorescent protein and other fluorescent proteins has yielded numerous benefits in optical probe design and efficiency. In the preceding decade, there has been significant progress in genetically encoded biosensors targeting chemicals associated with energy production, reactive oxygen species, and cyclic adenosine monophosphate (cAMP).

Similarly, cyclic guanosine monophosphate (cGMP) serves as a crucial signaling molecule and holds significance as a pharmacological target within the cardiovascular system [100]. Given these circumstances, researchers have successfully created biosensors based on Förster resonance energy transfer (FRET) to enable the visualization of cellular levels of cGMP, cAMP, and Ca^{2+}. Several of these sensors have high efficacy in primary culture and *in vivo* imaging of live cells. Several crucial elements have been successfully identified in developing sensors for live-animal imaging. The utilization of optimized methodologies, such as small-angle x-ray scattering for the development of calcium sensors and fluorescence resonance energy transfer probes for kinase sensing, is widely acknowledged as the most effective biosensor techniques in contemporary physiology in this manner, a few biosensors utilizing microbial and cell organelle systems were designed to detect and analyze specific targets [100]. As previously elucidated, electrochemical, electromechanical, and optical biosensors have been devised to detect miRNA more efficiently than alternative molecular methodologies. The development of living tissue imaging through the utilization of small chemical biological sensors has resulted in an improved knowledge of cellular activity and the finding of many molecules, such as DNA, RNA, and miRNA. The advancement in this domain necessitates the adoption of a comprehensive genomic methodology employing enhanced optical-based genetic biosensors. The current consensus in the scientific community is that optical-based biosensors, which utilize a mix of fluorescence and tiny molecules/nanomaterials, have demonstrated significant advancements in both their practical applications and sensitivity [101].

5.6 Microbial biosensors utilizing synthetic biology and genetic/protein engineering techniques

Current development in environmental monitoring and bioremediation involves the application of advanced technologies rooted in genetic/protein engineering and synthetic biology. These technologies enable the programming of microorganisms to exhibit desired signal outputs, sensitivity, and selectivity. For instance, the utilization of live cells possessing enzymatic activity for the degradation of xenobiotic substances holds significant potential for broader applications in bioremediation

[102]. In a similar vein, researchers have devised microbial fuel-based biosensors with the objective of monitoring levels of biochemical oxygen demand and assessing toxicity within the surrounding environment. Bacterial organisms can break down organic substrates and produce electrical energy through fermentation. The technology encompasses utilizing a bio-electrochemical apparatus that regulates the capacity of microbial respiration to transform organic substrates into electrical energy directly. Despite the potential advantages, microbial biosensors are constrained by limits related to their low power density, which affects both production and operational costs. There is a current focus on improving performance and reducing costs through novel systemic approaches. These approaches leverage technologies to create self-powered engineered microbial biosensors, which hold promise for considerable advancements. Microbial biosensors have demonstrated promising applications in detecting pesticides and heavy metals [91]. Eukaryotic microorganisms possess certain advantages over prokaryotic cells in this area. The primary reason for developing whole-cell biosensors is their ability to detect heavy metal selectively and sensitively and pesticide toxicity.

Moreover, eukaryotic microorganisms of increased complexity exhibit a broader range of sensitivity towards various hazardous compounds, hence bearing significance for higher organisms. The applications of microbial biosensors encompass a wide range of fields, including but not limited to environmental monitoring and energy production. Novel biosensors with heightened sensitivity, as opposed to selectivity, can be achieved by implementing innovative methodologies that involve utilizing microbial sources ranging from single cellular eukaryotic to modified prokaryotes. In the future, the utilization of microbial biosensors is expected to expand significantly, particularly in the areas of environmental metal pollution monitoring and sustainable energy production [103].

5.7 Technological comparison of biosensors

In the preceding sections, an examination was conducted on the many classifications of biosensors and their respective utilization. This section conducts a comparative analysis of biosensors concerning their technological aspects, specificity and detection limits, linear ranges, analysis durations, costs, and mobility. Electrochemical sensors have witnessed significant advancements in recent years, particularly in high-throughput methods. These methods have emphasized enhancing the detection limit, reducing analysis time, and improving portability [86]. As a result, there has been a notable expansion in the consumer market for affordable biosensors, specifically those designed for glucose monitoring and pregnancy tests. These biosensors employ immobilization strips with lateral-flow technology, which utilize anti-human chorionic gonadotropin. Utilizing polymers and nanomaterials for immobilizing analytes is crucial for enhancing sensitivity and improving the detection limit. This perspective highlights the utilization of lateral-flow technology to facilitate the targeted delivery of samples to a particular location, enabling specified interactions to occur, as opposed to random interactions [104]. Numerous biosensors mentioned earlier have utilized this approach, facilitating the advancement of biofabrication processes that leverage contact and non-contact-based structuring approaches. Using nanoparticles such as gold-, silver-, and silicon-based biofabrication has developed novel methodologies. Furthermore, using polymer coatings on these nanoparticles has led to a significant breakthrough in contact-based electrochemical detecting. The first advantage associated with electrochemical sensors of this nature is their high sensitivity and specificity, enabling real-time examination [105]. Nevertheless, the regeneration capacity or long-term viability of polymers and other materials remains restricted. Nonetheless, the lower cost associated with these electrochemical sensors renders them more economically accessible. The utilization of contact-based sensing for single-analyte detection offers significant benefits, such as the ability to do real-time measurements of molecules with a high degree of specificity. Both the sensitivity and the specificity of single-compound recognition have been enhanced through the development of various transducers, such as FRET (fluorescence resonance energy transfer) and luminous resonating transmitting energy, fluorescent-based transducers, and surface-plasma resonator-based transducers. Because of the overlap in the emitted signals, these methods are restricted in their ability to identify several analytes [106]. Nevertheless, resonance energy transfer techniques have often been used to detect numerous analytes. This is particularly valuable in clinical diagnosis due to the distinct biomarkers in patients and associated diseases. The use of micro- or nano-cantilevers as transducers in the biofabrication of electrochemical sensors shows promising prospects in identifying various analytes. Additionally, it has been noted that non-contact-based sensors using 3D bioprinting methods, such as inkjet or laser direct writing, provide improved results. However, these technologies have significant cost and customization stability limits. It is worth noting that most of these high-throughput biosensors have been integrated with electrochemical sensing techniques for targeted applications. Several highly significant amperometry electrochemical biosensors, characterized by their sensitivity, real-time capabilities, and portability, have been successfully developed for the purpose of disease diagnosis through the analysis of bodily fluids [107]. Electrochemical biosensors, when utilized in conjunction with biofabrication techniques, have a notable advantage in detecting single analytes with high specificity, real-time analytical capabilities, and cost-effectiveness, hence facilitating device portability. Optical-based biosensors represent a significant advancement in the field of biosensing, namely in the domain of fiber-optic chemistry. Hydrogel-based cross-linking is the preferred method for detecting single molecules, such as DNA or peptides, owing to its advantageous characteristics of high loading capacity and hydrophilicity. Subsequent advancements in optical biosensor technology have yielded enhanced capabilities for DNA measurement, hence expanding its utilization in the fields of biomedicine and forensic research. The incorporation of biological constituents, including enzyme groups, antibody and antigen combinations, and nucleic acids, has brought about substantial advancements in the realm of optical biosensor technology [108]. In addition, the biosensing system may be expanded to include microorganisms, animal or plant cells, and tissue sections. Optical fingerprint recognition systems were made possible by recent progress in molecular optoelectronics. The use of integrated optics technology allows for incorporating both passive and active optical components onto a single substrate, simplifying the development of compact sensing devices with diminished dimensions. This objective is accomplished by integrating several sensors onto a single microchip. In the present scenario, high-quality polymer compounds can fabricate hybrid assemblies for optical biosensors. Ongoing progress in surface anatomy studies has improved optic-based biosensor equipment using advanced methods like high-end electrons and atomic strength microscopy. Despite these factors, the detection limit of optical biosensors has not yet reached the femto level due to the high equipment cost and lack of device portability. To achieve this objective, recent advancements in optical technology have led to the development of nanomechanical biosensors that utilize microcantilevers and surface resonance technology [109]. These revolutionary biosensors have enabled the creation of DNA chips capable of conducting real-time analysis with high specificity and sensitivity. The advantages of optical biosensors primarily encompass rapid analysis, immunity to electrical or magnetic interference, and the ability to provide a wide range of information. However, a significant limitation of this approach is the substantial expense associated with specific instrumentation prerequisites. Additional challenges in optical biosensors include the complexity of immobilization, particularly in the context of biofabrication, as well as the crucial necessity for a sterile environment. These issues must be effectively addressed to fully harness the potential of optical biosensors. The utilization of biofabrication techniques in the development of mechanical devices yields superior outcomes in the context of mass-based biosensors. Both electrochemical and optical biosensors utilize this technology to develop advanced biosensors. Significant progress in micro- and nanofabrication technologies has facilitated mechanical devices' emergence using nanoscale dimensions components [110]. The capacity to generate these structures by implementing semiconductor processing techniques has effectively merged the principles of biophysics and bioengineering, leading to advancements in the development of practical biosensors at the micro- and nano-electromechanical scale, which can be manufactured in significant quantities. Fluorescence or gold nanoparticles have effectively labeled glass, silicon, and quartz materials. While the precision of these biosensors in detecting single molecules is higher, the feasibility of low-cost mass production is limited. Numerous obstacles still need to be addressed in the field of mass-based sensors, particularly in developing improved capture agents that can be fabricated at the nanoscale utilizing microelectronic fabrication techniques. These advancements are crucial for enabling high-throughput analysis. It is noteworthy to underline the significant potential applications of semiconductor materials and quantum dot technologies in this context. Nevertheless, existing biosensor innovations exhibit a deficiency in their capacity to conduct quantitative trials concurrently and instantaneously for extensive panels. However, micro and nano cantilevered fabrication can provide like capability [111].

One significant advancement in biosensors is the identification of genetically encoded or synthetic fluorescence biosensors, which enable the examination of molecular mechanisms underlying various biological processes. While the potential of these sensors for detecting single molecules and measuring specific analytes is significant, the methodology, probe preparation, and detection process pose challenges and necessitate the use of sophisticated instruments. When considering biomaterials, it is worth noting that microbial fuel-based biosensors provide notable characteristics such as high sensitivity and selectivity. However, developing a microbial strain for mass production and genetic engineering purposes necessitates intricate procedures and incurs significant costs. Microbial biosensors provide an additional benefit to their prospective application as tools for biological remediation, a field of study that bears considerable significance in ecosystem surveillance [112].

Nevertheless, submitting the advancement and dissemination of genetically modified varieties to thorough scrutiny in alignment with suitable legal frameworks and ethical standards is crucial to concurrently guarantee the efficient administration of cultivation expenses. It is essential to advance diverse micro and nano biosensor frameworks, including innovations based on galvanic or optically bio-electronic ideas, to attain devices with enhanced sensitivity and reduced size. It is recommended that these foundations include a synergistic blend of macromolecules or biological material polymers and nanoparticles [113]. A typical diagram of the progression of biosensor creation is shown in figure 5.14.

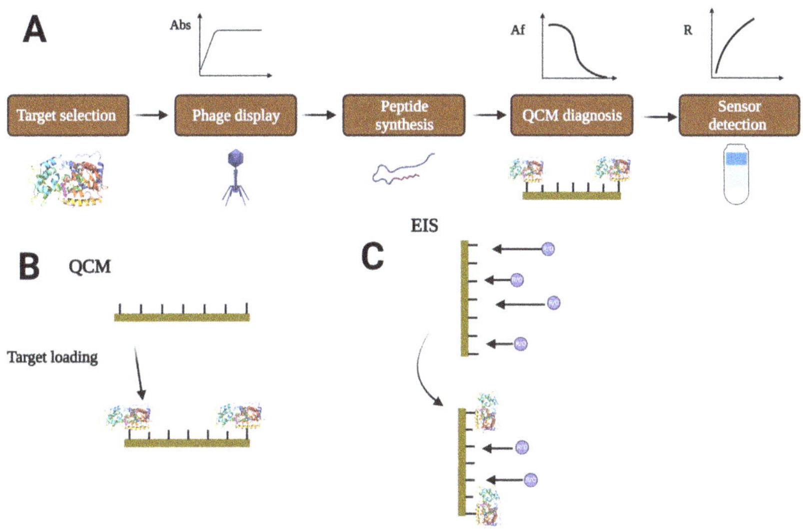

Figure 5.14. (A) schematic diagram depicting the typical progression of biosensor creation. (A) Flowchart outlining the steps involved in biosensor development: (1) Identification of the target protein, (2) Selection via phage display, (3) Synthesis of peptides, (4) Diagnosis using quartz crystal microbalance (QCM), (5) Detection via biosensors. (B) Explanation of QCM's fundamental principle, wherein the attachment of the target protein to immobilized peptides results in a frequency alteration in the oscillation of the quartz crystal. (C) Explanation of electrochemical impedance spectroscopy (EIS) principle, where the binding of the target protein to immobilized peptides leads to increased resistance to the reaction of an introduced redox couple.

5.8 Prospective challenges, and inherent limitations associated with biosensor technology

Contemporary methodologies used in exploring biological sensors include amalgamating several technological modalities, including electrochemical in nature, electromechanical in nature, and fluorescence-based biological sensors, incorporating mutated microorganisms. Specific biosensors exhibit significant potential for use in illness detection and therapy. The increasing demand and necessity for utilizing biosensors in rapid and cost-effective analysis necessitate the development of biofabrication techniques. These techniques will enable the identification of cellular to whole-animal activity with a high level of accuracy in detecting single molecules. Subsequently, directing the biosensors towards functioning under multiplex situations is essential. In the given scenario, it is necessary to employ both 2D and 3D detection techniques, utilizing advanced transducers, in order to effectively identify and measure minuscule analytes of significance [114]. Several significant discoveries were achieved in this study, involving patterning at various levels using both contact-based and non-contact-based methods. The subsequent stage of advancement should strive to uncover regenerative biosensors that possess enhanced durability for prolonged utilization. In this occurrence, there is potential for developing novel diagnostic biosensors that may be utilized in therapeutic applications. This advancement would offer significant benefits to both medical practitioners and those seeking treatment, as it would contribute to a more comprehensive comprehension of diseases and their corresponding therapies in the long term. Given these circumstances, it can be observed that using a biosensor based on fluorescence resonance energy transfer has proven to be a highly effective diagnostic method for evaluating the effectiveness of imatinib treatment in cases of chronic myeloid leukemia [115]. Using aptamers, affibodies, peptide arrays, and molecularly imprinted polymers represents conventional instances of potential study methodologies in this domain. Limited success is also attained with promising compounds for innovative medicinal, antibacterial, and drug delivery purposes. Advancements in this field have led to the rise of biosensors with electrochemical reactions as reliable analytical equipment for detecting bird influenza virus infections in complex matrices. A recent paper has elucidated the aptitude functions of affinity-based biosensors in sports medicine and doping control analysis. Recently, a diverse range of wearable electrochemical biosensors has been comprehensively examined. These biosensors have explicitly been evaluated for their ability to provide real-time and noninvasive analysis of electrolytes and metabolites in bodily fluids. This analysis aims to serve as an indicator of an individual's health state. Another intriguing application is evaluating meat and fish quality using hypoxanthine biosensors via manufacturing techniques [87]. Significant progress has been made in using biosensors to detect bacteria, viruses, and poisons used in biological warfare. Scholars have investigated the use of a wide range of biosensor devices, including but not limited to electrochemical, nucleic acid, optical, and piezoelectric sensors. The advancements possess significant potential for use within military, healthcare, defense, and security domains. Integrating nanomaterials and polymers with diverse biosensors will yield hybrid devices with improved application functionality.

Furthermore, the utilization of synthetic biology techniques in the development of microbial biosensors is expected to make a significant contribution to both environmental monitoring and the management of energy consumption [116]. The significance of employing microbial fuel cells for water treatment and, as the authors of this paper emphasized, power sources for environmental sensors. From a larger standpoint, we have emphasized categorizing biosensors, their prospective applications, and critical attributes such as their capacity for analyte detection, analysis time, portability, cost, and customization [117].

5.9 Grand challenges in biosensors and biomolecular electronics

In the field of multidisciplinary research that spans the fields of chemistry, physics, biological engineering, advanced materials, nanotechnologies, biotechnology, and medical science, the function that biosensors perform is essential. They are now in an established role because of the biomedical sciences and medicine. Given the persistent and ongoing impact of the COVID-19 pandemic on world health, the utilization of biosensors has emerged as an increasingly crucial component in health diagnostics and illness observation [118]. Technological advancements have greatly enhanced the development of biosensors in the interdisciplinary subject of chemistry. This is evident via the emergence of improved sensing technologies in both academic and industrial settings. The initial biosensor was devised during the 1950s specifically to detect oxygen. Since their inception, biosensors have significantly improved their sensing capabilities, modalities, flexibility, and applications.

In contrast to conventional biosensing platforms that operate on bulk surfaces, contemporary biosensors exhibit enhanced versatility and compatibility. These include disposable paper-based biosensing devices, printable biochips, wearable biosensors, implantable biosensors, ingestible biosensors, and biosensors assisted by artificial intelligence. The development of sophisticated biosensing platforms is facilitating the transition into the era of digital health, hence contributing to improved healthcare outcomes [119]. Moreover, a biosensor can achieve a degree of sensitivity to detect individual cells and even individual molecules. The nanopore technology currently available for detecting individual DNA or RNA molecules has achieved a noteworthy advancement in the field of biosensors and has played a crucial role in the efforts to combat the COVID-19 pandemic [120]. According to a recent study, using a mobile phone microscope has demonstrated the capability to identify a solitary molecule. This breakthrough discovery presents a significant potential for point-of-care diagnostics since it offers substantially improved sensitivity. Ordinary papers lateral circulation tests, once paired with the procedure known as Clustered Regularly Interspaced Short Palindromic Repeats/Cas enzymes (CRISPR/Cas), can detect SARS-CoV-2 infections. These assays demonstrate adequate sensitivity when used with CRISPR/Cas technology.

Furthermore, these assays can also be implemented in a wearable platform. The rising incidence of chronic and lifestyle diseases, such as diabetes, has led to an increased utilization of biosensors across multiple industries. In addition to widely utilized point-of-care equipment such as oximetry, pregnancy test strips, and glucose test strips, the market also offers continuous glucose monitoring systems. Biosensors have consistently exhibited efficacy in biological science and healthcare, owing to their appealing attributes, including notable sensitivity, exceptional specificity, convenient mobility, accessibility for end-users, prompt delivery of results, and compatibility with various technologies and devices [121]. The rapid expansion of the global biosensors market is primarily attributed to the enhanced functionality of biosensors and the escalating need for efficient and affordable point-of-care testing. Projections indicate a compound annual growth rate (CAGR) of 7.9% from 2021 to 2028. The advancement of biosensors holds promise for various applications in healthcare. However, the full integration of biosensors into clinical practice to enhance healthcare outcomes is still in the process of development. This is mostly owing to several significant hurdles that need to be addressed [122].

5.9.1 Sensitivity

Identifying substances, including cytokines that modify proteins after translation, and moving cells with cancer presents a notable obstacle owing to the considerable background signal in clinical specimens. Using nanomaterials-based amplifiers of signals is one of the most common ways to make something more sensitive. These methods use nanomaterials' big surface area to their advantage, which lets many biorecognition molecules stick to them [123]. Nanozymes have emerged as an exciting field, presenting benefits regarding stability, cost-effectiveness, sensitivity, and response speed. Nevertheless, more improvements are needed to increase their accuracy. Utilizing CRISPR/Cas technology in biosensors has emerged as an essential step forward since 2017, primarily due to its remarkable levels of precision and sensitivity in comparison to the commonly used nucleic acid-based signal amplification approaches to determining nucleic acids or another analyte. Using a CRISPR/Cas12a autocatalytic feedback amplification network enables the very effective identification of genomic DNA in clinical samples, resulting in unparalleled sensitivity within the molar range.

Furthermore, there are situations in which the process of sampling presents difficulty owing to the restricted quantities of bodily fluids, such as human breath, tears, and cerebrospinal fluid, in addition to the obstacles connected with the development of assays that are capable of detecting minute quantities of analytes [124]. Therefore, the collaboration between sampling, assay development, and device engineering is necessary to achieve optimal detection. Cytokines, tiny proteins, can be found in cerebral fluid in minimal quantities. The impact of cytokine-binding proteins, inhibitors, and soluble cytokine receptors on the behavior of cytokines inside biological systems has been observed. Interferences inside the matrix of biological samples can potentially induce erroneous positive results. Hence, to ensure precision in measurements, it is imperative to carefully consider and explicitly specify the procedures and conditions of sample collection and handling. To facilitate the acquisition of accurate data on cytokine levels within the brain or spinal cord, we have devised a portable apparatus capable of detecting cytokines with high sensitivity directly within these anatomical regions. This innovative technology eliminates the need for sample collection and enables real-time analysis of living organisms. In addition to implementing signal amplification methodologies in bioassays, the engineering of devices is crucial for enhancing sensitivity [125].

5.9.2 Multiplex capability

Multiplexing assays are of great significance in clinical practice for precision diagnostics since they ultimately depict disease characteristics and accurate biological markers. A multiplex assay offers the advantage of concurrently detecting many analytes, enabling high-throughput sample analysis. This approach decreases the time required for conducting the assay and the amount of sample input needed and minimizes the variances that may arise when performing single-plex assays. The use of multiplexed biological sensors has many obstacles, such as constrained signal readouts, interaction concerns, and restrictions in sensitivities [126]. Multiplex bead binding assays, specifically Luminex multiplex assays, are widely utilized in biomedical science and clinical research. They can do a concurrent analysis of many analytes inside a clinical sample. The driving force for advancing the subsequent iteration of bead-based multiplex analysis is achieving cost-efficiency and tests that do not need specialized instruments. The simultaneous measurement of more than three analytes without signal overlap poses a significant challenge for electrochemical biosensors. Optical biosensors offer enhanced capabilities for conducting multiple analyses by integrating various optical tags, including surface plasmon resonance (SPR), surface-enhanced Raman scattering (SERS), and upconverting nanoparticles. Furthermore, the progression of printing technologies has enabled the development of bioassays that can perform many tests simultaneously [127]. By leveraging advancements in microfluidic technology and assay development, a lateral-flow assay successfully identified seven pathogenic single nucleotide polymorphisms inside a solitary test strip, exhibiting a remarkable sensitivity of 0.04 pg ml^{-1}. While there are several potentials for multiplexed analysis, only a limited number of high-throughput platforms have been successfully applied in point-of-care detection. The main obstacles in this field are the insufficient reproducibility of detection, and the lack of robustness in the devices used [128].

5.9.3 Continuous monitoring *in vivo*

The provision of efficient healthcare services is contingent upon the utilization of technological advancements that enable the continuous monitoring of physiological parameters, hence ensuring the ongoing assessment of an individual's health status. Contemporary biosensing technologies necessitate integrating multiplexing capabilities, rapid reaction time, minimal sample volume and heightened sensitivity [129]. Furthermore, the achievement of *in situ* real-time monitoring poses an additional challenge for biosensors; that is, the improvements in electronic and microfabrication processes have substantially improved the employment of wearable devices and implanted chips for ongoing surveillance of numerous health conditions. The current trajectory in bioelectronics is focused on developing devices that possess biocompatibility, flexibility, and multimodality. In recent years, there has been a proliferation of commercially available wearable and implanted technologies designed for healthcare purposes. These technologies can monitor various physical signals, including heart rate, muscle movement, and electrocardiography, among others. The simultaneous measurement of physical qualities and underlying biological processes is of utmost importance for the functionality of biosensors.

A biosensing device that operates in real time can continuously detect and produce reversible signals in response to changes in analyte concentration [130]. Consequently, it can distinguish signals between the analyte and interferants within a complicated sample matrix. In addition, it can promptly deliver the analyte's real-time signal without the need for supplementary procedural actions. The current obstacle in utilizing biosensors for ongoing molecular monitoring is converting targeted analyte data into continuous output signals that can be measured within a living organism while mitigating any potential interference from background signal drift. The successful implementation of the detecting device necessitates the utilization of functional units. For instance, integrating a component on the sensing interface with antifouling capabilities can significantly mitigate nonspecific adsorption, hence improving the signal-to-noise ratio. In the context of continuous molecular monitoring *in vivo*, radiometric measurement is advantageous in mitigating background drifting, enabling the development of calibration-free biosensing systems [131]. The glucose continuous monitoring system is an illustrative instance of biosensors in continuous molecular monitoring. The objective of developing biosensors that do not require reagents and can provide continuous monitoring of various bioanalytics, including hormones, medicines, peptides, and proteins, in clinical samples for real-time healthcare applications has not been fully achieved. In addition to achieving continuous monitoring through chemical means, developing wireless and Bluetooth signal readout technologies is also crucial for enabling continuous *in vivo* monitoring. This project investigates the collaborative integration of many fields, including biological materials, biosensors, bioelectronics, biological engineering, and the web of things, intending to promote collaboration across disciplines [132].

5.10 The Implementation and commercialization of biosensing devices

The ongoing COVID-19 epidemic has led to a substantial surge in the need for cost-effective and dependable laboratory diagnostics, particularly in countries with low resources. Transitioning laboratory-developed biosensors for commercial application poses significant challenges due to the substantial disparity between scientific understanding and routine medical practice. Integrating assays and devices is crucial to enhancing their adaptability for practical applications. Two significant challenges hinder the transition of benchtop technologies from the laboratory to the market: there are two key processes involved in the progression of scientific advancements from laboratory-based technologies to clinical investigations and, subsequently, the translation of these clinical studies into practical applications within the field of medicine [133]. Contemporary scientific investigations prioritize successfully navigating the initial obstacle, which may be effectively addressed by optimizing laboratory technologies. The viability of the new assays/devices is contingent upon the market effect, as their acceptance by end-users and payers is crucial. Before being introduced into the marketplace, laboratory-developed tests or instruments are required to comply with regulatory requirements, which include the guidelines established by the US Food and Drug Administration (FDA). Ensuring laboratory findings' accuracy, reliability, and appropriateness is of utmost importance, regardless of the tested site. Techniques created in laboratories must meet specific performance criteria before they may replace FDA-approved or cleared diagnostic procedures. These criteria include a reported spectrum, quantitative sensibility, clarity, analytic preciseness, accuracy, and an adequate comparison interval [134]. To get past the second issue, it is vital to consider what the market wants and needs. In places with limited resources, the monitoring system needs to be accurate, reliable, easy for people to employ, and cheap for them. The reported spectrum, analytical sensibility, precision, analysis particulars, accuracy, and reference interval are only a few of the required performance criteria that laboratory-developed technologies must exhibit before they can be used as FDA-approved/cleared results [135]. To effectively surmount the second barrier, it is essential to consider the distinct prerequisites and expectations of the market. In contexts with limited resources, it is critical for a system for detection to exhibit accuracy, resilience, and ease of use while also being cost-effective for end-users. The desirability of simplified and integrated detection systems lies in their potential to facilitate the translation of sensing technologies into commerce. However, they encounter many obstacles and necessitate dependable standardization of assays and devices for these *in vitro* diagnostics. Therefore, it is imperative to foster collaborative endeavors among chemists, engineers, biologists, and clinicians to elucidate the intricate path from laboratory experimentation to practical implementation of biosensors in clinical settings [136].

5.10.1 Sustainability to the ecosystem

Disposable sensors are currently experiencing a surge in popularity due to their affordability and the increasing demand for prompt, convenient, and dependable health-related data in our interconnected society. In contamination prevention, the imperative for employing single-use sensors is paramount. Although disposable biosensors offer ease and rapidity, they also raise ecological problems. Incorporating electrical components is necessary to enhance the intelligence of biosensing devices. Achieving biodegradability in biosensors and biochips is significant [137]. The necessity to develop a biosensing system that is smarter, more user-friendly, cost-efficient, and environmentally friendly has been underscored by recent discoveries in the field of sustainable sensing systems. These discoveries include wearable devices, paper-based biochips, smartphone-based detection, and recyclable biosensors.

Researchers are committed to developing sustainable materials and methods for sensors. An instance of the development of distance-based biosensors on filter paper is observed, wherein these biosensors enable instrument-free semi-quantitative examination. In addition, paper-based devices provide several advantageous characteristics, including their affordability, flexibility, and capacity to conduct point-of-care testing with changeable signal reading [138]. Moreover, biodegradable silk or hydrogels have been extensively employed in biosensing devices. Developing a sustainable sensing system encompassing all desired qualities poses a significant challenge. To create advanced and intelligent biosensing devices or bioelectronics with optimal analytical performance, it is crucial to strike a balance that ensures sustainability within the ecosystem [139].

References

[1] Suekane M 1982 Immobilization of glucose isomerase *Z. Allg. Mikrobiol.* **22** 565–76

[2] Newman J D and Setford S J 2006 Enzymatic biosensors *Mol. Biotechnol.* **32** 249–68

[3] Rocchitta G *et al* 2016 Enzyme biosensors for biomedical applications: strategies for safeguarding analytical performances in biological fluids *Sensors* **16** 780

[4] Mulchandani A and Bassi A S 1995 Principles and applications of biosensors for bioprocess monitoring and control *Crit. Rev. Biotechnol.* **15** 105–24

[5] Clark Jr L C and Lyons C 1962 Electrode systems for continuous monitoring in cardiovascular surgery *Ann. N. Y. Acad. Sci.* **102** 29–45

[6] Updike S J and Hicks G P 1967 The enzyme electrode *Nature* **214** 986–8

[7] Hiratsuka A, Fujisawa K and Muguruma H 2008 Amperometric biosensor based on glucose dehydrogenase and plasma-polymerized thin films *Anal. Sci.* **24** 483–6

[8] Chambers J P *et al* 2008 Biosensor recognition elements *Curr. Issues Mol. Biol.* **10** 1–12

[9] Iqbal S S *et al* 2000 A review of molecular recognition technologies for detection of biological threat agents *Biosens. Bioelectron.* **15** 549–78

[10] Newman J D and Turner A P 1992 Biosensors: principles and practice *Essays Biochem.* **27** 147–59

[11] Habermüller K, Mosbach M and Schuhmann W 2000 Electron-transfer mechanisms in amperometric biosensors *Fresenius J. Anal. Chem.* **366** 560–8

[12] Pearson J, Gill A and Vadgama P 2000 Analytical aspects of biosensors *Ann. Clin. Biochem.* **37** 119–45

[13] Thévenot D R *et al* 2001 Electrochemical biosensors: recommended definitions and classification *Anal. Lett.* **34** 635–59

[14] Turner A P, Chen B and Piletsky S A 1999 In vitro diagnostics in diabetes: meeting the challenge *Clin. Chem.* **45** 1596–601

[15] Wang J 2008 Electrochemical glucose biosensors *Chem. Rev.* **108** 814–25

[16] Akyilmaz E, Yorganci E and Asav E 2010 Do copper ions activate tyrosinase enzyme? A biosensor model for the solution *Bioelectrochemistry* **78** 155–60

[17] Venugopal V 2002 Biosensors in fish production and quality control *Biosens. Bioelectron.* **17** 147–57

[18] Diviès C 1975 Remarques sur l'oxydation de l'éthanol par une électrode microbienne d'Acetobacter xylinum *Ann. Microbiol.* **126A** 175–86

[19] Rechnitz G 1978 Biochemical electrodes uses tissues slice. *Chem. Eng. News* **56** 16–21

[20] Wang J 1998 DNA biosensors based on peptide nucleic acid (PNA) recognition layers. A review *Biosens. Bioelectron.* **13** 757–62
[21] Scognamiglio V *et al* 2014 Biosensing technology for sustainable food safety *TrAC, Trends Anal. Chem.* **62** 1–10
[22] Leatherbarrow R J and Edwards P R 1999 Analysis of molecular recognition using optical biosensors *Curr. Opin. Chem. Biol.* **3** 544–7
[23] Zhang J *et al* 2002 Creating new fluorescent probes for cell biology *Nat. Rev. Mol. Cell Biol.* **3** 906–18
[24] Lippincott-Schwartz J and Patterson G H 2003 Development and use of fluorescent protein markers in living cells *Science* **300** 87–91
[25] Shaner N C, Steinbach P A and Tsien R Y 2005 A guide to choosing fluorescent proteins *Nat. Methods* **2** 905–9
[26] Tsien R Y 2006 Breeding and building molecules to spy on cells and tumors *Keio J. Med.* **55** 127–40
[27] Giepmans B N *et al* 2006 The fluorescent toolbox for assessing protein location and function *Science* **312** 217–24
[28] Ibraheem A and Campbell R E 2010 Designs and applications of fluorescent protein-based biosensors *Curr. Opin. Chem. Biol.* **14** 30–6
[29] Wu B *et al* 2011 Modern fluorescent proteins and imaging technologies to study gene expression, nuclear localization, and dynamics *Curr. Opin. Cell Biol.* **23** 310–7
[30] Aye-Han N-N, Ni Q and Zhang J 2009 Fluorescent biosensors for real-time tracking of post-translational modification dynamics *Curr. Opin. Chem. Biol.* **13** 392–7
[31] Zhao Z and Jiang H 2010 Enzyme-based electrochemical biosensors *Biosensors* **302** 1–22
[32] Weltin A, Kieninger J and Urban G A 2016 Microfabricated, amperometric, enzyme-based biosensors for *in vivo* applications *Anal. Bioanal. Chem.* **408** 4503–21
[33] D'costa E, Higgins I and Turner A 1986 Quinoprotein glucose dehydrogenase and its application in an amperometric glucose sensor *Biosensors* **2** 71–87
[34] Weibel M K and Bright H J 1971 The glucose oxidase mechanism: interpretation of the pH dependence *J. Biol. Chem.* **246** 2734–44
[35] Guilbault G and Lubrano G 1973 An enzyme electrode for the amperometric determination of glucose *Anal. Chim. Acta* **64** 439–55
[36] Jin W, Wollenberger U and Scheller F W 1998 PQQ as redox shuttle for quinoprotein glucose dehydrogenase *Biol. Chem.* **379** 1207–11
[37] Zayats M *et al* 2005 Reconstitution of apo-glucose dehydrogenase on pyrroloquinoline quinone-functionalized Au nanoparticles yields an electrically contacted biocatalyst *J. Am. Chem. Soc.* **127** 12400–6
[38] Raitman O A *et al* 2002 Electrical contacting of glucose dehydrogenase by the reconstitution of a pyrroloquinoline quinone-functionalized polyaniline film associated with an Au-electrode: an *in situ* electrochemical SPR study *Chem. Commun.* **2002** 1936–7
[39] Bartlett P N and Whitaker R G 1987 Strategies for the development of amperometric enzyme electrodes *Biosensors* **3** 359–79
[40] Bartlett P, Simon E and Toh C 2002 Modified electrodes for NADH oxidation and dehydrogenase-based biosensors *Bioelectrochemistry* **56** 117–22
[41] Gorton L and Domínguez E 2002 Electrocatalytic oxidation of NAD (P) H at mediator-modified electrodes *Rev. Mol. Biotechnol.* **82** 371–92
[42] Eggins B R 2008 *Chemical Sensors and Biosensors* (New York: Wiley)

[43] Chaubey A and Malhotra B 2002 Mediated biosensors *Biosens. Bioelectron.* **17** 441–56
[44] D'Orazio P 2003 Biosensors in clinical chemistry *Clin. Chim. Acta* **334** 41–69
[45] Bakker E and Pretsch E 2005 Potentiometric sensors for trace-level analysis *TrAC, Trends Anal. Chem.* **24** 199–207
[46] Caras S and Janata J 1980 Field effect transistor sensitive to penicillin *Anal. Chem.* **52** 1935–7
[47] Hafeman D G, Parce J W and McConnell H M 1988 Light-addressable potentiometric sensor for biochemical systems *Science* **240** 1182–5
[48] Mourzina Y *et al* 2001 Ion-selective light-addressable potentiometric sensor (LAPS) with chalcogenide thin film prepared by pulsed laser deposition *Sens. Actuators* B **80** 136–40
[49] Poghossian A *et al* 2001 Penicillin detection by means of field-effect based sensors: EnFET, capacitive EIS sensor or LAPS? *Sens. Actuators* **B 78** 237–42
[50] Xu G *et al* 2005 Cell-based biosensors based on light-addressable potentiometric sensors for single cell monitoring *Biosens. Bioelectron.* **20** 1757–63
[51] Kloock J P *et al* 2006 PLD-prepared cadmium sensors based on chalcogenide glasses—ISFET, LAPS and μISE semiconductor structures *Sens. Actuators* **B 118** 149–55
[52] Stein B *et al* 2004 Extracellular measurements of averaged ionic currents with the light-addressable potentiometric sensor (LAPS) *Sens. Actuators* **B 98** 299–304
[53] Lee C-S, Kim S K and Kim M 2009 Ion-sensitive field-effect transistor for biological sensing *Sensors* **9** 7111–31
[54] Schöning M J and Poghossian A 2002 Recent advances in biologically sensitive field-effect transistors (BioFETs) *Analyst* **127** 1137–51
[55] Jaffrezic-Renault N and Dzyadevych S V 2008 Conductometric microbiosensors for environmental monitoring *Sensors* **8** 2569–88
[56] Ghourchian H, Moulaie R A and Elyasvandi H 2004 A Conductometric urea biosensor by direct immobilization of urease on Pt electrode *Iran. J. Chem. & Chem. Eng.* **23** 55–63
[57] Spink C and Wadsö I 1976 Calorimetry as an analytical tool in biochemistry and biology *Methods Biochem. Anal.* **23** 1–160
[58] Grime J K 1985 *Analytical Solution Calorimetry* (Wiley)
[59] Mosbach K and Danielsson B 1974 An enzyme thermistor *Biochim. Biophys. Acta Enzymol.* **364** 140–5
[60] Danielsson B, Mattiasson B and Mosbach K 1981 Enzyme thermistor devices and their analytical applications *Applied Biochemistry and Bioengineering* (Amsterdam: Elsevier) pp 97–143
[61] Danielsson B and Mosbach K 1988 Enzyme thermistors *Methods in Enzymology* (Amsterdam: Elsevier) ch 16 pp 181–97
[62] Turner A, Karube I and Wilson G S 1987 *Biosensors: Fundamentals and Applications* (Oxford: Oxford University Press)
[63] Steiner M-S, Duerkop A and Wolfbeis O S 2011 Optical methods for sensing glucose *Chem. Soc. Rev.* **40** 4805–39
[64] Pickup J C *et al* 2005 Fluorescence-based glucose sensors *Biosens. Bioelectron.* **20** 2555–65
[65] Ligler F S and Taitt C R 2002 *Optical Biosensors: Present & Future.* (Gulf Professional Publishing)
[66] Lakowicz J R (ed) 2006 *Principles of Fluorescence Spectroscopy* (Berlin: Springer)
[67] Tan W 1998 Optical measurements on the nanometer scale *TrAC, Trends Anal. Chem.* **17** 501–13

[68] Lübbers D and Opitz N 1975 The pCO_2-/pO_2-optode: a new probe for measurement of pCO_2 or pO in fluids and gases (authors transl). *Z. Naturforsch. C, Biosci.* **30** 532–3
[69] Chudobova I *et al* 1996 Fibre optic biosensor for the determination of D-glucose based on absorption changes of immobilized glucose oxidase *Anal. Chim. Acta* **319** 103–10
[70] Weiss S 1999 Fluorescence spectroscopy of single biomolecules *Science* **283** 1676–83
[71] Analytical Chemistry 1960 New products *Anal. Chem.* **32** 102A–13A
[72] Shichiri M *et al* 1982 Wearable artificial endocrine pancreas with needle-type glucose sensor *Lancet* **320** 1129–31
[73] Tierney M J *et al* 2000 The GlucoWatch® biographer: a frequent, automatic and noninvasive glucose monitor *Ann. Med.* **32** 632–41
[74] Yao H *et al* 2012 A contact lens with integrated telecommunication circuit and sensors for wireless and continuous tear glucose monitoring *J. Micromech. Microeng.* **22** 075007
[75] Bhatia S, Naved T and Sardana S 2018 *Introduction to Pharmaceutical Biotechnology, Volume 2* (Bristol: IOP Publishing)
[76] Pohanka M 2017 The piezoelectric biosensors: Principles and applications *Int. J. Electrochem. Sci.* **12** 496–506
[77] Moina C and Ybarra G 2012 Fundamentals and applications of immunosensors *Advances in Immunoassay Technology* (InTech)
[78] Peña-Bahamonde J *et al* 2018 Recent advances in graphene-based biosensor technology with applications in life sciences *J. Nanobiotechnol.* **16** 17
[79] Soper S A *et al* 2006 Point-of-care biosensor systems for cancer diagnostics/prognostics *Biosens. Bioelectron.* **21** 1932–42
[80] Ahmed M U *et al* 2014 Personalized diagnostics and biosensors: a review of the biology and technology needed for personalized medicine *Crit. Rev. Biotechnol.* **34** 180–96
[81] Singh A *et al* 2021 Recent advances in electrochemical biosensors: applications, challenges, and future scope *Biosensors* **11** 336
[82] Turner A P 2013 Biosensors: sense and sensibility *Chem. Soc. Rev.* **42** 3184–96
[83] da Silva E T *et al* 2017 Electrochemical biosensors in point-of-care devices: recent advances and future trends *ChemElectroChem* **4** 778–94
[84] Bohunicky B and Mousa S A 2010 Biosensors: the new wave in cancer diagnosis *Nanotechnol. Sci. Appl.* **2011** 1–10
[85] Wang J 2006 Electrochemical biosensors: towards point-of-care cancer diagnostics *Biosens. Bioelectron.* **21** 1887–92
[86] Griffiths D and Hall G 1993 Biosensors—what real progress is being made? *Trends Biotechnol.* **11** 122–30
[87] Uniyal S and Sharma R K 2018 Technological advancement in electrochemical biosensor based detection of organophosphate pesticide chlorpyrifos in the environment: a review of status and prospects *Biosens. Bioelectron.* **116** 37–50
[88] Mehrvar M and Abdi M 2004 Recent developments, characteristics, and potential applications of electrochemical biosensors *Anal. Sci.* **20** 1113–26
[89] Carpenter A C, Paulsen I T and Williams T C 2018 Blueprints for biosensors: design, limitations, and applications *Genes* **9** 375
[90] Healy D A *et al* 2007 Biosensor developments: application to prostate-specific antigen detection *Trends Biotechnol.* **25** 125–31
[91] Vigneshvar S *et al* 2016 Recent advances in biosensor technology for potential applications —an overview *Front. Bioeng. Biotechnol.* **4** 11

[92] Yang P *et al* 2011 Phenol formaldehyde resin nanoparticles loaded with CdTe quantum dots: a fluorescence resonance energy transfer probe for optical visual detection of copper (II) ions *ACS Nano* **5** 2147–54
[93] Moreno-Guzman M *et al* 2015 Self-propelled enzyme-based motors for smart mobile electrochemical and optical biosensing *Anal. Chem.* **87** 12380–6
[94] Uttenthaler E, Kößlinger C and Drost S 1998 Quartz crystal biosensor for detection of the African Swine fever disease *Anal. Chim. Acta* **362** 91–100
[95] Heydari S and Haghayegh G H 2014 Application of nanoparticles in quartz crystal microbalance biosensors *J. Sens. Technol.* **2014**
[96] Pérez-López B and Merkoçi A 2011 Nanomaterials based biosensors for food analysis applications *Trends Food Sci. Technol.* **22** 625–39
[97] Lv M *et al* 2018 Engineering nanomaterials-based biosensors for food safety detection *Biosens. Bioelectron.* **106** 122–8
[98] Sutarlie L, Ow S Y and Su X 2017 Nanomaterials-based biosensors for detection of microorganisms and microbial toxins *Biotechnol. J.* **12**
[99] Eason M G *et al* 2020 Genetically encoded fluorescent biosensor for rapid detection of protein expression *ACS Synth. Biol.* **9** 2955–63
[100] Wang M, Da Y and Tian Y 2023 Fluorescent proteins and genetically encoded biosensors *Chem. Soc. Rev.* **52** 1189–214
[101] Niu W and Guo J 2013 Expanding the chemistry of fluorescent protein biosensors through genetic incorporation of unnatural amino acids *Mol. Biosyst.* **9** 2961–70
[102] Park M, Tsai S-L and Chen W 2013 Microbial biosensors: engineered microorganisms as the sensing machinery *Sensors* **13** 5777–95
[103] Hyeon J E, Shin S K and Han S O 2016 Design of nanoscale enzyme complexes based on various scaffolding materials for biomass conversion and immobilization *Biotechnol. J.* **11** 1386–96
[104] Pashchenko O *et al* 2018 A comparison of optical, electrochemical, magnetic, and colorimetric point-of-care biosensors for infectious disease diagnosis *ACS Infect. Dis.* **4** 1162–78
[105] Dziąbowska K, Czaczyk E and Nidzworski D 2018 *Application of Electrochemical Methods in Biosensing Technologies* (Rijeka: InTech)
[106] Hucklesby J J *et al* 2021 Comparison of leading biosensor technologies to detect changes in human endothelial barrier properties in response to pro-inflammatory tnfα and il1β in real-time *Biosensors* **11** 159
[107] Byfield M and Abuknesha R 1994 Biochemical aspects of biosensors *Biosens. Bioelectron.* **9** 373–99
[108] Ciminelli C *et al* 2019 Silicon photonic biosensors *IET Optelectron.* **13** 48–54
[109] Velasco-Garcia M N and Mottram T 2003 Biosensor technology addressing agricultural problems *Biosystems Eng.* **84** 1–12
[110] Welch E C *et al* 2021 Advances in biosensors and diagnostic technologies using nano-structures and nanomaterials *Adv. Funct. Mater.* **31** 2104126
[111] Full J *et al* 2021 Market perspectives and future fields of application of odor detection biosensors within the biological transformation—a systematic analysis *Biosensors* **11** 93
[112] Zhang Y *et al* 2022 Current technological trends in transdermal biosensing *Adv. NanoBiomed Res.* **2** 2200040

[113] Luka G *et al* 2015 Microfluidics integrated biosensors: a leading technology towards lab-on-a-chip and sensing applications *Sensors* **15** 30011–31
[114] Gupta N *et al* 2019 Cell-based biosensors: recent trends, challenges and future perspectives *Biosens. Bioelectron.* **141** 111435
[115] Bhalla N *et al* 2020 Opportunities and challenges for biosensors and nanoscale analytical tools for pandemics: COVID-19 *ACS Nano* **14** 7783–807
[116] Alfa A A *et al* 2021 Blockchain technology in IoT systems: current trends, methodology, problems, applications, and future directions *J. Reliab. Intell. Environ.* **7** 115–43
[117] Sharma V, Tripathi A K and Mittal H 2022 Technological revolutions in smart farming: current trends, challenges and future directions *Comput. Electron. Agric.* 107217
[118] Liu G 2021 Grand challenges in biosensors and biomolecular electronics *Front. Media SA. p.* **9** 707615
[119] Malhi G S *et al* 2017 The promise of digital mood tracking technologies: are we heading on the right track? *BMJ Ment. Health* **20** 102–7
[120] Alahnomi R A *et al* 2021 Review of recent microwave planar resonator-based sensors: techniques of complex permittivity extraction, applications, open challenges and future research directions *Sensors* **21** 2267
[121] Ramesh M *et al* 2022 Nanotechnology-enabled biosensors: a review of fundamentals, design principles, materials, and applications *Biosensors* **13** 40
[122] Richter T *et al* 2021 Machine learning-based behavioral diagnostic tools for depression: advances, challenges, and future directions *J. Pers. Med.* **11** 957
[123] Al Mamun M *et al* 2021 Electrochemical biosensors with aptamer recognition layer for the diagnosis of pathogenic bacteria: barriers to commercialization and remediation *TrAC, Trends Anal. Chem.* **145** 116458
[124] Darwish A, Ismail Sayed G and Ella Hassanien A 2019 The impact of implantable sensors in biomedical technology on the future of healthcare systems *Intelligent Pervasive Computing Systems for Smarter Healthcare* (Wiley) pp 67–89
[125] Hashem A *et al* 2021 Nanomaterials based electrochemical nucleic acid biosensors for environmental monitoring: a review *Appl. Surf. Sci. Adv.* **4** 100064
[126] Dargaville T R *et al* 2013 Sensors and imaging for wound healing: a review *Biosens. Bioelectron.* **41** 30–42
[127] Kim K B and Baek H J 2023 Photoplethysmography in wearable devices: a comprehensive review of technological advances, current challenges, and future directions *Electronics* **12** 2923
[128] Gupta S *et al* 2021 A comprehensive review on emerging constructed wetland coupled microbial fuel cell technology: potential applications and challenges *Bioresour. Technol.* **320** 124376
[129] Barbosa A *et al* 2021 Current nanotechnology advances in diagnostic biosensors *Med. Devices Sens.* **4** e10156
[130] Šumak B, Brdnik S and Pušnik M 2021 Sensors and artificial intelligence methods and algorithms for human–computer intelligent interaction: a systematic mapping study *Sensors* **22** 20
[131] Salehmin M N *et al* 2021 Pushing microbial desalination cells towards field application: prevailing challenges, potential mitigation strategies, and future prospects *Sci. Total Environ.* **759** 143485

[132] Di Nardo F *et al* 2021 Ten years of lateral flow immunoassay technique applications: trends, challenges and future perspectives *Sensors* **21** 5185
[133] Scognamiglio V *et al* 2010 Biosensors for effective environmental and agrifood protection and commercialization: from research to market *Microchim. Acta* **170** 215–25
[134] Yang B *et al* 2021 Wearable chem-biosensing devices: from basic research to commercial market *Lab Chip* **21** 4285–310
[135] Sezgintürk M K 2020 Introduction to commercial biosensors *Commercial Biosensors and Their Applications* (Amsterdam: Elsevier) pp 1–28
[136] Denmark D J *et al* 2019 Readiness of magnetic nanobiosensors for point-of-care commercialization *J. Electron. Mater.* **48** 4749–61
[137] Chapin III F S, Torn M S and Tateno M 1996 Principles of ecosystem sustainability *Am. Naturalist* **148** 1016–37
[138] Baird R 2005 On sustainability, estuaries, and ecosystem restoration: the art of the practical *Restor. Ecol.* **13** 154–8
[139] Lu Y *et al* 2015 Ecosystem health towards sustainability *Ecosyst. Health Sustainability* **1** 1–15

IOP Publishing

Introduction to Pharmaceutical Biotechnology, Volume 2 (Second Edition)

Enzymes, proteins and bioinformatics

Ahmed Al-Harrasi, Saurabh Bhatia and Ajmal Khan

Chapter 6

Biotransformation and enzymes

6.1 Introduction

Microorganisms have the tendency to enzymatically alter a wide range of organic compounds. Biotransformation (bioconversions or microbial transformations) widely refers to the processes in which microorganisms convert organic substances into structurally related products. Biotransformation deals with microbial (enzymatic) transformation of a substrate into a product with a limited number of (one or a few) enzymatic reactions. This is in comparison to fermentation which includes a number of reactions (often complex in nature). Although a number of biotransformations are recognized, only particular reactions are valuable for the production of commercially important products. The implication of bioconversion reactions becomes evident when the synthesis of a certain compound is either difficult or costly using chemical approaches. In addition, biotransformations are usually considered for chemical reactions because of substrate specificity, stereospecificity and mixed reaction conditions (pH, temperature, pressure). The environmental pollution due to biotransformation is virtually insignificant or negligible. Moreover, it is easy to apply rDNA technology to make suitable changes in biotransformations. Another practical benefit of biotransformations is that it is very easy to scale-up the procedures due to the restricted number of reactions.

6.2 Types of biotransformation reactions

Different types of chemical reactions occur during biotransformations, such as oxidation, reduction, hydrolysis, condensation, isomerization, formation of new C–C bonds, production of chiral compounds and reversal of hydrolytic reactions. Among these, oxidation, isomerization and hydrolysis reactions are more commonly observed in biotransformations. Other biotransformations involve more than one type of reaction. Some examples of significant biotransformation reactions along

doi:10.1088/978-0-7503-5387-8ch6

Table 6.1. A selected list of important biotransformation reactions.

Type of reaction	Example	Commonly used micro-organism(s)
Reduction	Benzaldehyde → benzyl alcohol nitropentachlorobenzol → pentachloroaniline	*Saccharomyces cerevisiae*, *Streptomyces aureofaciens*
Oxidation	Tryptophan → 5 hydroxytryptophan naphthalene → salicylic acid	*Bacillus subtitis*, *Corynebacterium* spp.
Hydrolysis	Anhydrotetracycline → tetracycline menthyl laureate → menthol	*Streptomyces aureofaciens*, *Mycobacterium phlei*
Condensation	Streptomycin → streptomycin-phosphate	*Streptomyces griseus*

with the microorganisms involved are listed in table 6.1. The conversion time required for biotransformation is related to the type of reaction, the substrate concentration and the micro-organism used. Usually, oxidation, hydrolysis and dehydration reactions are accomplished in a few hours.

6.3 Sources of biocatalysts and techniques for biotransformation

There are number of techniques available to enhance biotransformation and bioconversion processes, which may include immobilization techniques, genetic engineering and the use of biocatalysts that can tolerate organic solvents [1]. The utilization of enzymes to conduct biotransformation reactions is often challenging, as it faces difficulties such as:

- Reactant or product toxicity.
- Inhibition.
- High dilution.
- Conformational changes.
- Stability issues.
- pH and temperature dependence.

Nevertheless, biocatalysts are the only source for conducting biotransformation reactions [2]. Another challenge is its dependence on the substrate; if the selected substrate is toxic then it can kill the micro-organism and may further delay the biotransformation reaction. The micro-organism also utilizes the substrate as a nutrient and energy source, which can affect product recovery. Limitations related to process time and the choice of biocatalysts makes biotransformation more complicated in the manufacturing of a small molecule pharmaceutical [3]. Another challenge is our inadequate understanding of complex biological systems and the need to increase the yield of the desirable product. However, the slow action (in comparison to chemical transformation) and specific nature of enzymes makes them more suitable for biotransformation. An extensive range of biological catalysts is available for biotransformation reactions [4]. These include growing cells, resting cells, killed cells, immobilized cells, cell-free extracts, enzymes and immobilized enzymes. The most significant sources of biocatalysts and the protocol used for biotransformation are briefly described below.

6.3.1 Growing cells

Suitable cells are cultured in a suitable medium. As the desired growth of the cells occurs (6–24 h), a concentrated substrate is supplemented to the culture. Occasionally, supplementation of emulsifiers (Tween, organic solvents) is required to solubilize substrates and/or products, e.g. steroid biotransformation. The substrate transformation to the product can be examined by chromatographic procedures. Biotransformation can be stopped when the formation is optimum.

6.3.2 Non-growing cells

Non-growing cells are considered for biotransformation reactions for a number of reasons, such as:

- A very high concentration of substrate can be used (with high substrate concentration, growing cells stop their growth).
- The conversion efficiency of substrate to product is high.
- Cells can be washed and used and thus there will be no contaminating substances.
- Biotransformation can be optimized by creating specific environmental conditions (pH, temperature, etc). Product isolation and recovery are easy.

6.3.3 Immobilized cells

Biotransformations can be performed constantly by utilizing immobilized cells. Further, the same cells can be used again and again. Several bioconversion reactions with single or multistage reactions are in fact performed using immobilized cells, e.g. large-scale production of l-alanine and malic acid.

6.3.4 Immobilized enzymes

Immobilized enzymes are frequently used in biotransformation, due to a number of advantages, such as:

- Cell-free enzyme systems in the form of immobilized enzymes.
- There is no transport barrier across the cell membrane for the substrate or product.
- The isolation and recovery of the product is simpler and easier.
- The desired products are not degraded.
- There is no occurrence of undesirable side reactions.

Several immobilized enzyme systems have been established for biotransformations, such as glucose isomerase and penicillin acylase.

6.4 Product recovery in biotransformations

During most biotransformation reactions, the anticipated end-products are extracellular. The product may either be in a soluble or a suspended state. When whole cells are utilized, they have to be isolated and frequently washed (with water or organic solvent) as required. The extracted product can be recovered, using common techniques such as precipitation by salts, extraction with solvents, adsorption to ion-exchangers, etc. The volatile products can be recovered by direct distillation from the medium. A number of biotransformations are reported in the literature. Of these, only a selected few are significant for large-scale purposes. The major drawbacks with a number of biotransformations are low yields, expensive processes or very limited markets. Recently, an increase in the rate of biotransformations and product recovery was observed in a membrane bioreactor by using direct electric current. The amount of production of benzoic acid was found to be escalated by 42% when the current was applied. This type of process has immense potential in increasing productivity from biotransformations by means of a simultaneous enhancement in metabolic activity and *in situ* product recovery [5]. It was also observed that recovery of 3-methylcatechol produced in a biphasic system (aliphatic alcohol/water bioreactor) was 10–20 fold more than in an aqueous medium. This demonstrates the effectiveness of double-phase systems for this particular biotransformation [6]. Similarly, the recovery and productivity of vicinal diol was increased by using a biphasic system in a hollow fiber membrane bioreactor [7]. In 1998, a combined bioreactor–separator system was developed for simultaneous biotransformation and recovery of the product by crystallization in an immobilized l-aspartate beta-decarboxylase reactor system. An increase in the biotransformation rate and recovery of the isoflavones genistein and daidzein from industrial antibiotic fermentations was observed in 2013 [8].

6.5 Application of biotransformation in the production of pharmaceutical products

6.5.1 Biotransformation of steroids

The structure cyclopentanoperhydrophenanthrene is present in all steroids. In general, steroids are hormones that have an extensive range of therapeutic functions, e.g. cortisone is extensively employed in the treatment of rheumatoid arthritis and skin diseases; progesterone and estrogen derivatives are used as contraceptives. Some derivatives of cortisone (e.g. prednisolone) are more effective in their therapeutic action. Steroid production at the commercial level is an important endeavor, which has required the attention of many researchers. Cortisone production once involved 37 reactions and the cost of this product was approximately \$200 g^{-1} in 1950. With the help of biotransformation reactions, this lengthy procedure of 37 reactions was reduced to 11. This also decreased the cost of the product to just \$1 g^{-1} in 1980. Thus developments in biotransformation allow the shortening of lengthy reactions which can ultimately impact the cost of the final product.

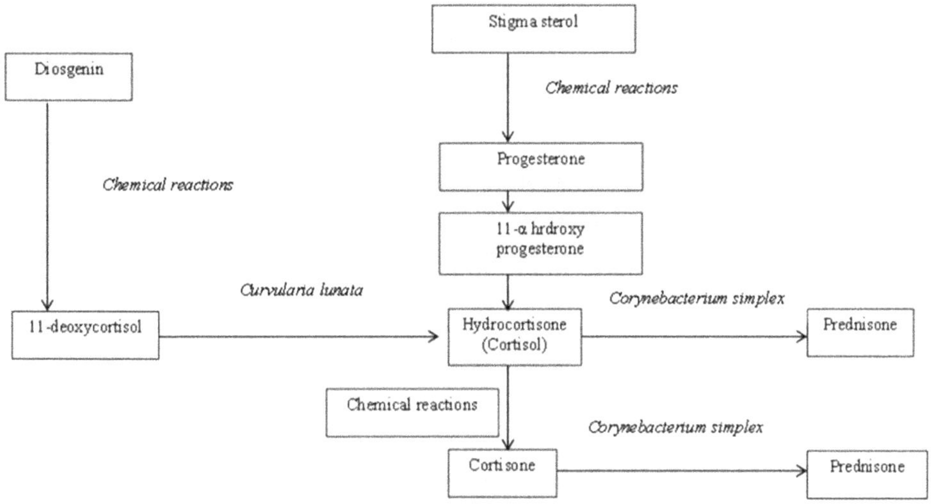

Figure 6.1. Biotransformation of commercially important steroids.

There are several reactions involved in the production of steroids, microbial transformation in particular mainly involves oxidation (introduction of hydroxyl groups, splitting of side chains, production of epoxides, etc), reduction (conversion of aldehydes or ketones to alcohols, hydration of double bonds), hydrolysis and ester formation. Steroid production exclusively by biotransformation reactions is not possible, thus in addition to microbial transformation, chemical reactions are required. Key steps involved in the biotransformation of steroids are shown in figure 6.1. There are a number of precursors available to initiate biotransformation reactions, such as stigma sterol extracted from soybeans or diosgenin isolated from the roots of the Mexican barbasco plant.

In steroid synthesis, stigma sterol can be chemically converted to progesterone, which is further subjected to biotransformation to ultimately produce 11 α-hydroxyprogesterone through microbial transformation (*Rhizopus nigricans*). Cortisol or hydrocortisone, derived from 11 α-hydroxyprogesterone by chemical reactions, is exposed to a microbe (*Corynebacterium simplex*) to produce prednisolone. In addition, product derived from cortisol can be subjected to biotransformation by a micro-organism (*C. simplex*) to synthesize prednisone. Once diosgenin is used as the precursor compound, substance S can be synthesized by chemical reactions, which can be further converted to cortisol by biotransformation with the help of *Curvularia lunata.* Biotransformation of steroids is generally achieved by batch fermentation. In addition, several immobilization techniques are emerging in this area, which may further encourage more efficient biotransformation reactions by using immobilized cells or enzymes. This is more profitable as the biotransformation is more efficient with a high substrate concentration, short conversion time and good product recovery. As not all steroids are water soluble, the microbial transformation reactions are always performed in an organic solvent (water-immiscible) system. However, organic solvents are toxic to microorganisms or enzymes. It is best to use a two-phase aqueous system for the biotransformation of steroids. Mibolerone is a synthetic anabolic and androgenic steroid utilized for the treatment of estrous in female dogs. Based on a recent report, microbial transformations of mibolerone with *Cunninghamella blakesleeana*, *Cunninghamella echinulata* and *Macrophomina phaseolina* led to production of 11β,17β-dihydroxy-7α,17α-dimethylestr-4-en-3-one of potential use [10]. Similarly, microbial transformation of drospirenone, an oral contraceptive drug, with *Cunninghamella elegans* was also reported recently, which helps in understanding the metabolism of this important drug and provide new analogs of drospirenone [9].

6.5.1.1 Biotransformation of cholesterol

Recently, many research activities have focussed on the importance of the lymphatic route in reversing cholesterol transport, as well as the biliary and the non-biliary pathways for removal of cholesterol from the body, which will help in understanding and preventing more of the causes of ischemic coronary heart disease [10]. Studies are also conducted to understand the role of cholesterol in multiple sclerosis (a progressive, neurodegenerative disease of the central nervous system) by specific modification in the mRNA and protein expression of key molecules involved in the maintainance of cholesterol homeostasis in the rat spinal cord. It was observed that modification in the regulation of cholesterol metabolism at onset can result in the progression of disease, whereas during the course of the recovery period it may have beneficial effects, contributing to the regeneration of myelin sheath and restoration of neuronal function [11]. The importance of cholesterol for normal brain function was also realized and it is understood that astrocytes produce most of the brain cholesterol which is important for brain functioning. During this study it was observed that sterol regulatory element-binding protein (a transcription factor decreased during diabetes which can ultimately lead to decrease in brain cholesterol synthesis) mediated cholesterol synthesis in astrocytes plays an important role in brain function and development [12]. Alteration in the expression of this transcription factor can significantly affect brain cholesterol synthesis which draws a relationship between diabetes and altered brain function. Similarly, the key importance of cholesterol in brain physiology and function, changes in cholesterol homeostasis and levels related to brain disorders and neurodegenerative diseases have been studied recently. It was observed that intracellular cholesterol pools in the compartments of mitochondria and endoplasmic reticulum play an important role in understanding the importance of cholesterol homeostasis disruption in neurodegeneration [13]. The above mentioned reports help in understanding the importance of cholesterol in our human body and its biotransformation. A number of commercially important steroids (e.g. androstendione, androstadiendione) can be synthesized directly from cholesterol by biotransformation (figure 6.2).

6.5.2 Biotransformation of antibiotics

One of the most important priorities of the pharmaceutical industry is the production of new antibiotics or modifications of existing ones for more effective

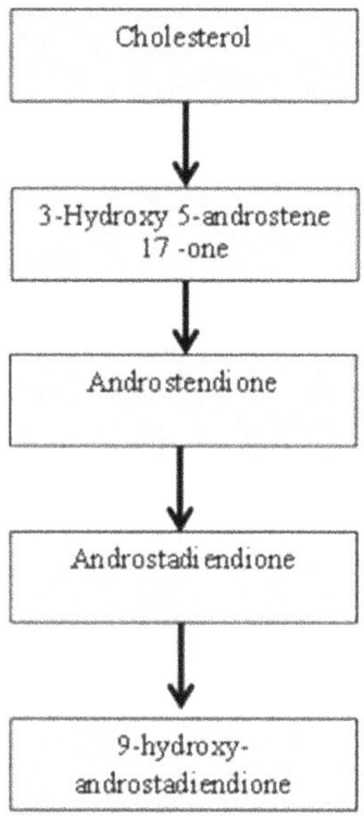

Figure 6.2. Biotransformation of cholesterol by mycobacteria to commercial products.

treatment against particular diseases or infections. In addition, antibiotics with a broad spectrum, minimum toxicity, minimal allergic reactions and decreased resistance are highly preferred [14]. The significant contribution of biotransformation allows the production of various new antibiotics. Based on recent reports it is well understood that modification in bacterial metabolism, e.g. those related to dormancy (metabolically inactive spores to survive harsh conditions) or biofilm formation, control bacterial susceptibility against antibiotics. This is called phenotypic resistance, presenting a connection between bacterial metabolism and antibiotic resistance (table 6.2)[15].

Adoption of new techniques such as miniaturization, nanotechnology, microdosing, chemometrics and high-throughput analysis helps in the exploration of new molecules. Alternatively, it can be produced by 'green chemistry', a novel synthetic approach resulting in reduced production of waste and the smallest environmental impact [16]. Since the discovery of penicillin by Sir Alexander Fleming, more than 20 000 types of antibiotic molecules have been produced using microorganisms, although only few are clinically useful. Reports also confirm a steep decline in the discovery of new molecules, in particular antibiotics [17]. During the last three decades, among the 28 new molecules discovered, only three semisynthetic molecules that have experienced chemical modifications have been approved for clinical use [28]. Even after advancement in synthetic chemistry, biotransformation is considered as the most cost-effective track to discover new molecules [18]. This requires a focus towards developing more approaches to produce a substantial number of molecules from microorganisms. This gives scope for considerable further

Table 6.2. Production of new antibiotics.

Organism	Antibiotics	Reference
White rot fungi (*Irpex lacteus*, *Panus tigrinus*, *Dichomitus squalens*, *Trametes versicolor* and *Pleurotus ostreatus*)	Biodegradation of fluoroquinolones (norfloxacin, ofloxacin and ciprofloxacin)	[16]
Streptomyces davawensis and *Streptomyces cinnabarinus*	Antibiotics (riboflavin analogs) roseoflavin and 8-demethyl-8-aminoriboflavin	[17]
Ligninolytic fungi (*Irpex lacteus*, *Dichomitus squalens*)	Flumequine (fluoroquinolone antibiotic)	[18]
Marine-derived fungus *Paecilomyces* spp.	Tetracycline, minocycline, chlortetracycline, oxytetracycline, doxycycline	[19]
Cystobacter fuscus	Myxobacterial antibiotic (cystothiazole A)	[20]
Streptomyces venezuelae strain	Rosamicin antibiotic into 10,11-dihydrorosamicin	[21]
Xylaria longipes	Danofloxacin	[22]
Spores of *Streptomyces griseus*	Acylation of chloramphenicol	[23]
Deoxystreptamine-negative mutant of *Micromonospora purpurea*	2,4,6/3,5-pentahydroxycyclohexanone and 2,4/3,5-tetrahydroxycyclohexanone	[24]

development biotransformation processes in the future [19]. However, there are still various challenges that need to be addressed, such as:

- Determining the relationship between structural changes and time and cost efficiency.
- Determining the relationship between the biological activity of products and the optimization of pharmacokinetic/pharmacodynamic properties and safety.
- The limited number of suppliers involved in large-scale drug production with good quality practices [30].

6.5.2.1 Direct biotransformation

Various reactions such as acylation and de-acylation, phosphorylation, adenylation and hydrolysis are involved in direct biotransformation, in particular during microbial transformation of antibiotics.

6.5.2.1.1 Biotransformation of penicillin G

The earliest extraction of penicillin G from *Penicillium chrysogenum* and its conversion into 6-aminopenicillanic acid and phenyl acetic acid was reported in 1992. In this study 6-aminopenicillanic acid was converted into ampicillin when a liquid membrane carrier system was electro coalescence [20]. Recent study related to the production of 6-aminopenicillanic acid has revealed production of penicillin G acylase from immobilized whole cells of *Escherichia coli*. Later, *E. coli* was utilized

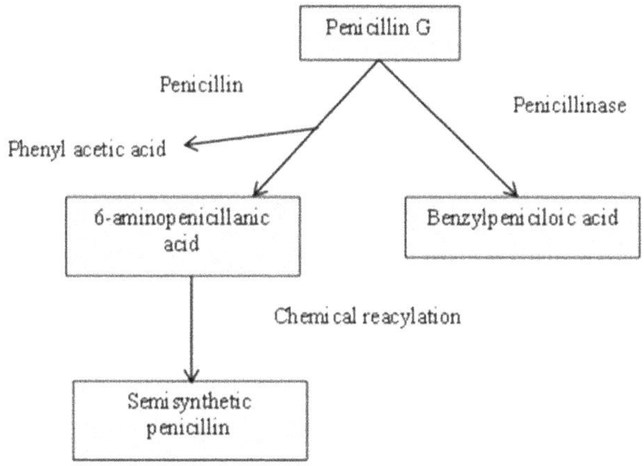

Figure 6.3. Biotransformation of penicillin G.

for the biotransformation of penicillin V to 6-aminopenicillanic acid to express a highly active penicillin V acylase [21]. In association with chemical synthesis, microbial transformation is usually used for the commercial synthesis of semisynthetic cephalosporins and penicillins. During this conversion, 6-amino-penicillanic acids derived from the enzymatic cleavage of penicillin by penicillin acylase is a very important reaction (figure 6.3). With the help of enzyme penicillinase (β-lactamase), penicillin G becomes inactivated by its conversion to benzylpenicilloic acid.

6.5.2.1.2 Biotransformation of narbomycin

During 1998, hydroxylation of narbomycin was achieved by the pikC (P450 hydroxylase) encoded cytochrome P450 in *Streptomyces venezuelae.* In this process hydroxylation of narbomycin to picromycin (by *Streptomyces* spp.) is performed with the help of P450 hydroxylase [22].

6.5.2.1.3 Biotransformation of macrolides

The macrolides are prodrugs and semisynthetic derivatives that are used in a variety of infections. The most important feature of macrolides is that they are frequently administered with other drugs, thus this may increase chances for pharmacokinetic interactions. The potential of macrolides to participate in the biotransformation of some other drugs has been extensively documented, typically with erythromycin and troleandomycin. Macrolides can induce their own hepatic biotransformation into nitrosoalkanes. Less active products are derived from de-acylation of macrolide antibiotics. These products can be used for the further synthesis of more efficient semisynthetic macrolides [23].

6.5.2.2 Indirect biotransformation

During antibiotic production, biotransformation reactions can often be controlled by the addition of certain inhibitors or modified substrates to the medium, or in other words the biosynthetic processes of antibiotics occur in a controlled fashion in indirect biotransformation.

6.5.2.2.1 Biotransformation of actinomycins

A good example of indirect biotransformation is biotransformation of actinomycins which involves the production of new actinomycins in the presence of 4-methyl-proline (a proline analog) in the medium by using the micro-organism *Streptomyces parvulus.* These actinomycins are more effective in their function as they have 4-methylproline in place of proline [24].

6.5.2.2.2 Biotransformation of ribostamycin

Ribostamycin, an intermediate during biosynthesis of neomycin, can be synthesized in large quantities by employing mutant strains of *Streptomyces fradiae.* Numerous other mutant strains of microorganisms have been produced by rDNA technology for the synthesis of modified antibiotics of aminoglycosides and rifamycins [25].

6.5.3 Biotransformation of arachidonic acid to prostaglandins

Prostaglandins are significant in pharmaceutical and therapeutic application, e.g. PGE_1 as a contraceptive, PGG_1 in the treatment of CHF and PGG_2 for relieving labor pains. Arachidonic acid (unsaturated fatty acid) is the starting compound for the biosynthesis of prostaglandins. Several reports based on biotransformation of arachidonic acid to PGE_1, PGE_2, PGF_1 and PGF_2 by using fungi area are available. It is assumed that prostaglandins with better efficacy will be synthesized by biotransformations in upcoming years [26].

6.5.4 Biotransformation for the production of ascorbic acid

Another common example of biotransformation includes the combination of chemical and microbial transformation processes for the commercial production of ascorbic acid (vitamin C).

6.5.5 Biotransformation of glycerol to dihydroxyacetone

Dihydroxyacetone is often employed in cosmetics and suntan lotions. By the process of biotransformation certain acetic acid bacteria can convert glycerol to dihydroxyacetone (figure 6.4). Sufficient oxygen supply, a temperature of 26 °C–28 °C and pH 6.0 are ideal for optimal biotransformation [27].

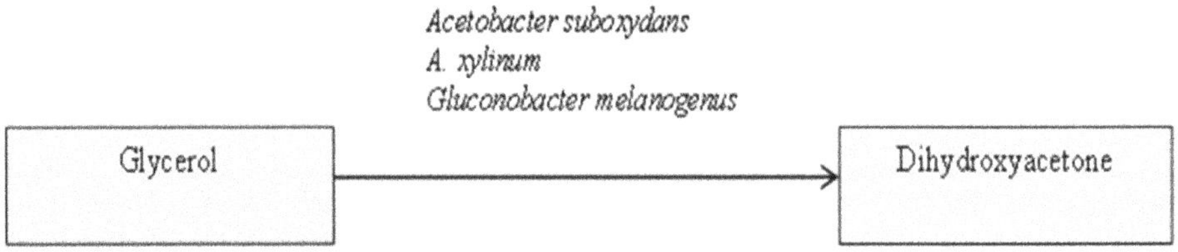

Figure 6.4. Biotransformation of glycerol to dihydroxyacetone.

6.5.6 Biotransformation for the production of indigo

By means of microbial transformation, indigo can be produced. This can be achieved by cloning a single *Pseudomonas* gene that encodes naphthalene dioxygenase in the creation of *E. coli.* The related reactions of biotransformation for the synthesis of indigo are represented in figure 6.5.

6.6 Mechanisms of enzyme action in biotransformation

Biotransformation is primarily a metabolic process occurring in the liver, aiding the excretion of both exogenous (outside the body) and endogenous (within the body) substances. Enzymes catalyze reactions altering these substances' chemical structures, potentially rendering the substrate inactive, active, or even toxic [28]. The action of enzymes in biotransformation can be broadly categorized into Phase I (functionalization reactions) and Phase II (conjugation reactions) as per the traditional understanding. This systematic categorization helps understand enzymes' different roles in modifying substances to facilitate their elimination or utilization within the body [29].

6.6.1 Enzyme kinetics and biotransformation

Enzyme kinetics is pivotal in understanding how enzymes interact with substrates and how their catalytic activities are modulated during biotransformation processes.

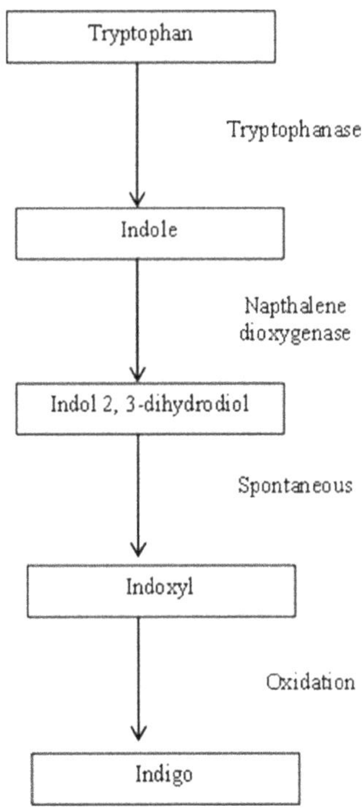

Figure 6.5. Microbial production of indigo.

In the context of biotransformation, enzymes act as biocatalysts, speeding up biochemical reactions without being consumed. They can be extracted from cells and catalyze a wide range of commercially important processes. Enzymes are known for their ability to direct groups controlling selectivity alongside acting as catalysts, making them invaluable in biotransformation processes.

In some biotransformation scenarios, enzymes exhibit synergistic catalytic activity. For instance, the combined action of different enzymes can lead to efficient biotransformation in a one-pot reaction, as demonstrated in a study where a hypothetical synergistic mechanism of two enzymes (CDase and MTSase) was proposed through analyzing enzyme reaction pathways [30].

6.6.2 Cofactors and coenzymes in biotransformation

Cofactors and coenzymes play a crucial role in facilitating enzymatic processes. Enzymes that rely on cofactors facilitate a diverse array of chemically valuable reactions. However, the need for cofactors presents significant economic and practical obstacles to effectively using these biocatalysts. Enzymes bind cofactors, either tiny molecules or metal ions, to aid in catalysis and activity. Approximately 50% of all enzyme activities need a cofactor, either a firmly attached prosthetic group or a loosely linked coenzyme [31]. Acetyl coenzyme A, nicotinamide adenine dinucleotide phosphate (NAD(P)+), and adenosine triphosphate (ADP) all play important roles in microbial metabolism3. These cofactors and coenzymes are essential in assisting enzymes in catalyzing reactions, highlighting their importance in biotransformation [32]. The general mechanism of the enzyme activation is shown in figure 6.6.

6.6.3 Enzyme inhibition and activation

Enzyme activity modulation through inhibition and activation plays a significant role in regulating cellular metabolism. Enzyme inhibition is often used in drug

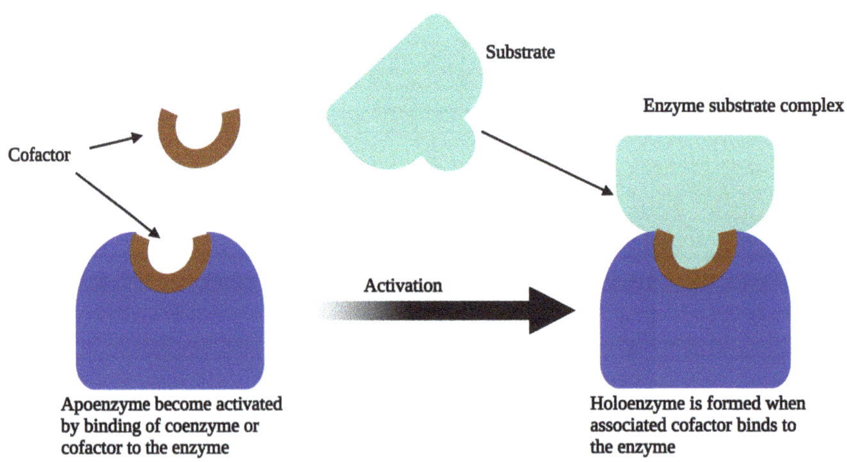

Figure 6.6. Enzyme activation mechanism: transition from apoenzyme to holoenzyme upon cofactor binding.

design to treat various conditions or elucidate mechanisms involved, with many drugs functioning through enzyme inhibition. On the other hand, enzyme activation aims to intensify reaction processes for higher yield quickly and can be utilized for various applications in biotransformation. Factors such as proinflammatory cytokines can modulate enzymatic activity, affecting an organism's response to medications. The balance between enzyme inhibition and activation is crucial for effective biotransformation processes [33].

6.6.4 Role of enzyme specificity and selectivity

Enzyme specificity and selectivity are crucial for achieving desired reactions in biotransformation. Specific enzymes highly catalyze reaction-specific and stereospecific reactions to synthesize compounds that cannot be produced by chemical means. Specificity is often assessed using the value of k_{cat}/K_m, which is more manifest in the rate at which a substrate reacts rather than the affinity of substrate binding [34]. Enzyme engineering can alter substrate specificity and product selectivity to enhance enzyme activity, illustrating the potential for optimizing biotransformation processes through enzyme engineering. Furthermore, the substrate specificity of enzymes has unavoidable physicochemical limits, underlining the importance of understanding enzyme specificity and selectivity in biotransformation [35]. An overview of the enzyme inhibition is given in figure 6.7.

6.7 Biotransformation in environmental applications

Biotransformation in environmental contexts primarily involves using microorganisms or enzymes to detoxify or mineralize chemical contaminants. This process is

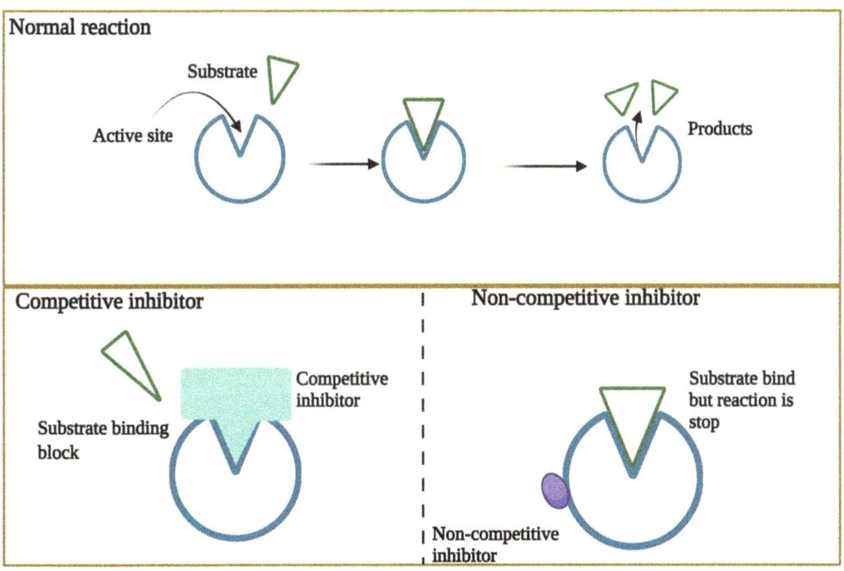

Figure 6.7. Comparative diagram of enzyme inhibition: normal reaction versus competitive and noncompetitive inhibition.

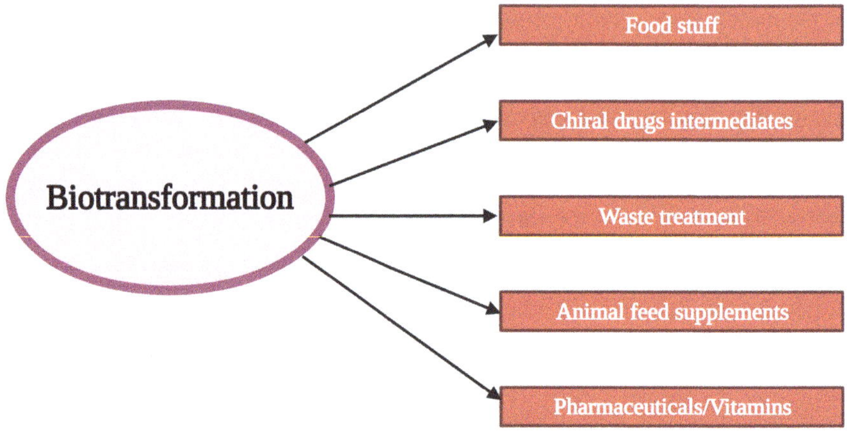

Figure 6.8. Diverse applications of biotransformation in producing food, feed supplements, pharmaceuticals, and environmental waste treatment.

instrumental in transforming harmful compounds into less active metabolites or complete mineralization, which is crucial for environmental remediation [36]. Over the past few decades, substantial knowledge has accrued regarding the biotransformation of major legacy contaminants like chlorinated solvents, BTEX (Benzene, Toluene, Ethylbenzene, and Xylenes), and explosives/munitions chemicals, primarily in a bioremediation context where these contaminants are metabolically degraded [37]. Several applications of the biotransformations are reported in figure 6.8.

6.7.1 Degradation of pollutants

The degradation of pollutants through biotransformation is a significant aspect of environmental remediation. Various strategies and methodologies have been developed to enhance the efficiency of this process. For instance: PAHs are a cluster of organic contaminants that pose environmental and human health risks. Biotransformation is an eco-friendly biological treatment solution for PAH remediation, with microbial remediation approaches being prominently utilized [38]. Biotransformation helps remove contamination from soil and water systems by transforming unwanted complexes into desired products. This process is achieved through microorganisms or enzymes, with recent research focusing on implementing biocatalysts to enhance the stability and efficiency of enzymes involved in this process [39]. Catalases play a crucial role in breaking down various contaminants, such as phenolic chemicals, insecticides, dyes, and poly-aromatic hydrocarbons. Furthermore, the utilization of catalase-based biosensors has been implemented to monitor hazardous waste, hence demonstrating the adaptability and potential of enzyme-mediated biotransformation in the realm of environmental applications [40].

Biotransformation of plastics and microplastics involves breaking these materials into simpler substances by biological agents. The entire procedure starts with plastic waste in an aqueous medium split into micro- and nano-plastics by ultraviolet (UV) radiation and the action of microbes. This is how the process starts. Over time, microplastics in the soil undergo transformations influenced by biotic and abiotic factors, which alter their morphology and particle size [41]. Biotechnological advancements such as biostimulation, bioaugmentation, and enzymatic biodegradation have been proposed for removing microplastics (MPs) by biodegradation and bioaccumulation processes [42].

Moreover, algae, fungi, and bacteria play significant roles in the biodegradation of microplastics, with biotechnological methods like gene editing tools and bioinformatics being utilized to enhance degradation processes. The review articles further discuss various microorganisms and enzymes capable of degrading synthetic plastics like polyethene, polypropylene, and polyvinyl chloride, among others. To provide an all-encompassing comprehension of the biotransformation procedure, a summary of the various microbial species, genes, biochemical reaction pathways, and enzymes involved in plastic decomposition has also been included [43].

Bioremediation uses biological agents, such as fungi and bacteria, to remove or reduce environmental pollutants. The metabolic and ecological features of fungi make them suitable for bioremediation and waste treatment processes. The synthesis of practical microbial taxa, including bacteria, fungi, and microalgae for hydrocarbon removal in marine systems has been reviewed, showcasing the importance of these organisms in bioremediation processes [44]. Additionally, fungi are deemed sustainable and green agents for the clean-up of contaminated sites due to their diverse metabolic capacities, which enable them to detoxify various toxic and recalcitrant compounds[8]. Bacteria and fungi have shown potential in bioremediation strategies, particularly in the environmental degradation of xenobiotic compounds[9]. The potential of bacteria and fungi, individually and in association with plants, has been critically examined, showing high metal tolerance and bioremediation potential up to 98% when associated with plants [45].

6.7.2 Enzymatic breakdown of pesticides

Enzymes play a crucial part in the process of pesticide biodegradation. The compounds in question play a crucial role in the biological aspects of numerous pesticides, impacting their methods of operation, environmental outcomes, and the development of resistance in target species. Specific enzymes are crucial in the degradation of certain pesticides, such as the enzymatic degradation of the organophosphate pesticide malathion [46]. Microbe-derived enzymes are considered excellent candidates for pesticide remediation, and screening elite microbial strains is crucial during biodegradation [47]. The significance of enzymes in mitigating environmental contamination resulting from pesticides has been the subject of numerous studies, highlighting their pivotal role in the biodegradation process. Furthermore, the focus has been placed on the remediation of chemical pesticides from polluted areas using possible microorganisms and their functional enzymes. This emphasizes this study area's potential opportunities and obstacles [48].

6.8 Emerging technologies in biotransformation

Emerging technologies in biotransformation involve novel methods and advancements that enable the conversion of substances through biological agents or systems. These advancements encompass various fields, including enzyme engineering, biocatalyst design, and precision biotransformation. Developing new and successful biotransformation processes in medicinal and pharmaceutical chemistry often entails creating new biocatalysts with improved or even new activities and selectivity [49]. Moreover, the emergence of precision biotransformation strategies has provided detailed insights into biotransformation pathways in natural environmental settings using high-accuracy quantum chemistry, particularly for emerging pollutants whose metabolites are easily overlooked but may cause idiosyncratic toxicity [50].

6.8.1 Enzyme engineering and directed evolution

Enzyme engineering and directed evolution are pivotal in modifying enzymes to meet industrial applications and research requirements. Enzyme engineering focuses on modifying the properties of enzymes to improve their performance for specific tasks. Engineering enzyme properties has facilitated the biocatalysis industry in performing highly selective chemical syntheses, which was achievable through the development of effective methods in enzyme engineering to overcome the limitations of naturally occurring enzymes. The field of enzyme engineering has seen a significant transformation, resulting in a remarkable increase in the range and potential uses of enzymes that have been modified or enhanced to possess specific physical and catalytic characteristics [51]. Directed evolution accelerates the organic process of evolution in biological molecules and systems inside a controlled laboratory environment. This is achieved through repeated rounds involving gene divergence and library screening/selection. In recent years, there has been a significant advancement in the utilization of this instrument for enhancing or creating new functionalities in enzymes and biocatalysts based on entire cells. Notable progress has been made in generating novel enzyme activities and establishing many practical strategies for directed evolution. The approach described herein entails emulating the inherent evolutionary mechanisms to attain specific enzyme characteristics, rendering it an indispensable technique in advancing enzymes for applications in industrial biocatalysis [52]. The integration of nanotechnology and biotechnology occurs through the manipulation of nanostructures, resulting in the modification of their inherent properties. This interaction influences the dispersion of particles and the biotransformation processes they induce. The biotransformation of nanomaterials like silver nanoparticles (AgNPs) is noted, where sulfidation dominates as a cellular detoxification pathway [53]. Though direct information on the integration with bioinformatics and computational biology was not obtained, it is reasonable to infer that nanotechnology, when coupled with these fields, can enhance data analysis and modeling, thus facilitating a better understanding and manipulation of biological systems at the nanoscale. Nanotechnology exhibits the potential to address a diverse range of issues within the domains of medical technology, biosensors, cancer therapy, bioimaging, pharmaceutical administration, precision agriculture, water treatment, and environmental remediation. Through a systems biology and metabolic engineering lens, nanotechnology can be utilized to develop systemic approaches for addressing environmental contaminants and health issues. For instance, bioremediation combined with nanotechnology has been explored to develop more systemic approaches for removing contaminants from environmental matrices [54]. This process within the food and beverage sector pertains to converting a given substance, denoted as A (substrate), into another substance, referred to as B (product), through a biocatalyst. This process can be carried out using purified and immobilized enzymes, growing cultures, resting or washed microbial cells, immobilized cells, or a combination of two sequential biotransformation steps catalyzed by different microorganisms. Here is a deeper dive into the sub-topic.

6.8.2 Production of flavors and fragrances

Enzymes play an imperative starring role in the biotransformation processes within the food and beverage industry. For instance, the beverage industry extensively uses amylases, pectinases, and cellulases to derive flavors and fragrances from natural substrates like grapes and other fruit [55]. Microorganisms are pivotal in biotransformation to produce enzymes and metabolites of industrial interest. For example, the role of microorganisms in brewers' spent grain (BSG) exploitation to produce enzymes and metabolites of industrial interest is well documented [56]. Biotransformation categories such as glycosidic cleavage, terpenol transformation, organic acid conversion, and thiol release are key to flavor and fragrance development in brewing. Glycosidic cleavage, for instance, can release aglycones, often aromatic compounds contributing to the flavor and aroma of the beverage [57]. The end goal of these biotransformations is often to enhance the consumer experience by improving the nutritional profiles and bioavailability of nutrients and creating appealing flavors and fragrances that connect with the consumers on an emotional level, enriching the overall sensory experience of the food or beverage product [58].

6.8.3 Biotransformation of lipids for healthy oils

The biotransformation of lipids to produce healthy oils involves modifying the structure and composition of fats and oils to enhance their nutritional profiles and meet consumer preferences for healthier fat options. Biochemical processing techniques alter the physicochemical and nutritional properties of natural fats and oils, enabling the production of health-promoting lipid products [59]. SLs are designed through the rearrangement or modification of fatty acids on a glycerol backbone, often targeting the incorporation of $n-3$ long-chain polyunsaturated fatty acids (LCPUFAs) which are known for their health benefits [60]. Enzymatic processes produce bioactive, SLs with improved nutritional characteristics. These processes utilize enzymes to modify lipids in fish oil, microalgal lipids, and new seed oils high in omega-3 fatty acids, enhancing their health-promoting properties [61]. Naturally occurring and synthetic ether lipids can be biotransformed in microorganisms, plants, or animal tissues, which can enhance or inhibit the effects of these lipids depending on the compounds involved in the biotransformation process.

6.8.4 Fermentation and enzymatic modification of food products

Fermentation and enzymatic modification are crucial processes in the food industry that enhance food products' nutritional, biochemical, and sensory qualities. Fermentation, driven by microorganisms and enzymes from raw ingredients, alters foods' nutritional and biochemical quality, creating complex ecosystems within fermented products. This process also contributes to food stability through physical and biochemical changes [62]. Enzymatic processes are suitable for converting food waste into valuable products, with potential biotechnological applications such as creating functional foods with probiotic properties. Microbial enzymes, including lipases produced by bacteria, fungi, and yeast, find extensive application in the food industry, contributing significantly to the global market of lipases. They are used in various industries, including food, biofuel, and others [63]. Enzymatic treatment, particularly employing non-*Saccharomyces* yeast with enzymatic activities, produces complex flavor profiles in fermented fruit-based products, aligning with new market trends and consumer preferences. The fermentation process also produces enzymes, organic acids, Baker's yeast, ethanol, vitamins, and other products, which are crucial for various industrial and food applications.

6.9 Biotransformation challenges and future perspectives

The challenges and prospects in biotransformation span across analytical, biotechnological, and industrial sectors. The advancement in biotransformation technologies is seen as a potent tool for addressing various environmental and industrial challenges. Current challenges in biotransformation are primarily analytical and biotechnological, with a specific mention of challenges associated with the bioconversion of tetracyclines by fungi, as an example, illustrating the need for research to advance technology for applications like wastewater and manure treatment [64]. Scalability issues are particularly significant when considering the industrial applications of biotransformation. An integrative approach involving the design of biocatalysts using enzyme engineering and metabolic engineering tools is suggested to enhance biocatalytic efficiency, making it a feasible tool for industrial and pharmaceutical applications. In another instance, the scalability of bioprocesses for the purification of stem cells was discussed, indicating the breadth of scalability challenges across different domains of biotransformation [65]. The necessity of overcoming technical challenges before large-scale implementation can be achieved in the biotransformation of carbon dioxide in bioelectrochemical systems, with recommendations on technical perspectives for successful implementation and future research directions being provided [66].

6.9.1 Scalability issues in industrial applications

Scalability issues in industrial applications of biotransformation technologies are a significant challenge. The transition from lab-scale or pilot-scale to industrial-scale operations often entails numerous challenges. Ensuring the process is optimized for large-scale operations, including the efficient design of biocatalysts and the utilization of suitable engineering tools. Ensuring that the scaled-up process is cost-effective and economically viable is critical for industrial adoption. Adequate infrastructure and equipment are necessary to handle large-scale biotransformation processes. Adhering to industrial standards and regulatory compliance is crucial, especially in pharmaceutical and food industry applications. Continuous technological advancements are needed to address the evolving challenges associated with scalability.

6.9.2 Regulatory and safety concerns

The regulatory and safety concerns surrounding enzymes, particularly food enzymes, primarily revolve around allergies, irritation, and potential toxic properties. There is a lack of consistency in the global regulatory landscape for enzymes despite authorities' familiarity with enzyme technology and its applications. The safety assessment of enzyme production strains is crucial and involves repeated toxicological testing to establish a safe strain lineage (SSL) when no adverse effects are identified from enzymes derived from the same strain lineage. Enzyme production and use regulation is overseen by three central bodies: the Joint Food and Agriculture Organization of the United Nations/World Health Organization Expert Committee on Food Additives, the European Food Safety Authority, and the US Food and Drug Administration [67].

6.9.3 Challenges in enzyme storage and stability

Enzyme stability during storage and operational usage is a critical aspect that impacts the efficacy and shelf-life of enzymes. The challenges include maintaining the enzyme's catalytic abilities from the point of manufacture to eventual use, known as storage stability, and ensuring the persistence of enzyme activity during operational stability. Various strategies for enzyme stabilization have been reviewed, although a practical approach towards this is often seen as lacking. This includes using certain chemicals and conditions to maintain enzyme activity over time. The stability of enzymes is a crucial issue, especially when implementing them as catalysts in industrial processes, which may involve extreme environmental conditions that can induce enzyme instability [68].

6.9.4 Future trends and emerging areas of research

Various emerging trends and prospects in enzyme technology have been identified. For instance, the application of enzyme technologies in developing 'future foods' is seen as a growing research area, focusing on creating healthier, more nutritious, and sustainable food options, although challenges with texture, nutrition, and flavor remain. Enzyme engineering is advancing to address limitations such as lower catalytic efficiency at ambient conditions and poor productivity in native microbial cultures. Additionally, the utilization of enzymes for environmental applications is expanding with the advent of recombinant DNA technology, protein engineering, and rational enzyme design. These emerging research areas aim to leverage various technologies, including gene shuffling, high throughput screening, and nanotechnology, to further the environmental applications of enzymes [69].

6.9.5 Biotransformation in biofuel production

The process of biotransformation plays a crucial role in the production of biofuels, namely in the conversion of lignocellulosic biomass into bioethanol, biodiesel, and biohydrogen through biological deterioration. A principal part of this process entails engineering microbial strains to optimize substrate utilization, sugar transportation, tolerance to inhibitory compounds, and increased metabolic fluxes for improved fermentation outcomes. Such engineered microbes help economically exploit metabolic pathways for biofuel production from lignocellulosic biomass. Metabolic engineering, a significant aspect of biotransformation, has been extensively utilized to alter biosynthetic pathways for desired product formation in native or engineered hosts. The challenges in this domain include the cost of enzymes required for biomass conversion and the optimization of diverse practices for most harvests. The integration of process engineering, fermenting technology, enzyme engineering, and metabolic engineering has significantly propelled the progress of the biofuel sector. The emergence of metabolic engineering and the proliferation of whole-genome sequenced organisms have facilitated the enhancement of microbial metabolic pathways and the synthesis of crucial molecules for biofuel production [70].

6.9.6 Biotransformation in the cosmetic industry

Biotransformation has found significant application in the cosmetic industry, contributing to developing more environmentally friendly products. There is a growing trend towards leveraging marine species to produce green and sustainable cosmetic products via biotransformation. Marine microorganisms, for instance, have been reviewed for their potential in various cosmetic applications owing to their natural products [71]. Moreover, advancements in recombinant DNA technology and genetic engineering have facilitated the large-scale production of bioactive molecules essential for cosmetics, addressing various ethical concerns traditionally associated with production. Dedicated symposia and discussions in academic and industrial circles emphasize biotransformation's widening scope in the pharmaceutical and cosmetic industries [72].

6.9.7 Specialized enzyme systems: lignin-modifying enzymes in biotransformation

Lignin-modifying enzymes (LMEs) are critical in acting upon lignin polymers through catalytic cleavage, depolymerization, and valorization processes. These enzymes are emerging as versatile biocatalysts, with applications extending to developing environmentally friendly products like lignin biopolymers, binders, and bio-vanillin, among others. Particularly, LMEs produced by white rot fungi are noted for their high specificity, which enhances the yield of biotechnological processes, ultimately aiding in the generation of biodegradable products and reducing waste. Genome-based engineering is being employed to modify and enhance the capabilities of ligninolytic enzymes, facilitating the breakdown of lignin into less complex molecules, which holds promise for various industrial applications [73]. Biotransformation is continuously evolving with advancements in molecular structures and metabolic pathways. The exploration of enzyme technology, especially in the context of lignocellulosic biomass, is considered a viable alternative for bioethanol production, although challenges related to pre-treatment requirements and economic considerations remain. Moreover, as drug molecules grow in complexity, the role of drug-metabolizing enzymes, a facet of biotransformation, is expanding, signifying the potential for further research and development in this area. Furthermore, the prospective trajectory of biotransformation research within the pharmaceutical sector suggests a significant need for specialist expertise, notably in drug metabolism and pharmacokinetics departments [74].

References

[1] Leresche J E and Meyer H-P 2006 Chemocatalysis and biocatalysis (biotransformation): some thoughts of a chemist and of a biotechnologist *Org. Process Res. Dev.* **10** 572–80

[2] Collins A M and Kennedy M J 1999 Biotransformations and bioconversions in New Zealand: past endeavours and future potential *Aus. Biotech.* **9** 86–94

[3] Woodley J M and Lilly M D 1994 Biotransformation reactor selection and operation *Applied Biocatalysis* ed J M S Cabral, D Best, L Boross and J Tramper (Chur: Harwood Academic) 371–93

[4] Mustacchi R *et al* 2005 Enhanced biotransformations and product recovery in a membrane bioreactor through application of a direct electric current *Biotechnol. Bioeng.* **89** 18–23

[5] Rojas A *et al* 2004 Biotransformation in double-phase systems: physiological responses of Pseudomonas putida DOT-T1E to a double phase made of aliphatic alcohols and biosynthesis of substituted catechols *Appl. Environ. Microbiol.* **70** 3637–43

[6] Gao P *et al* 2017 Enhancing productivity for cascade biotransformation of styrene to (S)-vicinal diol with biphasic system in hollow fiber membrane bioreactor *Appl. Microbiol. Biotechnol.* **101** 1857–68

[7] Takamatsu S and Ryu D D 1988 Recirculating bioreactor–separator system for simultaneous biotransformation and recovery of product: immobilized l-aspartate β-decarboxylase reactor system *Biotechnol. Bioeng.* **32** 184–91

[8] Weber J M *et al* 2013 Biotransformation and recovery of the isoflavones genistein and daidzein from industrial antibiotic fermentations *Appl. Microbiol. Biotechnol.* **97** 6427–37

[9] Siddiqui M *et al* 2017 Biotransformation of a potent anabolic steroid, mibolerone, with Cunninghamella blakesleeana, C. echinulata, and macrophomina phaseolina, and biological activity evaluation of its metabolites *PLoS One* **12** e0171476

[10] Baydoun E *et al* 2017 Biotransformation of drospirenone, a contraceptive drug, with Cunninghamella elegans *Steroids* **126** 30–4

[11] Wang H H *et al* 2018 Cholesterol and lipoprotein metabolism and atherosclerosis: recent advances in reverse cholesterol transport *Ann. Hepatol.* **16** 27–42

[12] Bauer A and Brönstrup M 2014 Industrial natural product chemistry for drug discovery and development *Nat. Prod. Rep.* **31** 35–60

[13] Lavrnja I *et al* 2017 Expression profiles of cholesterol metabolism-related genes are altered during development of experimental autoimmune encephalomyelitis in the rat spinal cord *Sci. Rep.* **7** 2702

[14] Zaks A and Dodds D R 1997 Application of biocatalysis and biotransformations to the synthesis of pharmaceuticals *Drug Discov. Today* **2** 513–31

[15] Arenas F, Garcia-Ruiz C and Fernandez-Checa J C 2017 Intracellular cholesterol trafficking and impact in neurodegeneration *Front. Mol. Neurosci.* **10** 382

[16] Ferris H A *et al* 2017 Loss of astrocyte cholesterol synthesis disrupts neuronal function and alters whole-body metabolism *Proc. Natl Acad. Sci.* **114** 1189–94

[17] Čvančarová M *et al* 2015 Biotransformation of fluoroquinolone antibiotics by ligninolytic fungi–metabolites, enzymes and residual antibacterial activity *Chemosphere* **136** 311–20

[18] Čvančarová M *et al* 2013 Biotransformation of the antibiotic agent flumequine by ligninolytic fungi and residual antibacterial activity of the transformation mixtures *Environ. Sci. Technol.* **47** 14128–36

[19] Suzuki Y, Ojika M and Sakagami Y 2004 Biotransformation of cystothiazole A, a myxobacterial antibiotic, into novel derivatives by the mother producer, Cystobacter fuscus *Biosci. Biotechnol. Biochem.* **68** 390–6

[20] Nguyen L H *et al* 2014 Biotransformation of rosamicin antibiotic into 10,11-dihydrorosamicin with enhanced *in vitro* antibacterial activity against MRSA *J. Microbiol. Biotechnol.* **24** 44–7

[21] Rusch M *et al* 2015 Biotransformation of the antibiotic danofloxacin by *Xylaria longipes* leads to an efficient reduction of its antibacterial activity *J. Agric. Food Chem.* **63** 6897–904

[22] El-Kersh T and Plourde J 1976 Biotransformation of antibiotics I. Acylation of chloramphenicol by spores of *Streptomyces griseus* isolated from the Egyptian soil *J. Antibiot.* **29** 292–302

[23] Daum S J, Rosi D and Goss W A 1977 Production of antibiotics by biotransformation of 2,4,6/3,5-pentahydroxycyclohexanone and 2,4/3,5-tetrahydroxycyclohexanone by a deoxystreptamine-negative mutant of *Micromonospora purpurea J. Am. Chem. Soc.* **99** 283–4

[24] Martínez J L and Rojo F 2011 Metabolic regulation of antibiotic resistance *FEMS Microbiol. Rev.* **35** 768–89

[25] Tucker J L 2006 Green chemistry, a pharmaceutical perspective *Org. Process Res. Dev.* **10** 315–9

[26] Solano D M *et al* 2012 Industrial biotransformations in the synthesis of building blocks leading to enantiopure drugs *Bioresour. Technol.* **115** 196–207

[27] Newman D J and Cragg G M 2012 Natural products as sources of new drugs over the 30 years from 1981 to 2010 *J. Nat. Prod.* **75** 311–35

[28] Phang-Lyn S and Llerena V A 2019 *Biochemistry, Biotransformation.*

[29] Kubiak-Tomaszewska G *et al* 2020 Molecular mechanisms of ethanol biotransformation: enzymes of oxidative and nonoxidative metabolic pathways in human *Xenobiotica* **50** 1180–201

[30] Parkinson A *et al* 2010 Human biotransformation *Biotransformation and Metabolite Elucidation of Xenobiotics* (Wiley) pp 1–77

[31] Kara S *et al* 2014 Recent trends and novel concepts in cofactor-dependent biotransformations *Appl. Microbiol. Biotechnol.* **98** 1517–29

[32] Brass E P 1994 Overview of coenzyme a metabolism and its role in cellular toxicity *Chem. Biol. Interact.* **90** 203–14

[33] Saboury A 2009 Enzyme inhibition and activation: a general theory *J. Iran. Chem. Soc.* **6** 219–29

[34] Pleiss J 2014 Systematic analysis of large enzyme families: identification of specificity-and selectivity-determining hotspots *ChemCatChem.* **6** 944–50
[35] Johnson K A 2008 Role of induced fit in enzyme specificity: a molecular forward/reverse switch *J. Biol. Chem.* **283** 26297–301
[36] Kosjek T *et al* 2007 Mass spectrometry for identifying pharmaceutical biotransformation products in the environment *TrAC, Trends Anal. Chem.* **26** 1076–85
[37] Birolli W G, Lima R N and Porto A L 2019 Applications of marine-derived microorganisms and their enzymes in biocatalysis and biotransformation, the underexplored potentials *Front. Microbiol.* **10** 1453
[38] Parales R E and Haddock J D 2004 Biocatalytic degradation of pollutants *Curr. Opin. Biotechnol.* **15** 374–9
[39] Petronella F *et al* 2017 Nanocomposite materials for photocatalytic degradation of pollutants *Catal. Today* **281** 85–100
[40] Khalid N *et al* 2017 Carbonaceous–TiO_2 nanomaterials for photocatalytic degradation of pollutants: a review *Ceram. Int.* **43** 14552–71
[41] Tarr M A (ed) 2003 *Chemical Degradation Methods for Wastes and Pollutants: Environmental and Industrial Applications* (Boca Raton, FL: CRC Press)
[42] Reineke W and Schlömann M 2023 Microbial degradation of pollutants *Environmental Microbiology* (Berlin: Springer) pp 161–290
[43] Verbruggen S W 2015 TiO2 photocatalysis for the degradation of pollutants in gas phase: from morphological design to plasmonic enhancement *J. Photochem. Photobiol.* C **24** 64–82
[44] Maqbool Z *et al* 2016 Perspectives of using fungi as bioresource for bioremediation of pesticides in the environment: a critical review *Environ. Sci. Pollut. Res.* **23** 16904–25
[45] Quintella C M, Mata A M and Lima L C 2019 Overview of bioremediation with technology assessment and emphasis on fungal bioremediation of oil contaminated soils *J. Environ. Manage.* **241** 156–66
[46] Riah W *et al* 2014 Effects of pesticides on soil enzymes: a review *Environ. Chem. Lett.* **12** 257–73
[47] Bose S *et al* 2021 Microbial degradation of recalcitrant pesticides: a review *Environ. Chem. Lett.* **19** 3209–28
[48] Munnecke D *et al* 2018 Microbial metabolism and enzymology of selected pesticides *Biodegradation and Detoxification of Environmental Pollutants* (CRC Press) pp 1–32
[49] Nunes V O *et al* 2022 Biotransformation of phytosterols into androstenedione—a technological prospecting study *Molecules* **27** 3164
[50] Fenner K *et al* 2021 Methodological advances to study contaminant biotransformation: new prospects for understanding and reducing environmental persistence? *ACS ES T Water* **1** 1541–54
[51] Deepa A and Mishra B K 2020 Microbial biotransformation of hexavalent chromium [Cr (VI)] in tannery wastewater *Microbial Bioremediation & Biodegradation* (Springer) pp 143–52
[52] Mamma D and Christakopoulos P 2014 Biotransformation of citrus by-products into value added products *Waste Biomass Valori.* **5** 529–49
[53] S, Ohadi Rafsanjani M *et al* 2012 Application of novel nanotechnology strategies in plant biotransformation: a contemporary overview *Recent Pat. Biotechnol.* **6** 69–79
[54] Sarai A *et al* 2005 Integration of bioinformatics and computational biology to understand protein-DNA recognition mechanism *J. Bioinform. Comput. Biol.* **3** 169–83

[55] Singh G B 2015 *Fundamentals of Bioinformatics and Computational Biology* (Cham: Springer International Publishing) pp 159–70
[56] Smitha M, Singh S and Singh R 2017 Microbial biotransformation: a process for chemical alterations *J. Bacteriol. Mycol. Open Access* **4** 85
[57] Pervaiz I *et al* 2013 Microbial biotransformation: a tool for drug designing *Appl. Biochem. Microbiol.* **49** 437–50
[58] Tong W-Y and Dong X 2009 Microbial biotransformation: recent developments on steroid drugs *Recent Pat. Biotechnol.* **3** 141–53
[59] Salter R *et al* 2019 Microbial biotransformation–an important tool for the study of drug metabolism *Xenobiotica* **49** 877–86
[60] Venisetty R and Ciddi V 2003 Application of microbial biotransformation for the new drug discovery using natural drugs as substrates *Curr. Pharm. Biotechnol.* **4** 153–67
[61] El Sayed K A 1998 Microbial biotransformation of veratramine *J. Nat. Prod.* **61** 149–51
[62] Monagas M *et al* 2010 Insights into the metabolism and microbial biotransformation of dietary flavan-3-ols and the bioactivity of their metabolites *Food funct.* **1** 233–53
[63] Choi Y J *et al* 2022 Microbial biotransformation of aqueous film-forming foam derived polyfluoroalkyl substances *Sci. Total Environ.* **824** 153711
[64] Sultana N 2018 Microbial biotransformation of bioactive and clinically useful steroids and some salient features of steroids and biotransformation *Steroids* **136** 76–92
[65] Pierron A *et al* 2016 Microbial biotransformation of DON: molecular basis for reduced toxicity *Sci. Rep.* **6** 29105
[66] Ariffin Z Z, Saat M N and Zulkifle N T 2022 A review on response surface methodology optimization in microbial biotransformation *Sci. Lett.* **16** 64–72
[67] Daud N *et al* 2020 Intestinal hydrolysis and microbial biotransformation of diacetoxyscirpenol-α-glucoside, HT-2-β-glucoside and N-(1-deoxy-d-fructos-1-yl) fumonisin B1 by human gut microbiota *in vitro Int. J. Food Sci. Nutr.* **71** 540–8
[68] Zeng W-L *et al* 2014 Microbial biotransformation of gentiopicroside by the endophytic fungus *Penicillium crustosum* 2T01Y01 *Appl. Environ. Microbiol.* **80** 184–92
[69] Abad M C *et al* 2002 The X-ray crystallographic structure of *Escherichia coli* branching enzyme *J. Biol. Chem.* **277** 42164–70
[70] Zhang Y P, Sun J and Zhong J-J 2010 Biofuel production by *in vitro* synthetic enzymatic pathway biotransformation *Curr. Opin. Biotechnol.* **21** 663–9
[71] Hwang K 2015 Application of biotransformation in cosmetic industry *Korean Society of Biological Engineering Conf.* 20–0
[72] Tinikul R *et al* 2018 Biotransformation of plant-derived phenolic acids *Biotechnol. J.* **13** 1700632
[73] Iram A, Berenjian A and Demirci A 2021 A review on the utilization of lignin as a fermentation substrate to produce lignin-modifying enzymes and other value-added products *Molecules* **26** 2960
[74] Lundell T K, Mäkelä M R and Hildén K 2010 Lignin-modifying enzymes in filamentous basidiomycetes—ecological, functional and phylogenetic review *J. Basic Microbiol.* **50** 5–20

Ahmed Al-Harrasi, Saurabh Bhatia and Ajmal Khan

Chapter 7

Introduction to genomics

7.1 Introduction

In 1910 several researchers first worked together to identify and map genes in organisms of interest. From then, efforts progressively focused on specific organisms, e.g. maize, mice, *Drosophila*, bacteria and yeast.

Genetic mapping involves three important steps:

- Identification of spontaneous mutations, or mutants induced by chemical or physical agents or identifying the locus accountable for variation.
- Sequencing the region in cases and controls to define causal mutation(s).
- Investigating the molecular and cellular variations causes and changes in the functions of the genes discovered.

For spontaneous mutations, DNA sequence analysis has revelaed the types of mutations that are responsible for several hereditary diseases. Many disorders are due to deletions or duplications, including repeated sequences. Multiple sources, such as errors in DNA replication, lesions, and transposable genetics and elements are responsible for spontaneous mutations. When this type of mutation exists it can be used for linkage studies and planning for linkage maps. It was observed by Drake *et al* in 1998 that the rate of occurrence of spontaneous mutation per genome is extraordinarily identical within extensive groups of organisms, but varies extremely among groups [1]. Physical mappings of genes in organisms such as *Drosophila* were also created. This strategy was effective and is extensively used in genetics. However, one of the major shortcomings of this method is that at least one mutation for the respective gene in the genome is essential. Attaining mutations of each gene is very difficult and also labor intensive. Moreover, the genetic mutation may also impact phenotype. Mutations frequently have a harmful outcome, making it practically impossible to map the mutated gene. In the mid-1980s, researchers began using

doi:10.1088/978-0-7503-5387-8ch7

recombinant DNA technology for investigation. In this method, a number of clones, called a genomic library, are established. These are paired together into overlapping sets and brought together they provide genetic material and physical maps for the complete genome. The clones are initially sequenced and thereafter all the genes in the genome are identified from this sequence.

7.2 Characterizations in genomics

In 1987, the word genomics was coined by the geneticist Thomas H Roderick, at the Jackson Laboratory, Bar Harbor, ME [2]. During that period, the term was considered to mean mapping and sequencing to examine the arrangement and organization of genomes. Currently, genomics comprises the sequencing of genomes, determination of the complete set of proteins encoded by an organism, and the functioning of genes and metabolic pathways in an organism. Thus genomics not only deals with the determination of the genetic information present in an organism, but also with understanding the mechanism by which this information is used by the organism. The word genome was presented by H Winkler in 1920. He used the word genome for the complete set of chromosomal and extra chromosomal genes found in an organism, including viruses. This term is used in a similar sense in modern genetics [3].

Vast amounts of information are available in genomics. Understanding and management of this amount of information requires advanced computers and specific software systems. Bioinformatics is a developing area which involves development and application of computer hardware and software to the procurement, storage, analysis and imaging of biological information. Databanks, which are necessary for the storage and examination of genetic information, have now become important tools for geneticists. Genomics also involves the investigation of the products encoded by genetic material, including the number of genes that are expressed, their period of expression, the kind and level of any post-translational modification of the gene product, the role of the encoded protein, and its site in various cellular compartments.

The field of genomics is divided into the following two areas:

- Structural genomics.
- Functional genomics.

In structural genomics the complete sequence of genetic material or the whole set of proteins produced by an organism is determined by different techniques. This can be achieved using the following steps:

- Assembling of high resolution genetic and physical maps.
- Genome sequencing.
- Evaluation of the whole set of proteins produced in an organism. Analysis is required to determine the protein's three-dimensional structure.

Functional genomics deals with the study of the functioning of genes and metabolic pathways. This means the patterns of genetic expression in an organism.

7.3 Historical background

In 1984, the concept behind genome sequencing was first presented in the scientific community. Later, in 1986, a scheme was set for sequencing of the human genome. The Human Genome Project was announced to the public on 1 October 1990 [4]. The aim of the genome projects is to collect information on the structure of DNA in human chromosomes and those of other organisms. The next objective is to develop novel skills to accomplish mapping and sequencing. European scientific communities explored a number of genome projects on yeast, bacteria, *Drosophila* and *Arabidopsis thaliana* in 1988, and in 1990 started a new two year program on the human genome [5]. In 1995, the genetic material of the gram-negative bacterium, *Haemophilus influenza* (which is naturally transformable), was the first to be sequenced. In 1997, the complete genetic material of Escherichia *coli* (a 4 639 221-base pair sequence) was sequenced [6]. Among eukaryotic organisms, genetic materials of yeast (*Saccharomyces cerevisiae*) and a worm (*Caenorhabditis elegans*) were the first to be sequenced in 1999. One year after this breakthrough, *Drosophila melanogaster* and *A. thaliana* were sequenced [6]. Finally, on 26 June 2001, a rough draft of the human genome was published.

Separate drafts were achieved by the public-funded Human Genome Sequencing Consortium and the private company Celera Genomics, established by Craig Venter. However, the draft sequence was published collaboratively after involvement by the US President.

7.4 Genome sequencing

Defining the arrangement of nucleic acid residues in living specimens is an essential part of an extensive range of research applications. A simplified procedure for the sequencing of the whole genome is depicted in figure 7.1. For almost 50 years, investigators have explored various techniques to sequence DNA and RNA molecules, which involve sequencing short oligonucleotides to millions of bases, interpretation of the coding sequence of a single gene, and rapid and extensively available complete genome sequencing [7]. Genome sequencing is a highly complicated and challenging procedure. In one attempt, a portion of 500–600 bp (at best, 1000 bp) can be sequenced easily, however, most genomes are exceptionally large such as 4.2×10^6 bp for *E. coli* and 3.2×10^9 for humans. Thus for sequencing, the sequence of a genome has to be acquired in a particularly large number of small fragments. These small fragments then have to be assembled into a sequence for the genome. For sequencing, fragments are synthesized by splicing the genomic DNA into fragments at different locations. Consequently the actual site of the fragment in the genome has to be experimentally evaluated. In addition, the fragments subsequently produced typically overlap other fragments at their ends. The derived fragments from an organism's genetic material are cloned in a desirable vector. Ultimately this produces a genomic library of the organism.

For sequencing, cloning of the fragments is necessary to generate a large number of copies of each fragment required. The following two methods are available for the sequencing of genomes:

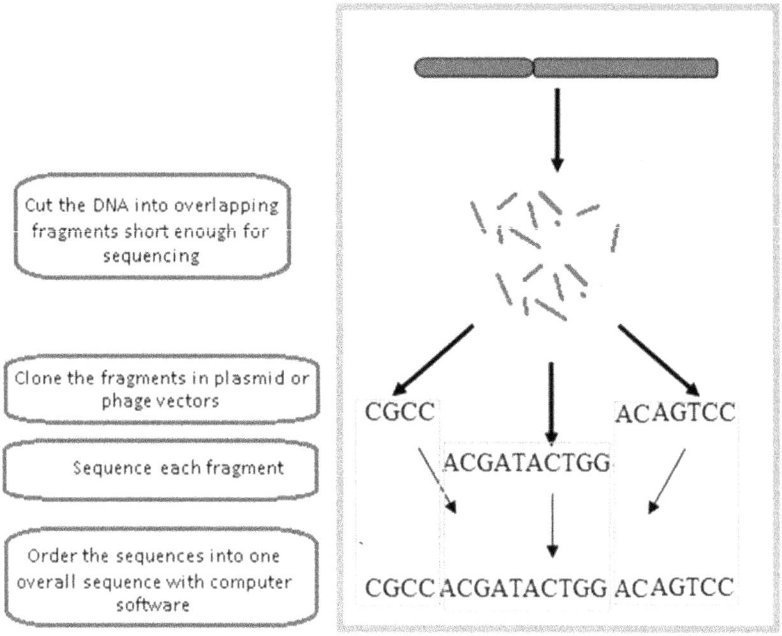

Figure 7.1. Sequencing of a complete genome.

- Shotgun sequencing.
- Clone-by-clone sequencing.

In both of these approaches, the principal step is to produce a genomic library for a particular chromosome.

7.4.1 Clone-by-clone sequencing

The basis of shotgun and clone-by-clone genome sequencing is the same, however, the difference iss that in clone-by-clone sequencing researchers create a DNA library of the pieces of DNA clones obtained from the sequence that was used in the first place. Data management and the mounting of DNA contigs (overlapping sequences) is a lot easier computationally speaking. In shotgun sequencing the same end is achieved but without cloning and libraries. Researchers directly mount contigs from sequenced genome pieces, therefore better computers are required. Shotgun strictly means the sequencing based on the random shearing and consecutive construction of contigs.

During clone-by-clone sequencing the genome or considered genetic material is fragmented or broken into large pieces (150 kb). The actual position of these fragments in the chromosomes is mapped to support assembling them after sequencing. The fragments are first aligned into contigs (overlapping sequence data, i.e., a cluster of sequences which is derived after the completion of the sequencing process, which eventually provides the sequence of a single fragment). These contigs form a physical map of the genome which is eventually used to guide sequencing and assembly. It is also called directed sequencing of BAC contigs. During the initial procedure, BAC clones (functional fertility plasmids) are introduced to the contigs and these a.e. then further introduced into a bacterial cell for growth. The fragments of DNA under consideration are copied each time the bacteria multiply to synthesize multiple duplicate copies. A BAC clone (80–100 kb) has a long DNA fragment duplicated into it. This piece is then further employed to produce cosmid clones and plasmid clones. These synthesized clones have progressively smaller DNA fragments. Now each individual chunk is 500 bp stretched; a more suitable size for sequencing. These synthesized fragments are incorporated into a vector that has a well-known DNA sequence. Then DNA fragments are sequenced, starting with an identified sequence of the vector and extending out into the unidentified sequence of the DNA. Following this type of sequencing even small chunks of DNA are joined together by exploring available overlapping locations to assemble the bulky chunks that were initially incorporated into the BACs. This assembly is done by processors (computers) which identify locations of overlap and assemble the DNA sequence. Using the map created during the initial phase, the large pieces can be arranged again into chromosomes as part of the whole genome sequence. This method was introduced during the 1980s and 1990s to initially sequence the genetic material of the *C. elegans* (the nematode worm) and *S. cerevisiae* (yeast). During the sequencing of Human Genome Project (2001), clone-by-clone sequencing was favored. There are a number of advantages to clone-by-clone sequencing: (1) each fragment of DNA is taken from a well-known region of the genome, so it is comparatively easy to regulate whether there are any gaps in the sequence; (2) as a genome map is followed this method offers more reliable assembly, so researchers know where larger pieces/fragments belong in relation to each other; and (3) as each and every piece of DNA is different, numerous people can work on the genome simultaneously.

7.4.2 Human whole-genome shotgun sequencing

The determination of the whole sequence of genes in a genome is required to understand the genetic basis of an organism. The sequencing of large numbers of gene fragments and even complete genomes is only possible with the development of tools for DNA sequencing. Novel significant tools such as physical mapping, DNA sequencing and sequence analysis have been established. To increase the output, robotic processes for sample preparation and novel software for sequence analysis have been applied [8]. A simplified representation of human whole-genome shotgun sequencing is illustrated in figure 7.2.

In 1997, Weber and Myers published a study entitled ‘Human whole-genome shotgun sequencing’. They contended, by means of computational models, that in the place of long reads, short reads would cover sufficient data to sequence the first human genome, which would not only be economical, but quicker than the Human Genome Project. This was so fiercely debated that Phillip Green published a review, describing why shotgun sequencing was not possible. Both studies were finally accepted and published side by side in the journal *Genome Research*.

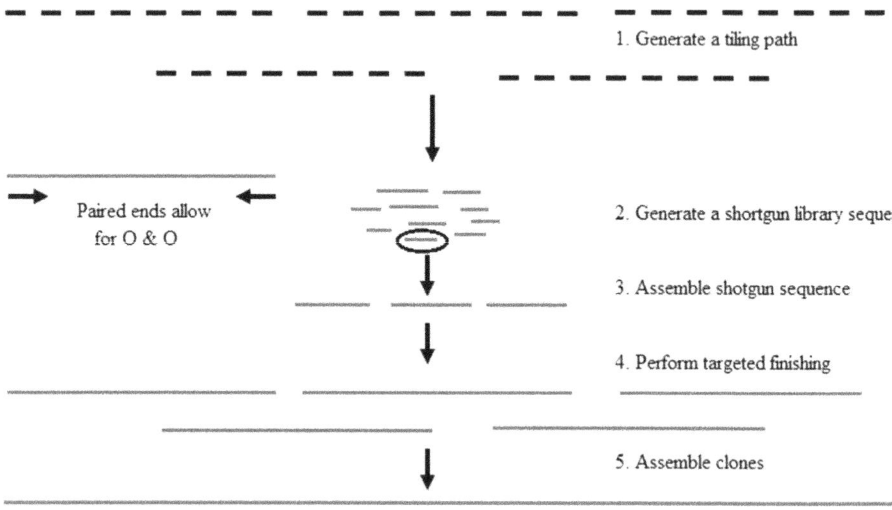

Figure 7.2. Human whole-genome shotgun sequencing.

Shotgun sequencing includes arbitrarily splicing of DNA sequences into numerous small fragments and then reconstructing the sequence by examining for regions of overlap. Because of their size and structural sophistication, large, mammalian genomes are the most problematic to clone, sequence and assemble [9].

For such genomes, the method known as clone-by-clone sequencing, although reliable and systematic, takes a very long time. With the development of cheaper sequencing techniques and more advanced computer databases, geneticists can thus rely on whole-genome shotgun sequencing to deal with large, complex genomes. Fred Sanger and co-workers initially used shotgun sequencing to sequence small genomes, for example, the genomes of viruses and bacteria. Complete genetic material shotgun sequencing avoids the long mapping and cloning steps that make clone-by-clone sequencing so gradual. During this procedure the complete genome is fragmented into small pieces of DNA for sequencing. These pieces are often of variable sizes, extending from 2–20 kb (2000–20 000 bp) to 200–300 kb (200 000–300 000 bp). Then these pieces are sequenced to examine the order and arrangement of the DNA bases (A, C, G and T). Subsequently, the sequenced fragments are collected together by computer databases that determine where fragments overlap. In analogy, this technique is akin to chopping several copies of a book (which is here the genome or genetic material), blending up all the pieces and at that point reuniting the original text (genome/genetic material) by finding fragments/pieces of DNA with text that overlaps and piecing the book back together based on these. This technique was used by Venter (founder of Celera Genomics) to sequence the human genome. Venter desired to sequence the human genome quicker than the reported goal, and considered shotgun sequencing to be the best approach. For assembly, Venter initially used the reported clone-by-clone data from the Human Genome Project. Currently, with advancements in computational technology, entire genome shotgun sequencing is being employed to further advance the accuracy of present genome sequences, for example, the reference human genome. This procedure can be utilized to eliminate errors, fill in gaps or rectify parts of the sequence that were initially assembled inaccurately (by clone-by-clone sequencing). Consequently, the reference human genome is continuously being developed to guarantee that the genome sequence is of the utmost high standard. There are number of merits to shotgun sequencing, such as:

- By eliminating the mapping steps, entire genome shotgun sequencing (EGSS) is a much quicker process than clone-by-clone sequencing.
- EGSS utilizes a piece of the DNA that clone-by-clone sequencing needs.
- EGSS is mainly effective if there is any available reference sequence against an unidentified genome. It is much more convenient to assemble the genome sequence by assembling it to a present reference genome.
- Shotgun sequencing is much quicker and economical than the procedures employed for genetic mapping.

However, there are still various disadvantages to shotgun sequencing, such as:

- An enormous amount of computing power and advanced and sophisticated software are necessary to align shotgun sequences together.
- For sequencing the genomic material of a mammal (billions of bases long), 60 million individual DNA sequence reads are required.
- Since a genetic map is not used, the possibility of error in assembly is greater. However, comparatively these errors are usually easier to resolve than in other procedures and are minimized if a reference genome can be used.
- EGSS assembly is very challenging without an existing reference genome to match it to.
- EGSS can also result in errors which must be determined by other, more labor-intensive types of sequencing, such as clone-by-clone sequencing.

7.4.3 Compilation of genome resources

Four main objectives were set out for the Genome Sequence Compilation [10]:

- To determine evolutionarily conserved sequence motifs, mainly outside protein-coding genes, which are accountable for regulatory and other critical genomic functions.
- To explore new models of human disease and heritable phenotypes.
- To offer a starting point for the evaluation of the expansion, contraction, and adaptation of gene families in different evolutionary lineages.
- To offer a outline for the reconstruction of genome organization, content and dynamics that have happened through the mammalian radiations.

Genome sequencing projects required the production of high throughput tools that produce desirable information quickly. This can be achieved by the employment of advance computers to manage this vast store of information. These computational tools have given birth to a new area called bioinformatics. Manual manipulation of gene data is time consuming, but bioinformatics can deal with the storage, examination, analysis and utilization of the information about biological systems. For example, it involves processes such as accumulating genome sequences, documentation of genes, assigning functions to the identified genes, planning of databases, etc. Different genetic compilers are available today. A software compiler is a way to use genetic information and provides a design platform allowing the geneticist to manipulate and design everything from single genes to whole genomes. So as to guarantee that the nucleotide sequence of a genetic material is complete and error-free, the genetic material is sequenced more than once, such as by using the shotgun method. The bacterial genome (*Pseudornonas aeruginosa*) was sequenced seven times to make the sequence accurate and free from faults. Stover and co-workers (2010) reported the complete genome sequence of *P. aeruginosa* PAO1. They suggest that the size and complexity of the *P. aeruginosa* genome reveals an evolutionary adaptation allowing it to flourish in various environments and limit the effects of a diversity of antimicrobial compounds [12]. However, the assembler software (a sequence assembler is innovative bioinformatics software for spontaneous DNA sequence assembly, contig editing, file format alteration, DNA sequence analysis and mutation recognition) identified 1604 regions that need further justification. These areas were reinvestigated and re-sequenced to successfully complete the genome sequence. The efficiency/accuracy of the shotgun technique was equated with the sequence derived from the clone-by-clone procedure of two extensively separated genomic regions of *P. aeruginosa.* These two considered areas together were 81 843 nucleotides long. The sequences derived by the two procedures were in perfect agreement. This assessment exposed the precision potential of the shotgun method of genome sequencing. This also demonstrates the safeguards to be considered during genome sequencing projects. This level of maintenance is not uncommon. Similar safety measures are employed in all genome projects. The Human Genome Project, an international scientific research project, sequenced the 3.2 billion bp of the human genome a total of 12 times. Celera Genomics (a private biotech company), using shotgun-cloning, used an approach of sequencing from both ends of DNA fragments. This project sequenced the human genome 35.6 times. While a rough draft of the human genome sequence is complete, some other objectives are yet to be accomplished. These include obtaining the remaining sequence and rectifying miscalculations (called proofreading the genome), filling in gaps and then sequencing the 7%–10% of the genome that comprise heterochromatin. This is present in ample amounts inside the cells that are less active or not active, whereas euchromatin is predominant inside cells that are vigorous or active in the transcription of several of their genes. Since they comprise low priority sections of repetitive DNA sequences, heterochromatic regions of the genome were not initially sequenced. Moreover, intially it was thought that the heterochromatin does not contain genes. However, the *Drosophila* genome sequence revealed that their heterochromatic regions contain a very small number of genes (around 50). Based on this discovery, the heterochromatic regions of the human genome must be sequenced to confirm that all genes in the human genome have been recognized. As soon as the genome of an organism is sequenced, compiled and proofread, the subsequent process of genomics, namely annotation, begins.

7.5 Understanding bioinformatics and sequencing

Advance computers and high-speed networks are compulsory to evaluate genome projects. Genetic data signify a potential source for investigators and organizations interested in how genes contribute to our health and wellbeing [11]. Nearly half of the genes identified by the Human Genome Project have no known function. Scientists, by means of bioinformatics, can identify genes, establish their roles and develop gene-based strategies for preventing, diagnosing and treating disease [12]. Simplified presentation of bioinformatics and sequencing is presented in figure 7.3.

Genome sequencing and investigation is an area that has developed very quickly over the last 10–20 years, in particular after publication of the final draft of the human genome sequence in 2003. From procuring a complete genome sequence from a characteristic individual or strain of a small number of species, the genomics community has moved on to recording and authenticating genetic assortment within species, with a special focus on human beings, and by sequencing the genomes of a quickly growing number of species. The introduction of economical, very high throughput sequencing tools has also made it promising to sample transcriptomes (the summation of all mRNA fragments expressed from the genes of an organism), genomic areas bound by proteins, bacterial populations, or sometimes even whole ecosystems, by means of sequencing methods. This has germinated an innovative generation of software techniques to manage the very large numbers of short sequences, often called reads, which are produced by the new machines, and has also moved the area of computational genomics into the territory of 'big data', requiring

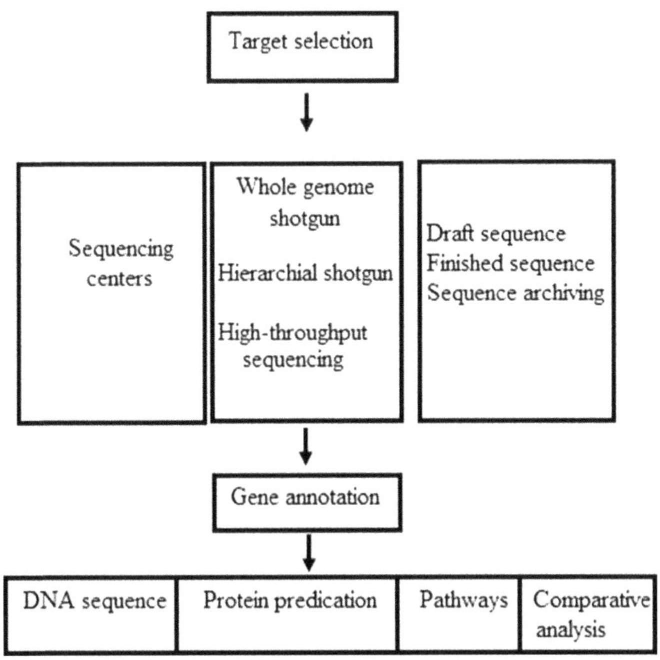

Figure 7.3. Bioinformatics and sequencing.

large and sophisticated computers for the organization and investigation of these sequences.

The entities that are selected for genome projects are those typically used in genetic and other systematic studies. Thus they are usually called model organisms. A model organism can be a prokaryotic or eukaryotic micro-organism, or an animal or plant, which is extensively investigated as it can be easily studied in the laboratory to understand biological processes. The Generic Model Organism Database project offers genetic researchers tools of open-source software machinery for imaging, interpreting, managing and procuring biological information. Model organisms include organisms such as *E. coli*, *Archaeoglobus fulgidus*, yeast (*Saccharorny cerevisiae*), *Bacillus subtilis, A. thaliana*, the fruit fly (*Droso melanogaster*) and nematide worm (*C. elegans*). The Human Genome Project focused on sequencing the whole human genome.

E. coli is, by far, the most extensively studied micro-organism. Various tools that are available currently were established for the *E. coli* genome project. The sequencing of the *E. coli* genome was accomplished in 1997 [13]. The *E. coli* K-12 genome contains 4408 genes (4288 protein-coding genes annotated) with a size of around 4.64×10^6 bp. *B. subtislis* is a gram-positive bacterium that settles over leaf surfaces and is significant for both production of enzyme and food supply fermentation. 'GRAS' is an acronym for the phrase Generally Recognized as Safe. GRAS is well suited for enzymes, given the general availability of scientific data supporting enzyme safety, and the generally recognized (peer-reviewed) methodology and decision trees for evaluating the safety of microbial enzymes used in food processing and in animal feed, respectively. It is usually named as safe (GRAS) with genome of 4.21×10^6 bp (4212 genes). The reference database SubtiList was exclusively created for the genome of *B. subtilis* 168, the paradigm of gram-positive endospore-forming bacteria [14]. Another example of a model organism is *Aracheoglobus fulgidus*, a strictly anaerobic archaebacterium with a genome size of 2.17 × 106 bp (2493 genes) [15] (1 563 423 bp, 1858 protein-coding, 52 RNA genes, according to the Genomic Encyclopedia of Bacteria and Archaea project) [16]. The yeast organism *S. cerevisiae*, so called because of its ability to ferment saccharose (sugar), is the most key fungal species used in biotechnological developments. In 1996 *the S. cerevisiae* genome was the first completely sequenced from a eukaryote. The current version, called 'S288C 2010,' was determined from a single yeast colony by means of advance sequencing tools and functions as the anchor for further innovations in yeast genomic science [16]. In 1989, genome sequencing of *S. cerevisiae* was accomplished. The yeast genome is 12.8×10^6 bp in size and contains 6548 genes. PlantGDB (http://www.plantgdb.org/) is a databank of molecular sequence data for all plant species with important sequencing efforts. The database arranges EST sequences into contigs that represent tentative unique genes. PlantGDB offers genome browsing abilities that integrate all accessible EST and cDNA reported for existing gene models (for *A. thaliana*, see the AtGDB site at http://www.plantgdb.org/AtGDB/) [16].

The first plant for which the complete genome was sequenced and published was *A. thaliana*. In 1907, it was first considered as a good organism for genetic investigations and has become a model plant for genetic investigations as it has the smallest genome of the higher plants. Furthermore, its genome contains only a small amount of repetitive DNA [17]. The genomic sequencing project of the *A. thaliana* genome began in 1990 and was completed in 2000. According to the sequencing results, the size of the *A. thaliana* rabidopsis genome is 130×10^6 bp and a predicted 26 000 genes [18]. The MIPS *A. thaliana* Database (MAtDB; http://mips.gsf.de/proj/thal/db) started out as a repository for genome sequence data in the European Scientists Sequencing *Arabidopsis* (ESSA) project and the *Arabidopsis* Genome Initiative. Another model organism, *C. elegans* (a free-living nematode) was completely sequenced in 1999 and was the first multicellular animal whose genome was sequenced. The *C. elegans* genome has 97×10^6 bp and has over 20 000 estimated genes. WormBase (http://www.wormbase.org) is a web-based resource for the *C. elegans* genome and its biology. It is based on the existing ACeDB databank of the *C. elegans* genome and offers data curation services, and a considerably extended scope [19].

D. melanogaster (the fruit fly) is often called the 'Queen of Genetics'. In 2000, the *Drosophila* genome was completely sequenced. It has 180×10^6 bp (16 000 genes). This breakthrough has offered a platform for further genomic research, as the number of genes present in the *Drosophila* genome is less than four times that of the bacterium *E. coli*. Since the human genome draft sequence was published in 2001, a number of observations have been made. Several significant features of the human genome are as follows:

- A minimum 50% of the genome is obtained from transposable elements.
- The genome sequences of individuals vary by less than 0.2% of their base pairs.
- It has approximately 35 000 genes.
- It encompasses over 3.2 billion base pairs.
- Only 5% of the genome encodes proteins.
- The genome contains gene-rich regions separated by gene poor regions, often called gene deserts.
- The largest gene is the gene encoding dystrophin (2.5×10^6 bp).

The majority of the variations in the human genome are present in the form of single-base differences in the sequence. A single-base difference is known as a single-nucleotide polymorphism (SNP), frequently called 'snips'. One SNP is present in roughly every 1000 bp of human genome. Approximately 85% of all variations in human DNA is due to SNPs. Advantages of genome projects include [20]:

- Better knowledge of human genetic diseases and their correlations should allow their management/cure.
- A number of methods have been established for genome sequencing projects.
- Information related to SNPs has become accessible; this may be beneficial in different ways.
- The complete genetic information existing in the genomes of various organisms can be determined.

- They have unlocked exciting opportunities for future research, e.g. functional genomics.
- They offer knowledge on why the individuals react differently to the same drugs (pharmacogenomics).
- They offer understanding of genome association and its evolution, and the most important mechanisms involved within that.
- Genome sequences allow the study of the many molecular interactions resulting in the normal development of organisms.
- Micro-organism pathogenicity can be better understood. This can offer protection from such diseases.
- The associations between genes can be studied with confidence.

7.6 Comparative genomics as a technique to understand evolution

The whole-genome sequence of an individual can be considered to be their final genetic map, in the sense that the heritable physical characteristics are encoded within the DNA and that the order of all the nucleotides along each chromosome is known. However, information on the DNA sequence does not tell us directly how these genetic data result in the observable traits and behaviors (phenotypes) that we want to understand. Identifying all the functional parts of genome sequences and using these data to improve the wellbeing of individuals and society are the focus of the next phase of the Human Genome Project [21]. Relative studies of genome sequences will be a major part of this effort. The investigation of variation and similarity in genomic structures and, in particular, their organization in various organisms is known as comparative genomics. The aims of comparative genomics are as follows:

- to recognize the route of evolution and
- to translate the DNA sequence data into proteins of known functions.

In order to equate the genomes of various organisms it is essential to understand the meaning of orthologues and paralogues. Orthologues are homologous genes present in different organisms and only encode proteins that have a similar function. Orthologues arise by direct vertical descent, and have deviated only by storing mutations. Comparatively, paralogues are homologous genes within similar organisms and always encode proteins that have interrelated but not similar functions. Paralogues have developed by gene duplication, followed by mutation accumulation, e.g. genes of the globin family.

7.6.1 The role of exon shuffling

Exon shuffling is a molecular tool for the development of new genes. It is a method by which two or more exons from diverse genes can be taken together ectopically (atypical gene expression in a cell, tissue, or at any developmental stage in which the gene is not typically expressed), or the same exon can be duplicated, to create a new exon–intron structure. Exon shuffling has been considered as one of the main development powers determining both the genome and the proteome of eukaryotes.

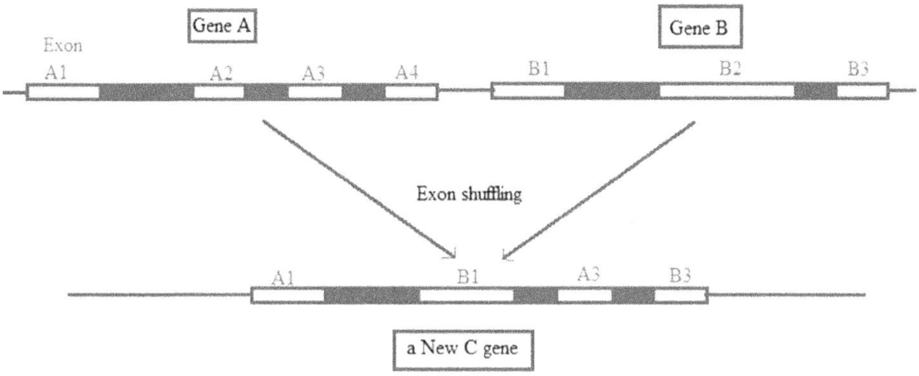

Figure 7.4. Exon shuffling. In this illustration the end gene is produced by shuffling exons from more than one gene.

This is vital in the formation of multidomain proteins throughout animal evolution, obtaining a number of functional genetic novelties [22]. A simple presentation of exon shuffling is depicted in figure 7.4.

Various proteins contain distinct domains. Such proteins are known as mosaic proteins, e.g. serine proteases responsible for blood coagulation. The majority of mosaic proteins are extracellular and are mainly present in metazoa. In addition, these types of proteins are also present in unicellular organisms.

The study of the genes that encode mosaic proteins explores the strong association between domain establishment and intron–exon structure. Each domain is inclined to be encoded by one or a combination of exons, which are synthesized by recombination within the intervening sequences; this is known as exon shuffling. This process synthesizes new genes that encode proteins with improved function. As introns are much longer than exons, the chances of crossovers in introns are greater than in exons.

7.6.2 Horizontal or lateral gene transfer

Horizontal gene transfer was first reported in 1928, in an experiment by Frederick Griffith. During this experiment, Griffith demonstrated that virulence was able to transfer from virulent to nonvirulent strains of *Streptococcus pneumoniae*, establishing that genetic information can be horizontally transferred between bacteria via a mechanism called transformation [23]. A schematic representation of horizontal and vertical gene transfer is presented in figure 7.5.

Horizontal or lateral gene transfer involves genetic transfer/exchange between organisms of different evolutionary origin/lineages (sequences of cells, genes, organisms or populations, linked by a continuous line of origin from ancestor to descendent) [24]. It is usually assumed that such gene transfers/exchanges have happened many times throughout the course of evolution. The following two approaches are employed for the discovery of those genes that are likely to develop by horizontal gene transfer:

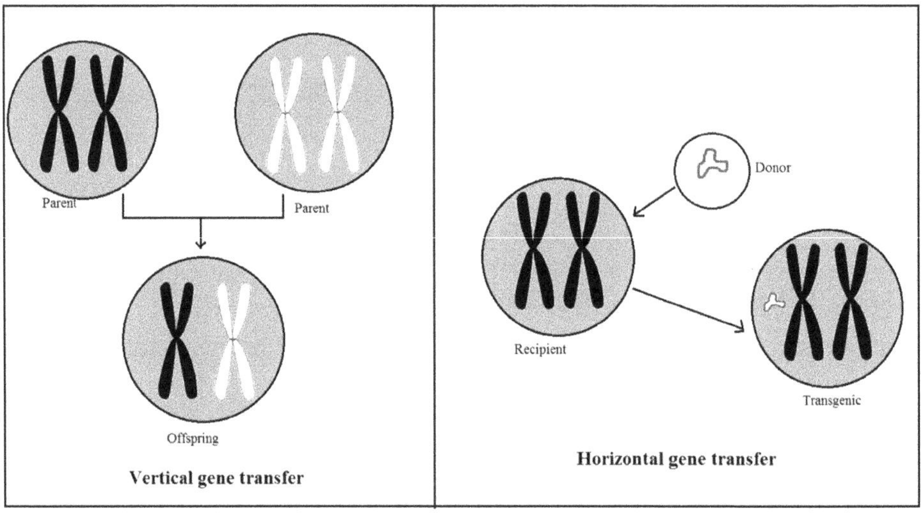

Figure 7.5. Horizontal and vertical gene transfer representation.

- Detection of genes having unusual base composition and bias in codon usage can also be used for the detection.
- Failure to find a similar gene in closely related species.

The accessibility of entire genome sequences has allowed the detection of such genes. It has been determined that hundreds (between 113 and 223) of human genes have been transferred directly from bacteria into the human genome rather than having developed from bacterial genes.

7.6.3 Genome similarity or homology

The sequence similarity searching tool is the most extensively used, and most reliable, approach for describing newly determined sequences. This tool can identify homologous proteins or genes by identifying a statistically significant similarity that reveals common ancestry [25].

Extensively used similarity searching databases are:

- BLAST [27].
- PSI-BLAST [27].
- SSEARCH [30].
- FASTA [28].
- HMMER3 [29].

These programs offer precise statistical evaluations, guaranteeing protein sequences that share considerable similarity also have similar structures. One of the amazing discoveries from the investigation of genome sequences of various organisms is as follows: organisms whose genomes are quite similar in appearance may look very different, for instance humans and mice.

These two organisms in fact have 97.5% of their DNA sequences in common that achieve the same genetic functions. It was also observed that humans and mice had a mutual ancestor some 100 million years ago. Since then, functional DNA has deviated only to a small extent, whereas the non-coding DNAs of the two species have deviated to a much greater extent. Likewise, it is estimated that human and chimpanzee genomes differ by only 1%–3% of their DNA sequence. It may be noticed that the organisms above are more closely related to each other than organisms such as yeast (a fungus) and the nematode worm (an animal). The nematode worm is estimated to have 19 000 genes, of which over 2000 encode proteins that have functional equivalents as in yeast.

7.6.4 SNPs

For the last few decades, the utilization of molecular markers, highlighting polymorphism at the DNA level, has contributed a great deal in the development of animal genetics [32]. Among all the techniques, microsatellite DNA markers have been the most extensively utilized. A new marker tool, the SNP (see above) [32], is now in the picture and has recently gained high recognition. It is just a single-base change in a DNA sequence, with a usual alternative of two likely nucleotides at a certain position [26].

SNPs, the most abundant type of genetic variation, are now the main raw material essential for most genetic investigations and databases. Variation comprising indels, copy number variants, microsatellites and epigenetic markers remain parameters to consider and can influence disease [27]. There are some reported 10 million SNPs in the human genome. The basic concept and types of SNPs are depicted in figures 7.6 and 7.7, respectively.

As mentioned above, SNPs are the most common type of genetic variant among people. Each and every SNP signifies a variance in a single DNA building block, known as a nucleotide. For example, an SNP can substitute the nucleotide cytosine with the nucleotide thymine in a specific stretch of DNA. SNPs usually take place throughout a person's DNA. They occur once in every 300 nucleotides on average, i.e., there are approximately 10 million SNPs present in the human genome. As a rule, these deviations are present in the DNA between genes. They can behave as biological markers, facilitating researchers to locate genes that are related to disease. Once SNPs occur inside a gene or in a promoter region closer to a gene, they might show an additional direct role in disease by influencing the gene's function. The majority of SNPs have no influence on health or development. Certain genetic differences, however, have been shown to affect human health. Scientists have discovered SNPs that may help to predict an individual's reaction to certain drugs, vulnerability against external environmental factors such as toxins and the threat of developing specific illnesses. SNPs may also be utilized to track the causes of disease, in particular the inheritance of disease genes inside families. Upcoming investigations will work to recognize SNPs linked to complex diseases, e.g. heart disease, diabetes and cancer. Various academic institutions and industries are currently involved in the development of large-scale SNP detection projects, and these projects introduced data on thousands of publicly available SNPs. The most common

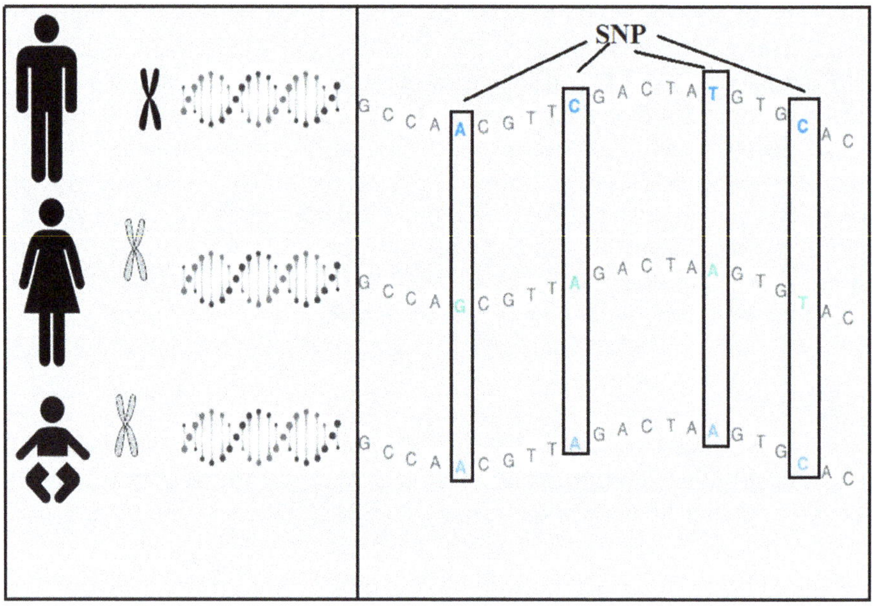

Figure 7.6. Representation of SNPs.

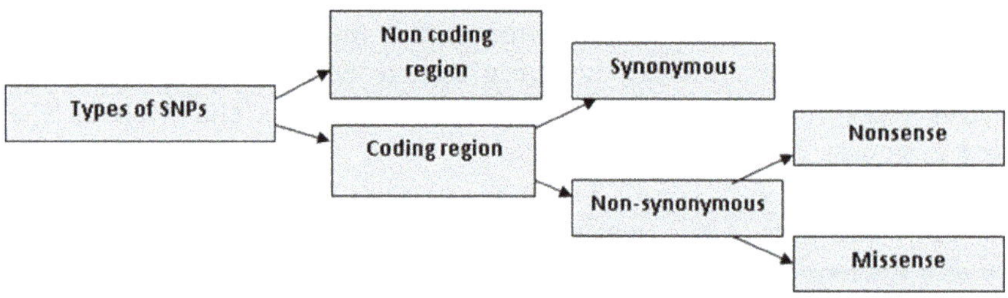

Figure 7.7. Types of SNPs.

example of these is the HGBASE database. It has been projected that 90% of sequence variation in humans is because of SNPs. Human genome is projected to contain 3–17 million SNPs. Out of these, 5% SNPs are likely to occur in genes. Thus each individual gene is likely to contain six SNPs. Therefore, SNPs offer a molecular marker that is present in the genome at a very high density. The SNPs can thus be utilized to map genes involved in human diseases. These genes are exceptionally difficult to map using other molecular markers as these latter markers are not distributed at an adequate density in the genome. Therefore, by using SNPs as markers, every gene in the human genome can be mapped. Additionally, it might be possible to identify all the genes involved in human diseases. An SNP might be present within the relevant gene or very near the gene which is tightly linked with the SNP. SNP1 and SNP2 are the two alleles of an SNP.

Some SNPs are situated in the recognition sequence of an endonuclease. They alter the recognition sequence (base sequence) and produce restriction fragment length polymorphism (RFLP). Some other SNPs are situated in the coding regions of genes. They are linked with definite phenotypes. The differences in the genetic sequences of individuals are understood to be responsible for the following:

- Disease susceptibility.
- Drug response.
- Normal development and aging.
- Reaction against environmental factors.

The field of study that is more concerned with the effect of genetic variation disease susceptibility and drug response is known as pharmacogenomics. Pharmacogenomics is the investigation of how genetic make-up regulates the response to a therapeutic intervention. Pharmacogenomics is likely to advance individualized treatments that will be safer and more effective [28]. Genetic variations may affect the drug reaction of an individual in the following ways:

- They may influence the metabolism of the drug itself.
- They may affect the action of the drug on its target molecule.

Pharmacogenomics aims to raise drug efficacy and safety by comparing drug properties to the genetic make-up of an individual. The response of the drug is expected to be influenced by various genes associated with drug metabolism, drug transport and creation of drug targets. Thus, various inputs have been made to employ SNPs to further map hundreds or thousands of genes that have an influence on the safety and efficiency of different drug treatments. These SNPs can be positioned on gene chips that can be employed to explore the genotype of those genes that are involved in responses to specific drugs. SNPs have the potential to describe the danger of an individual's susceptibility against numerous illnesses and reaction against various drugs. Biologically significant SNPs that are specifically related with the threat of disease need to be identified [29]. The identification and understanding of great numbers of these SNPs are essential before they can be used widely as genetic tools. Depending upon these data, more effective and safe treatment can be considered for these individuals, such as variants in the gene encoding apolipoprotein E (apoE), which were found to be associated with variation in the reaction to a drug used for treatment. apoE supports lipid transport and binds to cell surface receptors to facilitate lipoprotein uptake. It is the main apolipoprotein produced in the brain [37]. The apoE protein is present in three different isoforms (E2, E3 and E4) that are the outcome of two non-synonymous SNPs (rs429358 and rs7412) present in exon 4 of the APOE gene. Gene apoE is involved in vulnerability to Alzheimer's disease, and a cholinesterase inhibitor is employed to mitigate the symptoms of illness [30].

7.6.5 Inferences from comparative genomics

In the case of prokaryotes, the following genomes and characteristics have been considered:

- *Bacillus megaterium* is important in the *Bacillus* phylogeny, as an evolutionarily important species and, in particular, in understanding genome evolution, dynamics and plasticity in the bacilli. *B. megaterium* is a non-pathogenic commercially existing host for the biotechnological production of numerous substances such as vitamin B12, penicillin acylase and amylases. The genome sizes of bacilli vary significantly, such as from 0.58 × 106 bp (*Mycoplasma genitalium*) to 30 × 106 bp (*Bacillus megaterium*) [39, 41]. The gene density is, however, comparatively constant at one gene per kilo base pairs.

- *Vibrio cholerae* O1 is reported as an important causative agent for infectious diseases [41]. A number of bacteria like *V. cholerae* have two or more circular chromosomes in their genomes. As a minimum, one of these chromosomes is obtained from a plasmid.
- In the case of larger genomes such as *E. coli*, almost 50% of the ORFs (open reading frames, the portion of a reading frame that has the prospect of being translated) are of unidentified biological function [31].
- Around 25% of all ORFs are exclusive and do not have substantial sequence resemblance to any other available protein sequence. Therefore, there are some new protein families yet to be revealed. The incidence of paralogues (pairs of genes that develop from similar ancestral genes) ranges from 26% for *M. genitalium* (the smallest self-replicating organism and an effective human pathogen related to a variety of genitourinary diseases) to 75% for *Pseudomonas aeruginosa*. The incidence of paralogues increases with genome mass [32].
- In close relation with bacteria, chromosomal transposals are more likely to arise nearby the origin or terminus of replication. Several bacterial genomes present in the database comprise phage DNA incorporated into the bacterial chromosome. It is not uncommon for bacteria to hold several prophages in their chromosomes, which then establish a substantial part of the total bacterial DNA. Several prophages and prophage remnants litter many genomes [33]
- Since severe complete genomes have been sequenced, gene order conservation between diverse organisms is evolving as a revealing feature of genome [33]. Gene order conservation has been employed for forecasting the function and functional interactions of proteins, as well as for investigating the developmental relationships between genomes [34]. The explanations for gene order maintenance are still not well understood, since the association of the prokaryote genome into operons and adjacent gene transfer cannot perhaps be considered for all the examples of conservation found [45]. In fact, there is very small preservation of gene order between phylogenetically distant genomes. A statistically important preservation of gene order is most likely indicative of the related genes being organized into operons. This characteristic has been employed to explore a number of new operons and to allocate functions to the genes based on the prediction of operon function.
- Genes that are out of use for an organism are often called pseudogenes. In general, inactivated gene copies are characterized by interference to their reading frames due to frameshifts and premature stop codons. Pseudogenes take place in prokaryotic genomes [35].

In eukaryotes, the following features of genomes have been observed:

- The detection of orthologous groups is beneficial for genome annotation, investigations on gene/protein evolution, comparative genomics and the determination of taxonomically restricted sequences. The procedures effectively utilized for prokaryotic genome examination have, however, proved difficult to apply to eukaryotes, since larger genomes can hold multiple paralogous genes and sequence information is often inadequate. A great number of the proteins encoded by the human genome have orthologues in other eukaryotic genomes. For example, 60% of human proteins have sequence resemblances to yeast, fly, nematode or plant proteins.
- Ancient transposon copies are found more in the human genome, whereas the genomes of *Arabidopsis*, *Drosophila* and *Caenorhabditis* have transposons of more recent origin [51, 52]. Bennett *et al* reported on comparisons between *Caenorhabditis* (~100 Mb) and *Drosophila* (~175 Mb) using flow cytometry. This work showed the genome size in *Arabidopsis* to be ~157 Mb and therefore ~25% larger than the *Arabidopsis* Genome Initiative Estimate of ~125 Mb [36].
- Transcription factors control the expression of genes at the transcriptional level. *Arabidopsis* has not more than 20% transcription factors. These factors are zinc-coordinating proteins [53]. In contrast, in the fruit fly, yeast and nematode case, 51%–64% of the transcription factors are of this type.
- *Arabidopsis* transcription factors are represented by several genes and by the assortment of gene families matched with those of *D. melanogaster* or *C. elegans*. Around 50% of the genes recognized so far have unknown function [37].
- SINEs are retrotransposons that have appreciably significant reproductive success throughout the course of mammalian development, and have played an important role in shaping mammalian genomes [55]. Around 75% of the repetitive DNA in human genome is because of LINEs (long interspersed nuclear elements), these are sets of non-LTR retrotransposons [56] which are extensive in the genome of several eukaryotes and in SINE (short interspersed nuclear element) sequences. SINEs are sequences of non-coding DNA existing at high incidences in numerous eukaryotic genomes.
- As the genome size increases, gene density declines. It ranges from one gene per 2 kb in yeast to one gene per 10 kb in *Drosophila*, and one gene in 100 kb in humans.
- The beginning of the genomic era has unlocked the doors to the study of complete genome organization, not only in eukaryotes but also in prokaryotes, especially bacteria. Sufficient information on operon organization in *E. coli*, together with the completed chromosomal sequence of this bacterium, allowed the examination of the distances between genes and of functional interactions of adjacent genes in the same operon, as opposed to nearby genes in diverse transcription units. Bacterial genomes have distinguishing operons (a section of DNA that a repressor binds to); the *E. coli* genome has 600 operons [38].

- Approximately 15% of the ~20 000 *C. elegans* genes are present in operons, multigene clusters governed by a single promoter [39]. The *C. elegans* genome contains operons similar to those of bacteria, and they contain 25% of its genes.
- Eukaryotic genomes have relatively large amounts of repetitive DNA; this is a key reason for the variances in genome size.
- Transposable elements are found in the genomes of nearly all eukaryotes. The human genome has a much higher density of transposable elements (44.4% of the genome) than *A. thaliana* (10.5%), *D. melanogaster* (3.1%) or *C. elegans* (6.5%) [40].
- In plants such as maize and barley, genes are assembled in sections of DNA that can further be divided by long stretches of intergenic DNA. Earlier studies on the nuclear genomes of angiosperms showed that they are distinguished by a compositional compartmentalization and that the vast majority of genes derived from maize, rice, and barley are clustered in long DNA stretches that are separated by vast expanses of gene-empty DNA.
- Several human ailment networks are highly preserved in the fruit fly. Therefore, this insect can function as a model organism for the investigation of even complex human diseases, such as neurological disorders. *D. melanogaster* is a well-studied and highly tractable genetic model organism to explore the molecular mechanisms of human diseases. Various biological, physiological and neurological characteristics are maintained between mammals and *D. melanogaster*, and approximately 75% of human disease-causing genes are assumed to have an efficient homolog in the fly.
- The incidence of sole genes (having no paralogues in the genome) is highest (>70%) in yeast and fruit flies, and the smallest in *Arabidopsis* (35%).
- Variances in intron and exon structure are recognized in eukaryotic genomes; the *Arabidopsis* genome varies considerably. It has been reported that there are three basic patterns of exon–intron variation in eukaryotic genomes, and these patterns were consistently present in almost all 13 genomes analyzed [41]. There is a better degree of 'alternative splicing' in humans than in the other three eukaryotes. This facilitates more proteins to be encoded by each gene.
    1. Various eukaryotic proteins are mosaic proteins, i.e., they are made of a number of different domains. Around 90% of the domains known in human proteins are present in *Drosophila* and *C. elegans* proteins. Therefore, vertebrate development has been central for the creation of the few new domains [61]. Looking at both eukaryotes and prokaryotes, we have learned the following: certain bacterial species have more genes than lower eukaryotes.
    2. Certain genes are present in a wide variety of organisms. For instance, some of yeast genes have homologs among the human genes of unknown function.
    3. Unexpectedly, gene number does not essentially link with the complication of the organism or its evolutionary ladder.

Archaea is one of the three domains of life (alongside bacteria and eukaryotes). To date, 16 complete archaeal genomes have been sequenced, with a conserved core of

313 genes that are present in all sequenced archaeal genomes. The genomes of Archaea have similarities to eukaryotic genomes. For example, certain genes look like those of eukaryotes as they have histone genes and their DNA appears to be prearranged into chromatin [42].

7.6.6 Gene order comparisons (for phylogenetic inference)

Comprehensive information on gene maps or even complete nucleotide sequences for small genomes leads to the possibility of evolutionary interpretation based on the macrostructure of complete genomes. The mathematical modeling of development at the genomic level and the related inferential tools are, however, qualitatively different from the normal sequence comparison theory established to study evolution [43]. Equating gene order in dissimilar organisms is one of the techniques for developing molecular phylogeny. Once the gene instruction in a given region of the genome of two organisms is similar, they are called syntenic and the phenomenon is known as synteny. Gene order comparison in *S. cerevisiae* and *C. albicans* discloses numerous cases of inversions, around half of which are single gene inversions, in these two species separated by 140–330 million years [44]. Comparatively, inversions in prokaryotes tend to include much larger regions of genomes and are focused on the origin and terminus of replication. Additionally, the degree of inversion is much higher in eukaryotes than in prokaryotes. Furthermore, the path of transcription appears to have little effect on gene location. A number of regions of the human genome are highly conserved in dogs, cattle and sheep. One of the main benefits of synteny is that information on gene location from a highly mapped organism can be employed to locate the analogous gene in a poorly mapped relative.

7.6.7 Phylogenetic footprinting (computational method)

Phylogenetic footprinting is a process for the detection of regulatory elements in a set of orthologous regulatory regions from various species [45]. In other words, phylogenetic footprinting is a method employed to detect transcription factor binding sites (TFBS) inside a non-coding region of DNA of interest. This is done by equating it to orthologous sequences in different species. Scientists have discovered that non-coding pieces of DNA hold binding sites for regulatory proteins that direct the (spatiotemporal) expression of genes. A general representation of phylogenetic footprinting is shown in figure 7.8.

These TFBS or regulatory motifs are difficult to detect, mainly because they are very small in length, and can display sequence variation. Two main concepts on which phylogenetic footprinting rely are:

- Transcription factor functions and their DNA binding preferences are well-conserved between diverse species.
- Significant non-coding DNA sequences that are important for directing gene expression will display differential selective pressure. A more gradual rate of change occurs in TFBS than in others.

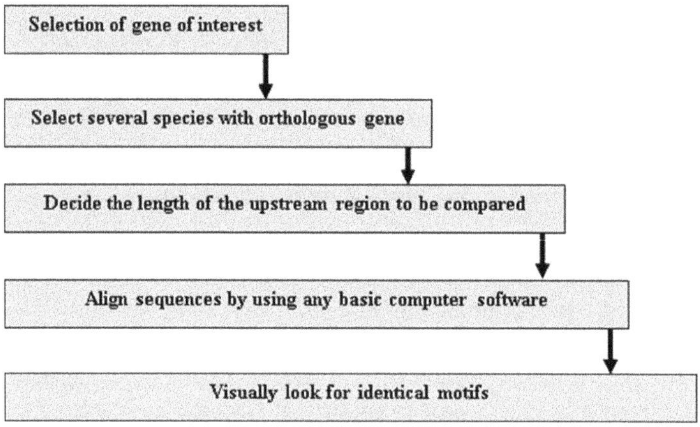

Figure 7.8. Phylogenetic footprinting.

7.6.8 Origins, evolution and phenotypic impact of new genes

The genetic code is shared, and the organization of the codons in the standard codon table is highly non-random [46]. The three main ideas on the origin and evolution of the code are the following:

- *Stereochemical theory*: In this theory codon assignments are dictated by physico-chemical affinity between amino acids and the cognate codons (anticodons);
- *Coevolution theory*: This postulates that the code structure coevolved with amino acid biosynthesis pathways.
- *Error minimization theory*: According to this theory selection to reduce the adverse effect of point mutations and translation errors was the principal factor of the code's evolution.

Thousands of genes present in eukaryotic genomes do not have complements in prokaryotes. Several 'new' genes are mostly regular prokaryotic genes that have been altered beyond recognition, such as domains involved in protein–protein interactions. Several 'new' eukaryotic domains are α-helical; these could have developed from the condensed coiled structures present in prokaryotes, which are now particularly abundant in eukaryotes. Certain other genes have arisen in completely unpredicted ways. For example, the hedgehog gene seems to have developed by gene fusion; during development an intein domain has fused with an extensively modified metalloprotease domain. However, the basis of several other genes remains unknown. A number of new genes might have risen from transposable elements. Among 13 799 human genes studied, 533 (4%) protein-coding regions comprised of transposable elements or sections of such elements were found. Such a transposable element could have incorporated into an exon. Otherwise, it may have initially first incorporated into an intron and then enrolled as an exon. This can become possible once the transposable element has possible splice sites. The incorporation of transposable elements into eukaryotic genomes could be one reason for the high incidence of alternative joining in human protein-coding genes. Therefore, incorporation of transposable elements into genes can produce new genes. For example, in their protein-coding regions, two mouse genes have one or numerous transposable elements, these genes have no human or rat orthologues.

7.6.9 The concept of minimum genome size

The 'minimal genome' method aims to estimate the smallest number of genetic elements adequate to create a modern-type free-living cellular organism. Or, in other words, the minimum genome size can be defined as the least number of genes essential to sustain life, and can at best only be predicted. A simplified scheme of the concept of minimum genome size is shown in figure 7.9.

For the following reasons, mycoplasma is considered a model organism for minimum genome size:

- It is a member of the mollicutes.
- It evolved by massive genome reduction.
- It lacks genomic redundancy.
- It is an obligate parasite.
- It has the smallest identified genome of any free-living organism capable of growing in axenic culture.
- It is wall-less.

Essential genes are considered important for its survival, e.g. genes that are encoding for protein that maintains the central metabolism, replicate DNA, translate genes into proteins, maintain a basic cellular structure, and mediate transport processes into and out of the cell. Some essential genes can tolerate mutations that are deleterious, but not wholly lethal, since they do not completely abolish the gene's function. Some of the essential genes, however, appear to perform non-essential functions, such as aging and cell death, while many of the non-essential genes play critical roles in cell survival. Essential genes can be difficult to study. If an essential

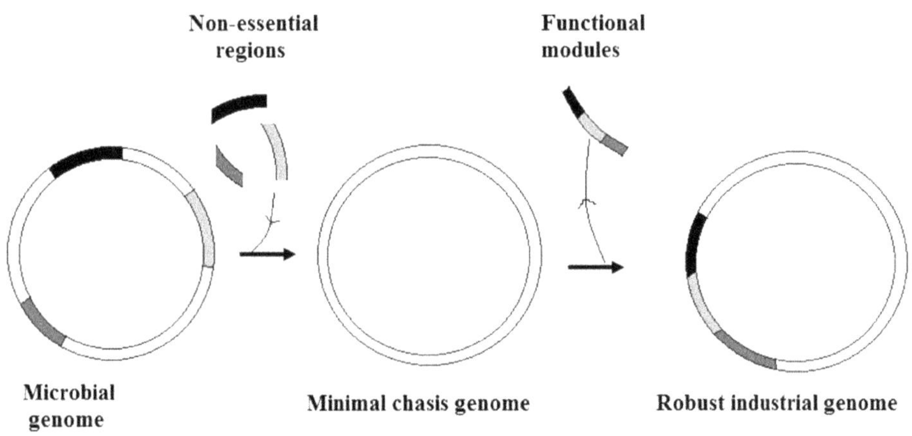

Figure 7.9. Concept of minimum genome size.

gene is disrupted in the macronucleus, it is unlikely that complete replacement of the wild-type copies with the selectable marker will ever be achieved. There are a number of different transposon-based approaches available for defining essential genes. There are two ways to identify essential genes or regions of the bacterial chromosome which can be based on the location of the transposon insertion: the 'negative' and the 'positive' approaches. A problem in trying to identify essential genes is that a knockout of an essential gene is lethal. Therefore, the use of the negative approach will help with the identification of many regions that are not essential and enable one to say with some certainty that regions in which transposon insertions are not observed are likely to be essential.

Whole-genome sequences are now available for a great number of assorted species [47]. Gene content quantification, expansion of the gene family, orthologous gene conservation and gene displacement are promising for the assessment of the minimal set of proteins adequate for cellular life.

The genes found in different organisms with the smallest genomes and their roles are matched carefully. Moreover, investigational findings are collected by deactivating specific genes of these organisms and measuring the outcome on the organism's survival. Based on these investigations, it has been estimated that living creatures need at least 250–350 genes. This minimum gene number is essential for the organisms to exist as autonomous, self-replicating organisms. The unicellular eukaryote minimum genome size was found to be 2.9×10^6 bp (the parasite *Encephalitozoan cuniculi*). *E. cuniculi* infects different mammals, including humans, and can be a source of digestive and nervous clinical syndromes in HIV-infected or cyclosporine-treated people [48]. The genome of *E. cuniculi* has very little repetitive DNA other than that for rDNA, and is expected to contain approximately 2000 genes [49]. Therefore, transformation from prokaryotes to eukaryotes has augmented the gene number by a factor of 7–8, however, the genome size has not grown remarkably. The minimum gene number in multicellular eukaryotes, e.g. *Drosophila*, *Arabidopsis*, etc, appears to be 16 000; this significant increase would be essential for development and growth, and for sufficiently reacting to environmental or other external factors. Despite its toxicity, *Fugu rubripes*, the pufferfish is widely consumed in Japan and considered the most delicious of all fish. Interest in *F. rubripes* is not only restricted to taste and toxicity, however. The smallest genome size for a vertebrate is that for the *F. rubripes*; it has only 4×10^8 bp DNA, but this genome has 35 000 genes, which is similar to that of the human genome [50]. The pufferfish genome has tightly packed genes, lacks repetitive factors and has single short intergenic and intronic sequences. This drop in genome size is attained by decreasing the sequences not involved in genetic functions to the minimum; it is known as genome compaction. Otherwise, genome size may be decreased by gene loss; this has happened in several parasites.

7.6.10 Comparative genomics analysis of mitochondria and chloroplasts

Comparative genomics investigation has offered new understanding of the origin of organelles by endosymbiosis and exposed the vast evolutionary dynamics of organellar genomes. Moreover, they have significantly assisted in elucidating phylogenetic relationships, particularly in algae and primary land plants with inadequate morphological and anatomical diversity [51]. The genomes of mitochondria are often circular but linear molecules also occur. A number of observations on mtDNA are as follows:

- Animal and fungal mitochondrial DNA (mtDNA) is very small (15–20 kb), compared to plant mtDNA (200–2000 kb) which is more complex than that of either animals or fungi.
- The greater genome size of plant mitochondria is mainly due to a greater amount of spacer DNA. For example, Arabidopsis mtDNA is almost 20 times larger than human mtDNA, but has less than twice the number of genes.
- The mtDNA of numerous species can be divided into two basic types: ancestral and derived DNA. Plant and animal mtDNAs are derived genomes. In the case of angiosperms, there has been extensive gene loss, however, the mtDNA has grown in size because of the duplication and capture of DNA from cpDNA and the nuclear genome.
- Mitochondria are thought to be derived from Rickettsia prowazekii, the agent responsible for epidemic, louse-borne typhus in humans [75]. The Rickettsia (alpha-proteobacteria) multiply in eukaryotic cells only. The organization, structure and gene content of this bacterium look exactly like the mtDNA of *Reclinomonas americana* [52].
- Seed plant mitochondrial genomes are exceptionally fluid in size, structure and sequence content, with the accumulation and activity of repetitive sequences underlying much of this variation. mtDNA genes have been transferred into the nucleus, as this transfer has stopped in animals, however, it continues to occur in the case of plants and protists [76]. For example, a gene from mitochondria, cox2, is still under the development of transfer in the case of legumes. In some legumes, cox2 is present in the mitochondria, whereas in other organisms it is present inside the nuclear genome, and in some it is present in both the nuclear and mitochondrial genomes [53].
- The three plant genomes gene types display differences in their evolutionary rates. Nuclear genes develop the fastest, followed by chloroplast genes and finally mitochondrial genes, in spite of the fact that the mitochondrial genome displays extensive reorganization of its structural organization. This gradual rate of evolution has made mitochondrial gene sequences unattractive to plant phylogenetic studies at the suborder and subfamily levels, but has proven to be valuable in inferring ancient phylogenetic relationships and in approximating the time of early diversification events in seed plants. There has been cross-species acquisition of DNA or horizontal gene transfer of genes by plant mitochondrial genomes such as the homing group I intron, introns that encode site-specific endonucleases to further catalyze their effective distribution from introns including alleles to intron-lacking alleles of similar gene in genetic crosses. This intron is present in the cox gene of some angiosperm species [54].

7.7 Gene estimation and counting

Annonation is a procedure which detects genes, and explores their regulatory sequences and promising functions. Annonation designates the non-protein-coding genes (those that do not encode protein sequences), e.g. coding genes for rRNA, tRNA and nuclear RNAs, mobile genetic elements (DNA segments that encode enzymes and other proteins that control the DNA movement inside genomes, called intracellular mobility or, between bacterial cells, intercellular mobility) and repetitive sequence families existing in the genome. The role of annonation begins only after the genome sequence has been attained. Gene estimation is a significant issue for computational science. There are numerous logarithms that can be employed for gene estimation by utilizing identified genes as a training data set which can be further utilized to form a model or to test (or validate) the built model. Gene counting is problematic until the actual locations of genes in a genome are determined. The occurrence of overlapping genes and splice variations makes the job more challenging as it becomes more difficult to forecast which region of DNA should be considered as the same or as many different genes.

Numerous genes in eukaryotes have an arrangement of exons (coding regions) trailed by introns (non-coding regions). Because of this, genes are not systematized as continuous ORFs (open reading frames). An ORF has a series of codons that require an amino acid sequence.

Also, eukaryotic genes are often widely spaced, thus there is a greater probability of finding false genes. However, novel methods of ORF scanning software for eukaryotic genes allow more effective scanning. It has been observed that approximately 99.8% of the 3.2 billion base pairs of two humans are identical and merely 0.2% are different. Of every 500 nucleotides, only one nucleotide varies between two individuals. It means that a difference in a few sites in the DNA sequence can result in severe disorders and dissimilar features in human beings.

7.7.1 Genome similarity, SNPs and comparative genomics

As discussed above, approximately 99.8% of every human genome is identical to any other human genome and 0.2% different, which indicates that two individuals vary only in 6 million locations out of 3.2 billion locations (figures 7.10 and 7.11). Two human beings will be similar if these locations have little influence. As already discussed, the human genome is closely related to that of chimpanzees (more than 98%). Therefore, variance in some locations in DNA results in a unique individual. One nucleotide among every 500–1000 nucleotides always differs between two individuals. The most considerable variations in individual genomes are SNPs, which have been detected in both coding and non-coding regions of genome [55]. SNPs as discussed above are fundamentally varied in a single base, i.e., A, C, G or T resulting in DNA variations which further result in the presence of different bases at such locations. With varying individuals the type of nucleotide or base existing at a given position on a chromosome can also vary. It has been observed that 90% of sequence variation among humans is because of the presence of SNPs. Thus SNPs offer a molecular marker that is present in high density. During DNA finger-printing

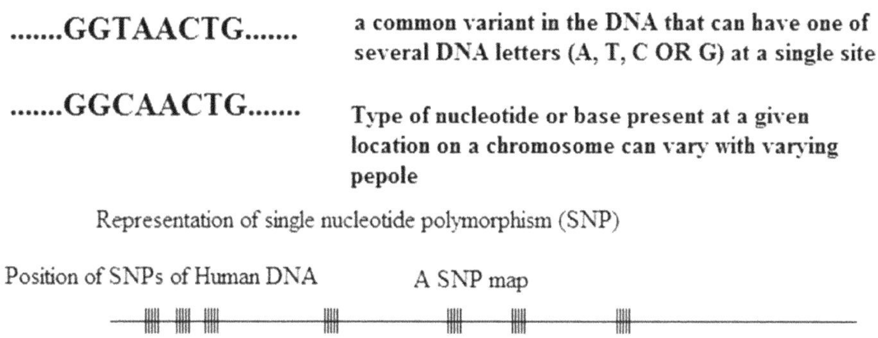

Figure 7.10. An SNP map.

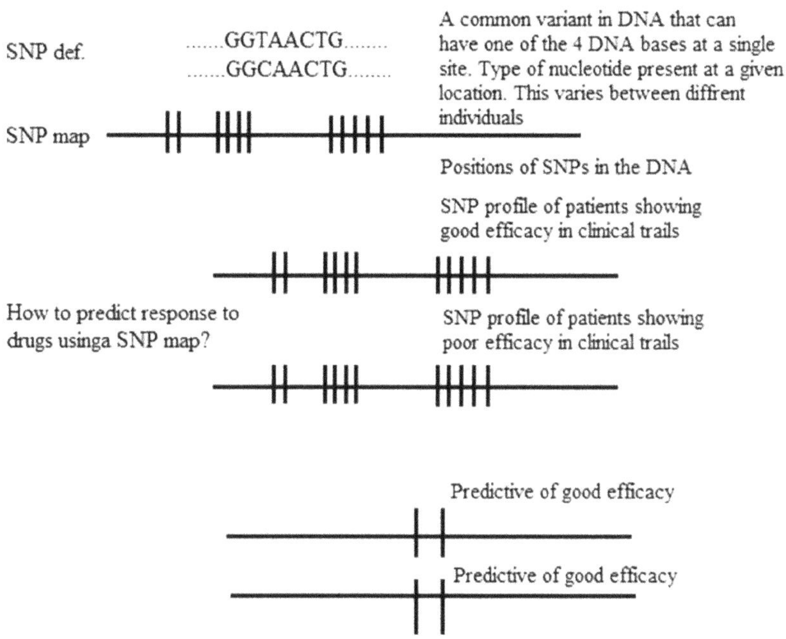

Figure 7.11. An SNP map to determine how patients are likely to respond to a particular drug.

in mainly non-coding parts of the genome, such genetic deviations among diverse human beings are used. These genetic variations are also accountable for the severity of disease and the reaction of the body to treatment.

7.8 Genomes: genome evolution

Genome trees are a way to contain the astounding amount of phylogenetic data that is found in genomes. Diverse formalisms have been presented to construct genome trees on the basis of various features of the genome [56]. On the basis of these characteristics, we divide genome trees into five classes:

- alignment-free trees based on statistical properties of the genome;
- gene content trees based on the presence and absence of genes;
- phylogenomics-based genome trees;
- trees based on average sequence similarity; and
- trees based on chromosomal gene order.

Despite their current advancement, genome tree approaches have already had some influence on the phylogenetic arrangement of bacterial species. However, their main impact so far has been on our understanding of the nature of genome evolution and the role of horizontal gene transfer therein [57]. Relative genome analyses disclose that most functional domains of human genes have homologs in commonly divergent species. These shared functional domains, however, are differentially shuffled among evolutionary lineages to create an increasing number of domain architectures. Combined with duplication and adaptive evolution, domain shuffling is accountable for the great phenotypic complexity of higher eukaryotes [83–85]. Mobile elements within genomes have determined genome evolution by different means. Mainly in plants and mammals, retrotransposons have been shown to establish a large fraction of the genome and have shaped both genes and the entire genome. Although the host can frequently govern their numbers, massive expansions of retrotransposons have been accepted during evolution. Currently, mobile elements are becoming valuable tools for learning more about genome evolution and gene function.

Based on paleological investigation, it was demonstrated that approximately 3.5 billion years ago, cells identical to bacteria existed on our planet. Based on this observation we can only accept that the genomes of these organisms or the organisms that evolved soon afterward contain double-stranded DNA molecules. According to previous findings (dated to about 1.4 billion years ago) the first eukaryotic fossils were similar to single-celled algae, which means that both prokaryotes and eukaryotes experienced variations in size, shape and complexity, thus their genomes also transformed vigorously. These variations were motivated by mutation, transposition, gene transfer and recombination, along with gene deletion and duplication. Through investigating and equating genomes of organisms that exist currently, we can gain understandings into how these mechanisms have shaped genomes.

7.8.1 Microbial genome reduction in bacteria

Once bacterial pathogens make the evolution from free-living life cycles to a permanent relationship with a host, they experience a significant loss of genes and DNA [86]. Complete genome sequences offer information on how significant genome reduction affects the developmental directions and metabolic capabilities of obligate pathogens and symbionts [58]. Reconstruction of the gene content and order of the last common ancestor of human pathogens can be achieved, for example in the case of *Mycobacterium leprae* and *Mycobacterium tuberculosis*. An understanding into which genes are the most indispensable for existence comes from equating the genomes of two related species of *Mycobacterium*: *M. tuberculosis*, which is responsible for tuberculosis and *M. leprae*, which is the causative agent of leprosy. As per reports, *M. tuberculosis* has 3959 protein-coding genes and a 4.41 Mb genome. In contrast, *M. leprae* has 1604 protein-coding genes and a 3.26 Mb genome. Therefore, during development or evolution, *M. leprae* has misplaced or lost approximately 2000 genes (more than 50% of its ancestral gene set). Several reasons can account for this, such as codon elimination or deletion and deterioration, through mutation and incorporation of transposable elements, which have disabled many genes. Consequently, metabolic functions vital for cell development have been abolished, and the bacterium develops very slowly; it multiplies once every 14 days. Moreover, genetic mutations for recombination and DNA repair are incapable of averting additional loss to the *M. leprae* genome. This blend of mutations may have comdemmed *M. leprae* to extinction, as epidemiologists have projected that the organism is at the limit of being able to sustain itself by infecting new individuals [59].

7.8.2 Role of duplications in the origin and evolution of the eukaryotic genome

Assessments of prokaryotic and eukaryotic genomes are providing indications of the lineages of the eukaryotic genome and by what means eukaryotes arose from prokaryotes. Several lines of inquiry, comprising amino acid analysis of proteins, gene sequences and metabolic pathways, determined that the eukaryotic genomes are actually mosaics that have notable contributions from both the Archaea and the Eubacteria. For example, the eukaryotic nuclear genome has few, if any, operons, and its genes encompass introns, both of which are features of the Archaea.

The mitochondrial genome of a eukaryotic looks very much like that of alpha-proteobacteria. To explain these observations, it has been suggested that eukaryotes arose as a result of a symbiotic relationship, or fusion, between an anaerobic archaebacterial host and an alpha proteobacterium (such as *Rickettsia*), which developed into the mitochondrion [90]. The monophyletic character of all eukaryotes suggests that this incident occurred effectively only once in the history of the Earth.

The duplication–divergence concept was suggested many decades ago, i.e., that new genes evolve from pre-existing ones via gene duplication and subsequent divergence of the extra copy to acquire a new function (figure 7.12). Based on this concept Susumu Ohno wrote the book *Evolution by Gene Duplication*. Since then, comparative genomics, genetics and biochemistry have clearly demonstrated that duplication–divergence mechanisms are a key contributor to the evolution of new genes. In contrast, the *de novo* origination model of new gene evolution is more recent and less supported. *De novo* origination of protein-coding genes takes place when genes arise from a nonfunctional DNA sequence that was formerly not a gene. It would seem highly questionable whether functional proteins could arise spontaneously from non-coding DNA, as the DNA must both be transcriptionally active and comprise a translatable open reading frame. Also, translation of any random ORF devoid of genes is anticipated to offer unimportant polypeptides rather than

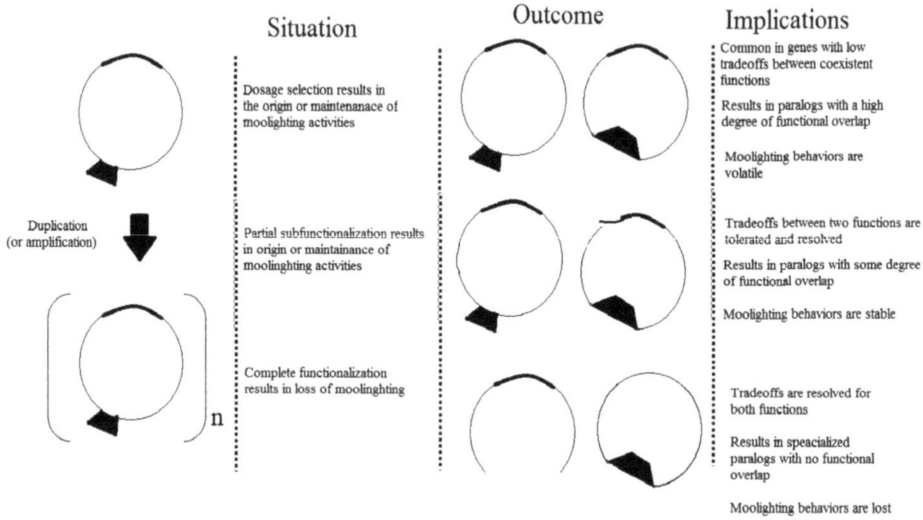

Figure 7.12. Role of duplications in the origin and evolution of the eukaryotic genome.

proteins with specific functions. Certainly it has been claimed that *de novo* origination of new genes is tremendously unlikely, however, irrespective of these reports, the arrival of large-scale sequencing and comparative genomics has delivered increasing proof that new genes have developed and continue to originate from non-coding sequences [60].

Gene duplication plays a significant role in the development of eukaryotic genomes, particularly their size and complexity. Susumo Ohno has predicted that complete genome duplications are a powerful development mechanism [91]. Examination of nucleotide sequence information from genome projects encourages the impression that a considerable portion of the difference in gene number that differentiates prokaryotes from eukaryotes arose from genome expansions. Currently, it is understood that a significant expansion in eukaryote genome size arose from a genome duplication event that accompanied the arrival of vertebrates in the fossil record. Genome duplications have also occurred at other times during eukaryotic development. A current investigation of the yeast genome displays traces of its earliest development by genomic duplication. The yeast genome has been determined to hold at least 55 duplicated regions encompassing 376 genes, which covers 5% of the genome. Of these 55 regions, 50 are in a similar comparative location on diverse chromosomes. For example, chromosomes XI and XIII comprise duplicated blocks of genes in which gene order and positioning relative to the centromere has been well-maintained. Additional chromosomes cover internal duplications, such as the region positioned on either side of the centromere on chromosome XII. Phylogenetic examination designates that this genome duplication incident took place around 100 million years ago. Examination of the human genome also displays proof of an early large-scale duplication, tracked by reorganizations and gene damage in certain duplicated regions. These duplications range

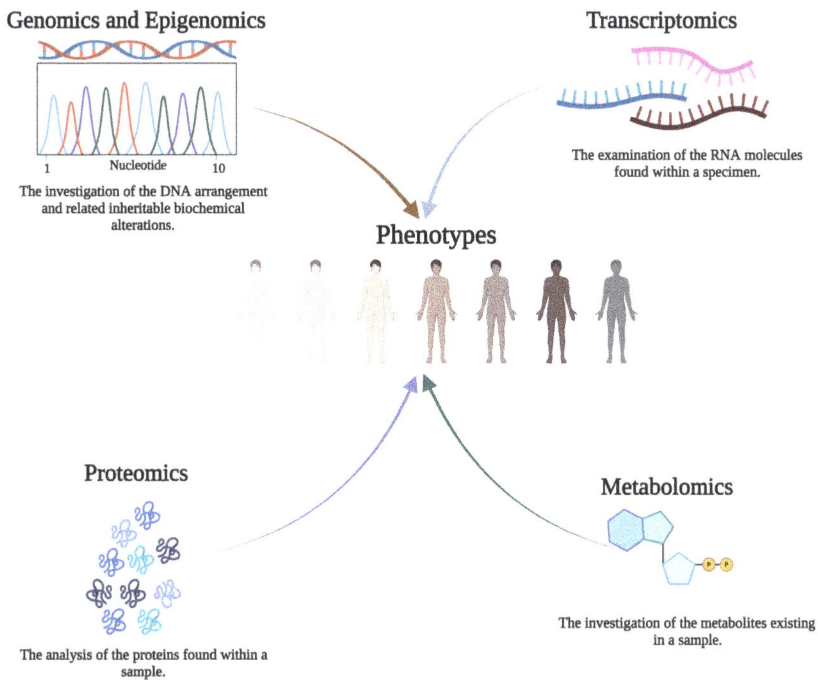

Figure 7.13. Functional genomics investigates the coordination among the genome, transcripts (genes), proteins, and metabolites to generate specific phenotypes.

from minor sections covering only few genes to great stretches that cover nearly a complete chromosome. The larger duplications date to the origin of the vertebrates, around 500 million years ago. Overall, there are 1077 blocks of duplicated regions in the human genome, covering 10 000 genes (around one-third of the genome). Such duplication includes chromosomes 18 and 20. Different potential areas covered under proteomics are presented in figure 7.13.

7.8.3 Gene duplications increase genetic diversity and complexity

Genome duplication is both a historic and continuing process in yeast, plants and animals. It was recently established that the yeast genus *Saccharomyces* experienced an ancient whole-genome duplication, and genome duplication is pervasive in plants. Numerous incidents of genome duplication have occurred during the divergence of angiosperms, including ancient polyploidization processes and the assembly of self-governing duplications in different ancestries. Although not as common as in plants, many genome duplications have also happened in independent lineages in metazoans. During chordate development, whole-genome duplications have occurred coincident with the origin of vertebrates gnathostomes, and teleosts.

Gene and genome duplications offer a basis of genetic material for mutation, drift and selection to act upon, making new evolutionary changes more likely. Thus, several researchers have claimed that genome duplication is a dominant factor in the evolution of complexity and diversity. However, a strong connection between a genome duplication incident and increased complexity and diversity is not conclusive, and there are variations in the patterns of diversity raised to support this claim. Remarkably, many studies of genome duplication processes in vertebrates show they are preceeded by numerous extinct ancestries, resulting in preduplication gaps in extant taxa.

Genomic nucleotide sequence information indicates that multigene families are found in the human genome, if not all genomes. In addition to genome-wide duplications, small chunks of genes and single genes can be duplicated by numerous mechanisms, including:

- unequal crossing over and
- replication errors.

Throughout replication of a template molecule, a slippage can cause the introduction of a short segment into the freshly produced strand. When produced, participants of multigene families may remain associated on a single chromosome or can scatter to other parts of the genome. Numerous mechanisms determine this procedure, such as inversions, translocations and transposition by mobile elements.

The ancestry and relationships among members of gene families have been recently established by several groups of molecular phylogeneticists. Among the most studied examples is the globin gene superfamily. Some 800 million years ago, duplication of a family gene encoding an oxygen transport protein occurred in this family. This has formed two sister genes, one of which developed into the modern day myoglobin gene. Myoglobin is an oxygen-carrying muscular protein, i.e., it is found in muscles. Around 500 million years ago, the ancestral globin gene duplicated to produce the prototypes of the α- and β-globin subfamilies. The α- and β-globin genes encode for the proteins that are present in hemoglobin, the oxygen-carrying molecule in red blood cells. Further duplications within the α- and β-globin genes occurred in the last 200 million years. Subsequent events dispersed members of this superfamily, and each is now on a separate chromosome. Similar patterns of development are reported in other gene families, including the trypsin-chymotrypsin family of proteases, the homeotic selector genes of animals and the rhodopsin family of visual pigments.

7.9 Algae bioinformatics

An alga is considered a unique source of various bioactive compounds and having significant biological activities. Algae bioinformatics, as the name suggests is the application of information technology to decipher more algae with the aid of computational tools and software. This emerging field, just like the other streams of bioinformatics employs computational or dry-lab techniques for applications in various areas such as gene prediction, comparative genomics, genome analysis, and functional genomics and so on. Algae bioinformatics cannot be performed without computer science, biology and genetics with a good-sized dollop of mathematics, statistics and other medical specialties thrown into the mix. There are many tools available for algae bioinformatics research, which are briefly discussed at the very end of this article.

7.9.1 Scope of algae bioinformatics

Algae bioinformatics is a valuable resource for geneticists, phycologists and other scientists who sequence algal genomes as a part of their wet-lab research. Therefore, there is an immense requirement for more reliable, sophisticated, computerized methods for examining this information bringing in the requirement of an algae bioinformaticist.

7.9.2 What is involved in algae bioinformatics

Algae bioinformatics involves the development of novel algorithms and statistics with which relationships among the different algal species can be measured. Examination and elucidation of different types of data and their related information is done. This data study involves DNA, RNA and protein sequences and structures. Development of various techniques allows the efficient access and management of different types of algal samples.

7.9.3 Role of algae bioinformatics

As discussed earlier, algae bioinformatics will only involve dry-lab research and it requires the use of RNA, DNA, protein sequence data. A series of wet-lab work is done so as to obtain the sequencing data and is subjected to bioinformatics analysis.

7.9.4 Steps involved in obtaining the data for analysis using bioinformatics

- Design of primers;
- Extraction of DNA, RNA;
- PCR amplification;
- Denaturizing gradient gel electrophoresis;
- Sequencing.

Nucleic acids are usually derived from the algal samples which are then utilized to synthesize and design primers and then PCR amplification is done. As the products of the PCR reactions are equivalent in their size, a denaturing gradient gel electrophoresis is done to identify variation between the sequences of the products. After this step algal bioinformatics work is performed. This can be achieved by making phylogenetic trees, BLAST searches for similar sequences, and annotation of the new sequences.

7.10 Functional genomics

Functioning genomics is an academic discipline that explores the relationship among a living thing's genetic composition, often termed the genome, and its discernible characteristics, known as an organism's phenotype. Recognizing the genetic processes that determine the operational dynamics and interaction of genes inside an individual is the fundamental goal. The study of gene expression, gene function, and research into the gene structure are all methods included in genomics with function [61]. An overview of functional genomics is presented in figure 7.13.

7.10.1 Introduction to functional genomics

The branch of research known as operational genomics seeks to understand the complex relationship that links the genome and its phenotype on a broad scale that encompasses the whole genome. The strategies used in this work include utilizing high throughput techniques to investigate genes' activation and interacting patterns. This facilitates the examination and comprehension of the actions performed by these genes and the cellular processes that govern their roles inside an organism.

7.10.2 Transcriptomics: studying the RNA molecules

Transcriptomics relates to the science of the field as it examines a transcriptome, which covers the totality of RNA molecules created by the genetic code during a specific time. The procedure involves the examination of the expression of gene designs, the recognition of transcription factors, and the exploration of functional elements inside the genome. The sequencing of RNA is the technique that is often used in the transcriptomics study. It gives us helpful information about how genes are expressed and how the genome is structured [62].

7.10.3 Proteomics: understanding the world of proteins

Proteomics is an extensive examination of peptides on a broad scale, focusing mainly on elucidating their functions and structural traits. The field of research being discussed has significance in understanding changes in metabolism under different conditions and assumes a pivotal role in the early detection of illnesses, forecasting their results, designing medications, and monitoring disease progression. Proteomics methods allow for in-depth analysis and characterization of its proteome at various stages of development and physiology by measuring protein expression, structure, function, interaction between molecules, and changes following translation [63].

7.10.4 Metabolomics: exploring cellular metabolites

Metabolomics is a contemporary field of study within the 'omics' sciences, focusing on the comprehensive analysis of metabolites, including qualitative and quantitative evaluations. These metabolites encompass essential intermediates and final products that arise from metabolic processes. The integration of high-throughput analytical techniques and bioinformatics enables the systematic identification and quantification of several metabolites, hence facilitating the comprehension of metabolic disruptions and the elucidation of underlying mechanisms associated with diverse diseases [64].

7.10.5 Interactomics investigating protein–protein interactions

Interactomics, as a sub-field within the discipline of systems biology, is primarily concerned with investigating protein–protein interactions and their consequential impact on phenotypic traits. Various methodologies are utilized to investigate and analyze the interactome, facilitating the comprehension of protein functionality and regulation. The utilization of interactomics encompasses biochemical and clinical domains, significantly contributing to understanding cellular signaling, disease pathogenesis and advancing therapeutic approaches [65].

7.11 Structural genomics

The primary objective of structural genomics is to get comprehensive insights into the spatial arrangement of all proteins encoded by genetic material. This discipline extends beyond conventional molecular genetics and biochemistry. To offer a more comprehensive comprehension of the genome. The main aims of this study are comprehensive genetic and physical mapping and sequencing of the entire genome. A crucial objective is elucidating the experimental structures of all potential protein folds. Structural genomics holds promise in offering a comprehensive comprehension of several facets of cellular existence, encompassing metabolic activities, DNA replication, transcriptional processes, protein synthesis, and protein folding [66]. The flow of structural genomics is represented in figure 7.14.

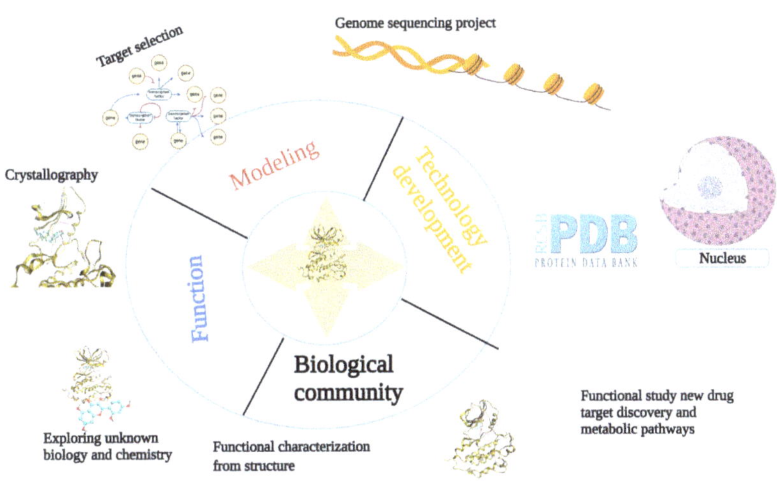

Figure 7.14. Structural genomics, facilitated by the National Institutes of Health (NIH) Protein Structure Initiative (PSI), established a collaborative network of research and resource centers. The primary objective was to comprehensively explore the structural aspects of proteins, particularly in the uncharted territories of the protein sequence space. A key challenge addressed by the PSI was elucidating the intricate connections between protein sequences and their respective structures. The ultimate aim was to enhance accessibility to structural data for the majority of proteins based on their gene sequences.

7.11.1 Introduction to structural genomics

Structural genetics may be seen as an extension of genomics that encompasses the domain that includes structural inquiry, aiming to uncover the features of genome architecture. High-throughput methods are used to determine the structural features of proteins across the whole genome. The insights gained by structural genomics are valuable in many fields, including medication creation and a molecular-level understanding of illnesses, since they allow for modifying genes and DNA segments. One of the main goals is to assign functional annotations to proteins whose activities have not yet been established, mainly by analyzing their structural properties [67]. The aim may be achieved using several methodologies, such as inferring distant homology relationships, identifying ligands, and characterizing electrostatic bands and cavities among a protein's structures. Genomic structural variants (SVs) are also studied in this field; chromosomal rearrangements affect at least 50 bp. Understanding structural variations is of the highest relevance owing to their ability to give valuable insights into mechanisms of evolution and the deep molecular foundations of illnesses such as varied forms of carcinoma and neurodevelopmental conditions [68].

7.11.2 The approaches used in the domain of structural genomics

Deciphering a three-dimensional (3D) structure that composes biological macromolecules, having a significant focus on certain peptide regions, is the goal of structural genomics. New methods have been created to find and analyze these combinations, which helps us learn more about the molecular and functional settings where these giant molecules work. The development of protein structure determination pipelines is mainly attributable to structural genomics, which has led to significant advances in identifying hitherto uncharacterized proteins. Notable advancements in protein production and the rapid identification of new protein structures have resulted from investigating proteins obtained from microbial dark matter and human diseases [68]. Crystallography using x-rays, NMR (nuclear magnetic resonance) spectral analysis, and cryo-electron microscopy (cryo-EM) are just a few examples of the many methods included in structural genomics and are essential to the field's overall goals and objectives. These techniques are often supplemented by other methodologies, including connecting mass spectroscopy, small angle scattering of x-rays (SAXS), and neutron diffraction. This collective approach offers a complete means of investigating biological macromolecules. The challenges encountered within structural genomics are manifold. The large volumes of data generated necessitate effective collection, display, and analysis protocols to maximize the value derived from such substantial investments [69]. Moreover, the quality of structures determined is a concern, particularly when resolution data are artificially limited, which might undermine the benefits of structural genomics endeavors.

7.11.3 Importance of structural genomics in drug design

Structural genomics holds significant promise for drug discovery. The growing repository of high-resolution structures of known and potential drug target proteins is poised to benefit future drug discovery programs substantially. When the target protein of a drug is known, structural genomics facilitates the rapid and efficient acquisition of ligand-bound structures, leveraging high-throughput x-ray crystallography and NMR [70]. In cases where the drug target is unknown, structural genomics provides purified proteins for numerous potential drug targets, thus supporting drug discovery efforts. The impact is already being felt in the early stages of drug discovery and target validation, with the contribution of new structures, complexes with ligands, and supportive protocols and reagents for additional structural work within drug discovery programs. The role of structural genomics in modern structure-based drug design is underscored by its ability to analyze many target proteins concurrently. While several structural genomics initiatives have been launched, a relative few have focused on integral membrane proteins, which represent a critical area for future exploration in drug design and discovery [71].

7.12 Epigenomics and epigenetics

Epigenomics is a sub-field of genomics that explores the comprehensive characterization and analysis of all epigenetic modifications across the genome. Epigenetics is the study of reversible, heritable changes in gene function that occur without altering the DNA sequence itself. DNA methylation is a hallmark epigenetic regulation mechanism [72]. Epigenomics is concerned with understanding the broader epigenetic landscape across the genome, focusing on modifications like DNA methylation, histone modifications, and chromatin remodeling that do not alter the DNA sequence but significantly impact gene expression, cellular function and phenotype. The conventional concept of epigenetics, articulated initially by Conrad Waddington during the 1950s, pertains to the investigation of enduringly inheritable phenotypic traits that arise from modifications to a chromosome without concomitant alterations to the DNA sequence [73]. Epigenetic alterations play a critical role in various biological processes, such as development, differentiation, and the ability to respond to environmental stimuli. The rapid acceleration of epigenetic research in the 21st century has generated excitement and hope, linking genetics to environmental factors and diseases [74]. DNA methylation, a pivotal epigenetic mechanism, involves adding a methyl group to the cytosine base of DNA, predominantly at CpG dinucleotides. DNA methylation patterns are established early in mammalian development and are maintained during somatic cell division, playing crucial roles in gene silencing, x-chromosome inactivation, genomic imprinting, and suppressing transposable element activity. These dynamic patterns can be altered in response to environmental stimuli and during different developmental stages. For instance, the review highlights the dynamic erasure and re-establishment of DNA methylation in embryonic, germline, and somatic cell development, emphasizing its significance in mice and humans. DNA methylation and demethylation processes also occur in the nervous system, associating with other epigenetic mechanisms like histone modifications and non-coding RNAs, showcasing the interplay between different epigenetic modifications [75]. The structure and distribution of CpG islands and the role of methylation in gene expression regulation, embryogenesis, ageing, and cancer development are also critical aspects of DNA methylation patterns. Histone modifications play a pivotal role in the regulation of genome functionality. They consist of post-translational modifications (PTMs) such as acetylation, phosphorylation, methylation, ubiquitination, and ADP ribosylation, which are carried out on the amino acid residues of histone proteins. These modifications can lead to a condensed or relaxed chromatin structure, thereby regulating gene expression. For instance, acetylation generally results in a more relaxed chromatin structure and, thus, enhanced gene expression. Furthermore, histone modifications can also have carcinogenic potential, with abnormal modification sites observed in various tumors. Some of these modifications are studied extensively, while others have been recently discovered, reflecting the complexity and ongoing research in understanding histone PTMs and their mechanistic implications in diseases like cancer [76]. Non-coding RNAs (ncRNAs) are instrumental in epigenetic regulation. They function in chromatin remodeling and regulation at both transcriptional and post-transcriptional levels. They modulate gene expression by interacting with other molecular entities like microRNA pathways, influencing various cellular processes. These ncRNAs play a role in vascular biology and mediate epigenetic modifications related to cardiovascular disease susceptibility [77]. Moreover, ncRNAs are key epigenetic factors that modulate cellular fate and gene expression patterns, thus playing a crucial role in the broader landscape of epigenetic regulation. The workflow of epigenetic regulation of gene expression is shown in figure 7.15.

7.12.1 Epigenetic inheritance and diseases

Epigenetic inheritance involves the transmission of gene expression patterns across generations lacking amendments in the DNA chain. There is a suggestion that

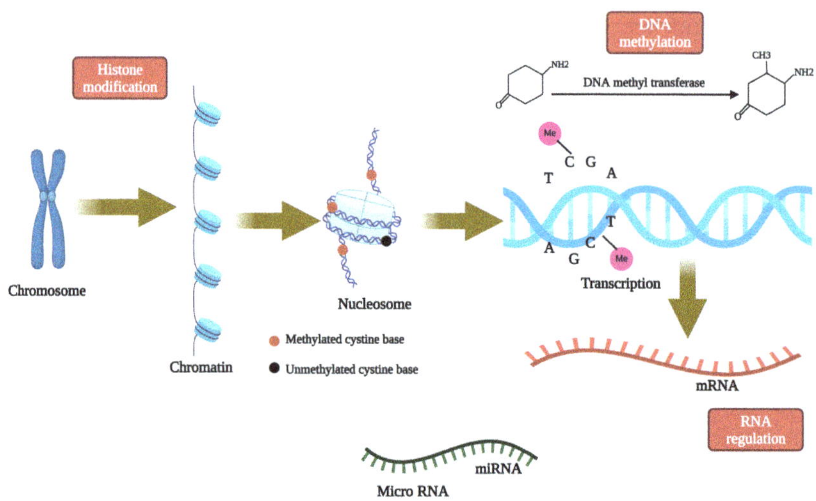

Figure 7.15. Epigenetic regulation of gene expression: interplay of histone modifications and DNA methylation in chromatin remodeling and RNA transcription.

epigenetic modifications triggered by environmental variables may influence the inheritance of illness vulnerability. These epigenetic alterations encompass DNA methylation, chromatin remodeling, histone modifications, and the activity of ncRNAs, all of which can lead to heritable phenotypic changes [78]. The disruption of gene expression patterns governed by epigenetics can result in various diseases, including autoimmune diseases and cancers. Moreover, epigenetics plays a significant role in disease etiology and understanding it better could unveil novel strategies for diagnosis and treatment of diseases. Some diseases are associated with mutations and epimutations in genes subject to genomic imprinting, a form of epigenetic regulation [79].

7.13 Pharmacogenomics

Pharmacogenomics is an interdisciplinary science that blends the principles of pharmacology and genomics to explore how an individual's genetic make-up influences their response to drugs. This field holds the promise of personalized medicine, where therapeutic strategies are tailored to everyone based on their genetic profile. Pharmacogenomics endeavors to understand the genetic underpinnings contributing to individuals' varied responses to drugs, encompassing efficacy and adverse effects [80]. This study examines the relationship between drugs and the genome, specifically investigating the impact of genetic variations, such as SNPs and copy number variations (CNVs), on drug absorption, distribution, metabolism, and excretion (ADME) processes. Additionally, it explores the influence of genetic variations on drug targets, including receptors and enzymes. Pharmacogenomics has advanced a long way from its infancy; the first pharmacogenomic recommendations for dosage had been released before the human genome was sequenced. The progression of pharmacogenomics in contemporary medicine has been characterized by the emergence of increasingly extensive dosage recommendations and genotyping technologies [81]. This evolution underscores the rapid growth and promise of pharmacogenomics in the field. Pharmacogenomics has a substantial influence on the realm of clinical practice. By knowing how genes affect drug response, doctors can choose the right drug in the right amount for each patient. This improves treatment results, lowers the risk of side effects, and improves patient care. Variations in drug metabolism are a clinically significant example because they can change how well or how dangerously a drug works [82].

7.13.1 The importance of personalized medicine

Personalized medicine encompasses a customized methodology that considers the unique interplay of genetic factors, environmental influences, and individual lifestyle choices for every individual. This idea aims to maximize the effectiveness of therapies while minimizing adverse side effects. In personalized medicine, the study of how a person's genes influence their reaction to medications is known as pharmacogenomics. This helps doctors craft individualized treatment plans for their

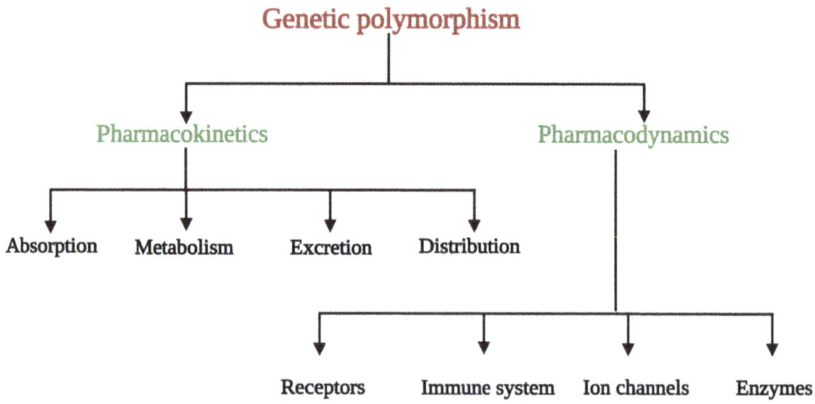

Figure 7.16. Influence of genetic polymorphisms on drug response: a schematic overview of pharmacokinetic and pharmacodynamic variations.

patients, improving care quality, safety, and the likelihood of positive outcomes [83]. The genetic polymorphisms on drug response overflow is shown in figure 7.16.

7.13.2 The impact of genetic variations on drug response

The observed disparities in medication responses among human populations can be attributed to the substantial influence of genetic variants. The discipline of pharmacogenomics aims to establish a correlation between genetic diversity and the variety observed in medication response. The focus of research in this field has transitioned from candidate gene studies to investigations of genetic diversity across entire genomes of human populations, encompassing individuals who display diverse responses to drugs [84]. The significance of genetic variants in drug-metabolizing enzymes is particularly pronounced, underscoring the necessity of incorporating both genotype and medication interaction data to enhance clinical results, particularly in neurology and psychiatry. Moreover, genetic variations can affect drug-related genes. For instance, a focused analysis revealed that the likelihood of a patient carrying germline variants in oncological drug targets is high enough to suggest that somatic alterations and germline variants could influence the response to antineoplastic agents [85].

7.13.3 Additional insights on pharmacogenomics

Pharmacogenomics, an evolving clinical tool for precision medicine, studies how an individual's genomic profile influences drug response. It aids in optimizing drug therapy by helping in drug selection and dosing, thereby reducing the risk of severe adverse effects from certain drugs. The field has rapidly developed, with the first pharmacogenomics dose recommendations published before human genome sequencing. This rapid evolution has brought about more comprehensive dosing guidelines and genotyping technologies, underlining pharmacogenomics's expansion and potential in modern medicine [86].

7.13.4 Pharmacogenomic tests in the market

Pharmacogenomic tests are designed to evaluate a person's genetic make-up to predict how they might metabolize or respond to medications, which is crucial in guiding healthcare providers in choosing the proper medications and dosing for individuals. These tests mainly include pharmacokinetic and pharmacodynamic genomic panels, which analyze how one's body affects a drug and how drugs affect the body, respectively. Pharmacogenomic testing is implemented in specialist academic centers worldwide, adopting a preemptive panel approach where patients are tested for multiple pharmacognosies on admission, and the results are integrated into the patient's electronic health records. Pharmacogenomic testing aims to maximize medication benefits while minimizing unintended adverse drug reactions by detecting genomic factors linked to drug response variability before treatment [87].

7.13.5 Challenges in implementing pharmacogenomics

The challenges in implementing pharmacogenomics are substantial and can be categorized broadly into two aspects. The first revolves around whether the testing should be performed, which relates to the sufficiency of available evidence and cost-effectiveness. The second pertains to integrating pharmacogenomic testing into clinical systems and workflows. One of the significant hurdles lies at the point of delivery into healthcare systems, requiring the modification of current clinical pathways and bridging a significant knowledge gap. The implementation challenges extend to the clinical practice setting, where there is a need for a clear understanding of how pharmacogenomic testing impacts clinical practices. In developing countries, identifying and overcoming challenges related to pharmacogenomics implementation, especially considering the experiences of early adopters and local experts, is crucial. Pharmacogenetic implementation initiatives are continuously explored, focusing on overcoming these challenges to improve drug safety and effectiveness [88].

7.14 Population genomics

Population genomics is a branch of genetics that analyses and compares genomic sequences within and across populations to understand genetic diversity, evolution, and the molecular basis of heritable traits and diseases. Population genomics takes a more comprehensive approach by analyzing the complete genomes of many people from various populations instead of studying individual genes or small sets of genes, as is common in classical genetics. The discipline of population genomics is primarily concerned with examining the effects of genetic diversity on the range of observable traits within populations while also seeking to comprehend the evolutionary processes that have shaped this diversity throughout time [89]. Using the concepts of population genetics on a genomic scale deepens our understanding of evolutionary processes, genetic adaptation, and the underlying genetic architecture of complex features. Evolution, biological conservation, and medicinal research may all benefit from population genomics due to its applicability across a wide range of species. Breakthroughs in technology, such as the development of technology for sequencing of the next generation (NGS), have significantly impacted the progression of population genomics. These technical developments have facilitated the generation of large volumes of genomic data at an economically feasible cost, enabling thorough exploration of genetic diversity on a vast scale. Using long-read sequencing technology has dramatically improved the detection of structural alterations, a common form of genetic diversity within species [90].

7.14.1 Studying genetic variation across populations

Understanding human evolution, migration patterns, and the genetic basis of diseases requires researching the genetic differences that exist across different populations. The examination of genetic diversity and allele frequencies across various populations worldwide is a fundamental application within the area of population genomics. This specialized branch of population genetics utilizes genomic data to achieve its objectives. This work is of great importance in examining evolutionary alterations, as shown by the analysis of population genetics, including 103 genomes of SARS-CoV-2. Even though the repercussions of these evolutionary shifts are still being researched, one study has demonstrated the presence of two fundamental lineages. Improved knowledge of evolution inheritance, molecular ecology, and biodiversity conservation may be achieved via population genomics, which identifies adapted molecular variation [91].

7.14.2 Population genomics techniques

Population genomics has seen significant progress, mainly due to the emergence of NGS technology. These tools have made a big difference in the field by letting scientists learn more about genome structure variation, the primary type of genetic diversity within species. For example, advances in long-read sequencing technology have made it easier to find structural changes, which has improved our ability to characterize the genetic landscape of different populations. Moreover, various analytical methods are employed to handle and interpret the voluminous data generated through genomic studies [92]. Zhang *et al* (2020) mention that multiple approaches must be used and compared in any population genomics project, underscoring the complexity and the multi-dimensional nature of the analyses required in population genomics [93].

7.14.3 Understanding human migration and evolution through population genomics

Population genomics provides a comprehensive lens through which human migration and evolution can be investigated. Established population genetics principles, applied with the advent of human genome sequencing projects, reveal intricate migration histories and population structures, especially in smaller ethnic populations. The dispersion of different human communities globally led to exposure to various infectious agents, hence creating a selection pressure that favored the adaptation to new environments by selecting beneficial genetic variants for the host. Advances in genomic sequencing and statistical analysis are now unveiling the links between past human migrations and present-day genetic differences governing traits like disease resistance, skin pigmentation, and tolerance to different environmental conditions [94]. The examination of genomic data derived from contemporary and historical populations enhances comprehension of genealogical connections, patterns of migration, instances of diversification, and genetic intermingling among diverse groups, augmenting our understanding of humanity's evolutionary history [95].

7.14.4 Conservation genomics in endangered species

The subject of conservation genomics is experiencing significant growth, utilizing genome-scale data to augment the abilities of resource managers in safeguarding species. Genetic methodologies have been extensively employed in the field of conservation research. The advent of genomics has facilitated the collection of extensive genome-wide information, which plays a pivotal role in efforts to preserve biodiversity. The field of advanced genomics encompasses a range of applications that contribute to the conservation of endangered species. These applications include studying demographic patterns, adaptive genetic variants, inbreeding, hybridization, introgression, and illness vulnerabilities in vulnerable biota. The investigation of threatened species' genomes that had previously been limited to the study of model organisms has become possible because of recent developments in genomics [96]. NGS methodologies and the collection of genome-wide data provide more extensive examinations of genetic diversity, population organization, and other crucial variables in species under threat. Furthermore, genetics is essential to finding 'conservation priors,' which are already set goals to help threatened species or groups that need to be saved immediately. This gives conservation plans a stronger foundation. The enhanced understanding of the genome composition and variability in endangered species has significant implications for population assessment, surveillance, administration, and the comprehension of phylogeography. These advancements can significantly contribute to managing wildlife health, identifying genetic disorder risk factors, and developing strategies for the demographic management of small populations in their natural habitats [97].

7.15 Microbiome genomics

The study of microorganisms or colonies of microorganisms found in a variety of habitats, such as the human body, has given rise to the multidisciplinary area of microbiota genomics. This discipline focuses on comprehending the interactions between microbial genomes, their host organisms, and their surrounding environment. This research uses a range of genomic methodologies to investigate the diversity, functionality, and dynamics of microorganisms at a genomic level. The expertise gained from gut microbiome genomics significantly improves our comprehension of how microbes coevolve, the diversity of microbes at the strain level, and the connections between specific genomic changes in the microbiome and common metabolic diseases, especially when it comes to human health [98].

7.15.1 Introduction to the human microbiome

The phrase 'human microbiome' refers to the vast community of microorganisms, such as bacteria, viruses, fungi, and other microbes, living inside and colonizing the human body. Microbial communities are of utmost significance in human health and illness. The bacteria under consideration possess a substantial amount of genetic material, as shown by calculations that propose a range of 2–20 million microbial genes associated with the human body. This amount is much higher than the roughly 20 000 human genes by a ratio of at least 1000-fold higher. The microbiome of humans is sometimes called the 'second genome' because of its substantial influence on our physiology and overall wellbeing [99]. The liver plays a crucial role in several vital processes, such as digestion, synthesis of nutrients, control of immunity, and defence against harmful microorganisms. It has also been shown that changes in the make-up and function of the human microbiome are associated with several metabolic diseases. The metagenome is the aggregate word for the genomes of these many microbial communities. It symbolizes the microbial genomic contribution to the mammalian halobiont, which is generated by the host and its microbial communities [100]. Recent technological advancements, specifically in NGS and metagenomics, have facilitated comprehensive investigation and comprehension of the human microbiome. This has provided an avenue for unraveling the intricate interplay between the host and its microbiome and the potential ramifications of these interactions on human health [101].

7.15.2 Techniques in studying microbial communities

Many different molecular approaches and sequencing methods are used to investigate microbial populations. One noteworthy methodology among these various approaches is NGS, which has demonstrated its efficacy in analyzing microbial populations through sequencing specific DNA targets. For instance, 16S ribosomal RNA gene amplified products can be sequenced to study bacterial populations, while the interior translated gap zones of ribosomal RNA genes can be sequenced to investigate fungal populations. Additionally, metagenomics can be employed using a shotgun approach to study viral populations. Fluorescence *in situ* hybridization FISH-2 is another molecular biological method that might be utilized to study microbes in anaerobic digesters. Additionally, new developments in molecular PCR-based methods have been discussed as a useful way to fully examine microbial communities, focusing on finding out their variety, identification, and abundance [102].

7.15.3 Role of microbiome in human health and disease

The human microbiome is critical in determining health and disease states. It comprises many organisms, such as bacteria, archaea, viruses, and eukaryotes, all playing essential roles in the body's metabolic and immunological processes. The microbiome plays a crucial role in digestion, acts as a protective barrier against harmful pathogens, contributes to the maturation of the immune system, and establishes communication with intestinal cells to uphold the overall wellbeing of the gastrointestinal tract. Disturbances in the microbiome have been linked to various ailments, including cancers and autoimmune and cardiovascular diseases. The composition of the gut microbiota, influenced by diet, stress, and medication, plays a significant role in health and disease [103].

7.15.4 Environmental microbiomes and their importance

Environmental microbiomes, comprising the microbiomes in the surroundings and those of animals in close contact, significantly impact the human microbiome and health outcomes. Microbiome transfer can occur in various settings like households and workplaces, affecting both the human microbiome and health. Environmental microorganisms, such as nitrogen, phosphorous, and carbon, play crucial roles in biochemical cycles, are central to Earth's systems and cycles. They adapt to external changes and are essential to agricultural practices, providing solutions to everyday needs through applied microbiology [104].

7.16 Synthetic biology and genome editing

Synthetic biology and genome editing are intertwined fields that blend engineering principles with biological systems to create novel functionalities or modify existing ones. Synthetic biology focuses on designing new biological parts, devices, or systems, embodying a modular and standardized approach that facilitates the creation of organisms with desired traits for applications in medicine, environmental remediation, and industrial processes. In contrast, genome editing encompasses the meticulous alteration of an organism's DNA via advanced technologies such as CRISPR-Cas9, ZFNs, TALENs, and base editing. This technique has enabled the treatment of genetic illnesses, the generation of genetically enhanced crops, and the engineering of microbes for use in various industrial applications. It has also opened new vistas in the field of medical research as well as agriculture and biotechnology. Despite ethical, technological, and accessibility concerns, both professions show potential in tackling some of society's most intractable problems [105]. As a field of study, synthetic biology combines ideas and methods from engineering and biology to create new living systems or change existing ones. The notion encompasses a wide array of strategies, technologies, and processes, intending to create customized solutions in several sectors like healthcare, industry, and the environment.

These are some key principles of synthetic biology and genome editing:

- **Modularity:** This views biological systems as discrete, interchangeable, and reusable components.
- **Standardization**: The standardization of biological components promotes uniformity and repeatability, allowing more people to share components and design ideas.
- **Abstraction:** It simplifies complex biological systems into understandable and manageable layers or modules.
- **Metabolic engineering:** Customizing microbial metabolic pathways to produce desired substances like biofuels or pharmaceuticals.

- **Gene circuits:** Designing gene circuits to control cellular behaviors predictably.
- **Genetic engineering:** Modifying organisms' genetic make-up to induce desired traits or behaviors.
- **Medicine:** Developing new therapies, diagnostics, and drug delivery systems.

7.16.1 Techniques like CRISPR/Cas9 in genome editing

CRISPR/Cas9, discovered by Doudna and Charpentier in 2012, revolutionized genome editing by providing a more effective, efficient, and accurate method to alter DNA in living cells across various disciplines. This system originates from a prokaryotic immune defence mechanism and has been adapted for genome editing in many organisms. It operates by guiding an endonuclease, Cas9, to a specific DNA sequence, which induces a double-strand break that can be repaired either imprecisely or precisely, enabling gene disruption or specific sequence alterations, respectively [106]. Genome editing, mainly through CRISPR/Cas9, holds immense promise across the biological fields: medical research aids in understanding, treating, or even curing genetic diseases; tailoring crops for better yield, nutritional value, or resistance to pests and diseases; engineering microorganisms for desired outputs like biofuels or chemicals. However, it brings about ethical concerns, particularly in human germline editing, which could have unforeseen consequences and raises issues of consent, equity, and societal acceptance. The irreversible nature of genome editing further emphasizes the need for careful consideration and robust regulatory frameworks [107].

7.17 Systems biology and genomics

Systems biology encompasses various disciplines and aims to explore intricate relationships and the collective dynamics occurring within a cell or an organism. The primary objective of this study is to gain a comprehensive understanding of biological systems, utilizing a wide array of methodologies that span from molecular biology to computational modeling. The goal is to unveil the intricate networks of interactions that drive biological processes and to develop an integrative understanding of how these interactions lead to the emergent properties observed in biological systems. Genomics, on the other hand, is the study of the genome, the complete set of DNA within a cell of an organism. It involves the sequencing and analysis of genome structures and the identification of genes. Genomics provides the raw material and often the initial insights that fuel investigations within systems biology [108]. Genomics and systems biology are often intertwined; genomics provides fundamental insights into the genetic basis of organisms, which systems biology leverages to understand the complexity of biological systems. The utilization of systems biology approaches, such as whole-genome sequencing, enhances the comprehension of gene function, hence facilitating the advancement of techniques for genetic manipulation. The interaction between genomics and systems biology is known as systems genomics or genomic systems biology. This term signifies the convergence of these two fields to leverage genetic data to gain insights into the underlying biological processes at the cellular or organismal levels [109]. Technological developments have significantly influenced the progression of systems biology and genomics. Using methodologies such as genome sequencing, bioinformatics, and high-throughput experimentation has facilitated the acquisition of extensive datasets. The datasets offer a thorough comprehension of intricate biological systems, enhancing the advancement of systems and synthetic biology. Automated DNA sequencing machines with high-throughput capabilities have significantly diminished the temporal and financial burdens associated with bacterial genome sequencing, expediting genomics research and its subsequent utilization in systems biology [110]. The field of systems biology endeavors to create innovative approaches for comprehensively understanding the functionality of biological systems. This statement provides insight into how bacteria adapt, evolve, and interact with other organisms. It also highlights the dynamics of RNAs, proteins, and metabolites, illuminating their intracellular relationships and revealing intricate regulatory networks. Synthetic biology, commonly regarded as a technological complement to systems biology, centers on developing artificial tools to accomplish specific functions. Microbes are particularly well-suited hosts for numerous essential applications in synthetic biology, including bioremediation, biodegradation, bioconversion, and bioproduction. The utilization of knowledge derived from systems biology informs the development of enhanced synthetic biology methods, facilitating the integration of these two disciplines and promoting progress in diverse areas such as energy, materials, and environmental applications [111]. In microbiology, there has been a notable convergence between systems biology and synthetic biology in recent times. As exemplified, engineered microorganisms have been widely employed in producing medicinal proteins, industrial enzymes, tiny molecular medicines, chemicals, biofuels, and materials. The utilization of synthetic biology tools in investigating and manipulating genomics, transcriptomics, proteomics, and metabolomics in microbial systems exemplifies the collaborative relationship between systems biology and synthetic biology. This partnership suggests the significant potential inherent in integrating these disciplines for studying and engineering microbes to carry out complex functions, such as the production of biofuels [112].

7.17.1 Integrative approaches in genomics

The goal of integrative genomics is to understand the intricate relationships that exist within biological systems by combining information from a variety of genetic datasets. It uses computational and statistical tools to analyse, interpret, and visualize genomic data. The molecular processes behind illnesses and other biological phenomena may be better understood with the help of integrated analysis. Methods include integrating information from numerous genomic datasets, such as gene expression, copy number variation, and methylation data, to characterize a biological system better. Multidisciplinary methods to comprehend the chemical processes that underlie diseases and the relevance of computational instruments in evaluating various genomic data [112].

7.17.2 Modeling biological systems and networks

The process of modeling biological systems and networks includes developing computer or mathematical models to gain insights into the intricate connections inside biological systems. These systems span a broad spectrum, ranging from molecular to ecological sizes. Models like this help us learn more about biological systems' structure, dynamics, and behavior by representing graphs. The behavior of biological systems under different situations may be simulated using methods including mathematical modeling, computer simulations, and probabilistic analyses [113].

7.17.3 Challenges and opportunities in systems biology

The field of systems biology faces challenges primarily due to the inherent complexity of biological systems. The burgeoning data from various omics technologies necessitates the development of robust computational tools to manage and interpret this data. Challenges also encompass the need for powerful computers and sophisticated software to handle complex biological data and models. However, with these challenges come opportunities. Through computational modeling and integrative approaches, systems biology can significantly contribute to medicine, pathology, and drug development by offering a systems-level understanding of diseases and drug interactions, enabling the development of personalized medicine strategies [114].

7.18 Genome-wide association studies (GWAS)

GWAS has brought about a revolution in understanding the genetic underpinnings of complex traits and diseases. The method entails a broad-scale examination of genetic variants in different individuals to find associations between genotypes (the genetic make-up) and phenotypes (observable characteristics). The successes of GWAS are numerous, encompassing identifying new disease susceptibility genes, understanding biological pathways, and transitioning these findings into clinical care. However, some criticisms surround GWAS, including concerns that the method might eventually associate the entire genome with disease predisposition and that many association signals might not have direct biological relevance to the diseases under study [115].

7.18.1 Introduction to GWAS

GWAS offers a crucial route for unbiased evaluation of the relationship between common genetic variants and disease risk. Recent advancements in comprehending human genetic variation and the technology to measure such variation have made GWAS a feasible approach. Many GWAS conducted over recent years have identified and replicated many associated variants, enriching the knowledge regarding the genetic basis of diseases. Some advocate for utilizing the results of GWAS for genetic testing, although the underlying mechanisms of many GWA study results remain unclear, and the findings explain only a limited amount of heritability. More detailed investigations are suggested to address these issues and clarify the potential value of genetic testing to public health. These could include analyses of less common variants, sequence-level data, and environmental exposure [116].

7.18.2 Techniques and platforms for GWAS

In GWAS, the techniques and platforms are essential for conducting these studies efficiently. The primary techniques employed in GWAS are based on high-throughput genotyping technologies that can efficiently process and analyze vast amounts of genetic data. These techniques aim to identify associations between genetic variants (primarily SNPs) and traits or diseases. Genotyping platforms capable of producing accurate high-density genotyping data are crucial for the success of GWAS. The popular genotyping methods are based on NGS and array hybridization. These platforms enable the identification and analysis of millions of genetic variants across many individuals to discern statistically significant associations with particular traits or diseases [117].

7.18.3 Challenges in interpreting GWAS results

Interpreting the results of GWAS can be pretty challenging. The primary challenges relate to false positives and negatives, which necessitate replication studies to confirm the associations. Only a limited number of variants are genuine risk alleles, so the importance of replication cannot be overstated. A significant challenge arises because many SNPs identified lie in non-coding genome regions, making it difficult to understand their functional relevance. Translating GWAS results into clinical care is also a significant challenge. The exact disease-causal variants and their functional implications must be understood better to translate the findings into actionable clinical insights [118].

7.18.4 Case studies: notable findings from GWAS

GWAS has led to numerous notable findings over the years. These studies have facilitated discoveries in population and complex-trait genetics and diseases' biology and paved the way towards new therapeutics. Thousands of loci associated with complex traits have been mapped, revealing molecular mechanisms altered in common complex diseases and identifying novel drug targets. GWAS has significantly impacted understanding of genetic variation's effect on the risk of many common cancers. For instance, a meta-analysis of GWAS provided insights into the genetic control of tomato flavor, demonstrating the utility of GWAS in agriculture as well. However, while GWAS has uncovered a wealth of information, it has also left several outstanding questions, particularly relating to the functional interpretation of the identified loci, most of which lie in non-coding regions of the genome [119].

7.19 Future of genomics

The trajectory of genomics is profoundly shaped by the fast progressions in genomic technologies, which have resulted in decreased expenses and time constraints associated with genomic sequencing. The advancement described facilitates the comprehensive examination of genomic data on a significant scale and is anticipated to further influence the discipline of genomics via enhanced accessibility and efficiency in genomic data analysis. In addition, developments in genetics are making personalized medicine, which adapts therapy to each patient's unique traits, a more realistic possibility. This personalized method will significantly alter the healthcare and illness management industries. Furthermore, there is a growing trend towards enhancing our comprehension and use of epigenomic, transcriptomic, and metagenomic data. This advancement will significantly contribute to a more holistic knowledge of biology and diseases [120].

7.19.1 Next-generation sequencing technologies

Over the last decade, there have been notable advancements in NGS technology, resulting in considerable enhancements in sequencing quality, output, cost, and time efficiency. NGS technology incorporates two essential concepts: short-read and long-read sequencing. The excellent accuracy and low cost of short-read sequencing make it a valuable tool for population-level studies and clinical variations detection. On the other hand, long-read sequencing exhibits considerable appropriateness for *de novo* genome assembly purposes and the thorough sequencing of whole isoforms [121]. Recent advancements have facilitated the proliferation of novel and varied technologies, facilitating the creation of hitherto unachievable applications. These include various scientific efforts, such as combining long-read and short-read sequencing methods, DNA sequencing in routine clinical settings, the continuous tracking of pathogen DNA, and large-scale initiatives to analyse whole populations [122]. NGS methods are widely used in investigating histone modifications. One prominent high-throughput technology in this field is chromatin immunoprecipitation-deep sequencing (ChIP-Seq), which combines chromatin immunoprecipitation with deep sequencing technology. The influence of NGS technologies is observable in genetics. These technologies have enabled the collection of large amounts of data, facilitating the development of a thorough understanding of the normal variations present in the human genome. This knowledge serves as a reference point against which the variations seen in individuals affected by genetic diseases may be assessed [123].

7.19.2 Ethical considerations in genomics research

The ongoing success of genomic research hinges on public trust. For this trust to be justified, robust stewarding and widespread engagement about the ethical issues inherent in such practices are crucial. Ethical considerations encompass the duty of researchers to disclose genomic research results to participants. Such disclosures can potentially cause anxiety or depression, significantly when results predict a risk of developing cancer or chronic diseases in the future. The capability to generate genomic data has surpassed our understanding of what these data signify. This gap presents challenges in best engaging with genomic data, especially in research contexts intertwined with clinical care. Issues of informed consent, results return, data sharing, privacy, and genetic determinism are among the ethical concerns in genomic research. These considerations are crucial for maintaining ethical standards across different areas of genomic research, including oncology.

7.19.3 The role of AI and machine learning in genomics

Significant advances in applying machine learning (ML) to genomics have been seen in variant calling, essential for understanding genetic variations and their implications in diseases [123]. AI and ML are instrumental in risk prediction and identifying causal SNPs, contributing to a deeper understanding of genetic predispositions and disease etiology. Responsible application of ML is crucial to navigate the challenges and realize the potential benefits in genomics and systems biology.

7.19.4 Personalized medicine and its potential impact

Personalized medicine offers tailored therapy based on individual genetic background and disease status, ensuring better patient care with optimal treatments, earlier diagnoses, and risk assessments [124]. It has the potential to significantly transform healthcare by providing practical, tailored therapeutic strategies based on an individual's genomic, epigenomic, and proteomic profile. This personalization promises to improve healthcare outcomes while potentially reducing costs [125]. The broader aim of personalized medicine is to move away from a 'one-size-fits-all' approach to a more individualized healthcare paradigm. This shift is driven by technological advancements in sequencing, bioinformatics, and a better understanding of omics (e.g., genomics, proteomics).

References

[1] Kuska B 1998 *Beer, Bethesda, and Biology: How 'Genomics' Came into Being* (Oxford: Oxford University Press)

[2] Lederberg J and McCray A T 2001 Ome SweetOmics—a genealogical treasury of words *Scientist* **15** 8

[3] Watson J D and Cook-Deegan R M 1991 Origins of the human genome project *FASEB J.* **5** 8–11

[4] Smith H O *et al* 1995 Frequency and distribution of DNA uptake signal sequences in the *Haemophilus influenzae* Rd genome *Science* **269** 538–40

[5] Blattner F R *et al* 1997 The complete genome sequence of *Escherichia coli* K-12 *Science* **277** 1453–62

[6] Heather J M and Chain B 2016 The sequence of sequencers: the history of sequencing DNA *Genomics* **107** 1–8

[7] Sterky F and Lundeberg J 2000 Sequence analysis of genes and genomes *J. Biotechnol.* **76** 1–31

[8] Weber J L and Myers E W 1997 Human whole-genome shotgun sequencing *Genome Res.* **7** 401–9

[9] Venter J C *et al* 1998 *Shotgun Sequencing of the Human Genome* (American Association for the Advancement of Science) pp 1540–2

[10] Lewin H A *et al* 2009 Every genome sequence needs a good map *Genome Res.* **19** 1925–8

[11] Lai K *et al* 2018 Artificial intelligence and machine learning in bioinformatics *Encyclopedia of Bioinformatics and Computational Biology: ABC of Bioinformatics* (Elsevier) vol 1 p 3

[12] Schicht S *et al* 2014 Whole transcriptome analysis of the poultry red mite *Dermanyssus gallinae* (De Geer, 1778) *Parasitology* **141** 336–46

[13] Moszer I *et al* 2002 SubtiList: the reference database for the *Bacillus subtilis* genome *Nucleic Acids Res.* **30** 62–5

[14] Dong Q, Schlueter S D and Brendel V 2004 PlantGDB, plant genome database and analysis tools *Nucleic. Acids Res.* **32** D354–9

[15] von Jan M *et al* 2010 Complete genome sequence of *Archaeoglobus profundus* type strain (AV18T) *Stand. Genomic Sci.* **2** 327–46

[16] Weigel D and Mott R 2009 The 1001 genomes project for *Arabidopsis thaliana Genome Biol.* **10** 1–5

[17] Goodman H M, Ecker J R and Dean C 1995 The genome of *Arabidopsis thaliana Proc. Natl Acad. Sci.* **92** 10831–5

[18] Pruitt R E and Meyerowitz E M 1986 Characterization of the genome of *Arabidopsis thaliana J. Mol. Biol.* **187** 169–83

[19] Sato S *et al* 1999 Complete structure of the chloroplast genome of *Arabidopsis thaliana DNA Res.* **6** 283–90

[20] Khromykh A and Solomon B D 2015 The benefits of whole-genome sequencing now and in the future *Mol. Syndromol.* **6** 108–9

[21] Collins F S *et al* 2003 A vision for the future of genomics research *Nature* **422** 835–47

[22] França G S, Cancherini D V and de Souza S J 2012 Evolutionary history of exon shuffling *Genetica* **140** 249–57

[23] Ravenhall M *et al* 2015 Inferring horizontal gene transfer *PLoS Comput. Biol.* **11** e1004095

[24] Hiramatsu K *et al* 2001 The emergence and evolution of methicillin-resistant *Staphylococcus aureus Trends Microbiol.* **9** 486–93

[25] Altschul S F *et al* 1997 Gapped BLAST and PSI-BLAST: a new generation of protein database search programs *Nucleic Acids Res.* **25** 3389–402

[26] Altschul S F and *BLAST* G 1997 and PSI-BLAST: a new generation of protein detabase search programs *Nucleic Acids Res.* **25** 3389

[27] Stein L *et al* 2001 WormBase: network access to the genome and biology of *Caenorhabditis elegans Nucleic. Acids Res.* **29** 82–6

[28] Snow J 1856 On the mode of communication of cholera *Edinb. Med. J.* **1** 668

[29] Snow J 1849 *On the Mode of Communication of Cholera* (John Churchill)

[30] Bekris L M *et al* 2008 Multiple SNPs within and surrounding the apolipoprotein E gene influence cerebrospinal fluid apolipoprotein E protein levels *J. Alzheimer's Dis.* **13** 255–66

[31] Mahley R W, Weisgraber K H and Huang Y 2006 Apolipoprotein E4: a causative factor and therapeutic target in neuropathology, including Alzheimer's disease *Proc. Natl Acad. Sci.* **103** 5644–51

[32] Huang Y *et al* 2004 Apolipoprotein E: diversity of cellular origins, structural and biophysical properties, and effects in Alzheimer's disease *J. Mol. Neurosci.* **23** 189–204

[33] Eppinger M *et al* 2011 Genome sequences of the biotechnologically important *Bacillus megaterium* strains QM B1551 and DSM319 *J. Bacteriol.* **193** 4199–213

[34] Pearson W R and Lipman D J 1988 Improved tools for biological sequence comparison *Proc. Natl Acad. Sci.* **85** 2444–8

[35] Kolisnychenko V *et al* 2002 Engineering a reduced *Escherichia coli* genome *Genome Res.* **12** 640–7

[36] Saikolappan S *et al* 2009 The *Mycoplasma genitalium* MG_454 gene product resists killing by organic hydroperoxides *J. Bacteriol.* **191** 6675–82

[37] Canchaya C *et al* 2003 Prophage genomics *Microbiol. Mol. Biol. Rev.* **67** 238–76

[38] Tamames J 2001 Evolution of gene order conservation in prokaryotes *Genome Biol.* **2** 1–11

[39] Liu Y *et al* 2004 Comprehensive analysis of pseudogenes in prokaryotes: widespread gene decay and failure of putative horizontally transferred genes *Genome Biol.* **5** 1–11

[40] Vanin E F 1985 Processed pseudogenes: characteristics and evolution *Annu. Rev. Genet.* **19** 253–72

[41] Vanin E F 1984 Processed pseudogenes: characteristics and evolution *Biochim. Biophys. Acta Gene Struct. Expression* **782** 231–41

[42] Mighell A *et al* 2000 Vertebrate pseudogenes *FEBS Lett.* **468** 109–14

[43] Goudet G *et al* 2008 Phylogenetic analysis and identification of pseudogenes reveal a progressive loss of *Zona pellucida* genes during evolution of vertebrates *Biol. Reprod.* **78** 796–806

[44] Makeyev A V *et al* 2005 HnRNP A3 genes and pseudogenes in the vertebrate genomes *J. Exp. Zool. A: Comp. Exp. Biol.* **303** 259–71

[45] Bulmer M 1986 Neighboring base effects on substitution rates in pseudogenes *Mol. Biol. Evol.* **3** 322–9

[46] D'Errico I, Gadaleta G and Saccone C 2004 Pseudogenes in metazoa: origin and features *Brief. Funct. Genomics* **3** 157–67

[47] Sisu C *et al* 2014 Comparative analysis of pseudogenes across three phyla *Proc. Natl Acad. Sci.* **111** 13361–6

[48] Logan I S 2017 Pseudogenization of the Humanin gene is common in the mitochondrial DNA of many vertebrates *Zool. Res.* **38** 198

[49] Li L, Stoeckert C J and Roos D S 2003 OrthoMCL: identification of ortholog groups for eukaryotic genomes *Genome Res.* **13** 2178–89

[50] Chen F *et al* 2007 Assessing performance of orthology detection strategies applied to eukaryotic genomes *PLoS One* **2** e383

[51] Blair J E, Shah P and Hedges S B 2005 Evolutionary sequence analysis of complete eukaryote genomes *BMC Bioinf.* **6** 1–10

[52] O'brien K P, Remm M and Sonnhammer E L 2005 Inparanoid: a comprehensive database of eukaryotic orthologs *Nucleic Acids Res.* **33** D476–80

[53] Kuzniar A *et al* 2008 The quest for orthologs: finding the corresponding gene across genomes *Trends in Genet.* **24** 539–51

[54] Tatusov R L *et al* 2003 The COG database: an updated version includes eukaryotes *BMC Bioinf.* **4** 1–14

[55] Haubold B and Wiehe T 2004 Comparative genomics: methods and applications *Naturwissenschaften* **91** 405–21

[56] Hane J K *et al* 2014 Genome sequencing and comparative genomics of the broad host-range pathogen *Rhizoctonia solani* AG8 *PLoS Genet.* **10** e1004281

[57] Miller W *et al* 2004 Comparative genomics *Annu. Rev. Genomics Hum. Genet.* **5** 15–56

[58] Cordoni G *et al* 2016 Comparative genomics of European avian pathogenic *E. coli* (APEC) *BMC Genomics* **17** 1–21

[59] Condon B J *et al* 2014 Comparative genomics of Cochliobolus phytopathogens *Genomics of Plant-associated Fungi: Monocot Pathogens* (Springer) pp 41–67
[60] Walkowiak S *et al* 2016 Whole genome sequencing and comparative genomics of closely related *Fusarium* head blight fungi: *Fusarium graminearum*, *F. meridionale* and *F. asiaticum* *BMC Genomics* **17** 1–15
[61] Hieter P and Boguski M 1997 Functional genomics: it's all how you read it *Science* **278** 601–2
[62] Schuler M A and Werck-Reichhart D 2003 Functional genomics of P450s *Annu. Rev. Plant Biol.* **54** 629–67
[63] Bouchez D and Höfte H 1998 Functional genomics in plants *Plant Physiol.* **118** 725–32
[64] Morozova O and Marra M A 2008 Applications of next-generation sequencing technologies in functional genomics *Genomics* **92** 255–64
[65] McCarthy F M *et al* 2006 AgBase: a functional genomics resource for agriculture *BMC Genomics* **7** 1–13
[66] Baxter I 2010 Ionomics: the functional genomics of elements *Brief. Funct. Genomics* **9** 149–56
[67] Mat-Sharani S *et al* 2019 Structural genomics *Encyclopedia of Bioinformatics and Computational Biology* (Elsevier)
[68] Teichmann S A, Chothia C and Gerstein M 1999 Advances in structural genomics *Curr. Opin. Struct. Biol.* **9** 390–9
[69] Bhattacharya A, Tejero R and Montelione G T 2007 Evaluating protein structures determined by structural genomics consortia *Proteins Struct. Funct. Bioinf.* **66** 778–95
[70] Lundstrom K 2006 Structural genomics: the ultimate approach for rational drug design *Mol. Biotechnol.* **34** 205–12
[71] Weigelt J *et al* 2008 Structural genomics and drug discovery: all in the family *Curr. Opin. Chem. Biol.* **12** 32–9
[72] Weigelt J 2010 Structural genomics—impact on biomedicine and drug discovery *Exp. Cell. Res.* **316** 1332–8
[73] Anderson W 2009 Structural genomics and drug discovery for infectious diseases *Infect. Disord. Drug Targets (Formerly Curr. Drug Targets Infect. Disorder.)* **9** 507–17
[74] Marsden B D and Knapp S 2008 Doing more than just the structure—structural genomics in kinase drug discovery *Curr. Opin. Chem. Biol.* **12** 40–5
[75] Ioerger T R and Sacchettini J C 2009 Structural genomics approach to drug discovery for *Mycobacterium tuberculosis* *Curr. Opin. Microbiol.* **12** 318–25
[76] Arcus V L *et al* 2006 The potential impact of structural genomics on tuberculosis drug discovery *Drug Discov. Today* **11** 28–34
[77] Musa T L, Ioerger T R and Sacchettini J C 2009 The tuberculosis structural genomics consortium: a structural genomics approachto drug discovery *Adv. Protein Chem. Struct. Biol.* **77** 41–76
[78] Bohacek J and Mansuy I M 2013 Epigenetic inheritance of disease and disease risk *Neuropsychopharmacology* **38** 220–36
[79] Whitelaw N C and Whitelaw E 2008 Transgenerational epigenetic inheritance in health and disease *Curr. Opin. Genet. Dev.* **18** 273–9
[80] Roden D M *et al* 2006 Pharmacogenomics: challenges and opportunities *Ann. Intern. Med.* **145** 749–57

[81] Whirl-Carrillo M *et al* 2012 Pharmacogenomics knowledge for personalized medicine *Clin. Pharmacol. Ther.* **92** 414–7
[82] Relling M V and Evans W E 2015 Pharmacogenomics in the clinic *Nature* **526** 343–50
[83] Issa A M 2007 Personalized medicine and the practice of medicine in the 21st century *McGill J. Med. MJM* **10** 53
[84] Dedov I *et al* 2012 Personalized medicine: state-of-the-art and prospects *Ann. Russian Acad. Med. Sci.* **67** 4–12
[85] Abrahams E and Silver M 2009 The case for personalized medicine *J. Diabetes Sci. Technol.* **3** 680–4
[86] Hamburg M A and Collins F S 2010 The path to personalized medicine *New Engl. J. Med.* **363** 301–4
[87] Ziegler A *et al* 2012 Personalized medicine using DNA biomarkers: a review *Hum. Genet.* **131** 1627–38
[88] Ginsburg G S and Willard H F 2009 Genomic and personalized medicine: foundations and applications *Transl. Res.* **154** 277–87
[89] Pokorska-Bocci A *et al* 2014 'Personalized medicine': what's in a name? *Pers. Med.* **11** 197–210
[90] Whitcomb D C 2012 What is personalized medicine and what should it replace? *Nat. Rev. Gastroenterol. Hepatol.* **9** 418–24
[91] Kashyap P C *et al* 2017 Microbiome at the frontier of personalized medicine *Mayo Clinic Proceedings* (Amsterdam: Elsevier)
[92] Hohenlohe P A, Funk W C and Rajora O P 2021 Population genomics for wildlife conservation and management *Mol. Ecol.* **30** 62–82
[93] Zhang Z *et al* 2020 Improved genome assembly provides new insights into genome evolution in a desert poplar *(Populus euphratica) Mol. Ecol. Resourc.* **20** 781–94
[94] Bourgeois Y X and Warren B H 2021 An overview of current population genomics methods for the analysis of whole-genome resequencing data in eukaryotes *Mol. Ecol.* **30** 6036–71
[95] Hancock-Hanser B L *et al* 2013 Targeted multiplex next-generation sequencing: advances in techniques of mitochondrial and nuclear DNA sequencing for population genomics *Mol. Ecol. Resour.* **13** 254–68
[96] Walters A D and Schwartz M K 2021 Population genomics for the management of wild vertebrate populations (Population Genomics: Wildlife) pp 419–36
[97] Sheppard S K, Guttman D S and Fitzgerald J R 2018 Population genomics of bacterial host adaptation *Nat. Rev. Genet.* **19** 549–65
[98] Johnson J S *et al* 2019 Advancing biogeography through population genomics *Population Genomics: Concepts, Approaches and Applications* (Springer) pp 539–85
[99] Young V B 2017 The role of the microbiome in human health and disease: an introduction for clinicians *Brit. Med. J.* **356** j831
[100] Ursell L K *et al* 2012 Defining the human microbiome *Nutr. Rev.* **70** S38–44
[101] Morgan X C and Huttenhower C 2012 Chapter 12: human microbiome analysis *PLoS Comput. Biol.* **8** e1002808
[102] Meisel J S and Grice E A 2017 The human microbiome *Genomic and Precision Medicine* (Amsterdam: Elsevier) pp 63–77
[103] Jovel J *et al* 2018 The human gut microbiome in health and disease *Metagenomics* (Elsevier) pp 197–213
[104] Blum H E 2017 The human microbiome *Adv. Med. Sci.* **62** 414–20

[105] Cox M J, Cookson W O and Moffatt M F 2013 Sequencing the human microbiome in health and disease *Hum. Mol. Genet.* **22** R88–94

[106] Rogers G 2015 The human microbiome: opportunities and challenges for clinical care *Int. Med. J.* **45** 889–98

[107] Memi F, Ntokou A and Papangeli I 2018 CRISPR/Cas9 gene-editing: research technologies, clinical applications and ethical considerations *Seminars in Perinatology* (Amsterdam: Elsevier)

[108] Gostimskaya I 2022 CRISPR–Cas9: a history of its discovery and ethical considerations of its use in genome editing *Biochemistry (Moscow)* **87** 777–88

[109] Plaza Reyes A and Lanner F 2017 Towards a CRISPR view of early human development: applications, limitations and ethical concerns of genome editing in human embryos *Development* **144** 3–7

[110] Baumann M 2016 CRISPR/Cas9 genome editing—new and old ethical issues arising from a revolutionary technology *NanoEthics* **10** 139–59

[111] Rossant J 2018 Gene editing in human development: ethical concerns and practical applications *Development* **145** 150888

[112] Emrani J *et al* 2020 Introducing chemistry students to emerging technologies in gene editing, their applications, and ethical considerations *J. Chem. Educ.* **97** 1931–43

[113] Coller B S 2019 Ethics of human genome editing *Annu. Rev. Med.* **70** 289–305

[114] Greenfield A 2021 Making sense of heritable human genome editing: scientific and ethical considerations *Prog. Mol. Biol. Transl. Sci.* **182** 1–28

[115] National Academies of Sciences, E. and Medicine 2017 *Human Genome Editing: Science, Ethics, and Governance* (National Academies Press)

[116] Yunta E R and Vaschetto L M 2022 Political, regulatory and ethical considerations of the CRISPR/Cas genome editing technology *CRISPR-/Cas9 Based Genome Editing for Treating Genetic Disorders and Diseases* (CRC Press) pp 71–84

[117] Schweikart S J 2019 Global regulation of germline genome editing: ethical considerations and application of international human rights law *Loy. LA Int'l Comp. L. Rev.* **43** 279

[118] Ayanoğlu F B, Elçin A E and Elçin Y M 2020 Bioethical issues in genome editing by CRISPR-Cas9 technology *Turk. J. Biol.* **44** 110–20

[119] Qiu R 2016 Debating ethical issues in genome editing technology *Asian Bioeth. Rev.* **8** 307–26

[120] Mathur R 2018 Ethical considerations in human genome editing—an Indian perspective *Asian Biotechnol. Dev. Rev.* **20** 47

[121] Ormandy E H, Dale J and Griffin G 2011 Genetic engineering of animals: ethical issues, including welfare concerns *Can. Vet. J.* **52** 544

[122] Turocy J, Adashi E Y and Egli D 2021 Heritable human genome editing: research progress, ethical considerations, and hurdles to clinical practice *Cell* **184** 1561–74

[123] De Lecuona I *et al* 2017 Focus: genome editing: gene editing in humans: towards a global and inclusive debate for responsible research *Yale J. Biol. Med.* **90** 673

[124] Segers S 2023 Heritable genome editing: ethical aspects of a developing domain *Hum. Reprod.* **38** 2055–61

[125] Mittal R D 2019 Gene editing in clinical practice: where are we? *Indian J. Clin. Biochem.* **34** 19–25

IOP Publishing

Introduction to Pharmaceutical Biotechnology, Volume 2
(Second Edition)
Enzymes, proteins and bioinformatics
Ahmed Al-Harrasi, Saurabh Bhatia and Ajmal Khan

Chapter 8

Basics of proteomics

8.1 Introduction

In 1995, the word 'proteomics' was coined and was defined as the characterization of the large-scale complete protein complement of a cell line, tissue or organism [1]. The main objective of proteomics is not only to recognize all the proteins in a cell but also to make a three-dimensional map of the cell representing where proteins are located. The first protein studies that can be considered proteomics began in 1975, when O'Farrell [2], Klose [5] and Scheele began mapping proteins from *Escherichia coli*, mice and guinea pigs, respectively, using two-dimensional gel electrophoresis (2DE). Although several proteins could be separated and visualized, they could not be identified. Despite these restrictions, soon thereafter a large-scale investigation of all human proteins was planned. The aim of this scheme, called the Human Protein Index, was to use 2DE and other approaches to sequence all human proteins [3]. However, a lack of funding and technical limitations prevented this project from continuing.

The proteome is defined as the whole set of proteins expressed in a cell's entire lifetime. In brief, it can also be described as the set of proteins expressed in a cell at a particular time. Proteomics is the investigation of the proteome; it uses tools varying from genetic analysis to mass spectrometry. Among all the genomes sequenced to date, several recently discovered genes have no known role, and others have only apparent functions determined by similarity to known genes. For instance, in two intensively studied organisms (*E. coli* and *Saccharomyces cerevisiae*), more than half of the genes encoded by their genomes have no known function. Such genes are frequently known as orphans or ORFans as they do not fit into any known gene family. The promising fields and basic procedures involved in proteomics are presented in figures 8.1–8.3.

doi:10.1088/978-0-7503-5387-8ch8

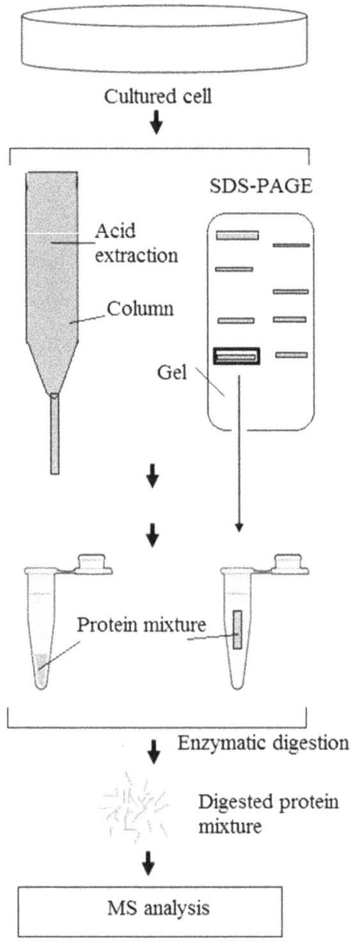

Figure 8.1. Basic protocol for proteomics.

8.2 Types of proteomics

8.2.1 Structural proteomics

In the postgenomic era, structural proteomics is one of the promising areas of investigation, and explains the structure–function relationships of uncharacterized gene products based on the three-dimensional protein structure (figure 8.4) [4]. It suggests the biochemical and cellular roles of unannotated proteins and thus classifies possible drug design and protein engineering targets [8]. Recently, several innovative groups in structural proteomics research have attained proof of structural proteomic theory by forecasting the three-dimensional structures of theoretical proteins that correctly recognized the biological functions of those proteins.

Structural proteomics can show the three-dimensional structure and nature of protein complexes present in a specific cell/organelle [5]. The final goal of structural proteomics is to form an organization of structural data that will assist in predicting

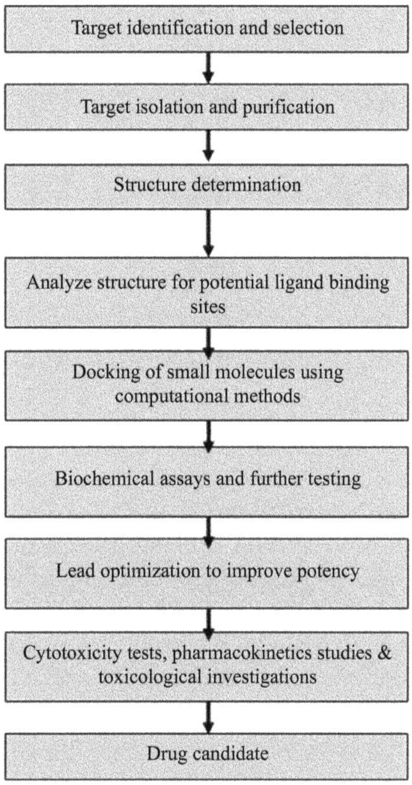

Figure 8.2. Basic procedure involved in proteomics.

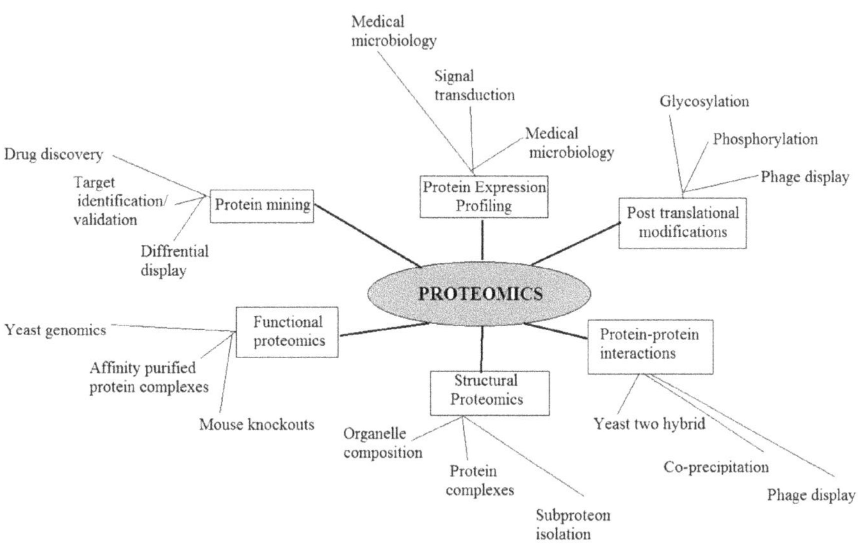

Figure 8.3. Different areas in proteomics.

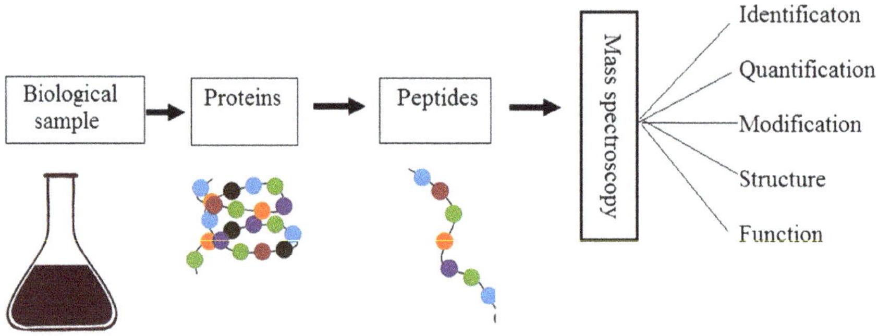

Figure 8.4. Basic procedure involved in structural proteomics.

the possible structure and possible function of virtually any protein from information of its coding sequence. This proteomics branch can also help in accumulating data about protein–protein interactions and about the construction of cells, to describe how the expression of certain proteins results in a cell's unique features. Recent mass spectrometry tools have offered a useful platform that can be combined with several procedures to examine protein structure and dynamics. Moreover nuclear magnetic resonance (NMR)-based structural proteomics coupled with x-ray crystallography can provide a comprehensive structural database to predict the basic biological functions of hypothetical proteins identified by genome projects.

8.2.2 Functional proteomics (strategy)

As the number of genome sequencing projects is increasing, there is a parallel exponential growth in the number of protein sequences whose function is still unidentified (figure 8.5) [6]. Functional proteomics is a developing research area in the field of proteomics whose methods are geared towards two main objectives: the interpretation of the biological function of unidentified proteins and the description of cellular mechanisms at the molecular level [7].

Functional proteomics uses proteomics tools to examine the features of the molecular protein networks involved in a living cell. Documentation and investigation of molecular protein networks involved in the nuclear pore complex in yeast is one of the recent accomplishments of functional proteomics. This accomplishment allows understanding of the translocation of molecules from the nucleus to the cytoplasm and vice versa [8].

8.2.3 Expression proteomics

Expression proteomics is the investigation of dysregulated proteins as a function of stimulation or condition (disease, time, drug, etc). In other words it is the quantitative investigation of protein expression between samples differing in a number of variables. It can also be defined as the examination of protein expression at a larger scale. The arrangement of expression of the entire proteome or a portion of it (a subproteome) between samples can be ascertained with the help of this

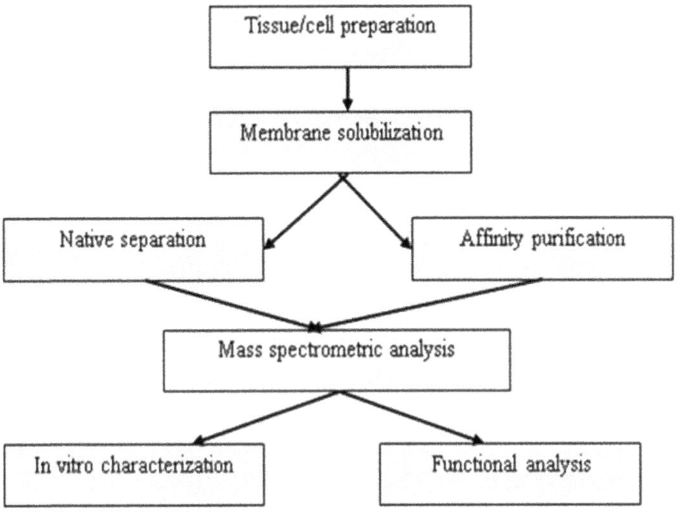

Figure 8.5. Functional proteomic analysis.

method. Expression proteomics is quite beneficial in finding disease-specific proteins. For example, over-expression or under-expression of proteins in cancerous cells and normal cells derived from a cancer patient and a normal individual, respectively, can be examined using several tools such as 2DE, mass spectrometry, microarrays, etc. This approach can recognize the growth of cancers and allows improvement of drugs in the management of cancer.

8.3 Basic techniques involved in proteomics

8.3.1 Sequence alignment (algorithms)

Fast emerging new sequencing tools offer information on an unparalleled scale. A principal challenge to the examination of these data is sequence alignment, wherein sequence reads must be matched to a reference [9]. An extensive variety of alignment algorithms and software have been developed over the past few years [9]. These techniques involve the study of the sequences of the DNA, RNA or protein to detect sites of resemblance that may be a result of functional, structural or evolutionary relationships between the sequences. Nucleotide or amino acid residues which are aligned sequences are characteristically presented as rows within a matrix. The residues gaps are incorporated between these, so that identical or similar features are associated in successive columns. The fastest way to allocate a new gene or cDNA is to perform pairwise assessment (a procedure of relating objects in pairs to judge which object is favored) with cDNA and EST sequences, and recognize gene sequences procured in databanks using alignment techniques such as BLAST (Basic Local Alignment Search Tool) or FASTA (a DNA and protein sequence alignment software package). However, this method is really only beneficial when there is >30% sequence uniqueness between the new gene and the databank sequence. If a similar gene/protein is found, it proposes the possible role of the product of new gene. However, additional experiments will be essential to determine the real *in vivo* function of the new gene product. To find resemblances below 30% sequence uniqueness, numerous sequence assessments are made by means of an algorithm such as PSI-BLAST (Position-Specific Iterated Blast). However, such a search may provide false positive findings. PSI-BLAST develops a position-specific scoring matrix or outline from the various sequence alignments detected above a given score threshold by protein–protein BLAST [10].

8.3.2 Protein structure (annotation resources)

An important reason three-dimensional protein structures are interpreted with supportive or derived data is to determine the molecular background of the protein function. In this endeavor, protein structure annotation databanks curate important evidence and explanations, based on community-accepted standards, for the ~100 000 three-dimensional investigational protein structures that allow further understanding of the structure–function relationship [11].

A method to control the function of an orphan gene is to inspect the three-dimensional structural arrangements of the protein, that the gene responsible for this protein is expected to encode; such a protein is called a theoretical protein. This three-dimensional structural arrangement is matched with the protein structures stored in databases. One of the bases for this method is the fact that the three-dimensional structures of proteins are better maintained than are their primary structures. For this reason protein function depends on the three-dimensional structure instead of the primary structure of the protein. It has been projected that 20%–30% of orphan genes could be allocated function by defining the three-dimensional structures of the proteins encoded by them, and equating these to protein structures in databanks. For example, the three-dimensional structural configurations of hemoglobin and myoglobin are very comparable, considering that they both are oxygen carriers. However, a BLAST search will fail to detect resemblance between myoglobin and α- or β-globin (both are hemoglobin polypeptides). Thus it has been projected that if a theoretical protein has a similar structure to a known protein, there is a 66% chance that it has a role related to that of the known protein. The structure of a theoretical protein can be evaluated in the following three ways:

- If this target sequence displays >25% resemblance to a sequence whose structure is already known (called a template sequence), relative modeling can be employed to forecast the structure of the target protein sequences.
- When the uniqueness is <25%, the sequence can be matched to known structures to examine the level to which the experimental data match the values anticipated by theory.
- The target sequence structure can also be examined from the primary data without reference to known structures. Protein structures are experimentally evaluated using x-ray crystallography and NMR spectroscopy. Both of these methods are slow, time consuming and require greater quantities (milligrams) of the purified protein. However, current developments in both procedures will allow their alteration for high throughput analyses.

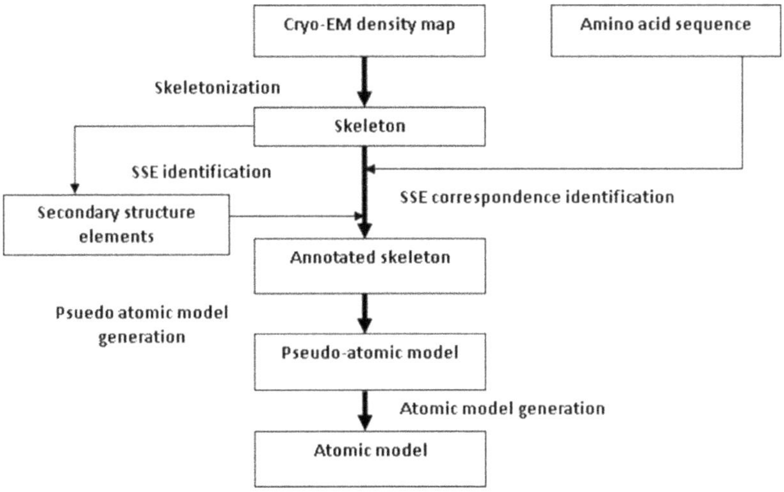

Figure 8.6. Procedure involved in protein structural investigation.

8.3.3 Protein structural investigation

Figure 8.6 provides a schematic representation of the process involved in protein structural investigation.

Structural investigation can often disclose the general function of a protein when sequence and structural assessments fail to suggest function. For example, protein surface scanning may disclose splits that may signify ligand-binding sites. A protein with a large split or cleft could be cautiously assigned the name 'enzyme'. A greater resolution in the description can be conceivable by comparing the shape of the split/cleft to a library of small molecular shapes using drug design software, e.g. DOCK and HOOK. These programs are capable of identifying possible ligands with binding sites present on protein surfaces. Scanning of the protein surface also facilitates identification of the domains most likely involved in interaction with other proteins. Knowing gene function involves more than recognizing the gene products. After they are produced, several gene products are altered by the breakdown of end groups (e.g. signal sequences, propeptides or initiator methionine residues), by the accumulation of chemical groups (such as methyl-, acetyl-, phosphoryl) or sometimes by adding linkages to sugars and lipids. In addition to the wide variety produced by the alternate splicing of mRNA, nearly a hundred mechanisms of post-translational modification are recognized. Therefore, the human genome, which may have 35 000–40 000 protein-coding genes, may offer over 350 000 different gene products. The main aim of proteomics is to provide data on each protein encoded in a genome, on its role, structure, cellular localization, post-translational modifications, associations (shared domains, evolutionary history) with other proteins and variants.

8.3.4 Two-dimensional gel electrophoresis in proteomics

Gel-based proteomics is one of the most multipurpose approaches for fractionating protein complexes [12]. Among these approaches, two-dimensional polyacrylamide

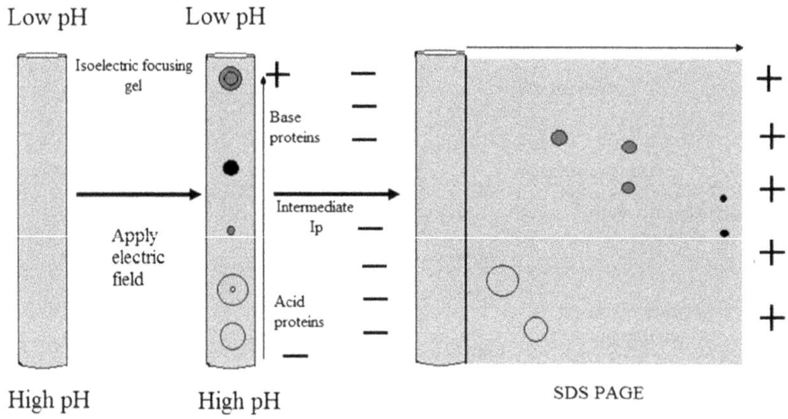

Figure 8.7. Two-dimensional gel electrophoresis.

gel electrophoresis (2DE) provides a key orthogonal method. It is commonly used to simultaneously fractionate, detect, and quantify proteins when coupled with mass spectrometric identification or other immunological tests.

The basic tools in proteomics include separation and identification of proteins that are isolated from cells. To achieve this, 2DE can be utilized. 2DE involves placement of the protein extract on a polyacrylamide gel after which an electric charge is applied across the gel to separate proteins based on their molecular weight (figure 8.7). Once this is complete, the gel is turned 90°, and through a second phase of electrophoresis, the proteins are separated in a second dimension based on their molecular mass. Once the gels are stained, the proteins are exposed as spots; different gels display 200–10 000 spots. To detect different proteins, spots are cut from the gel and are allowed to digest with enzymes, e.g. trypsin, to offer a characteristic set of fragments. These fragments are further studied by mass spectrometry, which is known as peptide mass fingerprinting. To recognize the proteins, the peptide's mass is matched with the masses predicted from data in genetic or protein databanks.

8.3.5 Domain fusion method (or rosetta stone method)

The examination of amino acid sequences from different individuals often provides results in which two or more proteins encoded for discretely in a genome also act as fusions, either in a similar genome or that of some other organism [13]. These fusion proteins, called Rosetta stone sequences, support the linkage of dissimilar proteins, and suggest the probability of functional interactions between the linked objects, creating local and global relationships within the proteome [14]. The domain fusion method searches for functionally active proteins that are distinct in a number of organisms, but are fused into a single protein, a Rosetta stone protein, in some other organisms. The basic principle of the Rosetta stone technique is as follows. The protein A sequence from an organism is utilized to search for a homolog in a different organism. This examination can recognize a single domain protein such as

A. However, in a number of organisms, it may recognize a Rosetta stone protein, such as A–B. As domains A and B are portions of a single protein, they are likely to be functionally related. Now the sequence of domain B is used to search for its homolog in the first organism. The homolog of the domain identified in this organism will be functionally related to protein A. Thus if the function of protein A were known, this strategy will reveal the function of protein/gene B, which was formerly an orphan gene.

8.4 Complete proteome of *Mycoplasma genitalium*

M. genitalium is the smallest member of the Mollicutes, has a genome size of 580 kb and the potential to express 480 gene products, and is thus an outstanding model to assess [15]:

- The minimum metabolism necessary for a free-living cell.
- Proteomic tools and the information derived by proteome analysis.

Wasinger and co-workers utilized proteomics to offer a portrait of what type of genes are expressed in the bacterium *M. genitalium* during exponential and stationary growth periods. *M. genitalium* is one of the simplest independent bacteria with a reduced genome. Using 2DE, the researchers explored 427 protein spots in exponentially growing cells. Of these, 201 were examined and recognized. The rest of the spots present in fragments derived from larger proteins, variants of similar proteins (isoforms) and post-translationally modified forms. The recognized proteins included enzymes involved in DNA replication, transcription, translation, delivery of materials across the cell membrane and energy metabolism. The study, however, could not cover 158 known proteins (33% of the proteome) and 17 unknown proteins. It was analyzed that there was a 42% reduction in the number of proteins synthesized during the transition from the exponential growth phase to the stationary phase. Moreover, a number of new proteins appeared, and additional proteins experienced intense variations because of nutrient exhaustion, enhanced acidity of the growth medium and other adaptations against environmental changes. In *M. genitalium*, a mere 33% of the proteome is expressed during maximal growth, and the remaining 67% of the proteome are the proteins to be expressed under different environmental conditions. Wasinger's examination of the *M. genitalium* proteome assisted in establishing the least number of expressed genes essential for independent existence and the modifications in gene expression that accompany the changeover from the exponential growth phase to the stationary phase. It was also noticed that the extensive range of information offered by proteome analysis cannot be derived only by genome sequencing.

8.5 Architecture and design of the nuclear pore complex

Three-dimensional examination of the nuclear pore complex discloses the fundamental, highly symmetric framework of this supramolecular assembly, how it is attached in the nuclear membrane and how it is constructed from many distinct, interconnected subunits [16]. The organization of the subunits within the membrane pore makes a large central channel, by which active nucleocytoplasmic transport is known to occur, and eight smaller peripheral channels that are probable routes for passive diffusion of ions and small molecules. The nuclear pore complex (NPC) is made up of proteins embedded in the nuclear membrane. This complex joins the cytoplasmic and nuclear compartments of the cell and permits transport of materials between the nucleus and the cytoplasm. As this transportation contains mRNA intended for the cytoplasm, nuclear pores are vital control points for regulating gene expression. Their structural and functional sophistication has been an obstacle in understanding their molecular organization. Genomics in association with proteomics has offered scientists techniques to investigate the three-dimensional construction of nuclear pores and to recognize their proteins. Depending on its size, the yeast nuclear pore complex contains around 200 different proteins. By using a rat genome databank as a resource, scientists were able to recognize potential nuclear pore complex proteins, also called nucleoporins, by means of sequence resemblance to already identified nuclear pore complex proteins from other organisms. In another example, proteomics was employed to outline the molecular construction of a nuclear pore complex. Accordingly, pore complexes were separated and purified, and then nucleoporins were detected by means of mass spectrometry on peptide digests of proteins purified from the NPCs. Yeast's NPC only includes around 30 different proteins, but with each protein present in multiple copies. The nucleoporins are prearranged into 16 subunits (eight on the pore's nuclear side and eight on its cytoplasmic side). Moreover, there are filament-base structures on both sides of the pore, formed into a bag on the nuclear side. Using multiple tools such as mutant analysis, microscopy and proteomics, the actual regions/sites of NPC proteins in the three-dimensional arrangement of the pore have been mapped. The majority of nucleoporins are proportionally distributed on the cytoplasmic and nuclear sides of the pore. Five proteins are present only on one side or the other, and seven are distributed more on one side than on the other. The function of nucleoporins in nucleocytoplasmic transportation or the regulation of transport can be studied by examining protein–protein interactions within the pore, as well as interactions of pore proteins with transport proteins, signal molecules and other cellular components.

8.6 Functional genomics and systems biology

Functional genomics is an efficient method for determining the roles of the novel genes revealed by complete genome sequences (figure 8.8) [17]. Such a method should take a hierarchical approach, as this will both bound the number of trials to be done and allow a closer and closer estimate of the function of any individual gene to be attained. Furthermore, hierarchical studies have, in their early stages, remarkable integrative power and functional genomics aims at a comprehensive and integrative view of the workings of living cells [18]. Functional genomics is an area where the function of a gene product is determined. This includes answers to the questions:

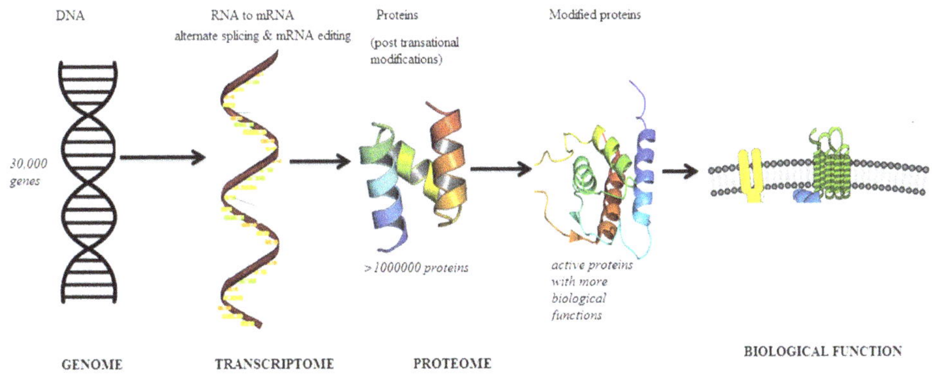

Figure 8.8. Schematic representation of functional genomics.

- How are genes expressed?
- How are the gene sequence and structure related to the end product, and its relationship with gene versus an individual from the same generation?
- Exactly how is a product associated with a sequence and structure, and how is it associated with the end products of other genes of similar organisms?
- What are the implications of the environment over a gene and how does this interaction help in understanding the rate of genetic variation? Gene–environment interaction helps in understanding genetic influences modeled as latent [19].

These questions can be answered by studying the following:

- Determining at what time and exactly at which place specific genes are expressed on a genomic scale (called expression profiling). This permits the identification of those particular genes that are over-expressed or under-expressed. This concept can be used to understand different biological processes in health and disease. This concept can also be utilized to study the expression in a particular tissue/organ at the molecular level. This type of gene-based profiling, and more specifically recent RNA sequence based profiling, can be used as an important tool for drawing correlations between gene activity and various physiological or developmental states. It also helps in creating collections of gene expression data across various cell types, development times, varied species and against different stimuli [20].
- The replacement of a particular natural gene with mutated gene under *in vitro* conditions to access its *in vivo* function (the knockout method) [21].
- The genetic relationship between proteins and other molecules (as first suggested by Archibald Garrod in 1902, who predicted that genes control the function of proteins during his study on patients suffering from alkaptonuria).

Functional genomics aims towards answering such questions thoroughly for most of the genes present in a genome, in comparison to classical strategies that report one gene at a time. Among potential branches of functional genomics, the field of transcriptomics helps in predicting and understanding the exact functions of genes and their respective products. High-throughput screening of gene transcripts in biological systems, through the development of the necessary bioinformatics analytical tools, has allowed scale-up of experiments classically performed with single genes to identify genetic variation at large scales. Functional genomics can be theoretically further categorized into gene-driven (dependent on genomic data to identify, clone and express genes in a genome) and phenotype-driven approaches (dependent on phenotypes from random mutation screens or naturally occurring variants to recognize and characterize genes for the phenotype, without having any previous information of the basic molecular mechanism or function). The most important aspect of functional genomics is that it explores the functional arrangement of all genomes, in particualr parts that are external to any coding gene sequences which play an important role in gene expression. The concept of the epigenome covers all the molecules and proteins which can affect DNA function, usually by turning genes on or off. Studies related with this field usually cover factors responsible for controlling development and differentiation against external changes. During this process epigenetic tags are made in the form of DNA methylation and covalent modifications of histones to determine the arrangements of cell- and tissue-specific gene expression, as described in figure 8.9. Epigenetic readers also help in determining gene expression. In certain cases, small RNA molecules are used to guarantee sequence specificity.

Overall, these studies of epigenetic modifications explain the forms of epigenetic 'flavors' (i.e., the existence of chromatin in different states). This means the presence of chromatin in heterochromatin (inactive, repressed) and euchromatin (potentially active), decides the tags and reads which may further decide flavors. In addition functional genomic studies also cover the complex organization of RNA molecules in the genome, i.e., well characterized coding RNA and non-coding RNAs. Functional genomic investigations include highly complex genome and proteome information which requires the development of potential computational and hardware tools. This discipline gave birth to an independent discipline called bioinformatics. Recent developments in bioinformatics have allowed collaboration between different disciplines, resulting in further new disciplines ending with the suffix '-omics', e.g. proteomics, genomics and metabolomics. All these disciplines have the common objective of computational analysis of sophisticated and vast information at each and every biological level; starting from the molecular level, i.e., genes and molecules, to cells, tissues and organs, and finally to the study of whole-body systems.

8.6.1 Gene expression profiling

As mentioned above, functional genomics is defined as the branch of genomics that predicts the functions of genes and gene products by high-throughput screening of gene transcripts in a biological system. Functional genomics has numerous applications in clinical medicine [22]. Functional genomics is a broad approach that allows the concurrent examination of mRNA levels for the complete human

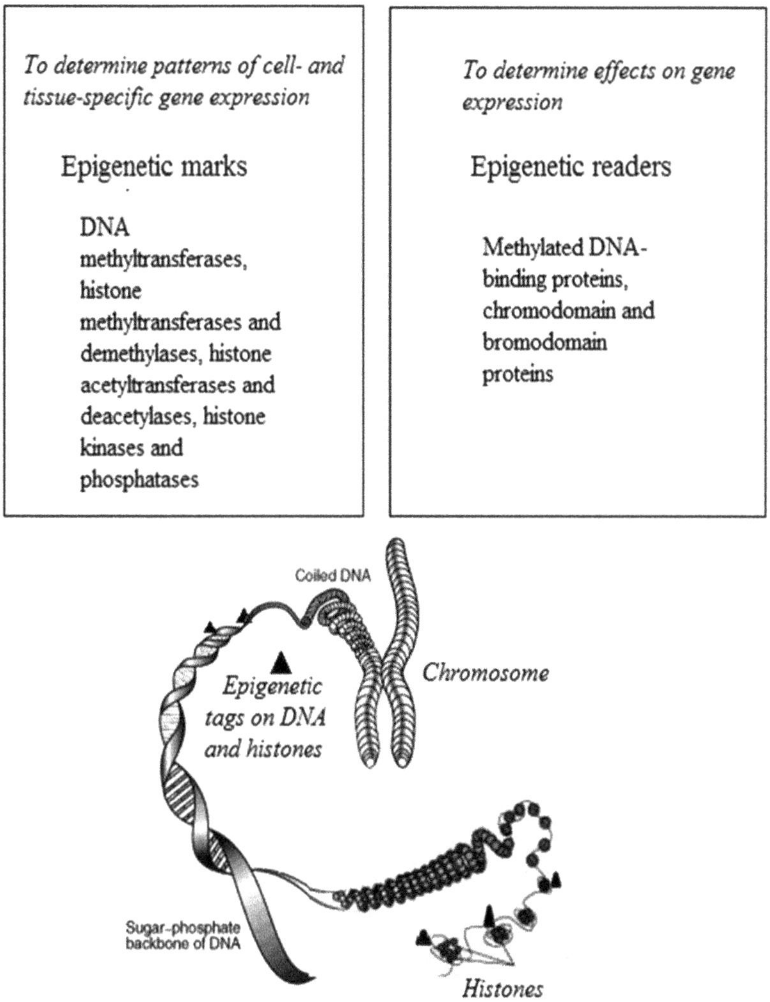

Figure 8.9. Epigenetic tags and reads.

transcriptome from as few as 1000 cells. Currently, functional genomics is employed to categorize the development of disease and survival in response to traumatic and burn injuries, sepsis and visceral ischemia, and reperfusion injury, as well as to designate patterns of gene expression in reaction to erratic microbial pathogens. Due to the number of new bioinformatics techniques emerging, functional genomics is providing a foundation to reveal the fundamental complexity of the biological response to a range of inflammatory diseases and is offering new methods for their exploration [23]. Functional genomics has now been developed as a standard tool in inflammation research to undo basic biological processes.

Expression profiling is a discipline that deals with the extent of expression of multiple genes at the same time, i.e., it attempts to determine the complete picture of cellular function at a molecular level. This can be achieved using certain tools, e.g. DNA microarrays, which help in measuring the relative expression of multiple genes and their correlation with already identified target genes. The microarray is an advanced tool to determine genetic expression by evaluating the actual amount of mRNA present in the sample. In addition to exploring the role of existing genes and their relevant association, microarrays also include genes with currently unknown functions. This can provide the prospect of new gene discovery, which in particular plays an important role in functional genomics, e.g. microarray based analysis of previously unknown genes selectively expressed in T-helper 2 type lymphocytes can offer new targets for asthma [24]. In addition, by using comprehensive arrays it is now possible to carry out deletion mapping to recognize selective areas of chromosomes whose genes are not present in a large microarray.

Functional genomics covers global expression profiling to study genes under epigenetic and transcriptional regulation to further study several forms of coding and non-coding RNA molecules. It is a branch that deals with the simultaneous examination of the expression pattern, usually of all genes present in the genome at the RNA level or at the protein level. In contrast to global expression profiling, traditional approaches are more focused on a single gene, which can restrict access to these complex interactions. Systematic investigation of gene expression profiling helps in interpreting the transcriptomes of consecutive developmental stages. This information is required to understand the developmental mechanism which can shed light on conservation and diversification at the molecular level. Thus functional genomics is directed towards studying global expression profiling at the RNA level (by nucleic acid arrays or direct sequence analysis) or at the protein level (by 2DE followed by mass spectrometry or protein arrays).

Global expression profiling is a valuable approach which can help in the identification of those particular genes that play an important role in development, and also help in understanding the complex behavior of a gene in a particular environment against different levels of stress or any other stimuli which can cause the onset of a disease, etc. Moreover, it also offers a unique method for characterizing cellular phenotypes and exploring novel drug targets which can help in developing potential drugs.

8.6.2 Transcriptome, proteome and genomes

The transcriptome is the initial product of genome expression. Basically, it is an assortment of RNA molecules obtained from those protein-coding genes whose biological information is essential for the cell at a specific time [25]. These RNA molecules further direct the production of the final product of genome expression, the proteome, the cell's repertoire of proteins, which stipulates the nature of the biochemical reactions that the cell is able to carry out. The transcriptome is created by the process known as transcription, in which individual genes are copied into RNA molecules.

Transcriptomic studies are part of integrative genomics, which includes the set of all RNA molecules from protein-coding (mRNA) to non-coding RNA, of a complete organism or a particular cell. As the name suggests, the transcriptome

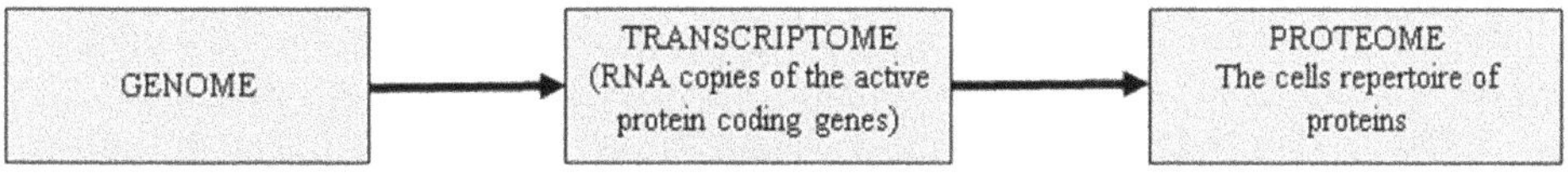

Figure 8.10. General overview of transcriptomes.

encompasses the complete set of transcripts (the copies of DNA or RNA) in a particular cell or tissue. Transcripts are complementary strands of DNA or RNA synthesized by the genome (figure 8.10). Thus the whole objective of transcriptome studies is to recognize genes differentially expressed under different environmental conditions. This may help in understanding genes or their associated pathways. To understand this more deeply we have to consider a eukaryotic system, in which genetic expression of a single gene results in the synthesis of more than one type of developed mRNA. This process of alternative splicing or differential splicing results in a single gene coding for multiple proteins, i.e., mRNA is directed to synthesize different proteins that may have different functions or properties. Alternative splicing involves elimination of introns (nucleotide sequences) from the gene (complementary RNA/DNA) and fixing exons together in the right direction to yield the final functional mRNA product. The information which is not of any use, i.e., non-coding sections of an RNA transcript, are removed and the coding sections (the code for proteins) are joined together to form the functional product in the form of mRNA. Alternative splicing can take place in different ways, but still results in well-defined patterns. This information helps in understanding the whole human genome project. For example, when a single human gene has undergone alternative splicing to produce functional RNA to further produce three different proteins, you can assume how many proteins the projected 35 000 human genes could create (the estimated number is 105 000 different proteins, i.e., different in their properties and functions). This diversity of proteins present inside the body helps in controlling the whole metabolism, structure, etc. A popular example of alternative splicing is seen in the case of the *Drosophila* gene Dscam [26]. Dscam is a (immunoglobulin superfamily) protein essential for the development of neuronal connections in *Drosophila*. By means of alternative splicing, Dscam can potentially develop 19 008 different extracellular domains associated with one of two alternative transmembrane segments, resulting in 38 016 isoforms. All these isoforms share the same domain structure, however, they encompass variable amino acid sequences within three Ig domains in the extracellular region [27]. A gene identified in this study produced approximately 40 000 different mRNAs. These functional mRNAs can be further translated in different receptor proteins. After the determination of the complete human genome sequence in 2001, it is now understood that only a small portion of the human transcriptome is translated into proteins. The rest of the residual transcripts have unidentified functions. It has been reported that a noticeable increase in transcriptional complexity is connected with organization of the transcriptional units in the genome. There are genomic regions that are highly enriched for transcripts which may be subjected to shared epigenetics regulatory control over larger regions. This complexity is due to the production of a manifold of functional mRNAs from each RNA transcript, which makes them more vulnerable to mutation. The multiple bioconversion steps, which involve the passage of large quantities of information from one molecule to another, and further the multiple copies made in the form of a functional message (mRNA) to synthesize different proteins, involve cascades of molecular events where each time elements are expose against different conditions, there is a chance of being mutated. The extent and nature of transcriptome varies from tissue to tissue because no tissue will express all of the genes. The genetic expression of the transcriptome always varies, which is why each tissue has its own transcriptome to synthesize unique proteins. This process is very selective in nature as genes expressed in a unique tissue will vary from those present in another tissue. Consequently, based on this variation it is obvious to discuss different transcriptomes, such as the human brain transcriptome, mouse liver transcriptome, etc

8.6.3 DNA arrays: a potential genomic tool

DNA microarray techniques are primarily used to determine the transcriptional levels of RNA transcripts derived from thousands of genes within a genome in a single experiment (figure 8.11). By using this approach we can relate physiological cell states to gene expression patterns for examining tumors, disease progression, cellular response to stimuli and drug target identification. Currently DNA

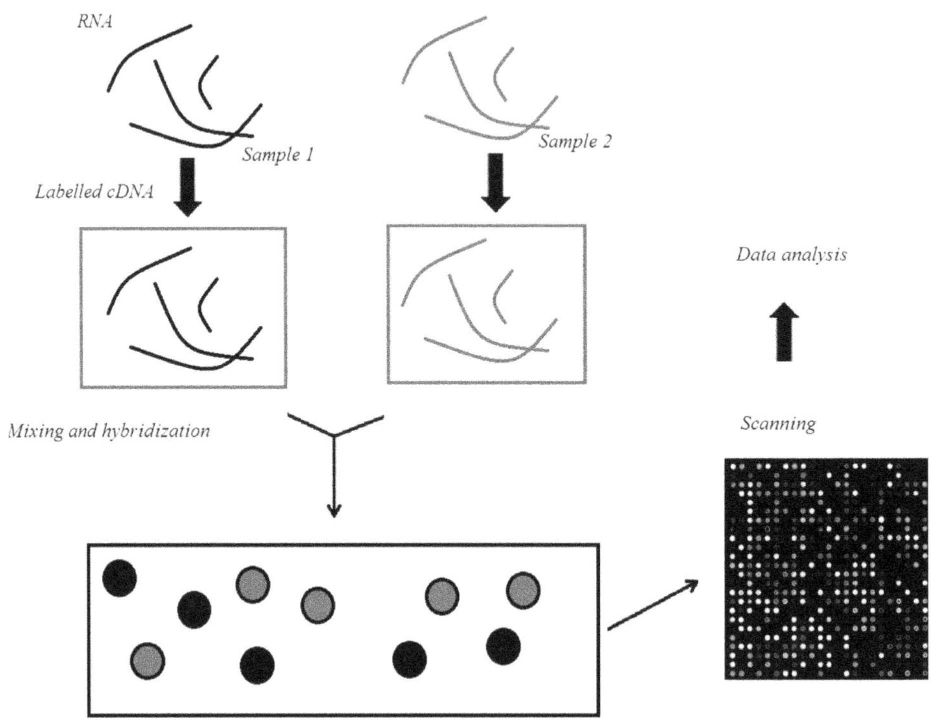

Figure 8.11. Schematic representation of DNA arrays.

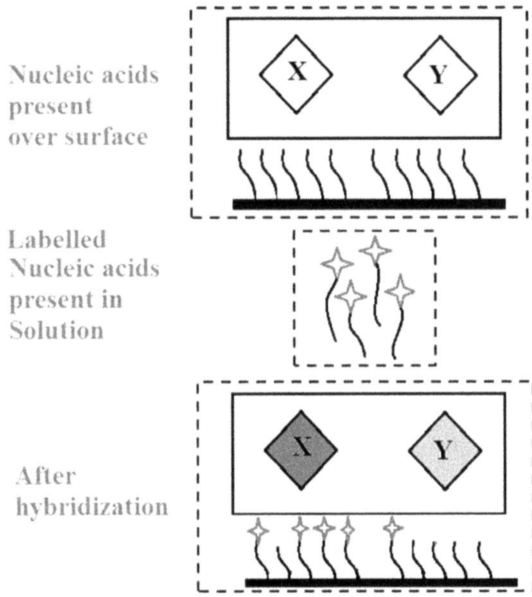

Figure 8.12. DNA array representing DNA on a solid surface before and after hybridization.

microarrays are not limited to gene expression, as they are also being used to detect the single nucleotide polymorphisms (SNPs) of the human genome (the Hap Map project), aberrations in methylation patterns, alterations in gene copy-number, alternative RNA splicing and pathogen detection [28].

DNA microarray or biochip techniques include synthesis of DNA sequences in two- or three-dimensional format. These sequences are synthesized such that the DNA sequences are covalently or non-covalently linked to the surface. In use, a DNA array allows the hybridization of targets (labeled nucleic acids) to the probes present on the array to evaluate the relative amount of nucleic acid present in a given solution, as shown in figure 8.12.

Generally, during this process small sequences of nucleic acids are immobilized or fixed on an appropriate solid support such as a glass chip, silicon chip or nylon membrane.

DNA arrays are available in three types:

- Spotted arrays on glass.
- *In situ* synthesized arrays.
- Self-assembled arrays.

Spotted arrays on glass. Spotted DNA arrays allow high-density DNA arrays (10^6–10^9 double-stranded DNA molecules with dense spots up to 5000 spots per cm^2) to fix over glass substrates [29]. Polylysine coated glass microscope slides are used for immobilizing DNA and for spotting a robotic spotter can be utilized. This robotic spotter spots various glass slide arrays with DNA from microtiter dishes. These small fragments of DNA are derived from genomic libraries, in particular from cDNA clones or by PCR

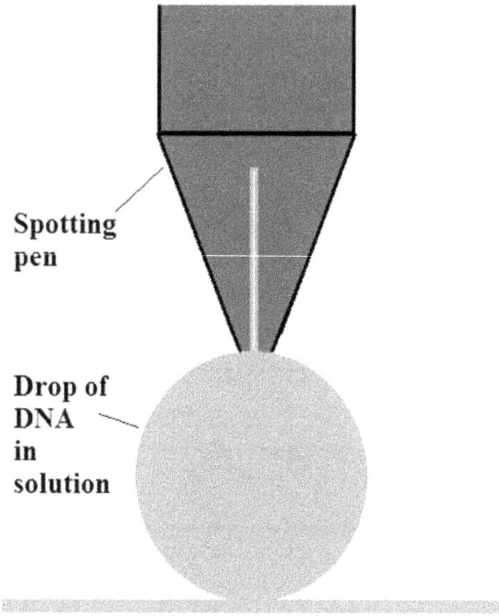

Figure 8.13. Spotting arrays. A glass fountain-pen-like structure (usually multiple pens are present) is allowed to dip into solutions containing DNA and this is then deposited on glass slides.

amplification. This robotic spotter contains slotted pins which are quite similar to fountain pens in design (figure 8.13). During this process a single dip is made in the DNA solution, which can then be used over numerous slides. This robotic facility also allows one to fluorescently label the samples for fluorescence based detection, which offers greater sensitivity and a broad dynamic range, and can provide different colored labels, which can further help in their detection after hybridization. Flourescent labels are also cheaper than radioactive or chemilluminescent labels. Spotting is done in such a manner that each individual spot or dot signifies a separate gene, i.e., the spots are not characterized by repetition. Spotting can be studied using confocal scanning [30].

In situ synthesized arrays. Fodor first suggested, in 1991, that single-stranded oligonucleotides are synthesized in the presence of light on a solid substrate (the process is called photolithography) [31]. Initially, ten amino acid peptides were synthesized using di-nucleotides, and later 256 different octa-nucleotides were synthesized. During 1995, Affymetrix array technology was utilized to determine the variation in the reverse transcriptase and protease genes of the highly polymorphic HIV-1 genome and also to determine mutation in the human mitochondrial genome. Affymetrix technology has been used to produce an extensive set of DNA arrays for use in expression analysis [48, 49], genetic characterization and gene sequencing [32]. *In situ* synthesized arrays can be synthesized by two approaches:

- Inkjet oligosynthesis methods.
- Photolithographic methods (e.g. Affymetrix).

Self-assembled arrays. Another method to construct arrays was initially suggested by David Walt at Tufts University [33]. This technique was later licensed to Illumina (a

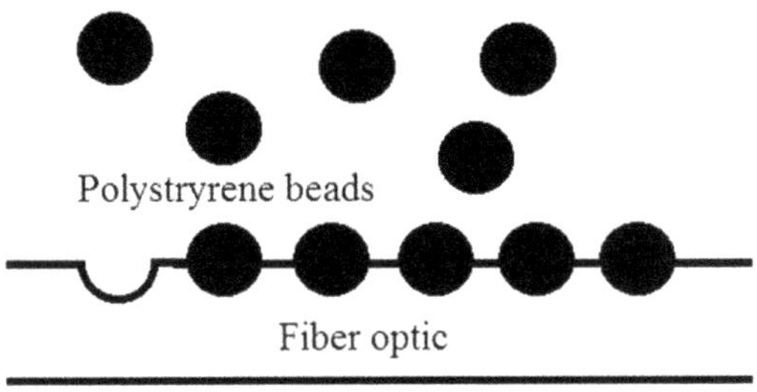

Figure 8.14. Self-assembled arrays.

sequencing and array technology company in San Diego, CA). In this method small DNA strands are synthesized on small polystryrene beads. Ultimately these DNA coated beads are deposited on the ends of a fiber optic array (figure 8.14). The fibers are engraved to provide a well which is larger than a single polystryrene bead. The beads are optically encoded with different fluorophores so as to identify which oligonucleotide was in which position on the array. This method is called an optical sensor array.

Small single-stranded strands of oligonucleotide (20–25 base pairs) are synthesized and fixed (printed) over a solid matrix with the light-directed printing technique known as photolithography, to form a printed oligonucleotide chip. Oligonucleotides are directly synthesized over the matrix. To reduce the chance of false positive outcomes, each fragment sequence is described by multiple oligonucleotides (20 non-overlapping oligonucleotides). A high density of oligonucleotides over the matrix (64 000 cm^{-2}) offers more accurate results for investigating gene expression patterns. One of the most interesting applications of a microarray is to establish the association between the gene expression patterns of two cell types (e.g. cancerous tissue and normal tissue). Microarrays have potential applications in transcriptomics, because the whole concept is based on the synthesis of complementary strands (cDNA) or probes from mRNA. For the development of probes, targeted cells must first be identified to isolated mRNA, e.g. to study the genetic variation between normal and cancerous cells mRNA from both is isolated. However, since RNA is not very stable and can be quickly degraded, using reverse transcriptase mRNA is converted into complementary DNA (cDNA). By using the RNA molecule, an enzyme known as reverse transcriptase copies strand to synthesize a new complementary template DNA. This newly formed cDNA is labeled with suitable fluorescent dyes (fluors, for short). These labeled cDNA are typically called probes. Labeling of target molecules (cDNA or cRNA) is s crucial step in a microarray as it helps to determine the amount of mRNA indirectly through the labeled molecules. In the case of investigating the genetic variation between normal and cancerous cells, cDNA derived from both types of cells is labeled with a different fluor that will yield fluorescence of different colors. Now, the amount of cDNA from each sample signifies the amount of mRNA present in that sample, i.e., the amount of cDNA in the probe will be comparable to that of the mRNA in the cell. These cDNA are allowed to hybridize with cDNA probes.

Each labeled cDNA molecule will hybridize with the DNA molecules of that dot of the microarray to which it is complementary. Since at this stage some strands are labeled and some are not, the strands utilized in hybridization can be identified by their respective fluorescence pattern. So, because of the fluor existing on the cDNA probe, these can be identified by their colored spots, however, those spots that do not have complementary cDNA in the probe will not fluoresce and will appear as a blank. Fluorescence intensity also helps in the identification of regions of blot paper where hybrid strands are present. This will indirectly determine the relative amount of mRNA present in the cell. To compare the genetic expression between cancerous and normal cells, cDNA probes of both are used concurrently for hybridization under same DNA array conditions. In such cases two different fluors are employed. The information based on fluorescence imaging (spots) of the two fluors can be accessed using suitable software. This software helps in establishing the relationship between the intensities of the images and the amount of mRNA. The examination of a microarray such as that described above will offer data on the following:

- The genes that are expressed in both normal and cancerous cells.
- The genes that are expressed in normal cells but are not expressed in cancerous cells.
- Those genes that are expressed only in cancerous cells. This information would allow the identification of cancerous cells, and also to devise suitable drugs to selectively target such cells.

8.6.4 Gene function determination from sequence information

Scientists have synthesized a vast number of genome sequences from different organisms. The available databases, such as GenBank at the NCBI, store many of these sequences. These databases can be potentially utilized for studying comparative biology [34]. Not only do the databases store the genome sequences, but also information about the function (if it is known) of the genes. By making comparisons between known genes in the database, GenBank can be used to identify unknown genes. In database, one program exclusively used for this purpose is BLAST (Basic Local Alignment Search Tool). BLAST is a sequence similarity searching algorithms, which is based on the principle that if two sequences are similar then they are possibly homologous (that is, they share a common evolutionary ancestor). By means of this database, one can understand the function of an unknown gene by discovering similar sequences of known genes and proteins. BLAST is an advanced program, in that it searches at the nucleotide level, as well as making assessments at the amino acid level, offering much greater sensitivity. Thus, if one is mainly interested in the DNA sequence itself, it is better to hunt for genes using proteins. In addition to whole proteins, similarity searches can find protein motifs. A motif is a characteristic arrangement of amino acids, stored across many proteins, which offers a particular function to the protein [35].

The primary objective of classical functional genomics is to regulate the function of specific genes. Initial gene cloning is followed by mutation under *in vitro* conditions and finally reincorporation of the mutated gene into the host organism to examine its expression or any other effect. This approach has its limitations, as the process is complicated, slow and has a low success rate. The applications of a combination of the experimental approach to functional genomics and high-throughput sequencing analysis are as follows:

- To identify the gene accountable for specific biological phenotypes and diseases.
- To help in determining the function of gene.
- To facilitate the rapid identification of genes.
- To enable the discovery of genes that participate in other biological processes.
- To mutate every gene in the genome and accumulate the mutant strain to create genome-wide mutant libraries.

The last point, establishing genome-wide mutant libraries in several organisms such as bacteria, yeast, plants and mammals, is called mutational genomics. A mutational genomics based library can be established using one of the following two approaches.

The systematic approach. To establish a library, the systematic mutation of individual genes in the genome at one time should be studied, which allows the development of a bank of specific mutant strains. This can only be attained if the complete genome sequence is known. In this method, homologous recombination (which functions in the repair of DNA double-stranded breaks and inter-strand crosslinks) is utilized to accommodate a selectable marker gene (which helps in the selection of the targeted gene) inside the gene of interest. Usually, the insertion of the gene of interest in a selectable marker disturbs the selectable marker function, which can be further checked against the expression of normal selectable marker gene. However, in contrast, here homologous recombination allows the selectable marker to integrate into the gene of interest, which allows the dislocation of the targeted gene. The whole process is called gene knockout. By using suitable sequences from or around the target gene the selectable marker gene is flanked to attain homologous recombination. So it is essential to recognize the sequences of the gene of interest [36]. After the employment of suitable vectors, integration performed by homologous recombination may possibly occur up to 90% in prokaryotes. However, the opposite is the case for plants and animals, the rate of integration by homologous recombination is only 0.001% of the entire integration process. Homologous recombination or integration in the case of embryonic stem cells derived from mice has a rate up to 0.1%, which is much lower than that of yeast, which has 6200 genes and a rate of homologous integration of up to 90%. Knockout investigations have allowed knockouts of almost 85% of yeast genes. The mutants produced by this approach are studied to determine the functions of the missing genes. It is probable that a similar mutagenesis procedure might be considered for *Drosophila* in the near future.

The random approach. In contrast to the systematic approach, in random integration the gene is randomly mutated and this can be functional for any species. Random insertional mutagenesis can be achieved by the addition or deletion of nucleotides from a target gene sequence. This type of insertion or deletion results in overall change in the sequences of the gene of interest, primarily a new region of assortment that cannot be achieved by only point mutation. Insertional mutagenesis is often studied during gene transfer by the *Agrobacterium* strain. In this process a gene of interest is inserted into a transposable element called T-DNA. This T-DNA of *Agrobacterium*, whenever it is introduced into the genome, results in the disruption and loss of gene function. It clearly suggests the scope of T-DNA in the transfer of a gene of interest. The gene of interest is labeled before its insertion into T-DNA, which can facilitate its isolation from the place where it is positioned. Thus this approach is often called signature-tagged mutagenesis. The incorporated DNA sequence after labeling is called a tag. Inserted labeled DNA sequences in the form of tags can be further employed as probes in hybridization or to synthesize PCR primers. These primers can be utilized to isolate the DNA sequences located on either side of the tag or labeled gene of interest [37]. They can further be connected to the DNA sequence with a genomic cDNA clone and used to identify its function, etc. The tool called BLAST can be utilized for this in databases. In the case that this random insertion results in a mutant phenotype, the gene can be assigned a tentative function. Moreover, the incorporated sequence or gene of interest can be altered into a gene trap vector (the process known as gene trapping is a high-throughput approach) by introducing insertional mutations to ultimately offer and generate the data regarding the gene it interferes with. Gene trap mutations are present in equal numbers to the insertional targeted mutations, as long as the trapped gene is known. During gene trapping, the incorporated element covers a selectable marker gene such as lac Z (responsible for β-glucosidase synthesis) or gus A (responsible for β-glucuronidase synthesis) situated in a splice acceptor site. The selectable marker gene is, thus, triggered only if this element is introduced within the transcribed region of a gene. This approach facilitates a convenient assortment for incorporation inside genes, and is valuable in all organisms.

In this strategy, a number of tools are employed to prevent the expression of genes. These tools produce variations in phenotype, which means the organisms with a similar appearance are mutants; however, they have the typical variant form of a given gene. High throughput tools to explore protein and gene function *in situ* are still necessary to exploit these emerging advances in gene and protein discovery and in order to validate these identified targets. High-throughput target-selected gene inactivation in zebrafish was reported in 2011 [56]. High throughput functional inactivation of genes can be attained by various approaches such as virus-induced gene silencing for plants and RNA interference. In the case of animals, short double-stranded RNAs are being considered as a potential approach for gene silencing [38].

8.6.5 Protein interactions

The identification of genetic fusion across genomes can be used for the prediction of functional interrelationships of proteins, including physical interactions or complex formation. These predictions are obtained by the detection of resemblance between pairs of 'component' proteins and 'composite' proteins [28]. The most important criterion is how the gene functions, which can reveal the actual performance of the encoded proteins. This performance can be understood as multiple interactions between different proteins, and among proteins and molecules. For example, the drugs usually employed to treat disease act by modifying protein interactions in a positive manner. The process of investigating protein interactions is as follows. Let us say, for example, the function of protein A is unknown. Protein A is found to resemble proteins B and C, which contribute to RNA splicing [39]. This type of relationship between proteins would suggest that protein A is involved in RNA splicing. Before the genomics age, communication between proteins was investigated on an individual basis by means of a range of approaches, including suppressor mutations and co-immunoprecipitation (to study protein–protein interactions). These tools are very useful, however, they are not suitable for high throughput investigation. Moreover, they do not offer an easy way to link the proteins to their respective genes.

Different types of protein–protein interactions are involved in all cellular processes. For systems biology, the mapping of these interaction networks to explain the organization of the proteome into functional units is essential [29–32]. Several approaches have been developed for screening protein interactions. One of the most traditional approaches is copurification (also called affinity purification or co-immunoprecipitation) of protein complexes, which requires *in vitro* handling of protein extracts. In addition, this approach also has the limitation of restricted sensitivity and bias towards high affinity interactions [29–32]. When a partner has been identified, detection by mass spectrometry (MS) is usually straightforward, although expensive [40]. Cloning of the resultant cDNA may be time consuming, but clone repositories, e.g. RIKEN or IMACE, can provide a suitable alternative. Currently, surface plasmon resonance has been reported for screening protein–protein interactions. In this procedure purified cellular extracts are introduced onto a sensor chip covered with an immobilized binding partner. The tool arrangement combines the capture of the binding partner with a quantitative readout of the binding event, such that the putative partners can be eluted and detected by using MS An additional method for interaction screening uses 'cDNA-expression' libraries, such as phage display or yeast two-hybrid (Y2H) methods, for which genomic scale, highly parallel and automated processes are necessary. However, only a few detection approaches for protein–protein interactions can be effortlessly adapted for high-throughput approaches. These include, in particular, the Y2H method and affinity purification coupled with MS (AP/MS).

The Y2H method is a protein–protein interaction assay to determine if two proteins are interacting. In this procedure, a 'bait' protein is attached to half of a protein such as GAL4 that is attached to a reporter gene promoter [41]. To settle on the promoter and activate transcription of the reporter gene, the 'prey' protein interacts with the 'bait', which will bring the other half of the GAL4 protein together (figure 8.15). This approach is discussed further below.

Protein interactions are investigated by means of high-throughput tools. For efficient screening of many proteins some library-based protein interaction mapping is required to assess their interactions by *in vitro* or *in vivo* assays. Such mapping helps in establishing relationships between proteins and genes, or the complementary

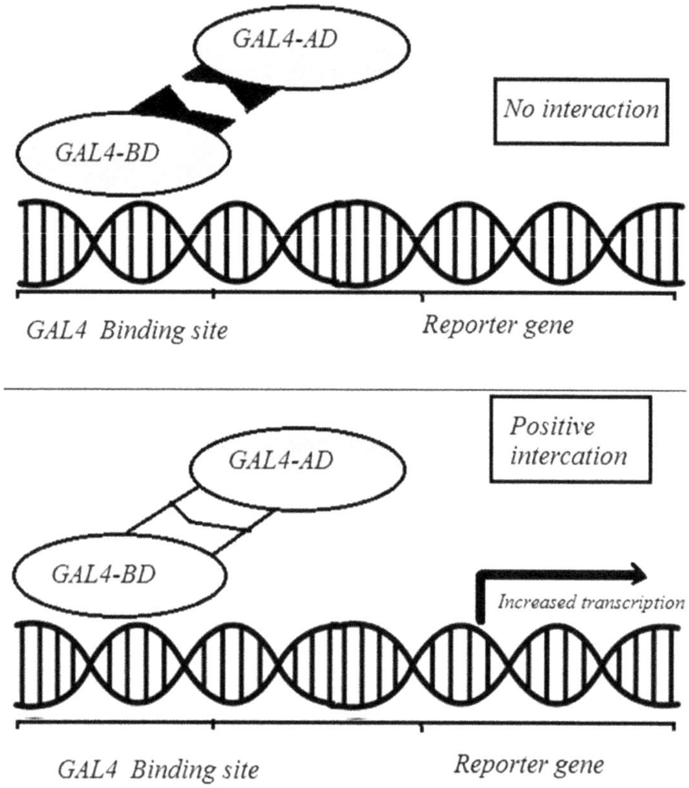

Figure 8.15. The Y2H hybrid method.

DNAs that encode them. To assess their biological potential *in vitro* examination is essential, which can be based on standard expression library. Based on expression cloning, an expression library is composed of clones, where each clone presents its own protein. This library helps in screening for suitable features and clones of interest, which can be recovered for further examination. Thus an expression library contains a variety of clones that carry cDNA derived from an organism which can be further incorporated in an expression vector to produce their protein products (figure 8.16).

As mentioned in figure 8.16, the last step of protein screening, i.e., identification of desirable proteins, can be achieved by immunological assays (antigen–antibody interaction). Other tools include the protein detection tools western blot and ELISA and protein characterization by mass spectrometry, and the function of the proteins can be assessed by functional protein analysis with HaloTag Technology. The identification of proteins is a crucial step which requires its respective antibody (the antibody functions as a probe) for its effective screening. Moreover, various proteins such as transcription factors can also be employed to recognize their interacting partners. For example, for the transcription factor c-Jun, also known as AP-1, is encoded by the JUN gene.

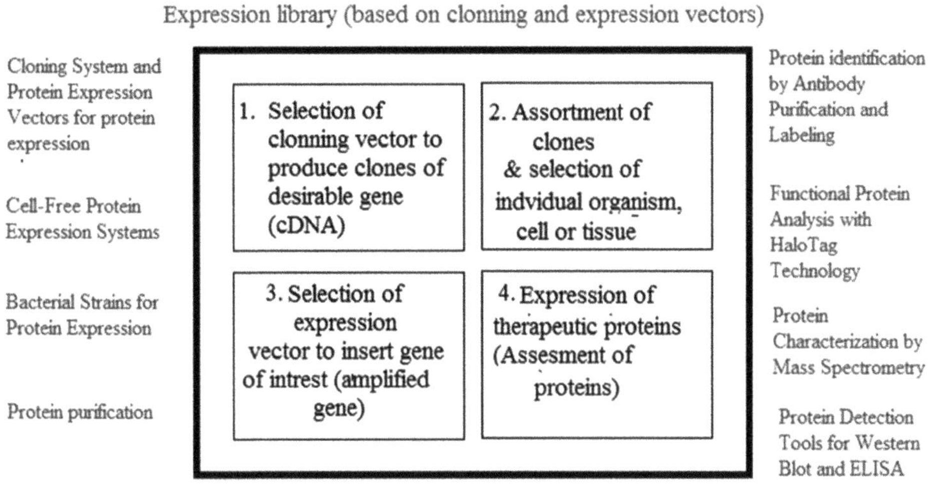

Figure 8.16. An expression library.

Another high-throughput approach is the phage display method, which offers a means to identify target-binding proteins from a library of millions of various proteins without the requirement of screening each molecule independently. Phage display is an approach to produce and screen a high number of novel therapeutic proteins and polypeptides by introducing a gene of interest into a gene responsible for the expression of a surface protein of a bacteriophage [42]. This allows the expression of a display of proteins of our own choice over the surface coating of the phage. One of the most important advantages of phage display is the manipulation and testing of biological activity. As mentioned above, in this method the proteins considered for screening are allowed to express as fusion proteins (e.g. virus coat proteins) in such a manner that they are accessible to the surface of the bacteriophage particle (figure 8.17). This probe protein is further immobilized over a matrix or support available in the form of a microtitre plate or membrane. Since the phage genetic material is responsible for the synthesis of surface proteins, this approach is based on the idea that phage phenotype and genotype are physically associated with each other. Certainly, the gene encoding the displayed molecule is packed as a single-strained DNA. Proteins that are synthesized in the form of displayed proteins are expressed in fusion with phage coat protein. Several genes are expressed in a bacteriophage library in the form of fusion proteins in the bacteriophage coat protein, for their display over the surface of the virus particle. Now at this point the proteins displayed over the surface resemble the genetic sequence within the phage [43]. Expression libraries containing phage displays have been created for screening with the probes (figure 8.17). This is done for the selection of particles that can efficiently interact with the probe.

After screening of the phage display with the probe, the surface particles that can efficiently interact with the probes are selected and further utilized to re-infect colonies of *E. coli*. Phage particles obtained after this are again selected to meet

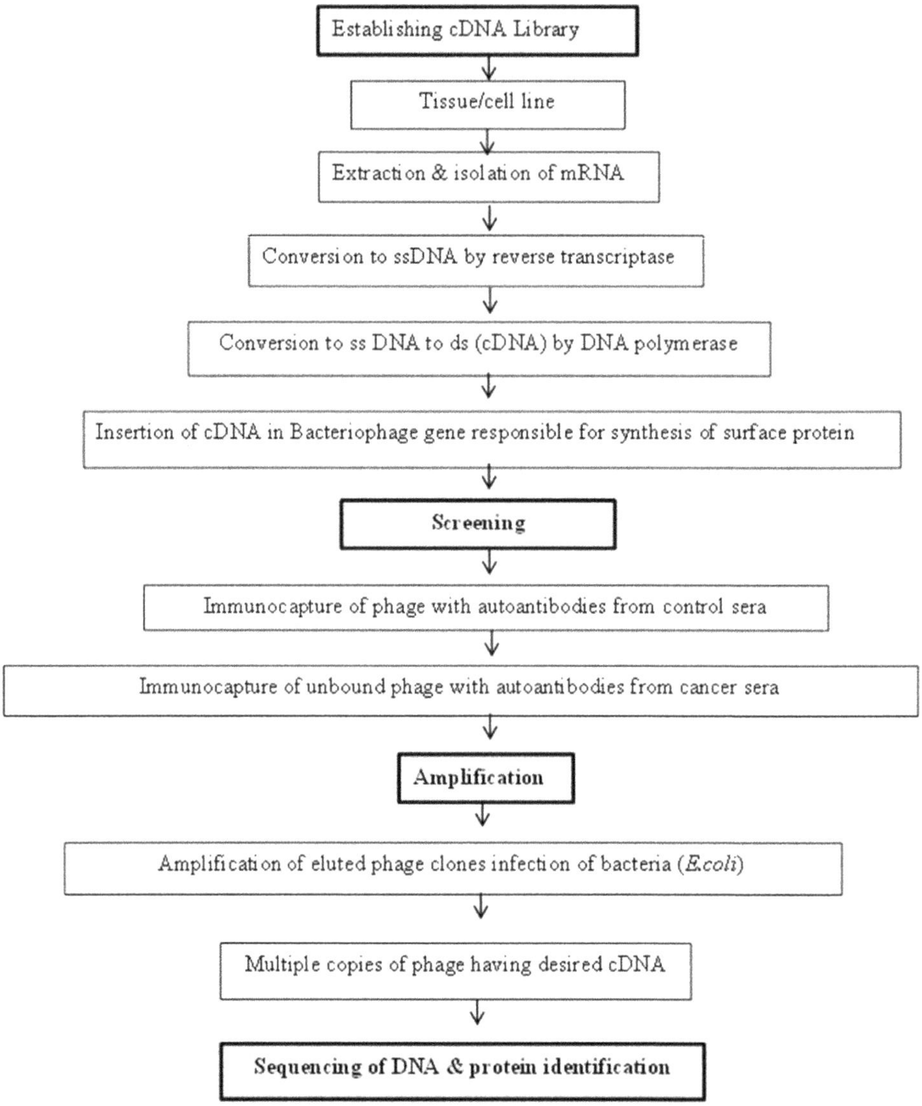

Figure 8.17. Important steps in creating a phage display based genomic library.

the requirements and this is repeated again until the desired expression of proteins is achieved (or not, as the case may be). During the last step the recovered phages are selected to isolate the interactive protein and the gene is responsible for their expression. Genomic libraries compiled using the phage display approach are found to be of great complexity. Thus more efficient screening tools in the array setup are required to allow the selection of suitable proteins with different probes. However, this strategy is yet to be used for genome-scale interaction investigations.

Yeast two-hybrid (Y2H) screening (introduced above) is a well established *in vivo* genetic approach for protein interaction studies, and is currently the most sensitive high-throughput method for interactomics research. This approach has offered the basis for a variety of interaction networks formed by different components, primarily proteins. One of the major applications of the hybrid system is to understand transient and dynamic protein–protein interactions. By using the yeast cell system we can test whether interaction between two different proteins takes place or not. The yeast cell system contains DNA which further contains transcription activator binding sites, along with the gene of interest which allows the expression of the desirable reporter protein [43]. So to produce reporter protein, the transcription activator should be activated. This can only be achieved when the target protein makes a complex with the transcription activator protein, which will further bind with the transcription activator site and transfer a signal to the cell to start the transcription of the desired gene, which will lead to the production of desired reporter protein, which ultimately confirms interaction between two proteins. In this case both proteins, i.e., the transcription activator protein and the target protein, contain binding sites in the form of the transcriptional activation domain and DNA-binding domain (figure 8.18), which are also known as

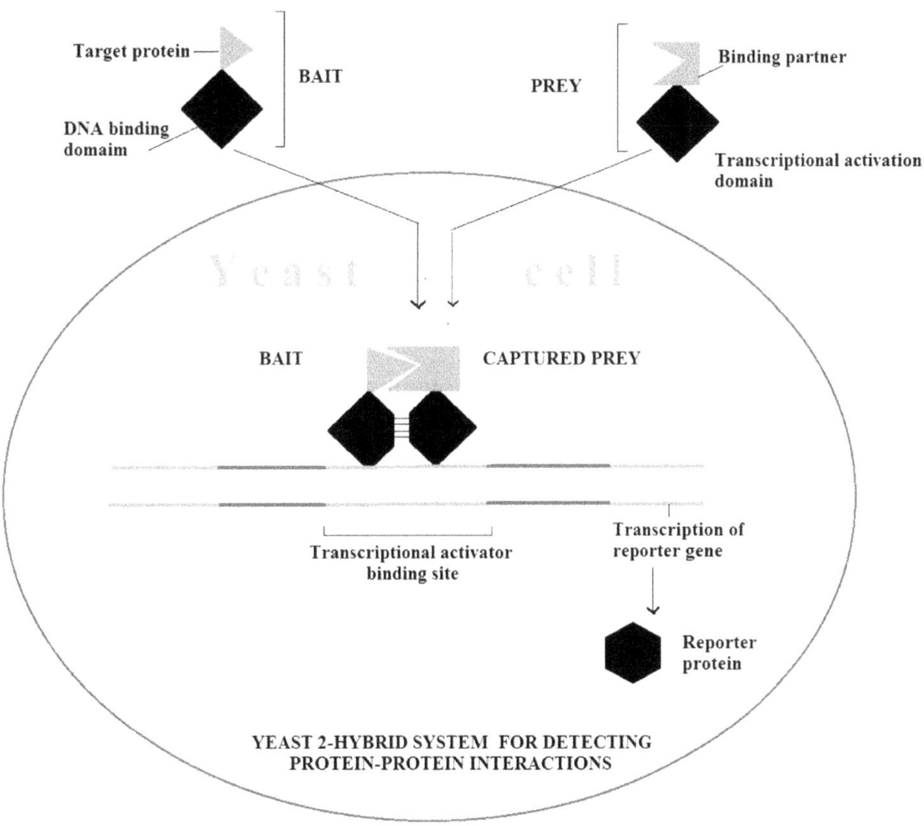

Figure 8.18. The Y2H system for detecting protein–protein interactions.

functionally self-governing domains. These domains interact with each other by covalent or noncovalent association. In addition, they both ('bait' and 'prey') contain their own interactive proteins called the target protein and binding partner (figure 8.18). Their interaction allows the formation of a complex which can bind with the transcriptional activator binding site to yield a reporter protein.

So, if this complex does not bind with the transcription binding site it will not produce the reporter protein, and the response for protein production will be suppressed or halted. Thus if there is no interaction between two proteins then no complex will form in the form of a dimer, and consequently the transcription activator gene will not be activated to activate the gene for protein production. To understand this more deeply we have to understand one concept, that an active transcription factor is only produced if independently expressed DNA-binding and activation domains are allowed to interact (figure 8.18). The approach for the Y2H system is as follows: the target protein is allowed to express as a fusion protein along with the DNA-binding domain (known as the 'bait') and diverse proteins are allowed to express as binding proteins with the activation domain (known as 'prey') [44]. The ultimate goal of Y2H system is to produce a protein by a reporter gene, which is only transcribed when it is activated by the complex formed by the 'bait' with the 'prey'. During the genome-wide mapping of protein interactions, complete libraries of 'baits' and 'preys' are produced. These libraries are assessed for protein interactions using the following:

- the matrix method.
- the random library approach.

Y2H, however, tends to give a high incidence of false positive and false negative outcomes. Another approach is known as GST (glutathione-S-transferase)-pull down. GST is a bacterial enzyme with a high affinity for its substrate glutathione. In particular, the 'bait' protein is expressed as fusion with GST. The proteins that interact with the 'bait' can be copurified, i.e., dragged down from a cell lysate by passing the lysate through a glutathione–sepharose column. This approach is functional on a genomic scale. Protein interaction data from different sources are integrated in databases [40]. Numerous bioinformatics based techniques have been advanced to derive data from such databanks. One of the main challenges is to discover a simple approach to present protein interaction information in an easily available format and in a consistent structure.

8.7 Synthetic genomics

One of the first aims of synthetic genomics is to design new organisms and biological systems to satisfy human needs [33]. In synthetic biology, the aims is to model and create biological components, functions and organisms that do not actually exist in nature or to redesign already existing biological systems to execute new functions. On the other hand, synthetic genomics involves tools for the production of chemically synthesized whole genomes or larger parts of genomes, allowing the simultaneous engineering of numerous changes to the genetic material of organisms (figure 8.18) [45].

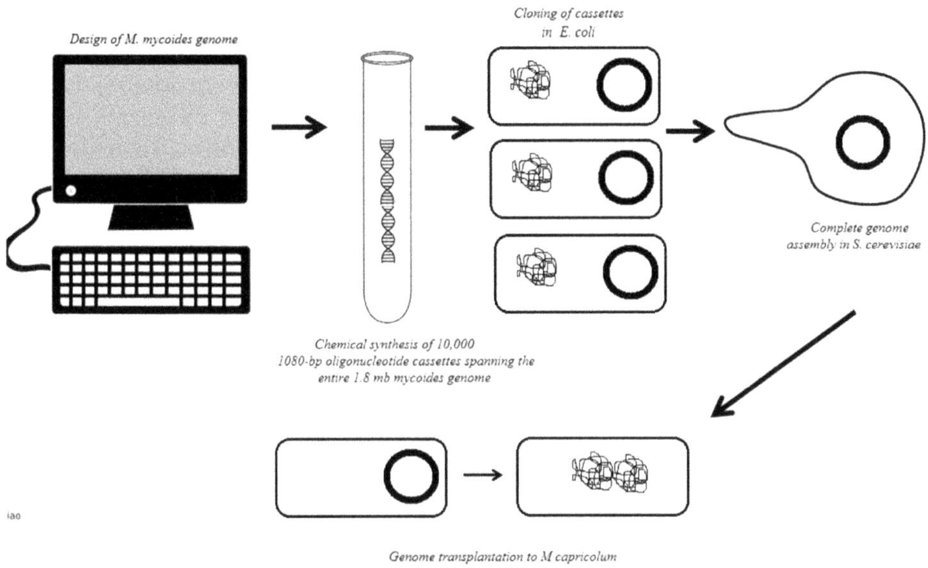

Figure 8.19. Creating a synthetic genome in a bacterial strain.

Synthetic genomes (artificial gene production to produce new DNA or complete live forms) can be defined as a genome assembled from smaller precursor molecules derived by either PCR amplification or chemical synthesis (figure 8.19). Viral genomes were the first to be produced. In 2002 a virus was reconstructed from its chemically synthesized genomes. Itaya and co-workers (2008) synthesized the mouse mitochondrial and rice chloroplast genomes. During the same period Gibson and co-workers produced the complete genome (0.58 million base pairs) of *Mycoplasma genitalium*, which has the smallest genome among the known culturable free-living organisms [46]. The synthetic genome function was assessed by incorporating it into *M. genitalium* cells and transferring their native genomes. Again Gibson and co-workers utilized the *M. genitalium* genome sequence to chemically produce a great number of oligonucleotides, demonstrating the complete genome. Exact chemical synthesis was achieveable for fragments of only up to 100 bases. By means of *in vitro* ligation, these small fragments were suitably arranged to produce 101 minimally overlapping DNA molecules 5–7 kb in length (overlapping 'cassettes'). During the following step, these DNA molecules were ligated successively to produce larger and larger genome segments. Assembly of the genome segments was then performed together, initially in *E. coli* and later in *S. corevisiae*, to derive the entire circular genome of *M. genitalium* (582 970 bp) [47]. To guarantee that the created genome had precisely the same base sequence as the original *M. genitalium*, the sequence used for chemical synthesis, a rough sequence confirmation of the precursor molecules at every stage was performed.

The tomato fruit and leaf are promising for investigating the evolution of gene regulation and the underlying development of different organs. Itaya and colleagues identified over 350 and 700 small RNAs from the tomato fruit and leaf, respectively, and further established a website (http://ted.bti.cornell.edu/digital/sRNA/) for public, searchable access to all of the small RNA sequences, their expression patterns in respective tissues, and their matching genes or predicted target genes [48].

With the help of PCR, Itaya and colleagues generated DNA fragments comprising the entire mouse mitochondrial and rice chloroplast genomess. To design PCR primers that encouraged the amplification of overlapping DNA fragments for the entire genome, they used the genome sequence information. By means of their serial integration into the genome of *Bacillus subtilis*, these precursor DNA fragments were assembled. The genome was removed from the *B. subtilis* genome and purified when the entire set of precursors was incorporated into the *B. subtilis* genome. Synthetic genomes offer several applications. They can allow the regeneration of already vanished organisms, if their genome sequences are known. They will allow documentation of the set of genes vital for cellular life by examining a diversity of minimal genomes. New discoveries in biology may be enabled by designing, synthesizing and examining genomes of different specifications. Synthetic genomes may also allow the complete restructuring of industrial microbes, producing inexpensive, better and even new products. However, numerous technical improvements/developments are required to attain these goals. It should be noted that so far only existing genomes have been reconstructed—designing a functional genome is yet to be accomplished.

8.8 Advanced techniques in proteomics

Advanced techniques in proteomics capture a range of methodologies aimed at the comprehensive analysis of proteins, which is pivotal in understanding biological and pathological processes. The rapid evolution of proteomic methods, stimulated by technological advancements and computational innovations, has significantly broadened the scope of protein analysis. High-throughput proteomics, including next-generation tissue microarrays single-cell and single-molecule proteomics, are at the top, enabling the exploration of the proteome at an unprecedented depth and speed. Mass spectrometry (MS) and its tandem version (MS/MS) remain the foundation for protein identification, quantification, and characterization [49]. Furthermore, quantitative proteomics using mass spectrometry has opened opportunities for comparative analysis of protein abundances across different biological conditions. Besides, advanced separation and prefractionation techniques and protein microarrays provide robust platforms for exploring protein interactions and function. These advancements are helpful in solving the molecular mechanisms causing diseases, discovering novel biomarkers, and developing personalized medicine approaches. Through integrating proteomics with other 'omics' technologies, a more in depth knowledge of cellular dynamics is achievable, propelling the biomedical research field towards more profound discoveries [50, 51].

8.8.1 Mass spectrometry in proteomics

The use of MS is essential for determining the identity and quantity of proteins as well as the post-translational modifications (PTMs) they undergo. MS may reveal a complete

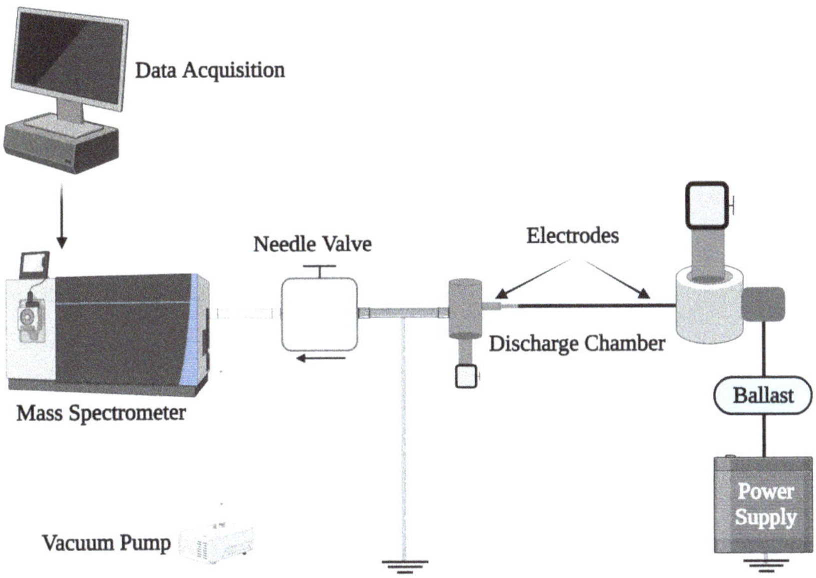

Figure 8.20. Schematic diagram of a mass spectrometer instrumentation system with data acquisition, vacuum, and ionization components.

protein or a subset of composite peptides, expanding the capabilities of classic immunoassays, which find it difficult to do this job. The accuracy and yield of protein identification is improved by MS by the integration of separation and prefractionation methods such as two-dimensional polyacrylamide gel electrophoresis (2D-PAGE) and liquid chromatography (LC). Because it enables continuous separation of proteins from complicated mixtures, the hybrid technique known as liquid chromatography–mass spectrometry (LC–MS) is especially renowned for improving output. In order to expand the dynamic range of measurements, MS is often combined with reversed-phase liquid chromatography (RPLC), which is a typical kind of separation platform based on LC [49]. A schematic diagram of MS is shown in figure 8.20.

8.8.2 Tandem mass spectrometry

MS/MS is a two-stage process where ions are selected based on their mass-to-charge ratio in the first stage, fragmented, and the pieces are then analyzed in the second stage. This technique is invaluable for sequencing peptides and identifying PTMs, thus advancing the protein characterization endeavor. MS/MS is also pivotal for validating the results obtained from high-throughput proteomics studies and significantly impacts quantitative proteomics as well [52]. The general workflow of MS/MS is shown in figure 8.21.

8.8.3 Quantitative proteomics using mass spectrometry

Quantitative proteomics aims to measure the relative or absolute abundance of proteins, which is central to understanding biological systems. MS-based

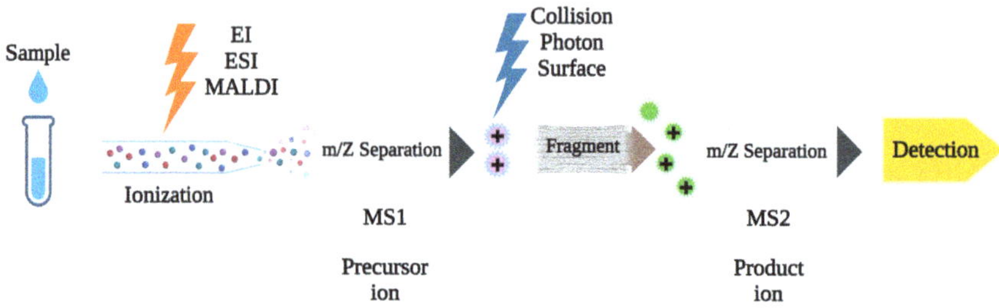

Figure 8.21. MS analysis flow: ionization methods, mass-to-charge (*m*/*z*) separation, and tandem MS for precursor and product ion detection.

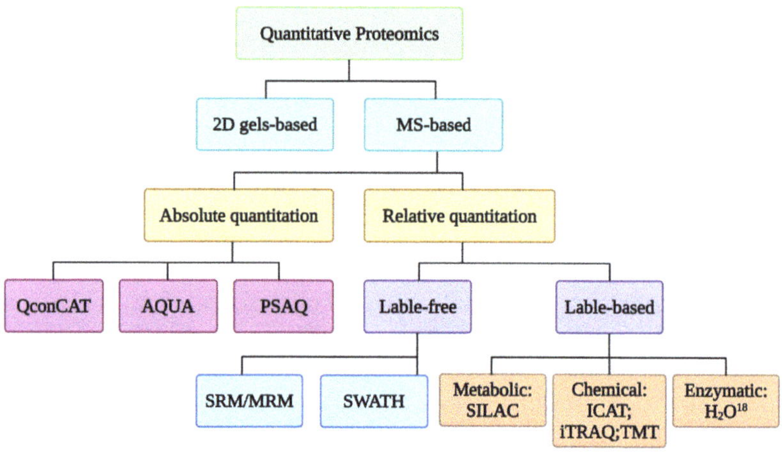

Figure 8.22. Quantitative proteomics techniques: from 2D gel and MS-based approaches to label-based and label-free quantitation methods.

quantitative proteomics methods include label-free quantification, isobaric tags for relative and absolute quantitation (iTRAQ), and tandem mass tags (TMTs). These techniques enable the comparison of protein abundances across different samples, thus facilitating the discovery of proteins associated with diseases and other biological phenomena [53]. Different techniques used in quantitative proteomics are shown in figure 8.22.

8.8.4 Other advanced techniques in proteomics

High-throughput proteomics methods include single-cell proteomics (SCP), next-generation tissue microarrays, and single-molecule proteomics. These approaches help to speed the analysis while also improving the accuracy and depth of proteome coverage. Methods of this kind are very useful throughout the discovery, network analysis, and clinical proteomics stages of the research process. They contribute to the determination of amino acid sequences, unknown protein structures, putative biomarkers, and the creation of clinical tests [49]. Protein microarrays advanced techniques involve antibody microarrays for labeling proteins with captured antibodies, functional microarrays for analyzing purified proteins, and reverse-phase protein microarrays for probing target proteins from cell lysates. They are key in exploring protein–protein interactions, and other protein functionalities [50]. Separation and prefractionation techniques such as 2D-PAGE and LC are critical for separating proteins based on properties like electrical charge and molecular weight, facilitating the subsequent MS analysis. They are essential for handling complex protein mixtures and integral to bottom-up and top-down proteomics approaches [51]. Protein–protein interaction networks (PPIs) are crucial for understanding an organism's biological functionality and intricacies. These networks, also known as interactomes, provide insights into the dynamic interplay among proteins, which is fundamental for numerous biological processes. The interactome, referring to the entirety of protein interactions within a cell, is far more complex than individual protein entities. MS-based proteomics has significantly contributed to deciphering these networks, offering a peek into the interaction dynamics, thus aiding in identifying potential drug targets and understanding disease mechanisms [54]. PTMs significantly diversify the proteome by altering the properties of proteins post-synthesis. These modifications include phosphorylation, acetylation, glycosylation, and methylation. PTMs regulate protein function, signaling, and responses to cellular perturbations. Various proteomic techniques, prominently MS, have become the preferred methods for identifying and quantifying PTMs due to their ability to measure changes in protein abundance and modifications simultaneously [55]. This novel approach combines oligonucleotide barcoding of proteins from individual cells, cell pooling to increase sample size, bulk gel electrophoresis to separate proteins and their PTM isoforms and sequencing related oligonucleotides to determine abundances. This method was used to examine the variations in H2B ubiquitination over the cell cycle in single yeast cells by measuring H2B and its monoubiquitination isoform [56].

8.8.5 Chromatography in proteomics

Proteomics relies heavily on chromatography, a basic method for separating intricate mixtures of proteins and peptides that is necessary since biological systems are diverse and complicated. Proteins and peptides may be separated using chromatographic techniques according to different features, which enables MS to be used for identification and quantification afterward. LC is the main chromatography used in proteomics because it can manage the complexity of proteome samples [57].

8.8.5.1 Liquid chromatography–mass spectrometry (LC–MS)

Combining the physical separation skills of LC with the mass analysis capabilities of MS, LC–MS is a well-respected analytical chemistry method. Proteomics uses LC–MS to detect and quantify individual peptides from complicated peptide mixtures (produced from protein digests). LC is helpful in identifying low-abundance species like post-translationally changed proteins because of its speed, resolution, and sensitivity when separating macromolecules. Proteome characterization and quantification may be achieved by the use of LC for separation and MS for mass analysis [58].

8.8.5.2 Multi-dimensional protein identification technology (MudPIT)

Multi-dimensional protein identification technology (MudPIT) is an advanced proteomics technique that uses 2D chromatographic separation and MS to identify proteins in complex mixtures. Peptides are first separated based on their charge in the first dimension using strong cation exchange chromatography. Reversed-phase chromatography, which divides peptides based on how hydrophobic they are. The resulting peptide mixture is then analyzed by tandem mass spectrometry for protein identification and quantification. MudPIT, which has been used in several proteomic research, facilitates the exploration of complicated protein mixtures. MudPIT is designed to separate peptides in a mixture so that MS can identify and measure individual peptides more accurately [59].

8.9 Proteogenomics

Using the complementing nature of genomic and proteomic data, proteogenomics is an emerging area at the confluence of proteomics and genomics that intends to increase our knowledge of cellular processes and disease pathways. This multi-disciplinary field seeks to supplement proteomic studies with genomic and transcriptome data. By merging many data sources, it is feasible to develop more complete and accurate models of the biological systems under investigation. Integrating genomic and proteomic data is a distinguishing element of proteogenomics, and it has the potential to shed light on previously undiscovered components of both healthy and sick physiologies. Utilizing genetic and transcriptome data, proteogenomics generates individual protein sequence databases. For the identification of new peptides with MS-based proteomic data, these specialized databases are required in the absence of reference protein sequence databases [60]. New proteins may be discovered when genomic and transcriptome data are combined with high-throughput methods like MS-based proteomics. A typical example of how proteogenomics can unmask new proteins is its ability to identify novel biomarkers that may be implicated in various diseases or biological processes, thereby enhancing our understanding and treatment options [61]. Proteogenomics is instrumental in examining the ramifications of genomic abnormalities. For instance, in cancer research, integrating proteins and their post-translational modifications with genomic, epigenomic, and transcriptomic data allows one to investigate deeper into the molecular underpinnings of malignant transformations and therapeutic outcomes. The proteogenomic analysis furnishes a more profound and quantitative characterization of tumor tissues, the potential drivers of the disease and possible therapeutic interventions [62]. The integration process demands robust computational tools and strategies to handle, analyze, and interpret the vast swathes of data generated. Various tools have been developed to handle the challenges associated with integrative proteogenomic approaches, in navigating the complex nature of proteogenomic data [63].

8.9.1 Proteogenomics role in precision medicine

Proteogenomics, a discipline converging proteomics and genomics, is rapidly evolving in precision medicine, mostly due to its capacity to provide a more complete view of cellular functions and disease mechanisms. Proteogenomics facilitates a high-throughput analysis of genes, mRNA, proteins, and metabolites present in biological samples, which are the foundations of genomics, transcriptomics, proteomics, and metabolomics. This amalgamated 'omics' approach is essential for unlocking novel drugs, biomarkers, early diagnosis possibilities, and therapeutic targets in biomedicine [64]. Through proteogenomics, the massive characterization of genetic content within a cell is feasible, either for investigating specific genes or for exploring the coding sequences in whole genomes from minimal DNA amounts. Concurrently, proteomics, a component of proteogenomics, enables a comprehensive characterization of a cell at the protein level, thereby permitting the development of a full-fledged quantitative map of a species' proteome [64]. The divergence between mRNA levels and the encoded protein levels in a cell underscores the significance of proteogenomics. For instance, certain post-translational modifications like glycosylation, phosphorylation, acetylation, or ubiquitinylation significantly impact protein stability, adding layers of complexity to the protein component of a cell, which cannot be deduced from genomics analysis alone. The Human Proteome Project aims to provide a map relating to cell molecular architecture based on human body proteins, which is integral for advancing precision medicine. Advancements in MS and protein microarrays augment the sensitivity for identifying and evaluating proteins in a high throughput format. Proteogenomics provides a unified vision for understanding cellular functions globally, which is vital for accurate diagnosis, therapy, and solving the underlying mechanisms of various conditions like antibiotic resistance and tumor microenvironments [65].

8.9.2 Novel peptide identification in proteogenomics

Novel peptide identification is a critical aspect of proteogenomics. Proteogenomics employs genomic and transcriptomic information to generate customized protein sequence databases. These databases are instrumental in identifying novel peptides not present in reference protein sequence databases from MS-based proteomic data [60]. In proteogenomics, MS data is typically matched against existing mapped peptides in a reference protein database, facilitating the discovery of novel peptides. This cross-referencing aids in the enhancement of genomic annotation and characterizes the protein-coding potential of genomes [66]. SCP is an expanding field that aims to elucidate the proteome of individual cells to grasp the inherent cellular heterogeneity within a population of cells. This endeavor has been enabled by significant advancements in technologies tailored for single-cell analysis. Before diving into individual cells proteome, isolating target cells from a heterogeneous population is imperative. The strategies for this isolation are dependent on several factors, such as the study's aim, the cell's source, the target cell's character, and potential contaminants in the source [67]. The efficiency of western blotting, facilitated by microfluidic devices, enabled single-cell western blotting (scWB). These devices create micrometer-scale polyacrylamide channels, which facilitate the quantification of minimal amounts of protein, eventually yielding single-cell measurements [68]. Advancements in next-generation sequencing or MS have significantly contributed to the progress in SCP, enabling more precise protein identification and quantification at a single-cell level [69]. The advancement in SCP was boosted by advancements in various aspects of MS-based proteomics, encompassing instrument design, sample preparation, chromatography, and ion mobility. The field is approaching a milestone where it can quantify a minimum of 5000 proteins from a single cell. This is a significant step forward, especially for applying SCP on biologically relevant samples instead of cultured cell standards. The advancements in MS instrumentation have significantly elevated the speed, sensitivity, and resolution, pushing the field to a new level [70].

SCP has emerged as a significant asset in the disease diagnostics and treatment model due to its ability to solve the complex cellular heterogeneities inherent within complex diseases like cancer. The critical points elucidating the importance of SCP in disease diagnostics and treatment include: SCP technologies have progressed to a stage where over 1000 proteins from individual mammalian cells can be quantified, offering a new level of coarseness in understanding biological systems. This depth of analysis is vital for delineating the unique molecular signatures of diseased versus healthy cells, thus aiding in accurate disease diagnosis and understanding disease progression. By enabling a mechanistic comprehension of how gene products interact to form cellular phenotypes, SCP holds promise in revealing the cellular complexity of diseases. This is particularly relevant in conditions where cellular heterogeneity is critical in disease manifestation and progression [68]. SCP facilitates a comprehensive assessment of system immunity and tumor microenvironment, which is crucial for effective and safe cancer therapy. By enabling system-wide profiling of protein levels in numerous single cells within the immune system and tumor, SCP provides insights integral for developing more effective immunotherapies [71]. In oncology, SCP is evolving to provide more accurate diagnoses based on the detailed molecular features of cells within tumors. Technologies within SCP allow for the collection of complex data from single cells and highlight methods adaptable to routine cancer diagnostics, thus propelling the field toward more precise and personalized diagnostic and therapeutic strategies [72].

8.10 Single-cell proteomics

SCP is a rapidly advancing field that focuses on analyzing the proteome (the entire set of proteins expressed by a cell) at a single-cell level. Conventional proteomics often looks at cell populations, which may obscure essential differences in proteins' expression, alteration, and function across individual cells. SCP offers more excellent knowledge of the processes behind various diseases by examining cellular heterogeneities which is a critical step in identifying disease subtypes and comprehending the biological course of different illnesses. SCP, which makes it possible to analyze protein expression at the single-cell level, has proven to be a useful tool for drug development and biomarker identification. It makes it possible to validate treatment techniques and identify new pharmacological targets. Creating personalized medicine techniques, whereby therapies are customized based on the distinct proteome profiles of individual patients' cells, depends heavily on the knowledge gathered from single-cell proteomic analysis. SCP can also play a role in therapeutic monitoring by providing detailed insights into how individual cells respond to treatment, thereby aiding in treatment optimization [73].

8.10.1 Technologies enabling single-cell proteomics

The advancements in SCP have been via improvements in mass spectrometric techniques and sequencing-based methods, which are now capable of characterizing single-cell proteomes. Recent enhancements in sample processing, separations, and MS instrumentation now enable the quantification of more than 1000 proteins from individual mammalian cells [74]. Continuous advancements in multiplexing, throughput, resolution, and accuracy in single-cell multi-omics technologies have significantly contributed to a more comprehensive understanding of the genetic landscape of a cell [75]. The methodological and technological advancements now allow for simultaneous genome, epigenome, transcriptome, and proteome profiling within single cells. This multi-omics approach has been facilitated by technologies such as laser capture microdissection (LCM), robotic micromanipulation, fluorescence-activated cell sorting, or microfluidic platforms, which enable the isolation of single cells into individual compartments for detailed analysis. Techniques such as single-cell antibody-based proteomics, RNA transcript detection, single-cell PTM, and proteomic-detection methods using antibody complexes have been developed better to understand proteomic profiles at a single-cell level. The importance of SCP in disease diagnostics and treatment is emerging as a critical component in personalized medicine and understanding of disease mechanisms at a cellular level [75].

The study of cancer using SCP is a developing subject that has the potential to deliver more precise diagnoses based on the specific cellular and molecular characteristics of cells that are found inside tumors. Conventional diagnostics often depend on histological examination, identification of mutations, and clinical imaging. However, it is possible that these old approaches are not always immediately transferable to established treatment tactics, which makes it difficult to forecast how a patient will respond to therapy. The cellular states that are disclosed via disturbed intracellular signaling pathways can discover functional mutations that are common in subgroups of cancer, which improves diagnostic accuracy [72]. SCP could be validated through clinical trials where serial samples before and during treatment can reveal excessive clonal evolution and therapy failure. This field is anticipated to ignite a diagnostic revolution that better aligns diagnostics with the current biological understanding of cancer, thereby refining therapeutic strategies [72]. The discovery of disease-specific, phenome-specific, and therapy-specific diagnostic biomarkers and therapeutic targets is of great value and could be significantly propelled by the advancements in SCP technologies. The rapidly advancing single-cell protein analysis tools provide insights into protein collections with great relevance to cell and disease biology. This deeper understanding is critical for explaining the underlying mechanisms of various diseases at a molecular level [76]. SCP allows for a coarse understanding of biological systems, thereby transforming biomedical research. This is crucial for tailoring treatment plans according to individual patients' unique cellular and molecular profiles, marking a significant stride towards personalized medicine [74].

8.11 Clinical and diagnostic proteomics

Clinical and diagnostic proteomics relies heavily on identifying biomarkers, proteins or protein networks that may be used to assess disease status, predict disease development, or track therapeutic efficacy. The discovery and validation of biomarkers are crucial milestones in clinical and diagnostic proteomics. For this, methods like protein microarrays and MS are often used. Protein microarrays make high-throughput investigation of protein interactions and activities possible, whereas MS is very effective at detecting and quantifying proteins. To effectively treat diseases, early diagnosis using biomarkers is essential. For instance, particular protein biomarkers may identify the existence of malignancies at an early stage. Keeping an eye on certain biomarker levels may assist medical professionals in determining how well a treatment plan works. Additionally, biomarkers may be utilized to estimate the course of a disease and assist in adjusting treatment strategies. The complexity and variability of the human proteome make it challenging to identify reliable biomarkers. The heterogeneity in protein expression may originate from genetic, epigenetic, and environmental variables [77]. To prove their validity and relevance, putative biomarkers must be verified in more significant, more varied groups once they are discovered. By combining proteomics data with transcriptomics and genome data (a multi-omics approach), disease causes may be better understood, and reliable biomarkers can be found. Further progress in biomarker discovery is anticipated to be driven by ongoing improvements in proteomics technology, such as more sensitive and accurate mass spectrometers and improved computational tools for data processing. A vast quantity of genetic data that may be examined to find possible therapeutic targets has been made available by the completion of the human genome project. Proteomic analysis serves a similar purpose by identifying proteins implicated in disease processes that may be targeted by pharmaceuticals. To find chemicals with a specific biological function quickly, high-throughput screening (HTS) techniques are utilized. This can potentially result in the discovery of novel pharmacological targets [78]. By studying big datasets and predicting which proteins would be feasible targets, computational technologies such as database analysis and machine learning can assist in identifying new drug targets [79]. Potential targets must be verified to confirm their importance in the disease process once they have been discovered. Several experiments may be used, such as *in vitro* and *in vivo* tests. Technological innovations like mice knockout models and short interfering RNA (siRNA) may verify the function of putative therapeutic targets in disease processes. Clinical trials are used to determine whether treating human patients with drugs targeting specific proteins results in the expected outcomes [78]. The development of therapeutic proteins is predicated on comprehending pathogenic pathways. Therapeutic proteins that target these molecules may be developed due to the discovery of essential proteins in disease processes. To put a therapeutic protein through its pace and put it to use in patients, it must be manufactured in large enough numbers. To guarantee the accurate and pure production of the proteins, sophisticated bioprocessing processes are required. Much like other medications, therapeutic proteins need extensive testing to guarantee their safety and efficacy. Preclinical research, clinical trials, and regulatory approval procedures fall under this category. Diseases as diverse as cancer, autoimmunity, and infection may all be treated using therapeutic proteins. They are a rapidly developing and crucial category of medications in contemporary medicine [80].

8.12 Metaproteomics

Metaproteomics is a developing area that comprises the large-scale identification and quantification of proteins from microbial communities, therefore supplying direct insights into the phenotypes of microorganisms at the molecular level. This method not only facilitates the identification of *in situ* carbon sources of community members and the absorption of labeled substrates but also allows the measurement of per-species biomass, the assessment of community structure, and the identification of microbial community members [81]. Metaproteomics contributes to direct knowledge of the molecular characteristics of microbial communities through the large-scale identification and quantification of proteins from microbial communities. To determine the composition of a community, scientists have developed advanced metaproteomic methods that enable the measurement of species-specific biomass. The expressed metabolism and physiology of microbial community members are analyzed using this method, which aids in the functional analysis of microbial communities [82]. Metaproteomics provides information on population equilibration, interactions between microbial species within a community, and stability of microbial communities [83].

In the past ten years, environmental materials such as ocean water, activated sludge, acid mine drainage biofilms, and plant or animal tissues have all been examined using metaproteomics [84]. The metabolic pathways and signaling activities of the gut microbiota have been investigated by examining their taxonomy and functional diversity using metaproteomics [85]. The gut microbiota is the most complex microbial community in the human body, and it may be possible to employ metaproteomics to understand its taxonomy and function better. The interaction between the host and the bacteria in the gut may significantly affect the state of health or illness. Next-generation sequencing (NGS) has made it much more practical to study the gut microbiota, improving our knowledge of the microbiome's function in health and disease [85]. The microbiota that resides in the human gut is vital to human health for its involvement in vitamin production, management of the immune system, and providing support for the digestive system. Researchers study the functional properties of gut microbiota using metaproteomics to understand how it contributes to health. This method involves analyzing proteins to uncover the roles of microbial communities in maintaining human health [86]. Dysbiosis, also known as the disturbance of the microbiota in the gut, has been related to several disorders, some of which include problems with mental health, diabetes, obesity, and gastrointestinal problems. Metaproteomics is what makes the study of the functional activities of microbiota feasible. It also sheds light on how variations in microbiota may contribute to disease states [87].

Increased use of metaproteomics in clinical settings has resulted from recent advances in the field, allowing for more accurate monitoring of microbiome health and perhaps facilitating the detection and treatment of disorders related to microbiome imbalances. Microbial communities' intricacy and dynamic character provide several computational hurdles for the metaproteomics study. The large-scale identification and quantification of proteins from microbial communities generate massive data. Analyzing this data to extract meaningful insights requires advanced computational tools and methods. Metaproteomic analyses' success relies heavily on the availability and completeness of protein databases against which the acquired data can be matched. Incomplete or outdated databases can significantly hinder the analysis. There is a need for more advanced algorithms capable of handling the complexity of metaproteomic data, including the identification and quantification of proteins, as well as the analysis of microbial community structure and function. Integrating metaproteomic data with other omics data (genomic, transcriptomic) to obtain a complete understanding of microbial communities requires sophisticated computational approaches [85].

8.13 Emerging topics in proteomics

8.13.1 Data-independent acquisition (DIA)

Data-independent acquisition (DIA) proteomics is a newly established global MS-based proteomics method. In DIA methods, precursor ions are separated and fragmented within preset isolation windows. Following fragmentation, each window's ions are examined using a high-resolution mass spectrometer [88]. DIA is an appealing alternative to the conventional shotgun proteomics methodologies, particularly for quantitative research. This method has a variety of applications, some of which include the proteome investigation of enzymes and transporters involved in drug metabolism [88]. The digital proteome maps generated by the next-generation proteomic technology DIA-MS are permanent and allow for highly reproducible backwards investigation of cellular and tissue specimens. Proteomics employing DIA–MS has evolved, and so have the tools available for evaluating the data it generates [89].

8.13.2 Top-down proteomics

Bottom-up proteomics, the standard method used in the field, necessitates the digestion of proteins into peptides before any analysis can be performed. However, it is possible to study proteins operating from the outside in. This method provides a more realistic image of the biological processes under investigation since PTMs are examined in their natural environments [90]. Moreover, top-down proteomics aids in finding protein isoforms and sequence variants, both of which are crucial to a comprehensive understanding of the proteome's numerous activities and features. This approach provides a more accurate description of protein structures and interactions, which helps the molecular mechanisms underpinning a broad range of biological and pathological events. Top-down proteomics is becoming increasingly popular as a method for understanding complex biological systems and improving proteome research because of these advantages [91].

8.13.3 Targeted proteomics and selected reaction monitoring (SRM)

Targeted proteomics is being recognized as a reliable protein quantification technique in clinical practice and biomedical research systems biology. This is because certain protein classes may be zeroed in on using focused proteomics. The basic methodology in targeted proteomics is called selected reaction monitoring (SRM), while another term for this method is multiple reaction monitoring (MRM) [92]. Targeted MS, or SRM, is a different method for proteomics than the more prevalent 'shotgun' technique. This approach out performs in searching several samples for the same set of proteins, such as those found in cellular networks or potential biomarkers [92]. Surface resonance microscopy, often also known as SRM, performed on triple quadrupole mass spectrometers was the quantitative approach considered to be the gold standard for the study of small molecules for many years. SRM has recently been identified as having utility in proteomics as a good device for quantitative analysis [93].

8.13.4 Proteomics in plant research

Proteomics based on MA has contributed much to our knowledge of plant biology in recent years. Proteomics has evolved from an ideal discipline into a powerful resource for the biological sciences, contributing to our understanding of plant resistance mechanisms and the methods by which organisms carry out their functions [94]. Proteomics has not yet reached its full potential in plant biology, nevertheless. The challenges include analyzing orphan plant species, small and resistant proteins, PTM research, and interactions with other proteins, DNA, RNA, and metabolites [95]. Increased agricultural productivity and plant resilience to stress are two areas where proteomics has made a difference. Proteomics has seen a rise in popularity during the 1990s, with the development of more sensitive MS instruments and the availability of genomic data for more species. The proteomics study focuses on protein entities since these molecules drive all biochemical and physiological processes [96]. A thorough knowledge of plant responses to biotic stress requires an understanding of protein PTMs and subcellular localization. Because it can analyze complex protein mixtures, LC–MS technology is the primary approach for spatial proteomics and PTMs. This technical development contributes to the knowledge of protein–protein interactions, cellular signaling networks, and the molecular processes underlying the response to biotic stress [97].

8.14 Ethical and data management issues in proteomics

Proteomics is just one area of medicine that has seen a dramatic surge in the use of human-origin products over the last several decades. Many moral and legal questions are raised by its widespread use in cancer, genetic diseases, and other therapeutic fields. Consent, anonymity, privacy, and secondary use of data are all critical ethical issues. When dealing with human samples, frameworks are urgently needed to control data exchange, access, and general management of proteomic data [98]. Proteomics data is growing at an accelerated pace, which brings both benefits and problems. Robust data management systems are necessary for processing large-scale proteomic data, often incorporating biological materials like cells, organelles, or fluids. To further research in this discipline, these platforms must guarantee data integrity, accessibility, and repeatability. Additionally, discovering new disease biomarkers and possible treatment targets depends on efficient data management techniques [99]. The advancement of proteomics, the confirmation of discoveries, and the promotion of joint initiatives depend on data exchange. However, there are moral concerns when dealing with a human being's data. Issues include handling secondary data uses, keeping data anonymous, and getting informed permission from participants. To solve these problems, we need robust protocols and platforms for exchanging data which comply with applicable regulations. Mainly, when working with proteomic data obtained from human samples, privacy is a significant problem. It is essential to protect the privacy and confidentiality of the people whose data is being shared or examined. This calls for reliable de-identification methods, safe data transmission and storage protocols, and stringent access restrictions. People should also be fully informed about the procedures to preserve their privacy, who will access their data, and how it will be used [100].

Bioinformatics resources and data repositories, alongside open-source platforms for proteomic analysis, are quintessential for the proficient management, analysis, and sharing of proteomic data. Proteomic data, being large and complex, necessitates the use of specialized bioinformatics resources and repositories. Many publicly available data repositories support protein-related information management, hypothesis generation, and biological knowledge discovery. Key characteristics of these repositories include well-documented resources, peer-reviewed or selected by reputable consortia like the UniProt consortium, and well-maintained databases. The guidelines for data submission, file format standardization, and submission systems are provided by repositories such as ProteomeXchange. These repositories are further categorized into archives that are responsible for data submission and resources for peptide and protein identification. These resources may include information about variants, mutations, or PTMs [101]. Repositories store a wide range of data types and use a variety of data submission mechanisms. They support numerous formats and provide data mining and visualization capabilities, often enumerating the data contents of model organisms for each resource. On the other hand, the public deposition and storage infrastructure for MS-based proteomics data lags behind that of genomics. The intrinsic complexity of proteomics data and the multiplicity of data types and experimental procedures involved are ascribed to this difference. These present difficulties in standardizing data input and retrieval protocols, impeding the creation of strong archives similar to those created in genomics [92, 102].

8.14.1 Open-source platforms for proteomic analysis

Open-source platforms facilitate the analysis and interpretation of proteomic data. Various tools and packages are available, tailored to different aspects of proteomic analysis.

- Tidyproteomics aims to streamline the analysis of quantitative proteomics data using MS through data standardization and facilitating data exploration across different platforms, catering to various R programming skill levels [103].
- Visualize is a free, multi-functional tool for proteomics data analysis, offering compiled executable files for Windows and Mac OS X alongside the complete PERL source code [104].
- Amica is web-based software that simplifies high throughput data analysis in quantitative proteomics, particularly for users with limited background knowledge [105].
- ProteoWizard facilitates the development of proteomic data analysis tools and format conversion through an open-source software platform [106].
- Informed-Proteomics is a software suite targeted at top-down proteomics analysis, encompassing a range of tools like an LC–MS feature finding algorithm (ProMex), a new database search algorithm (MSPathFinder), and an interactive results viewer (LcMsSpectator) [107].
- MaxQuant is a comprehensive software suite for analyzing large mass spectrometric datasets, mainly aimed at high-resolution MS data analysis and capable of handling extensive proteomic datasets [108].
- OpenMS is an open-source framework offering tools for processing MS data, including proteomic and metabolomic data analysis [109].
- PeptideShaker is an open-source software that interprets proteomics identification results from multiple search engines [110].
- SearchGUI is an open-source graphical user interface for configuring and running proteomics identification search engines [111].
- Skyline is a free and open-source program that helps develop quantitative methodologies and analyze mass spectrometer data, making it ideal for focused proteomics experiments [112].
- The Perseus software architecture allows for the interactive study of massive datasets, making it ideal for proteomics research [113].
- Pyteomics is a set of Python modules for analyzing proteome data, including parsing proteomics data files, manipulating data, and doing statistical analysis [114].

8.15 Cellular and molecular dynamics

Proteins are fundamental entities in molecular biology, orchestrating the functions of organisms. Their behaviors are far from static; instead, they exhibit dynamic characteristics essential for their functionality [115, 116]. Protein dynamics are intimately intertwined with their functions. The 3D structures of proteins are foundational to their function, but the dynamics, including conformational changes, enable proteins to interact with other molecules and carry out their roles [115]. The dynamism of proteins spans a field from fast vibrational states to folding/unfolding events. These conformational changes are crucial for many biological functions, allowing proteins to adapt to different molecular interactions and cellular environments [116]. The protein folding process, where a protein acquires its functional structure from a linear chain of amino acids, is a fundamental aspect of protein dynamics. The correct folding of proteins is crucial as it directly impacts their functionality. On the other hand, protein misfolding is associated with a broad range of diseases and may lead to dysfunction when proteins do not acquire or maintain their proper structure. Plaques occur in the cells of many neurodegenerative diseases, including Parkinson's and Alzheimer's. These plaques may be the result of misfolded proteins aggregating and forming. Numerous substances, including other proteins, nucleic acids, and small molecules, may interact to affect the folding and misfolding of proteins. The cellular environment, which may be very important due to chaperone proteins, may also be very important in ensuring correct protein folding or reducing the effects of protein misfolding [116].

8.15.1 Molecular mechanisms of protein function

Protein function is inherently complex, regulated by a variety of molecular mechanisms. Protein kinases are enzymes that modify the structure of other proteins by adding phosphate groups (a chemical modification) to them via phosphorylation. In contrast, phosphatases are responsible for the elimination of these phosphate groups, which is referred to as the dephosphorylation process. A proper balance between the activity of kinases and phosphatases is crucial to properly functioning proteins and, by extension, cells [117]. When a molecule, also known as a ligand, attaches to a specific site on a protein, the protein's function may be dramatically changed. This region, also known as the ligand-binding site, often has a cavity formed by a particular arrangement of amino acids. The protein's function may be altered due to conformational changes induced by ligand interaction. Phosphorylation, in which a phosphate group is transferred from a donor molecule (such as ATP) to a protein, is an example of a reversible process. The protein's shape may vary due to this insertion, affecting its function by changing its interactions with other proteins or subcellular localization [118].

8.15.2 Protein degradation pathways

Protein degradation is a process that cells go through to maintain their protein homeostasis. Proteasomes are protein complexes that use the process of proteolysis to break down damaged or superfluous proteins. A chemical process called proteolysis breaks down peptides into their constituent amino acids. A significant pathway called the Ubiquitin-Proteasome System, or UPS, involves the proteasome first destroying the proteins marked for death by the ubiquitin protein, which is a small protein. Lysosomes are membrane-bound organelles that contain enzymes to degrade waste materials and cellular debris. They are responsible for degrading long-lived proteins, insoluble protein aggregates, and even entire organelles through processes like endocytosis, phagocytosis, or autophagy [119]. The endosomal pathway is part of the lysosomal pathway, where proteins are sorted and sent to lysosomes for degradation. Post endocytosis, some cell surface proteins are recycled, while others are marked for degradation and sent to the lysosomes [119].

8.15.3 Post-translational modifications and protein function

PTMs are crucial molecular alterations that occur on proteins after their biosynthesis, significantly affecting their function, stability, and interactions with other cellular entities. PTMs refer to modifications on proteins' amino acid side chains occurring after their biosynthesis. Over 400 different types of PTMs have been identified, each potentially impacting various aspects of protein function. These modifications are indispensable molecular regulatory mechanisms arranging diverse cellular processes [120]. Protein PTMs significantly expand proteins' capabilities by adding new functions and dynamically regulating protein activity. They are able to do this by adjusting the interactions between molecules. Reversible attachments to nucleophilic functional groups on amino acid side chains are the common conception of protein-tyrosine modifications, with the polypeptide backbone remaining mostly unchanged [121]. A key regulatory mechanism for managing protein function, expression, location, and interactions with other biological components is protein PTM. Proteins have amino acid residues that either have chemical groups added to them or removed from them. Common types of PTM include phosphorylation, ubiquitylation, methylation, and acetylation. PTMs play a broad range of biological activities, which serves as an example of their significance in molecular and cellular biology [122]. PTMs need proteolytic cleavages, the formation of S-S cystine bonds, and the formation of asparagine-linked carbohydrate chains. Each of these events has a distinct impact on the protein's function and structure [123].

8.15.4 Cellular signaling pathways

The proper functioning of cellular signaling is essential for the appropriate control of cellular activity and the preservation of cellular integrity. In order to trigger a reaction from inside the cell, signals must be sent from the cellular membrane to the interior of the cell. Signaling pathways, like the Ras/MAPK and PI3K/AKT/mTOR pathways, are implicated in many cellular processes and are often thought to be involved in diseases like cancer [124]. The JAK/STAT signaling pathway is another pivotal signaling route at cellular, molecular, and genomic levels, involved in transmitting information received from extracellular signals to the nucleus, resulting in DNA transcription and expression of specific genes [125]. A conserved repertoire of intercellular signaling pathways enables communication between animal cells. These pathways are well-studied from a molecular perspective, although an operational understanding to control cellular behaviors rationally often lacks [126]. Multiple cellular processes, including as proliferation, differentiation, growth, and cell-cycle transition, as well as neurotransmission and pathogen-sensing, are governed by cellular signaling [127].

8.15.5 Proteomic analysis of signaling networks

The proteomic analysis of signaling networks involves studying the proteome to understand cell signaling pathways and networks. Critical regulators of biological activities, kinases, and phosphatases are integral parts of protein phosphorylation signaling networks. Proteomics, inherently a systems science, investigates individual proteins and their expressions and goes into the interplay of proteins, protein complexes, signaling pathways, and network modules. This field has seen a rapid accumulation of data in recent years [128]. MS has become an essential technique in the research of several aspects of cell signaling since it can be used to identify and quantify PTMs, characterize protein–protein interactions, and analyze changes in protein expression. Progress in the proteomic technique, especially in computational proteomics, has made it feasible to characterize a whole proteome quantitatively. Stable isotope labeling of amino acids in cell culture (SILAC) and isobaric tagging for relative and absolute quantification are two of the most widely used methods for MS-based measurement of proteins and PTMs (iTRAQ). Hundreds of phosphorylation and acetylation sites have been accurately determined by means of high-resolution quantitative MS. This has paved the way for both targeted functional analysis of specific proteins and broader 'systems-wide' investigations. Global signaling networks, as well as the dynamics of these networks in response to different cellular perturbations, that have been illuminated by the use of high-resolution quantitative MS bioinformatic proteomic data analysis may provide light on the origins and evolution of signaling networks, as well as the global kinase–substrate interactions [129].

8.15.6 Signaling pathway dysregulation in disease

Signaling pathways are intricately connected to numerous diseases due to their crucial role in maintaining cellular function and communication. Dysregulation in these pathways can lead to a multitude of diseases. Examples of factors that contribute to the oncogenesis and heterogeneity of lymphoid malignancies include dysregulated oncogenic signaling pathways and aberrant genomic changes. Disease pathophysiology may be better understood, and tailored therapeutics can be developed by focusing on the underlying processes of these dysregulated signaling pathways and the potential value of pathway-related biomarkers [130]. Furthermore, minor phenotypic changes in signaling pathways are implicated in causing significant human diseases such as hypertension, heart disease, diabetes, and various psychiatric illnesses. Such phenotypic remodeling alters the behavior of cells, disrupts their usual functions, and results in disease. Specific signaling pathways, like the mTOR signaling pathway, play intricate roles in cellular functions, and their dysregulation is associated with several diseases, particularly neurodegenerative disorders [131].

8.15.7 Targeting signaling pathways in drug discovery

Targeting signaling pathways for drug discovery is a promising strategy for developing novel therapeutics for various diseases. The Hippo pathway, for instance, has been explored across biological processes and diseases, and recent studies have shed light on its potential as a therapeutic target in cancer, fibrosis, and wound healing. Likewise, the Transforming Growth Factor-β (TGFβ) signaling pathway, implicated in disorders like cancer, fibrosis, and inflammation, has emerged as an attractive target for drug development [132]. The process of targeting signaling pathways extends to identifying crucial strategies, targets, and opportunities in drug discovery, enabling therapeutics to be developed to modulate these pathways for disease treatment. Recent advances in cancer drug discovery, for instance, have led to the development of signaling-based cancer therapies. Synthetic lethality is employed to target 'undruggable' proteins and treat drug-resistant cancers by perturbing specific signaling pathways, thus highlighting the potential of targeting signaling pathways in drug discovery [132].

8.15.8 Crosstalk between signaling pathways

Crosstalk between signaling pathways is a fundamental aspect of cellular signaling networks, facilitating the integration and coordination of multiple signaling inputs to ensure appropriate cellular responses. Molecular biologists and geneticists have spent the better part of the past two decades dissecting intracellular signaling networks in individual cells, revealing extensive crosstalk across crucial signaling pathways, especially in animals. Despite the apparent integration of several signals at gene promoters, reports of this crosstalk in plants are few [133]. One manifestation of crosstalk is observed in nuclear receptor signaling, where coupled nuclear receptor-induced signaling pathways exhibit either a direct or an indirect interplay, which could be additive or antagonistic. This crosstalk is essential for achieving precise control over cellular responses [134]. The Mitogen-Activated Protein Kinase (MAPK) cascades are well-known for the crosstalk between their constituent classical signaling pathways, such as ERK1/2, c-Jun N-terminal kinase (JNK), p38, and ERK5. These sub-pathways allow for the successive transmission of phosphorylation events by transporting signals across a chain of proteins. Phosphorylation events provide interaction and mutual influence across different signaling pathways, guaranteeing accurate signal transmission and manipulation. Cancer, which is characterized by the interplay of numerous signaling pathways to either promote or hinder tumor formation, is a prime example of the importance of crosstalk in the setting of sickness. Understanding the interplay between various signaling pathways may help develop novel therapeutic approaches. For instance, new avenues in the fight against cancer have been explored by exploring strategies to build anti-CSC medicines that target the crosstalk between signaling pathways in cancer stem cells (CSCs). The hope is that by adopting this approach, we may find better ways to treat cancer [135]. Cells can now react correctly to disruptions in homeostasis due to the development of crosstalk across signaling pathways. The connections that are made between significant signaling channels offer a feedback mechanism. This system makes it easier for cells to remain intact and enables a coordinated response to various stimuli [136].

8.16 Membrane proteomics

Membrane proteomics is a subdiscipline of proteomics, a larger area of research that focuses on the detailed examination of proteins present in membranes. Numerous cellular processes depend on these proteins, such as nutrition transport, bioenergetic activities, cell adhesion, and signal transduction [137]. Due to the challenges of solubilizing, isolating, and identifying membrane proteins, the area of membrane proteomics has generally been understudied. Since it is estimated that more than 30 percent of all proteins in Nature are located in membranes, membrane proteomics research has been mostly neglected. Recent developments in membrane proteomics have made major contributions to our knowledge of the intricate relationships between lipids and proteins that are necessary for healthy cell function [138].

8.16.1 Techniques for membrane protein analysis

Multiple methods and tools have been developed to investigate membrane proteins and their dynamic properties. The use of computer modeling and machine learning has been used to study protein membrane structures. In addition to extending to a wide variety of structural properties, such as lipid interactions, allostery, and structure prediction, these computational methods may be utilized to sidestep challenges associated with experimental characterization [139]. The essentials of building and evaluating membrane and membrane protein simulations have been addressed. These simulations may be carried out by following the precise instructions provided in earlier sources. The three most common single-molecule techniques used on membrane proteins are fluorescence correlation spectroscopy, single-particle tracking, and atomic force microscopy, and their principles are explained here. These approaches have greatly aided the area of membrane protein research by offering insights into the behavior of specific membrane proteins. Understanding the structure and function of membrane proteins requires efficient production, solubilization, and analysis. The amphipathic structure of membrane proteins makes them challenging to investigate, although numerous approaches have been devised to circumvent this obstacle [140].

8.16.2 Membrane protein structure and function

Membrane proteins are essential to a wide variety of biological functions because they act as conduits for information exchange between the inside and outside of the cell. Understanding the relationship between membrane protein structure and function is crucial for elucidating the function of membrane proteins in cellular physiology. How a protein binds to the lipid bilayer provides a valuable categorization scheme for membrane proteins. Proteins in membranes may be classified as either integral (crossing the whole membrane) or peripheral (associating with the surface but not penetrating the membrane) [141]. Furthermore, membrane proteins often have two regions: a hydrophilic portion that interacts with water and a hydrophobic region that interacts with the lipid bilayer. Both of these areas aid the movement of the protein across the membrane. The movement of ions and larger solutes across membranes, the promotion of intracellular communication, and the catalysis of chemical reactions are just a few of the functions membrane proteins perform. They are also engaged in cell adhesion, which aids in cell attachment to the extracellular matrix or neighboring cells, and signal transduction, where they may start intracellular signaling cascades in response to external signals. They aid in cell adhesion by assisting cells in sticking to the extracellular matrix, and they may begin intracellular signaling cascades in signal transduction [142]. The communication between proteins and lipids is crucial to the membrane's function. As a result, ion transport and other membrane protein functions may be altered by the lipid milieu in which they are embedded [143].

8.16.3 Membrane proteins in disease

Mutations or improper regulation of membrane proteins may result in a wide range of disorders. Mutations in membrane proteins have been linked to a number of diseases. One such mutation causes congenital hyperthyroidism and is designated V509A in the thyrotropin receptor. Hereditary deafness, Charcot–Marie–Tooth disease, and Dejerine–Sottas syndrome are also associated with mutations in membrane proteins [144]. Diseases can also arise from misassembling membrane proteins, where incorrect interactions in the folding and assembly of integral α-helical membrane proteins lead to functional aberrations. Membrane proteins play a significant role in oncology, especially those regulating the proliferation of tumor cells and affecting the immune response. Understanding the function and regulation of membrane proteins can aid in developing novel therapeutic strategies for cancer treatment [145].

8.16.4 Drug targeting of membrane proteins

Membrane proteins (MPs) are crucial targets in drug discovery due to their central roles in cellular processes and interactions with the extracellular environment. Membrane proteins are crucial drug targets across various fields of medicine due to their many important functions, which include transport, signaling, and serving as gatekeepers to the cell [146]. They are implicated in numerous human ailments and can be accessed by small- and large-molecule drugs from their location at the cell surface. The lack of reliable methods for creating functional variants of membrane proteins has historically been a significant barrier in the drug development process [146]. The amphipathic nature of membrane proteins, having both hydrophilic and hydrophobic regions, complicates their analysis and targeting. Advances in targeted protein degradation (TPD) technology, such as proteolysis-targeting chimeras (PROTACs) and lysosome-targeting chimeras (LYTACs), have emerged as significant breakthroughs in drug discovery. LYTACs, designed to degrade extracellular proteins, address some limitations of PROTACs, which are mainly restricted to the degradation of intracellular proteins. Drugging previously undruggable membrane proteins and modulating cellular signaling are now possible because of recent technological advances. These developments enable the regulation of protein–protein interactions, ion transport, and molecule transport in membranes, thereby increasing the number of potential therapeutic targets. Various strategies have been employed in drug discovery targeting membrane proteins. For instance, strategies for expressing, stabilizing, and formulating recombinant multipass MPs as potential small molecule medicines have been suggested [147].

8.17 Subcellular proteomics

Subcellular proteomics is an area of study focused on understanding the protein compositions within various subcellular structures or organelles of a cell. The eukaryotic cell is segmented into several subcellular locations, some of which include membrane-bound organelles and others that do not. Since proteins localize to specific places to perform their functions, it is conceivable for many biological processes to occur simultaneously. Understanding the functions of these subcellular structures, as well as the cellular processes and disorders associated with protein mislocalization, requires an understanding of the location, distribution, and abundance of the proteins contained inside. Hybridization techniques are only one of the numerous methods developed to quantify cellular data. These techniques can potentially advance our understanding of cellular structure and function by facilitating research into organelle composition [148].

8.17.1 Organelle-specific proteomics

Organelle-specific proteomics investigates further into the subcellular level by focusing on the protein compositions inside specific organelles. This approach enables the identification of novel diseases and molecular mechanisms by utilizing techniques to investigate specialized organelles like cilia, affinity proteomics, genetics, and cell biology are all useful tools. For instance, tagging human ciliary proteins helped establish a landscape of proteins, interactions, and complexes unique to this organelle, illuminating hitherto unsuspected complexes and interactions that are only present in the cilium. This detailed analysis linked various cellular components and processes to ciliary signaling and proteostasis, discovering the molecular mechanisms underlying ciliary diseases [149]. Imaging-based spatial proteomics, which requires a proteome-wide library of affinity reagents, a complete collection of cell lines expressing tagged proteins, and setups for high-throughput microscopy, is one of the methodologies used in organelle-specific proteomics. Organellar profiling is another approach that helps to create organellar maps through proteomic profiling, providing a conceptual guide for understanding the spatial distribution of proteins within organelles. In addition, low-abundance, organelle-specific proteins may be better understood with integrated analysis of data obtained from many organelles, which can show common molecular components engaged in coordination across distinct cell compartments [150].

8.17.2 Protein localization and trafficking

Protein localization and trafficking are integral to cellular functionality and organismal health. Proteins must be correctly localized within cellular compartments to perform their functions efficiently. The trafficking of proteins ensures that they are transported to their correct locations post-synthesis. Certain proteins, like G-protein coupled receptors (GPCRs), have their activity, trafficking, and localization regulated by interacting proteins. This regulation is pivotal for the proper functioning of GPCRs and, by extension, the signaling pathways they are involved in. Protein subcellular localization and trafficking studies, particularly those focusing on endomembrane system organelles, make use of current methodologies and organelle markers. These approaches, however, have drawbacks when it comes to studying protein colocalization [151]. Subcellular trafficking is greatly aided by the PTM of proteins by palmitoylation. It plays a role in cellular protein location and function. Measuring protein trafficking's efficacy, kinetics, and processes may be tricky. Protein trafficking across cellular compartments may be studied with the use of a number of technologies that allow for the spatial and temporal monitoring of protein distribution [152].

8.17.3 Proteomics of cellular compartments

The proteomics of cellular compartments investigates into understanding the protein composition within different cellular locations. Understanding the subcellular localizations and dynamics of proteins, or the spatial proteome, is essential for a comprehensive understanding of cell biology. Mature proteome-wide analyses of spatial cellular regulation have resulted from major advances in MS, microscopy, and machine learning algorithms for data interpretation. A few of the features that have come to light from the study include single-cell variations, dynamic protein translocations, developing interaction networks, and proteins localizing to different compartments [153]. Quantitative MS, via organellar profiling or interactomics, may reveal subcellular protein networks, while high-throughput imaging can reveal all proteins inside a cell or a compartment of interest in spatial proteomics. The current approaches in spatial proteomics and transcriptomics are directly compared in order to provide a comprehensive overview of the available tools. Among these methods are those that rely on imaging and sequencing to provide light on the location of proteins inside individual cell compartments [148].

8.17.4 Techniques for subcellular proteomic analysis

It is crucial to comprehend their distribution among the distinct subcellular compartments to obtain insight into the function of proteins and the associated cellular processes. Numerous alternative approaches have been established to analyze the subcellular proteome, each of which comes with its pros and limitations. Subcellular proteomes are often studied by performing cellular fractionation followed by proteomic analysis. Biological components are initially divided into subcellular proteomics according to the variations in their physical or chemical characteristics. Proteomic methods are then used to assess the protein composition of the isolated fractions [154]. Density gradient centrifugation is a dependable method for achieving cellular fractionation. Cellular components are separated using this centrifugation technique based on the buoyant densities of each component. Isolating organelles and other subcellular structures using this approach is common in subcellular proteomics. Fluorescence-assisted organelle sorting is a relatively new technology that employs fluorescence to sort and isolate certain organelles for proteome research. This method makes it possible to extract very pure organelles, which significantly facilitates the following analysis of their proteome. There are a number of spatial proteomics approaches that may be used to analyze protein distribution, abundance, and localization in different cellular compartments. Fluorescent imaging, protein proximity tagging, organelle purification, and cellular-wide biochemical fractionation are all examples of such techniques. The spatial organization of proteins inside a cell may be seen in a variety of ways, depending on the method used [155]. It is crucial to assess and confirm the results of the subcellular proteome analysis utilizing methods such as multiple reaction monitoring, RNA interference, and microscopy. These validation processes aim to confirm the accuracy and dependability of the results obtained from the subcellular proteomic analysis [156].

References

[1] Anderson N G and Anderson N L 1996 Twenty years of two-dimensional electrophoresis: past, present and future *Electrophoresis* **17** 443–53

[2] Wasinger V, Cordwell S J, Cerpa—Poljak A *et al* 1995 Progress with gene—product mapping of the mollicutes: *Mycoplasma genitalium Elcetrophresis* **16** 1090–4

[3] Wasinger V, Duncan M W, Harris R, Williams K L, Humphery-Smith I *et al* 1995 Progress with gene-product mapping of the Mollicutes: *Mycoplasma genitalium Electrophoresis* **16** 1090–4

[4] Wilkins M R *et al* 1996 Progress with proteome projects: why all proteins expressed by a genome should be identified and how to do it *Biotechnol. Genet. Eng. Rev.* **13** 19–50

[5] O'Farrell P H 1975 High resolution two-dimensional electrophoresis of proteins *J. Biol. Chem.* **250** 4007–21

[6] Klose J 1975 Protein mapping by combined isoelectric focusing and electrophoresis of mouse tissues: a novel approach to testing for induced point mutations in mammals *Humangenetik* **26** 231–43

[7] Scheele G A 1975 Two-dimensional gel analysis of soluble proteins. Charaterization of guinea pig exocrine pancreatic proteins *J. Biol. Chem.* **250** 5375–85

[8] Shin J, Lee W and Lee W 2008 Structural proteomics by NMR spectroscopy *Expert Rev. Proteom.* **5** 589–601

[9] Vinarov D A and Markley J L 2005 High–throughput automated platform for nuclear magnetic resonance–based structural proteomics *Expert Rev. Proteom.* **2** 49–55

[10] Ab E *et al* 2006 NMR in the SPINE structural proteomics project *Acta Crystallogr. Sect. D: Biol. Crystallogr.* **62** 1150–61

[11] Robinette D *et al* 2006 Photoaffinity labeling combined with mass spectrometric approaches as a tool for structural proteomics *Expert Rev. Proteom.* **3** 399–408

[12] Sali A *et al* 2003 From words to literature in structural proteomics *Nature* **422** 216–25

[13] Donnarumma D *et al* 2016 The role of structural proteomics in vaccine development: recent advances and future prospects *Expert Rev. Proteom.* **13** 55–68

[14] Hyung S J and Ruotolo B T 2012 Integrating mass spectrometry of intact protein complexes into structural proteomics *Proteomics* **12** 1547–64

[15] Date S V 2008 The Rosetta stone method *Bioinformatics: Structure, Function and Applications* (Springer) pp 169–80
[16] Suhre K 2007 Inference of gene function based on gene fusion events: the rosetta-stone method *Comparative Genomics* (Springer) pp 31–41
[17] Zhang X *et al* 2006 Joint learning of logic relationships for studying protein function using phylogenetic profiles and the Rosetta Stone method *IEEE Trans. Signal Process.* **54** 2427–35
[18] Van Brabant B *et al* 2008 Laying the foundation for a Genomic Rosetta stone: creating information hubs through the use of consensus identifiers *OMICS A J. Integr. Biol.* **12** 123–7
[19] Bucklin A *et al* 2010 A 'Rosetta Stone' for Metazoan zooplankton: DNA barcode analysis of species diversity of the Sargasso Sea (Northwest Atlantic Ocean) *Deep Sea Res. Part II* **57** 2234–47
[20] Williams T A, Wolfe K H and Fares M A 2009 No Rosetta Stone for a sense–antisense origin of aminoacyl tRNA synthetase classes *Mol. Biol. Evol.* **26** 445–50
[21] Marusyk A, Janiszewska M and Polyak K 2020 Intratumor heterogeneity: the Rosetta Stone of therapy resistance *Cancer cell* **37** 471–84
[22] Wasinger V C, Pollack J D and Humphery-Smith I 2000 The proteome of *Mycoplasma genitalium*: chaps-soluble component *Eur. J. Biochem.* **267** 1571–82
[23] Balasubramanian S *et al* 2000 Proteomics of *Mycoplasma genitalium*: identification and characterization of unannotated and atypical proteins in a small model genome *Nucleic Acids Res.* **28** 3075–82
[24] Wasinger V C *et al* 1995 Progress with gene-product mapping of the mollicutes: *Mycoplasma genitalium Electrophoresis* **16** 1090–4
[25] Ali S *et al* 2021 Proteome wide vaccine targets prioritization and designing of antigenic vaccine candidate to trigger the host immune response against the *Mycoplasma genitalium* infection *Microb. Pathog.* **152** 104771
[26] Ferrer-Navarro M *et al* 2006 Proteome of the bacterium *Mycoplasma penetrans J. proteome Res.* **5** 688–94
[27] Benedetti F *et al* 2019 Proteome analysis of *Mycoplasma fermentans* cultured under aerobic and anaerobic conditions *Transl. Med. Commun.* **4** 1–14
[28] Martínez-Torró C *et al* 2021 Functional characterization of the cell division gene cluster of the wall-less bacterium *Mycoplasma genitalium Front. Microbiol.* **12** 695572
[29] Jaffe J D *et al* 2004 The complete genome and proteome of *Mycoplasma mobile Genome Res.* **14** 1447–61
[30] Roachford O S E, Nelson K E and Mohapatra B R 2017 Comparative genomics of four *Mycoplasma* species of the human urogenital tract: analysis of their core genomes and virulence genes *Int. J. Med. Microbiol.* **307** 508–20
[31] Lluch-Senar M *et al* 2013 Comprehensive methylome characterization of *Mycoplasma genitalium* and *Mycoplasma pneumoniae* at single-base resolution *PLoS Genet.* **9** e1003191
[32] Cordwell S J, Basseal D J and Humphery-Smith I 1997 Proteome analysis of *Spiroplasma melliferum* (A56) and protein characterisation across species boundaries *Electrophoresis* **18** 1335–46
[33] Khalid K *et al* 2022 Vaccinomics-aided development of a next-generation chimeric vaccine against an emerging threat: *Mycoplasma genitalium Vaccines* **10** 1720
[34] Whisstock J C and Lesk A M 2003 Prediction of protein function from protein sequence and structure *Q. Rev. Biophys.* **36** 307–40

[35] Schneider T D 1997 Information content of individual genetic sequences *J. Theor. Biol.* **189** 427–41
[36] Braslavsky I *et al* 2003 Sequence information can be obtained from single DNA molecules *Proc. Natl Acad. Sci.* **100** 3960–4
[37] Skolnick J, Fetrow J S and Kolinski A 2000 Structural genomics and its importance for gene function analysis *Nat. Biotechnol.* **18** 283–7
[38] Ofran Y and Rost B 2003 Predicted protein–protein interaction sites from local sequence information *FEBS Lett.* **544** 236–9
[39] Jones S and Thornton J M 1996 Principles of protein-protein interactions *Proc. Natl Acad. Sci.* **93** 13–20
[40] Berggård T, Linse S and James P 2007 Methods for the detection and analysis of protein–protein interactions *Proteomics* **7** 2833–42
[41] Oncley J *et al* 1952 Protein–protein interactions *J. Phys. Chem.* **56** 85–92
[42] Marcotte E M, Xenarios I and Eisenberg D 2001 Mining literature for protein–protein interactions *Bioinformatics* **17** 359–63
[43] Fields S and Song O-k 1989 A novel genetic system to detect protein–protein interactions *Nature* **340** 245–6
[44] Rao V S *et al* 2014 Protein-protein interaction detection: methods and analysis *Int. J. Proteom.* **2014** 147648
[45] Wang L *et al* 2018 Synthetic genomics: from DNA synthesis to genome design *Angew. Chem. Int. Ed.* **57** 1748–56
[46] Luo Z and Dai J 2017 Synthetic genomics: the art of design and synthesis *Sheng wu gong cheng xue bao= Chin. J. Biotechnol.* **33** 331–42
[47] Thi Nhu Thao T *et al* 2020 Rapid reconstruction of SARS-CoV-2 using a synthetic genomics platform *Nature* **582** 561–5
[48] Schindler D 2020 Genetic engineering and synthetic genomics in yeast to understand life and boost biotechnology *Bioengineering* **7** 137
[49] Cui M, Cheng C and Zhang L 2022 High-throughput proteomics: a methodological mini-review *Lab. Invest.* **102** 1170–81
[50] Zubair M *et al* 2022 Proteomics approaches: a review regarding an importance of proteome analyses in understanding the pathogens and diseases *Front. Vet. Sci.* **9** 1079359
[51] Zhang Z *et al* 2014 High-throughput proteomics *Annu. Rev. Anal. Chem.* **7** 427–54
[52] Nesvizhskii A I, Vitek O and Aebersold R 2007 Analysis and validation of proteomic data generated by tandem mass spectrometry *Nat. Methods* **4** 787–97
[53] Sechi S and Oda Y 2003 Quantitative proteomics using mass spectrometry *Curr. Opin. Chem. Biol.* **7** 70–7
[54] Elhabashy H *et al* 2022 Exploring protein-protein interactions at the proteome level *Structure* **30** P462–75
[55] Holtz A, Basisty N and Schilling B 2021 *Quantification and Identification of Post-Translational Modifications Using Modern Proteomics Approaches Proteomics approaches, in Quantitative Methods in Proteomics* (Berlin: Springer) pp 225–35
[56] Zhang Y *et al* 2020 Detecting protein and post-translational modifications in single cells with identification and quantification separation (DUET) *Commun. Biol.* **3** 420
[57] Dupree E J *et al* 2020 A critical review of bottom-up proteomics: the good, the bad, and the future of this field *Proteomes* **8** 14

[58] Shi Y *et al* 2004 The role of liquid chromatography in proteomics *J. Chromatogr.* A **1053** 27–36

[59] Zhang X *et al* 2010 Multi-dimensional liquid chromatography in proteomics—a review *Anal. Chim. Acta* **664** 101–13

[60] Nesvizhskii A I 2014 Proteogenomics: concepts, applications and computational strategies *Nat. Methods* **11** 1114–25

[61] Tariq M U *et al* 2020 Methods for proteogenomics data analysis, challenges, and scalability bottlenecks: a survey *IEEE Access* **9** 5497–516

[62] Mani D *et al* 2022 Cancer proteogenomics: current impact and future prospects *Nat. Rev. Cancer* **22** 298–313

[63] Ruggles K *et al* 2017 Methods, tools and current perspectives in proteogenomics *Mol. Cell. Proteom.* **16** 959–81

[64] Roehrl M H, Roehrl V B and Wang J Y 2021 Proteome-based pathology: the next frontier in precision medicine *Expert Rev. Precis. Med. Drug Dev.* **6** 1–4

[65] Joshi S K *et al* 2024 Mass spectrometry–based proteogenomics: new therapeutic opportunities for precision medicine *Annu. Rev. Pharmacol. Toxicol.* **64** 455–79

[66] Campbell M 2019 The power of proteogenomics in precision medicineGenom. Res. *March 27* https://www.technologynetworks.com/genomics/articles/the-power-of-proteogenomics-in-precision-medicine-317341

[67] Santra T S and Tseng F-G 2022 *Handbook of Single Cell Technologies* (Berlin: Springer)

[68] Vistain L F and Tay S 2021 Single-cell proteomics *Trends Biochem. Sci.* **46** 661–72

[69] Bennett H M *et al* 2023 Single-cell proteomics enabled by next-generation sequencing or mass spectrometry *Nat. Methods* **20** 363–74

[70] Matzinger M and Mechtler K 2023 *Improving Single Cell Proteomics Experiments: How Can We Best Utilize Latest-Generation Data Acquisition and MS Instrument Architecture?* (London: Taylor and Francis)

[71] Li L *et al* 2018 Single-cell proteomics for cancer immunotherapy *Adv. Cancer Res.* **139** 185–207

[72] Gavasso S *et al* 2016 Single-cell proteomics: potential implications for cancer diagnostics *Expert Rev. Mol. Diagn.* **16** 579–89

[73] Ctortecka C and Mechtler K 2021 The rise of single-cell proteomics *Anal. Sci. Adv.* **2** 84–94

[74] Kelly R T 2020 Single-cell proteomics: progress and prospects *Mol. Cell. Proteomics* **19** 1739–48

[75] Baysoy A, Bai Z, Satija R, Fan R *et al* 2023 The technological landscape and applications of single-cell multi-omics *Nat. Rev. Mol. Cell Biol.* **24** 695–713

[76] Labib M and Kelley S O 2020 Single-cell analysis targeting the proteome *Nat. Rev. Chem.* **4** 143–58

[77] Lindsay M A 2003 Target discovery *Nat. Rev. Drug Discovery* **2** 831–8

[78] Hughes J P *et al* 2011 Principles of early drug discovery *Br. J. Pharmacol.* **162** 1239–49

[79] Shangguan Z 2021 A review of target identification strategies for drug discovery: from database to machine-based methods *J. Phys.: Conf. Ser* **1893** 012013

[80] Emmerich C H *et al* 2021 Improving target assessment in biomedical research: the GOT-IT recommendations *Nat. Rev. Drug Discov.* **20** 64–81

[81] Kleiner M 2019 Metaproteomics: much more than measuring gene expression in microbial communities *Msystems* **4** e00115–19

[82] Kleiner M *et al* 2018 Metaproteomics method to determine carbon sources and assimilation pathways of species in microbial communities *Proc. Natl Acad. Sci.* **115** E5576–84
[83] Shrestha H K *et al* 2021 Metaproteomics reveals insights into microbial structure, interactions, and dynamic regulation in defined communities as they respond to environmental disturbance *BMC Microbiol.* **21** 17
[84] Maseh K *et al* 2021 Metaproteomics: an emerging tool for the identification of proteins from extreme environments *Environ. Sustain.* **4** 39–50
[85] Wang Y *et al* 2020 Metaproteomics: a strategy to study the taxonomy and functionality of the gut microbiota *J. Proteomics* **219** 103737
[86] Salvato F, Hettich R L and Kleiner M 2021 Five key aspects of metaproteomics as a tool to understand functional interactions in host associated microbiomes *Advances in Clinical Immunology, Medical Microbiology, COVID-19, and Big Data* (Jenny Stanford Publishing) pp 647–60
[87] Henry C *et al* 2022 Modern metaproteomics: a unique tool to characterize the active microbiome in health and diseases, and pave the road towards new biomarkers—example of Crohn's disease and ulcerative colitis flare-ups *Cells* **11** 1340
[88] Li J, Smith L S and Zhu H-J 2021 Data-independent acquisition (DIA): an emerging proteomics technology for analysis of drug-metabolizing enzymes and transporters *Drug Discov. Today: Technol.* **39** 49–56
[89] Zhang F *et al* 2020 Data-independent acquisition mass spectrometry-based proteomics and software tools: a glimpse in 2020 *Proteomics* **20** 1900276
[90] Catherman A D, Skinner O S and Kelleher N L 2014 Top down proteomics: facts and perspectives *Biochem. Biophys. Res. Commun.* **445** 683–93
[91] Kelleher N L 2004 Peer reviewed: top-down proteomics *Anal. Chem.* **76** 196 A–203 A
[92] Picotti P and Aebersold R 2012 Selected reaction monitoring–based proteomics: workflows, potential, pitfalls and future directions *Nat. Methods* **9** 555–66
[93] Gallien S, Duriez E and Domon B 2011 Selected reaction monitoring applied to proteomics *J. Mass Spectrom.* **46** 298–312
[94] Komatsu S and Jorrin-Novo J V 2021 Plant proteomic research 3.0: challenges and perspectives *Int. J. Mol. Sci.* **22** 766
[95] Jorrin Novo J 2021 Proteomics and plant biology: contributions to date and a look towards the next decade *Expert Rev. Proteomics* **18** 93–103
[96] Komatsu S *et al* 2013 *Application of Proteomics for Improving Crop protection/Artificial Regulation* (Frontiers Media SA) p 522
[97] Liu Y *et al* 2019 Proteomics: a powerful tool to study plant responses to biotic stress *Plant Methods* **15** 1–20
[98] Reymond M A *et al* 2003 Ethical and regulatory issues arising from proteomic research and technology *Proteomics: Int. Ed.* **3** 1387–96
[99] Huang H *et al* 2007 Challenges and solutions in proteomics *Curr. Genom.* **8** 21–8
[100] Shi T *et al* 2016 Advances in targeted proteomics and applications to biomedical research *Proteomics* **16** 2160–82
[101] Perez-Riverol Y 2022 Proteomic repository data submission, dissemination, and reuse: key messages *Expert Rev. Proteom.* **19** 297–310
[102] Perez-Riverol Y *et al* 2015 Making proteomics data accessible and reusable: current state of proteomics databases and repositories *Proteomics* **15** 930–50

[103] Jones J *et al* 2023 Tidyproteomics: an open-source R package and data object for quantitative proteomics post analysis and visualization *BMC Bioinf.* **24** 1–14
[104] Halligan B D and Greene A S 2011 Visualize: a free and open source multifunction tool for proteomics data analysis *Proteomics* **11** 1058–63
[105] Didusch S *et al* 2022 amica: an interactive and user-friendly web-platform for the analysis of proteomics data *BMC Genom.* **23** 817
[106] Kessner D *et al* 2008 ProteoWizard: open source software for rapid proteomics tools development *Bioinformatics* **24** 2534–6
[107] Park J *et al* 2017 Informed-Proteomics: open-source software package for top-down proteomics *Nat. Methods* **14** 909–14
[108] Tyanova S, Temu T and Cox J 2016 The MaxQuant computational platform for mass spectrometry-based shotgun proteomics *Nat. Protoc.* **11** 2301–19
[109] Röst H L *et al* 2016 OpenMS: a flexible open-source software platform for mass spectrometry data analysis *Nat. Methods* **13** 741–8
[110] Vaudel M *et al* 2015 PeptideShaker enables reanalysis of MS-derived proteomics data sets *Nat. Biotechnol.* **33** 22–4
[111] Vaudel M *et al* 2011 SearchGUI: an open-source graphical user interface for simultaneous OMSSA and X! Tandem searches *Proteomics* **11** 996–9
[112] MacLean B *et al* 2010 Skyline: an open source document editor for creating and analyzing targeted proteomics experiments *Bioinformatics* **26** 966–8
[113] Tyanova S *et al* 2016 The perseus computational platform for comprehensive analysis of (prote) omics data *Nat. Methods* **13** 731–40
[114] Goloborodko A A *et al* 2013 Pyteomics—a Python framework for exploratory data analysis and rapid software prototyping in proteomics *J. Am. Soc. Mass. Spectrom.* **24** 301–4
[115] Cherney M M and Bowler B E 2011 Protein dynamics and function: making new strides with an old warhorse, the alkaline conformational transition of cytochrome C *Coord. Chem. Rev.* **255** 664–77
[116] Miller M D and Phillips Jr G N 2021 Moving beyond static snapshots: protein dynamics and the protein data bank *J. Biol. Chem.* **296** 100749
[117] Shah N H and Kuriyan J 2019 Understanding molecular mechanisms in cell signaling through natural and artificial sequence variation *Nat. Struct. Mol. Biol.* **26** 25–34
[118] Vieira R C, Pinho L G and Westerberg L S 2023 Understanding immunoactinopathies: a decade of research on WAS gene defects *Pediatr. Allergy Immunol.* **34** e13951
[119] Zhao L *et al* 2022 Targeted protein degradation: mechanisms, strategies and application *Signal Transduct. Target. Ther.* **7** 113
[120] Ramazi S and Zahiri J 2021 Post-translational modifications in proteins: resources, tools and prediction methods *Database* **2021** baab012
[121] Müller M M 2018 Post-translational modifications of protein backbones: unique functions, mechanisms, and challenges *Biochemistry* **57** 177–85
[122] Li Y, Zhang R and Hei H 2023 Advances in post-translational modifications of proteins and cancer immunotherapy *Front. Immunol.* **14** 1229397
[123] Duan G and Walther D 2015 The roles of post-translational modifications in the context of protein interaction networks *PLoS Comput. Biol.* **11** e1004049
[124] Yip H Y K and Papa A 2021 Signaling pathways in cancer: therapeutic targets, combinatorial treatments, and new developments *Cells* **10** 659

[125] Hu X *et al* 2021 The JAK/STAT signaling pathway: from bench to clinic *Signal Transduct. Target. Ther.* **6** 402
[126] Antebi Y E, Nandagopal N and Elowitz M B 2017 An operational view of intercellular signaling pathways *Curr. Opin. Syst. Biol.* **1** 16–24
[127] Nair A *et al* 2019 Conceptual evolution of cell signaling *Int. J. Mol. Sci.* **20** 3292
[128] Wu X, Hasan M A and Chen J Y 2014 Pathway and network analysis in proteomics *J. Theor. Biol.* **362** 44–52
[129] Choudhary C and Mann M 2010 Decoding signalling networks by mass spectrometry-based proteomics *Nat. Rev. Mol. Cell Biol.* **11** 427–39
[130] Sun R-F, Yu Q-Q and Young K H 2018 Critically dysregulated signaling pathways and clinical utility of the pathway biomarkers in lymphoid malignancies *Chronic Dis. Transl. Med.* **4** 29–44
[131] Movahedpour A *et al* 2022 Mammalian target of rapamycin (mTOR) signaling pathway and traumatic brain injury: a novel insight into targeted therapy *Cell Biochem. Funct.* **40** 232–47
[132] Akhurst R J and Hata A 2012 Targeting the TGFβ signalling pathway in disease *Nat. Rev. Drug Discovery* **11** 790–811
[133] Vert G and Chory J 2011 Crosstalk in cellular signaling: background noise or the real thing? *Dev. Cell* **21** 985–91
[134] De Bosscher K *et al* 2020 Nuclear receptor crosstalk—defining the mechanisms for therapeutic innovation *Nat. Rev. Endocrinol.* **16** 363–77
[135] Bhal S and Kundu C N 2023 Targeting crosstalk of signaling pathways in cancer stem cells: a promising approach for development of novel anti-cancer therapeutics *Med. Oncol.* **40** 82
[136] Prahallad A and Bernards R 2016 Opportunities and challenges provided by crosstalk between signalling pathways in cancer *Oncogene* **35** 1073–9
[137] Kongpracha P *et al* 2022 Simple but efficacious enrichment of integral membrane proteins and their interactions for in-depth membrane proteomics *Mol. Cell. Proteom.* **21** 100206
[138] Zafra F and Piniella D 2022 Proximity labeling methods for proteomic analysis of membrane proteins *J. Proteomics* **264** 104620
[139] Almeida J G *et al* 2017 Membrane proteins structures: a review on computational modeling tools *Biochim. Biophy. Acta Biomembr.* **1859** 2021–39
[140] Boulos I *et al* 2023 Exploring the world of membrane proteins: techniques and methods for understanding structure, function, and dynamics *Molecules* **28** 7176
[141] Levental I and Lyman E 2023 Regulation of membrane protein structure and function by their lipid nano-environment *Nat. Rev. Mol. Cell Biol.* **24** 107–22
[142] Reis R and Moraes I 2019 Structural biology and structure–function relationships of membrane proteins *Biochem. Soc. Trans.* **47** 47–61
[143] Cournia Z *et al* 2015 Membrane protein structure, function, and dynamics: a perspective from experiments and theory *J. Membr. Biol.* **248** 611–40
[144] Schwake M, Schröder B and Saftig P 2013 Lysosomal membrane proteins and their central role in physiology *Traffic* **14** 739–48
[145] Dosedělová L *et al* 2018 Importance of membrane proteins in the treatment of tumor diseases and the possibilities of their further study *Klin. Onkol.: Casopis Ceske a Slovenske Onkologicke Spolecnosti* **31** 32–40
[146] Gulezian E *et al* 2021 Membrane protein production and formulation for drug discovery *Trends Pharmacol. Sci.* **42** 657–74

[147] Yin H and Flynn A D 2016 Drugging membrane protein interactions *Annu. Rev. Biomed. Eng.* **18** 51–76
[148] Christopher J A *et al* 2022 Subcellular transcriptomics and proteomics: a comparative methods review *Mol. Cell. Proteomics* **21** 100186
[149] Boldt K *et al* 2016 An organelle-specific protein landscape identifies novel diseases and molecular mechanisms *Nat. Commun.* **7** 11491
[150] Agnetti G, Husberg C and Van Eyk J E 2011 Divide and conquer: the application of organelle proteomics to heart failure *Circ. Res.* **108** 512–26
[151] Zhu D *et al* 2020 Protein trafficking in plant cells: tools and markers *Sci. China Life Sci.* **63** 343–63
[152] Aicart-Ramos C, Valero R A and Rodriguez-Crespo I 2011 Protein palmitoylation and subcellular trafficking *Biochim. Biophys. Acta Biomembr.* **1808** 2981–94
[153] Lundberg E and Borner G H 2019 Spatial proteomics: a powerful discovery tool for cell biology *Nat. Rev. Mol. Cell Biol.* **20** 285–302
[154] Drissi R, Dubois M L and Boisvert F M 2013 Proteomics methods for subcellular proteome analysis *FEBS J.* **280** 5626–34
[155] Christopher J A *et al* 2021 Subcellular proteomics *Nat. Rev. Methods Primers* **1** 32
[156] Lee Y H, Tan H T and Chung M C 2010 Subcellular fractionation methods and strategies for proteomics *Proteomics* **10** 3935–56

IOP Publishing

Introduction to Pharmaceutical Biotechnology, Volume 2 (Second Edition)

Enzymes, proteins and bioinformatics

Ahmed Al-Harrasi, Saurabh Bhatia and Ajmal Khan

Chapter 9

Bioinformatics

9.1 Introduction

According to the *Oxford Dictionary*, bioinformatics involves conceptualizing biology in terms of molecules and applying informatics techniques to understand and organize the information associated with these molecules, on a large scale. In brief, bioinformatics is a management information system for molecular biology and has many practical applications.

Bioinformatics analysis involve:

- the assembly of sequenced data (directly from environmental samples) in order to construct contiguous sequences (contigs and scaffolds);
- the prediction of genes (and putative proteins) based on the assembled data; and
- prediction of domains, functions and pathways for the putative proteins.

Bioinformatics is a discipline related to the exploitation and application of computer hardware and software to the procurement, storage, investigation and imaging of biological material (figure 9.1) [1]. Scientific developments in recent years have encouraged marked progress in understanding the genetic basis of phenotypes. With these advances, genomics has tremendously transformed the scope of biological problems at a genome-wide scale, exploring vast data and opening numerous possibilities [2]. However, the enormous amount of information that has been produced increases the challenges that must be overcome for storage (Moore's law) and the processing of biological information. Bioinformatics and computational biology have been pursued to overcome such challenges [3]. A general scheme of the process of bioinformatics is shown in figure 9.2.

Bioinformatics has the following three main components:

doi:10.1088/978-0-7503-5387-8ch9

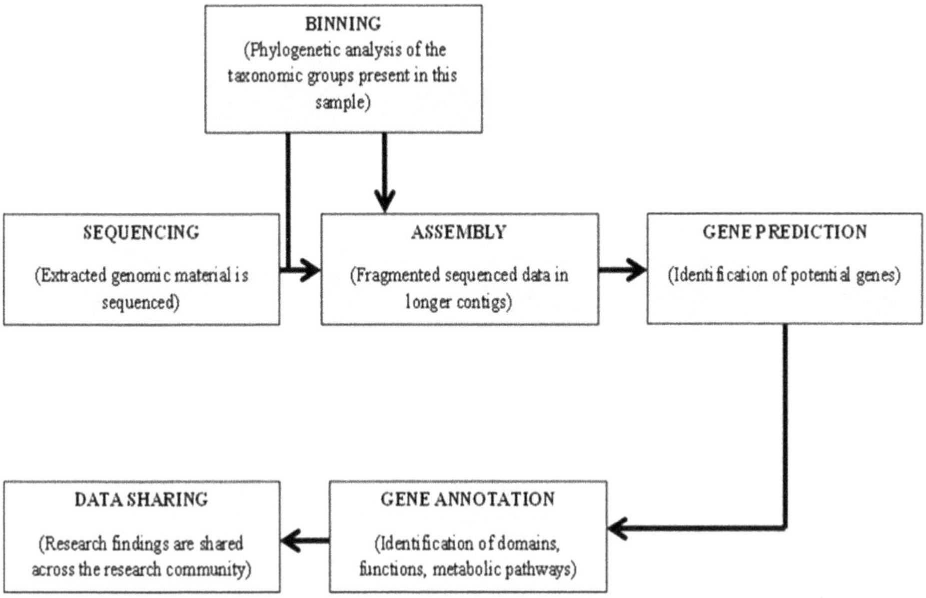

Figure 9.1. Bioinformatics: genomic material is sequenced and processed using assembly, gene prediction and gene annotation tools. Finally, the results are pooled by scientific groups around the world.

- New algorithms and statistics production for evaluating the connections among large sets of biological data, e.g. DNA sequence data.
- Application of these techniques for the examination and understanding of different biological data, including nucleotide sequences, amino acid sequences, etc.
- The production of systems for effective storage, access and management of a large body of varied biological information.

The field of bioinformatics first developed for the production of amino acid sequences of proteins and nucleotide sequences of DNA. Zuckerkandl and Pauling (1962) predicted that the amino acid sequences of proteins could be employed to investigate the evolutionary relationship between different organisms [4]. This suggestion was based on the evidence that the amino acid sequences of homologous proteins, i.e., proteins having similar functions, were related. This started a new area of investigation known as 'molecular evolution'. Subsequent studies have allowed inferences of evolutionary relationships from the relative analysis of amino acid sequences of functionally related proteins. These investigations became possible due to the development of quantitative procedures for sequence comparisons.

9.2 History of bioinformatics

The first complete assortment of amino acid sequences was collected in the *Atlas of Protein Sequence and Structure* by the National Biomedical Research Foundation (USA). This assortment was modified by Margaret Dayhoff in 1965–78 [2]. Dayhoff

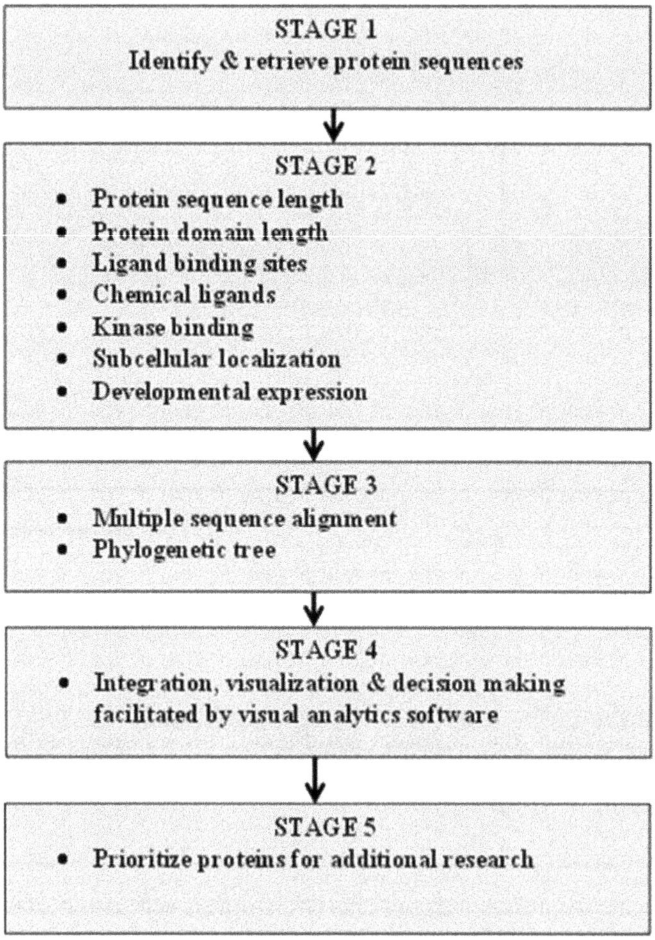

Figure 9.2. Basic process of bioinformatics.

and colleagues also made considerable contributions to the assessment of amino acid sequences by means of exploring applications of computer software in the identification of remotely related sequences, deducing evolutionary relationships, etc. In 1990, the European Molecular Biology Laboratory established their data library to collect, arrange and allocate nucleotide sequence data and associated information.

This task is now carried out by the European Bioinformatics Institute (Hinxton, UK). In the early 1980s, the National Centre for Bioinformatics Information (NCBI) was established in the USA. NCBI works as a main information databank and source for other information. It is one of the leading databases and provides search engines for diverse information in the field [5]. The DNA Data Bank was later established by Japan. In 1984, the National Biomedical Research Foundation established the Protein Information Resource. This assists investigators in the detection and elucidation of protein sequence information. These large databases function in close association with each other and frequently exchange data. These

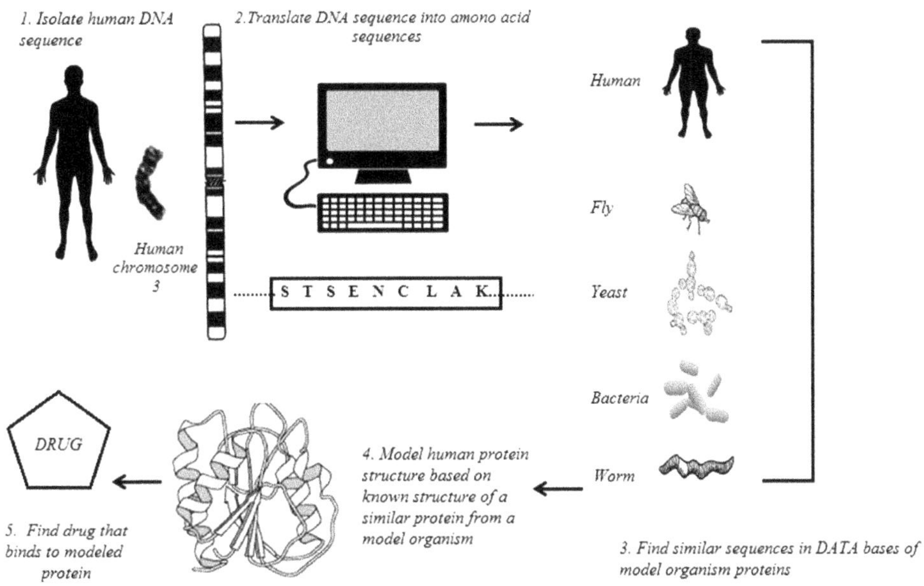

Figure 9.3. A schematic depiction how of bioinformatics can aid in analytical drug discovery.

databanks are a key resource for all scientists involved in the study of biological phenomena, predominantly the molecular aspects of biologic sciences [6]. The organization and investigation of the rapidly accumulating sequence data require advanced computer software and statistical procedures. This has resulted in the involvement of teams of researchers from computer science and mathematics in the development of the discipline of bioinformatics. Diverse procedures and techniques have now been established that allow the organization, utilization and dissemination of biological information [7]. In bioinformatics, we can design compounds that bind specifically with an expressed protein, or perhaps more importantly, a transcription regulator can cause changes in expression levels, as shown in figure 9.3.

9.3 Sequences and nomenclature

The incorrect use of sequence analysis techniques may result in numerous errors in genome annotation. In bioinformatics, sequence examination is the process of exposing a DNA, RNA or peptide sequence to any of an extensive range of analytical approaches to recognize its features, function, structure or evolution [7]. The procedures employed in sequence analysis include sequence alignment and searches in biological databases. With the development of approaches of high-throughput production of gene and protein sequences, the rate of addition of new sequences to databases has increased exponentially. Such a collection of sequences does not, by itself, increase the scientist's understanding of the biology of organisms. However, equating these new sequences to those with known functions is an important approach to understanding the biology of an organism. Therefore, sequence examination can be employed to allocate functions to genes and proteins through the study of the similarities between the compared sequences. Currently, there are numerous tools and techniques that offer sequence comparisons (sequence alignment) and examine the alignment of the product to understand its biology. One of the major difficulties of bioinformatics is the arrangement of the vast data in a well-organized and easily comprehensible format [8]. The nucleotide and amino acid sequences are easily reduced to digital data by using single letter codes. The nomenclature system accepted in bioinformatics is founded on the protocols set out by IUPAC, which allow the understanding and utilization of the data produced by different individuals or research groups.

9.3.1 DNA sequences

The key symbols employed to signify DNA sequences are denoted by single letters A (adenine), C (cytosine), G (guanine) and T (thymine). However, sequence data often encompass doubts as to which of the four bases is present at several locations. These doubts in DNA sequences are addressed by frequent sequencing of the related DNA segments. The base sequences of the two complementary strands of a DNA molecule are signified by means of identical symbols. Even those locations that display uncertainty can be represented by this system of symbols. The base sequence of only one strand is registered in databanks [9]. This sequence runs from the 5′ to the 3′ direction, i.e., the 5′-end is at the left-hand extreme and the 3′-end is at the right-hand extreme of the sequence. The base sequence of the complementary strand is effortlessly obtained either manually (for short sequences) or by means of a suitable software package. Exclusively in the case of RNA sequences, the symbol U (for uracil) takes the place of T.

9.3.2 Amino acid sequences of proteins

Amino acids are usually represented by three-letter symbols, e.g. Ala (alanine), Val (valine), etc. However, in bioinformatics, they are represented by single letters, such as A (alanine), C (cysteine), D (aspartic acid), etc. However, a number of locations in protein sequences have uncertainties; this situation is comparable to that for DNA sequences. For example, it can be unclear whether a site has glutamine or glutamic acid; such a site is denoted by the symbol Z. Similarly, B represents either asparagine or aspartic acid. The character X is used to show that the position may have any amino acid. The protein synthesis usually initiates at the N-terminus and ensues to the C-terminus. The amino acid sequences in databanks are thus listed from the N-terminus (at the extreme left of the sequence) to the C-terminus (at the extreme right) of the polypeptide [10].

9.3.3 Types of sequences in nucleotide sequence databases

The databanks of DNA sequences comprise a variety of sequence types. A short explanation of each of these sequence types is provided in the following.

cDNA sequences. A cDNA molecule is derived by reverse transcription of an RNA molecule. The cDNA sequences thus represent that part of the genome that is transcribed into RNA. If the cDNA is derived from mRNA, it will represent only the exon sequences of the genes expressed in the cell/tissue/organism of interest [11].

Genomic DNA sequences. These sequences signify the complete genome of the organism, regardless of whether it is expressed or not. Once the genome sequence is complete, it will encompass the sequence of the complete genome of the organism. In prokaryotes, the genome typically entails a single chromosome, whereas in the case of eukaryotes the genome comprises the nuclear DNA.

Expressed sequence tag (EST) sequences. ESTs are mRNA sequence fragments resulting from single sequencing reactions executed on randomly selected clones from cDNA libraries [12]. To date, almost 45 million ESTs have been produced from over 1400 different species of eukaryotes. Usually EST projects are used to either match existing genome projects or as low-cost options for purposes of gene discovery. However, with developments in accuracy and coverage, they are starting to find applications in fields such as phylogenetics, transcript profiling and proteomics [13]. These sequences are derived by sequencing only a portion of the cDNA molecules made using mRNA [4]. These sequences are dubbed 'tags' as they can be utilized as probes for the isolation of the related genes from the genomic DNA. This strategy was used by Venter and colleagues for deriving the sequence of the expressed portion of the human genome. The EST sequences method produced massive amounts of sequence data that allowed the assembly of a preliminary transcript map of the human genome. Large numbers of EST sequences have been assembled in an EST databank, dbEST. One of the challenges with ESTs is duplication; long genes may be represented by two or more ESTs. For example, one major databank has over 1300 ESTs for a single gene. This results as an EST has to be short enough to signify a single exon or its part, and long genes have many exons [14].

9.3.3.1 Genome sequence tag (GST) sequences

A genes-first approach to genome sequencing has been described which efficiently generates GSTs from genomic DNA [5]. GSTs were first produced to recognize the genes of *Plasmodium falciparum*. It was noticed that the enzyme mung bean nuclease (Mnase) cuts *P. falciparum* genomic DNA between genes. GSTs are produced by sequencing the DNA fragments on either side of the points of cuts generated by Mnase [5]. Examination of gene sequence tags prepared from mung bean nuclease-digested *P. falciparum* DNA demonstrates that this technique has numerous advantages over the popular cDNA expressed sequence tag approach. So far, 673 sequence tags containing over 215 kb of sequence have been generated from 400 clones [15].

9.3.3.2 Organellar DNA sequences

Mitochondria and plastids are membrane-bound organelles that translate energy from foodstuffs or sunlight into cellular energy. Organelles have their own independent genome that encodes a range of genes directly related to producing energy for the cell. Organellar DNA is the DNA existing in mitochondria (mtDNA) and chloroplasts (cpDNA) [16]. The sequences of these are stored in databanks.

Mitochondria and chloroplasts are thought to have developed from bacteria that formed a symbiotic relationship with ancestral cells containing a eukaryotic nucleus. The majority of the genes initially within these organelles have been transferred to the nuclear genome over evolutionary time, leaving different genes in the organelle DNAs of different organisms [17].

9.3.3.3 Sequences of other molecules

In addition to the DNA sequence databases, sequences of molecules such as tRNA, small RNAs, etc, are also collected in databanks.

9.3.4 Databases

Various database and software resources have reported and applied within the fields of medicine, biology and bioinformatics [18]. Up-to-date information on existing databases and software would be a valuable resource [19]. Previous efforts have been made to preserve accurate lists of available bioinformatics resources, however, most have not been adequately completed due to the slow process of manual curation, or specialized requirements for resource inclusion. There are three public domain bioinformatics services:

- The National Centre for Biotechnol Information (NCBI), located in the USA.
- The European Bioinformatics Institute (EBI), located in the UK.
- GenomeNet (the Japanese Bioinformatics Service), located in Japan.

These organizations develop databases as well as suitable analysis techniques. These computational tools and databases are essential for the organization and management of the vast amounts of biological data. A database/databank is a huge assortment of information relating to a specific topic, such as nucleotide sequence, protein sequence, etc, maintained in an electronic environment. Databanks are at the core of bioinformatics. The amount of data is growing rapidly.

9.3.4.1 Nucleotide sequence databases

The EMBL Nucleotide Sequence Database (http://www.ebi.ac.uk/embl/) incorporates, organizes and distributes nucleotide sequences from all available public sources [20]. The database is located and maintained at the European Bioinformatics Institute (EBI) near Cambridge, UK. In an international collaboration with DNA Data Bank of Japan (DDBJ) and GenBank, data are exchanged amongst the collaborating databases on a daily basis to achieve optimal synchronization [11]. The main nucleotide sequence databanks are thus GenBank, maintained by NCBI, the DDBJ and the Nucleotide Sequence Database maintained by EMBL. These, and several other nucleotide sequence databases that have been created, are listed in the following:

- *E. coli*: This databank, established by NCBI, has nucleotide sequences of the *Escherichia coli* genome.
- Mito: This databank contains sequences of mitochondrial genomes and is held at NCBI.

- GenBank: This is the key nucleotide sequence databank created by NCBI. This databank comprises nucleotide sequences of genomic DNA.
- dbEST: This database contains EST entries from the GenBank, EMBL and DDBJ databases. This databank is likely to have sequencing errors, contamination by heterologous sequences and the presence of transcribed repetitive elements. The database is maintained by NCBI.
- EMBL: This is a complete nucleotide (DNA and RNA) sequence database held at EMBL and compiled from numerous sources. It is in partnership with the GenBank and the DDBJ. EMBL connects with GenBank and DDBJ on a regular basis and to exchange data and update its contents.
- Kabat: This databank is maintained at NCBI. It has nucleotide sequences that are useful from the immunological point of view.
- Yeast: This NCBI database comprises the nucleotide sequence data of the yeast genome.
- The International ImmunoGenetics Database (IMGT): This databank holds the nucleotide sequences of immunologically important genes, such as T-cell receptors, B-cell receptors, etc.

9.3.4.2 Protein databases

Protein databases have now become an important part of modern biology. Vast amounts of information on protein structures, functions and, mainly, sequences are being generated. Examining databases is often the initial step in the study of a new protein. Comparisons between proteins or between protein families offer information about the association between proteins within a genome or across various species, and therefore offer much more information than can be acquired by reviewing only an isolated protein [21]. Moreover, secondary databases obtained from new databases are also extensively available. These databases rearrange and annotate the data or provide predictions. The utilization of multiple databases often helps scientists to understand the structure and function of a protein [22]. Although certain protein databases are well known, they are far from being fully utilized in the protein science community:

- The Protein Data Bank (PDB): This databank has protein sequences whose three-dimensional structures are already identified. It is maintained at Brookhaven National Laboratory, USA. The records are predominantly nonredundant. The databank is also held ay NCBI's PDB mirror site MMDB, and at the PDB mirror site of EBI, UK.
- Swiss-Prot Database: This is a nonredundant protein sequence databank, held at the University of Geneva, Italy, and maintained by EBI, UK. It is an adaptation of the Protein Identification Resource (PIR) databank of NCBI. NCBI also offers Swiss-Prot, which has the most releases of protein sequence entries from the Swiss-Prot Database of EBI.
- Yeast: This NCBI databank contains yeast protein sequences.
- Kabat: This databank is maintained by NCBI. It has protein sequences that have immunological relevance.

9.3.4.3 Other databases

A number of other types of databanks have been generated, such as the Radiation Hybrid Database (RHdb), which comprises experimental conditions and radiation hybrid records from the human and mouse. The radiation hybrid score vectors can be employed to create chromosome maps that are an alternative to the genetic map. The Kyoto Encyclopedia of Genes and Genomes (KEGG) comprises data on metabolic pathways in numerous microorganisms. It is part of the GenomeNet (Japan) database system [23].

9.3.5 Search engines and analysis tools

The exploitation of several databases requires the use of suitable search engines and analysis tools. These tools are often called database mining tools and the process of database utilization is known as database mining.

9.3.5.1 The basic local alignment search tool (BLAST)

A method for rapid sequence comparison, BLAST directly estimates alignments that optimize an amount of local similarity, the maximal segment pair (MSP) score [24]. Current mathematical findings on the stochastic characteristics of MSP scores permit an examination of the performance of this technique as well as the statistical implications of the alignments it generates. The basic algorithm is simple and robust; it can be applied in different ways and in a variety of contexts comprising straightforward DNA and gene identification searches, protein sequence database searches, motif searches and in the examination of multiple regions of similarity in long DNA sequences [25]. BLAST is a sequence similarity search program that can be employed to rapidly search a sequence database for matches to a query sequence. A number of variants of BLAST exist to compare all combinations of nucleotide or protein queries against a nucleotide or protein database [26]. In addition to performing alignments, BLAST provides an 'expect' value, statistical information about the significance of each alignment.

BLAST is a family of easy to use sequence similarity search techniques available on the Internet. BLAST is maintained by NCBI. This technique is intended to recognize possible homologs for a given sequence. It can examine both DNA and protein sequences. Documentation of homologs permits the prediction of possible roles and demonstration of the three-dimensional structure. A local arrangement finds the ideal alignment between subregions or local regions of particular sequences. A local alignment search engine discovers the sequence motifs, domains, etc, in the database that are homologous to the submitted sequence motif, domain, etc. Various BLAST programs have been explored [27]. Each of them functions for specific purpose. The newest BLAST programs are known as BLAST 2.0. A variety of BLAST programs are listed in the following:

- BLASTn: This program links a sample nucleotide sequence with a nucleotide sequence database.
- BLASTp: This program matches a sample protein sequence to a protein database.

- BLASTx: This program interprets a sample nucleotide sequence into an amino acid sequence and compares the latter with a protein database.
- tBLASTn: This program translates a sample protein sequence into a nucleotide sequence and compares it with a nucleotide sequence database.
- tBLASTx: This program interprets a sample nucleotide sequence as well as the nucleotide sequence database into amino acid sequences and examines for homology between the two.

As an example, a scholar has created a nucleotide (DNA/RNA) or amino acid (protein) sequence and needs to compare this sequence with those contained in a database with a view to detect homologous sequences. The BLAST search engine carries out the assessment by means of algorithms. Simply, the logic used by BLAST programs is as follows:

- The sequence submitted by researcher is compared base-per-base or amino acid-per-amino acid with the database sequences.
- A replacement scoring matrix is employed by the BLAST programs. Each counterpart is conferred a specified score, while each divergence is penalized by a particular negative score.
- The sequence alignment is then allocated a complete score, which is the summation of scores allocated to each of its paired amino acids/nucleotides.
- Top scoring alignments are rated according to set standards. These measures differentiate between a similarity due to an ancestral relationship and that due to random chance.
- Discovered homologies or counterparts are further studied by means of data available through ENTREZ and other search engines.

The BLAST engine can be accessed online (www.ncbi.nlm.nih.gov). The steps users have to take are as follows:

- The sequence for which homology is to be examined is initially submitted into the 'input sequence' box of the BLAST interface. This sequence has to be in a appropriate format, i.e., the FASTA format.
- A suitable BLAST program is designated depending on the type of assessment to be made.
- The suitable database from which homologous sequences are to be searched has to be selected. The default database used by BLAST is the NR database of NCBI. The NR protein database maintained by NCBI as a target for their BLAST search services is a composite of Swiss-Prot, Swiss-Prot updates, PIR, PDB.
- The sequence is now submitted to the BLAST server.
- The outcomes of the search can be accessed either by email or via the BLAST interface.

9.3.5.2 Entrez search and taxonomy browser

The NCBI Taxonomy database is a curated set of names and classification for all the organisms represented in the gene bank. There are two main tools for viewing the information, the Taxonomy Browser and Taxonomy ENTREZ. Both systems allow the searching of the databases for names and links to relevance sequence data [28].

ENTREZ is the text-based search and retrieval system used at the NCBI for all of the major databases, including PubMed, nucleotide and protein sequences, protein structures, complete genomes, taxonomy and many others [29]. ENTREZ is simultaneously an indexing and retrieval system, a collection of data from many sources and an organizing principle for biomedical information [30].

ENTREZ is one of the most standard search tools in the field. The ENTREZ engine explores bibliographic citations and biological information from a range of reliable databases, e.g. Swiss-Prot, PDB, GenBank, EMBL, etc. It uses PubMed's bibliographic database for bibliographic or citation search. ENTREZ provides a range of criteria for searching, and is an extremely useful and compliant search engine. It can be used to explore diverse information, e.g. all potential citations from a specific author in a given area, standard names for given genes, a specific sequence in the databases, etc. There are several database retrieval tools such as ENTREZ, LocusLink, Taxonomy Browser, etc.

The NCBI Taxonomy database (www.ncbi.nlm.nih.gov/taxonomy) is the standard nomenclature and classification repository for the International Nucleotide Sequence Database Collaboration (INSDC), comprising the GenBank, ENA (EMBL) and DDBJ databases. The diversity of organisms is such that millions of species are known. This search engine offers taxonomic information on different species. The Taxonomy databank of NCBI has data (including scientific and common names) on all organisms for which some sequence data are known (over 79 000 species) [31]. The engine offers genetic data and the taxonomic relations of the species in question. The Taxonomy Browser has links with the other servers of NCBI, e.g. Structure and PubMed. The browser supports two different kinds of web page hierarchies, which present the familiar indented view of the taxonomic classification, and taxon-specific pages, which summarize all of the information that we associate with a particular taxonomic entry in the database [32].

9.3.5.3 NCBI's LocusLink

The LocusLink and RefSeq databases were started to report data-access issues ensuing from significant increases in both sequence data and the number of web sites relating to information about genes [33]. LocusLink offers a single point-of-access to a variety of gene-specific information sources including web resources.

LocusLink is an NCBI project to link information applicable to specific genetic loci from several disparate databases. LocusLink covers data about genes, comprising their official names. Moreover, it permits one to search for genes homologous to a specific gene, and to derive data about these genes. For example, one can effortlessly obtain data about mouse genes that are homologous to given human genes. One can also search for homologs of a specific gene in numerous other organisms [34]. The LocusLink website is www.ncbi.nlm.nih.gov/LocusLink/.

9.3.5.4 Prosite

PROSITE contains entries describing protein domains, families and functional sites, as well as associated patterns and profiles to identify them [18–21]. It is complemented by ProRule, a collection of rules based on profiles and patterns, which increases the discriminatory power of these profiles and patterns by providing additional information about functionally and/or structurally critical amino acids [35]. PROSITE is mainly used for the annotation of domain features of UniProtKB/Swiss-Prot entries. Among the 983 (DNA-binding) domains, repeats and zinc fingers present in Swiss-Prot (release 57.8 of 22 September 2009), 696 (~70%) are annotated with PROSITE descriptors using information from ProRule. In order to allow better functional characterization of domains, PROSITE developments focus on subfamily specific profiles and a new profile building method giving more weight to functionally important residues [18–21]. In other words the PROSITE database consists of a large collection of biologically meaningful signatures that are described as patterns or profiles. Each signature is linked to documentation that provides useful biological information on the protein family, domain or functional site identified by the signature. The PROSITE web page has been redesigned and several tools have been implemented to help the user discover new conserved regions in their own proteins and to visualize domain arrangements [36].

PROSITE has an assortment of active sites and sequence patterns present in various proteins. Entries in PROSITE are usually associated with Swiss-Prot and other significant databases. The PROSITE file comprises the sequence entries that share the matched sequence motif-of-interest. The characterized motifs are well documented to minimize redundancy. PROSITE has search engines for comparing patterns/motifs. The PROMOT search engine can be employed to compare a sequence against the PROSITE database. PROSEARCH is another search engine to explore the Swiss-Prot and Tremble databases for a specific motif [37].

9.3.6 Various indian databases

9.3.6.1 GM crops database

This database, based at the National Research Centre on Plant Biotechnology, New Delhi, is an active web resource storing data on the biosafety of transgenics (released in India), comprising over 800 publications on the subject. For example, a total of 139 transgenic lines using four genes (crylAb, crylAb, cry2Ab and vip3A) and a single promoter (CaMV 35S) have been established.

9.3.6.2 Vanshanudhan

The Vanshanudhan database (http://125.18.242.23:8080/genome/Login.jsp) allows searches based on complete genome data comprising genes, cDNA and protein sequences. Currently, the Vanshanudhan data are based on rice pseudomolecule version 3.0, released from Michigan State University with a unique gene nomenclature, e.g. 01-0001, which defines the chromosome number as well as gene number. This database has been established by the NRC on Plant Biotechnology researchers as an result of an Indian rice genome initiative [38]. It covers information on the 56 298 rice genes.

9.4 Investigation by means of bioinformatics tools

Bioinformatics based engines have been established for distribution of the large amount of biological data being produced at a very rapid rate. For example, when a long piece of DNA has been sequenced, the first objective is to regulate if it contains any genes. This objective is comparatively simple in the case of prokaryotes, but the search for eukaryotic genes is quite difficult [39].

9.4.1 Identification of genes

With the increase in genomic and functional genomics information, approaches for disease gene identification are rapidly being developed [40]. Databases are now indispensable to the process of selecting candidate disease genes. Relating positional information with disease characteristics and functional information is the normal approach by which candidate disease genes are selected. Enrichment for candidate disease genes, however, depends on the skills of the operating researcher [41].

Prior to genome sequencing, gene identification used approaches based on transcript mapping. The genomic clone of interest was exposed to zoo blot hybridization, i.e., hybridization with the whole genomic DNA of a range of species. It has been discovered that coding sequences are strongly conserved during development. Thus, a clone that tested positive in a zoo blot is possible to characterize as a gene. The clone of interest can be hybridized with cDNA libraries or employed for northern blot or reverse northern blot assays. A constructive assay identifies a gene as only genes are transcribed. CpGProD is an application for identifying mammalian promoter regions associated with CpG islands in large genomic sequences [24]. Detection of CpG islands in the clone suggests it to be a gene as about 50% of human genes have related CpG islands. CpG islands are short stretches of G. C-rich DNA often found in association with vertebrate genes. Other methods of gene identification included cDNA selection, cDNA capture and exon trapping. These methods provide research that is appropriate for individual gene identification but unsuitable for genome annotation. Consequently, the correct reading frame is identified by carrying out a six-frame translation of the DNA sequence. The accurate reading frame is predicted to be the longest frame uninterupted by a stop codon (TGA, TAA or TAG); this type of reading frame is known as an open-reading frame (ORF). The longer this ORF, the better is the probability that it represents a gene. Locating the 3′-end of an ORF is relatively easier than locating its 5′-end, although the 5′-end may be indicated by an ATG. However, more tools are required to locate the 5′-end of an ORF, such as the presence of a Kozak sequence (CCGCCA UGGG) flanking the AUG codon. Investigation of codon usage may also be supportive, and the presence of CpG islands may designate the 5′-end of numerous vertebrate genes. However, determination of ORFs may be hindered by sequencing errors. The most significant single progress in genome annotation is the use of PCs to predict genes from DNA sequences. Identification of genes may achieve using one of the following two approaches. In the first technique, sequences of known genes, cDNAs, ESTs and proteins present in databases are equated with the genome sequence; this is achieved by homology search techniques, such as BLAST. In the second method, specific software is employed to identify genes [42].

In prokaryotes, programs such as GenMark (a modified GeneScan algorithm) and Glimmer can identify all the genes, including overlapping genes, present in the genome.

Numerous sophisticated software programs have been developed for gene prediction in eukaryotes, e.g. Genie, GeneScan, Grail, GeneFinder, HMM Gene, etc. These programs required training with information or need to be provided with a set of rules. Grail can be employed with human, mouse, *Arabidopsis*, etc, genome sequences, but Genie has only been trained on human and *Drosophila* sequences. However, no single program is 100% perfect at identifying genes. An algorithm trained with the DNA sequence of one organism, *Caenorhabditis elegans*, will not execute suitably with that of another organism, e.g. a plant, without being retrained [43].

The gene prediction programs search for gene-specific characteristics, e.g. promoters, splice sites and polyadenylation sites, or for pertinent gene content such as ORFs. The currently available gene search programs are associated with different search criteria and their sensitivities vary widely. The identification of ORFs, usually exceeding 300 nucleotides, is sufficient to find most genes in prokaryotic genomes. However, such a simple search criterion will miss smaller genes and overlapping genes. These problems are resolved by using algorithms that consider differences in base composition between genes and noncoding DNA, e.g. in GenMark. The gene prediction programs used in eukaryotes use the output of several algorithms to generate a whole gene model. In this model, a gene is defined as a series of exons that are coordinately transcribed. The various features of eukaryotic genes recognized during gene detection include transcriptional and translational controls, e.g. the TATA box, cap site, Kozak consensus and polyadenylation sites. But problems arise as the TATA box is missing in 70% of human genes, and polyadenylation signals can differ considerably from the consensus sequence AATAAA. Moreover, these sequences recognize only the first and the last exons of a gene. Thus, additional features have been encompassed in modern gene search tools; these features include 5′- and 3′-splice sites, differences in base composition between coding and noncoding DNA (typically, comparison of hexamer base composition), etc.

9.4.2 Identification of the function of a new gene

A convenient approach to detect the function of a new gene is as follows. The gene sequence is translated into the amino acid sequence and thus the protein it is anticipated to encode. This protein sequence is then compared with a protein database. A program such as tBLASTx will execute both these functions. If the encoded protein is homologous to a protein in the databank, it allows identification of the new gene and also suggests the function of the new gene [44]. The FASTA and HMMER programs are slower than BLAST, but they are more sensitive.

9.4.3 Identification of functional domains

Several bioinformatics techniques for the detection of protein motifs and protein domains have been explored. Among these tools are PRINTS, PROSITE, SMART, BLOCKS, etc.

9.4.4 Detection of noncoding RNA

A number of RNAs are noncoding, such as rRNA, tRNA, small RNAs, etc. Of these, rRNAs are the easiest to find; this is done by sequence similarity search. The program tRNAScanSE searches for aRNA sequences [44].

9.4.5 Genome annotation

After the detection of a gene and prediction of its functions, suitable experiments have to be devised to authenticate these findings. This information is then employed for genome annotation. Standard genome annotation languages have become extensively accepted [45]. GAME is a program for describing investigational confirmation to support annotation. Likewise DAS (the distributed annotation system) is mainly useful for indexing and visualization. Several software programs such as BioPerl 2001, BioJava 2001, etc, are employed for storing, manipulating and imagining the genome annotations [46].

9.4.6 Molecular phylogenetics

DNA and protein sequence statistics can be employed to examine the development of genes and their protein products; this is called molecular phylogeny. Bioinformatics techniques are employed to define phylogenetic relationships, which may be accessible in the form of either a phylogenetic tree or a dendogram. While the two depictions look different, they depict exactly the same relationship [47].

9.5 Computational approaches in bioinformatics

9.5.1 Algorithm development

Sequence alignment is a crucial task in bioinformatics, which provides the groundwork for several applications, such as functional annotation, structure prediction, and phylogenetics. The main goal of sequence alignment is to arrange DNA, RNA, or protein sequences to find comparable sections that may result from functional, structural, or evolutionary links between the sequences. Sequence alignment may be roughly classified into multiple sequence alignment (MSA) and pairwise alignment [48]. Two sequences align in pairwise alignment, while three or more sequences align in multiple-sequence alignment [49]. The Needleman–Wunsch technique [50] for global alignment and the Smith–Waterman algorithm [51] for local alignment are two popular pairwise alignment algorithms. The goal of global alignment, which works best for equal-length sequences, is to align every residue in every sequence. Local alignment, on the other hand, finds comparable sections within lengthy sequences that are often distinct overall. Algorithms like MUSCLE [52] and ClustalW [53] are widely used in multiple sequence alignment. MSA is crucial for phylogenetic analyses and identifying conserved domains across species. It is more complex than pairwise alignment due to the increased computational demands and the complexity of optimally aligning multiple sequences. A fundamental aspect of sequence alignment algorithms is the scoring system, which uses substitution matrices to score alignments based on the substitution, insertion, or deletion of residues. Gap penalties are a crucial part of the scoring system, imposing penalties for opening and extending gaps, which is essential for managing indels (insertions or deletions) [54]. Various algorithmic strategies are employed in sequence alignment. Dynamic programming is a common approach used in both the Needleman–Wunsch and Smith–Waterman algorithms to ensure the optimality of the alignment. However, due to the computational intensity of dynamic programming, empirical methods are often employed to accelerate the alignment process at the cost of optimality, with BLAST (Basic Local Alignment Search Tool) [55] and FASTA being prime examples [56]. In the case of multiple sequence alignment, a progressive alignment strategy is often employed, where pairwise alignments are extended to multiple alignments by aligning the most similar sequences first. Advancements in computing have also impacted the field of sequence alignment. Parallel computing, for instance, has significantly reduced the computational time required for alignment tasks, making real-time analysis of large datasets feasible. Additionally, the integration of machine learning techniques has emerged as a promising avenue to improve alignment accuracy and predict novel alignments, signifying a blend of traditional bioinformatics approaches with modern computational methods [57].

9.5.2 Phylogenetic tree construction algorithms

Phylogenetic tree construction is fundamental for understanding evolutionary relationships among species or sequences. Various algorithms have been developed to implement this method, and they fall into different categories based on their approach [58]. A schematic diagram representing the structure and flow of the phylogenetic tree is shown in figure 9.4.

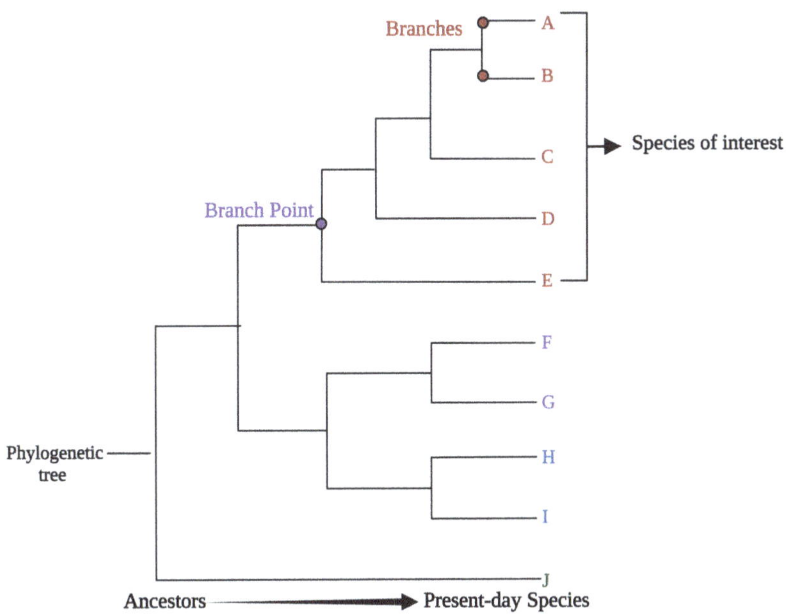

Figure 9.4. Phylogenetic tree representation: mapping evolutionary relationships and ancestral lineages of present-day species.

9.5.2.1 Distance-based algorithms

Neighbor-Joining (NJ) [59] and UPGMA (Unweighted Pair Group Method with Arithmetic Mean) are distance-based algorithms [60]. These algorithms begin by computing a matrix of pairwise distances between sequences. NJ is a widely used method due to its efficiency. It iteratively joins the nearest neighboring taxa into a tree, updating the distance matrix in each iteration to reflect the newly formed clusters. The UPGMA assumes a constant rate of evolution (molecular clock hypothesis) across different lineages, which may not always hold, thus limiting its accuracy in some scenarios [61].

9.5.2.2 Character-based algorithms

The character-based algorithms include maximum parsimony [62] and maximum likelihood. The maximum parsimony method seeks to find the tree that explains the data with the fewest evolutionary changes. Maximum likelihood estimates tree topologies and branch lengths based on a probabilistic model of sequence evolution, aiming to find the tree that maximizes the likelihood of observing the given data [63].

9.5.2.3 Bayesian phylogenetics

The Bayesian phylogenetics approach employs Bayesian assumption to estimate the posterior probabilities of different tree topologies given in the data, incorporating *a priori* knowledge through prior distributions [64].

9.5.3 Machine learning algorithms in bioinformatics

Machine learning (ML) encompasses various algorithms applied to various bioinformatics tasks. Support Vector Machines (SVM) are used for classification tasks like distinguishing between disease and healthy samples based on gene expression data. Random Forests are ensemble learning methods used for classification and regression tasks, providing feature importance scores that can be insightful in bioinformatics. Unsupervised learning includes K-means clustering [65]. It is employed for grouping data into clusters based on feature similarity, like clustering genes based on expression profiles. Hierarchical clustering is useful for generating a dendrogram of clustered data, often employed in gene expression analysis. Convolutional neural networks (CNNs) have shown to be very beneficial in image analysis applications, such as histopathology image analysis, within the field of deep learning. Since recurrent neural networks (RNNs) are good at processing sequential data, they are often used for sequence analysis tasks [66]. Drug discovery process optimization may benefit from reinforcement learning, a subfield of ML in which a method learns how to act in a given environment to maximize some concept of cumulative reward [67].

9.5.3.1 Structural bioinformatics algorithms

Structural bioinformatics focuses on studying and predicting biological macromolecules' three-dimensional (3D) structures. Homology modeling, sometimes called comparison modeling is a technique used to predict the 3D structures of proteins and nucleic acids based on the known structures of similar molecules. It is based on the idea that even when protein sequences differ dramatically, the tertiary structures of the proteins remain constant throughout evolution [68]. There are four primary phases in the process:

1. Template identification is used for searching databases for known structures that share sequence similarity with the target molecule.
2. The target sequence is aligned with the template structures to identify corresponding residues in the sequence alignment phase.
3. In the model-building phase, a 3D model is generated for the target based on the template structures, often using spatial restraints derived from the templates.
4. Finally, the model refinement and validation of the model to improve its stereochemical quality and validate it using various structural and statistical checks.

The 3D protein structure homology modeling program MODELLER is frequently used. It creates models by comparing the modeled sequence to similar sequences [69]. Molecular docking aims to determine which orientation of two molecules will result in the most stable combination. Predicting how compounds will react with their intended targets is essential in the drug design process [70]. Necessary procedures in molecular docking include:

1. Preparing the receptor and ligand structures, including adding hydrogen atoms, defining rotatable bonds, and assigning charges.
2. Defining scoring functions to evaluate different binding orientations and conformations.
3. Employing algorithms to explore possible binding modes, including stochastic or deterministic search methods.
4. Ranking the predicted binding modes based on scoring functions and analyzing the results to understand the binding interactions.

AutoDock is a suite of automated docking tools designed to predict how small molecules, such as substrates or drug candidates, bind to a receptor of known 3D structure [71]. *Ab initio* modeling, or *de novo* modeling, predicts protein structures solely from their amino acid sequences without using any template structure. It is beneficial when no suitable template is available for homology modeling [72, 73]. The *de novo* modeling process often requires:

1. Building protein conformations by assembling short fragments from a library of known structures.
2. Employing computational methods to find low-energy conformations that are likely close to the native structure.
3. Using statistical mechanics techniques to explore conformational space and find the global minimum energy conformation.

Rosetta is a software suite for predicting and designing protein structures, folding, and protein–protein interactions from amino acid sequences, using a fragment-based approach when no homologous templates are available [74].

Alpha-helices, beta-sheets, and twists are all examples of local protein structures that can be predicted using just the amino acid sequence [75]. The main procedures in secondary structure method are:

1. Statistical techniques use the known structures statistics to predict secondary structure elements.
2. Machine learning techniques like neural networks are used to predict secondary structures based on patterns in training data.
3. The profile-based methods are used in multiple sequence alignments to generate profiles and predict secondary structures based on conserved patterns.

PSIPRED is a technique that uses neural networks to accurately predict secondary structure components like alpha-helices and beta-sheets from amino acid sequences [76].

9.5.4 High-performance computing (HPC) in bioinformatics

High-performance computing (HPC) has become vital in bioinformatics, enabling large-scale biological and genomic data processing and analysis [77]. The advent of next-generation sequencing (NGS) technologies and the surge in publicly available biological data have made modern biological experiments both data and computationally intensive [77]. HPC provides the computational power necessary to handle the 'Big Data' challenges posed by bioinformatics, facilitating the extraction of knowledge from raw data through larger computational platforms known as supercomputers [78]. Parallel computing is a type of computation in which many calculations or processes are carried out simultaneously. Bioinformatics accelerates the analysis of large datasets and complex computational tasks [79]. The HPC in bioinformatics is particularly used in the following areas:

- **Sequence alignment:** Parallel algorithms can drastically reduce the time required to align large or multiple sequences [80].
- **Phylogenetic analysis:** Constructing phylogenetic trees from large datasets is computationally demanding, and parallel computing can significantly accelerate this process [81].
- **Structural modeling:** Parallel computing enables faster processing in structural bioinformatics, such as molecular docking and homology modeling.

The background in the high-performance computing area, including parallel computing, opens up significant opportunities for simulating relevant biological systems and applications in bioinformatics, computational biology, and computational chemistry [82]. A schematic workflow of HPC and how it works is shown in figure 9.5.

9.5.5 Cloud computing in genomics

Cloud computing provides a flexible and scalable environment for storing, managing, and analyzing a gigantic amount of genomic data. It has emerged as

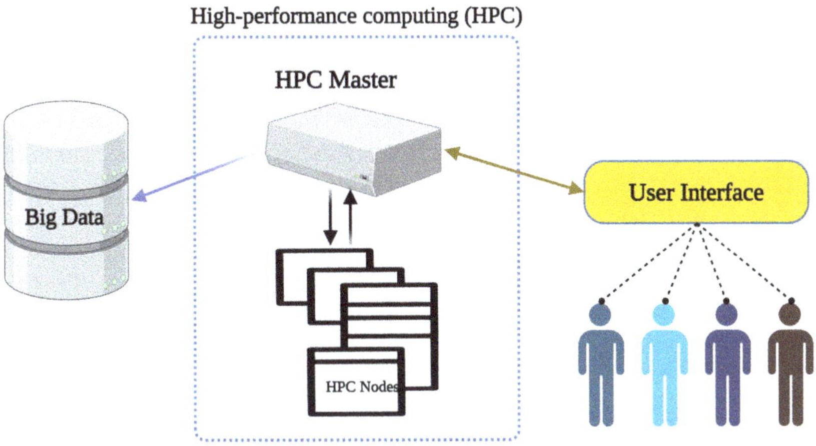

Figure 9.5. HPC framework: data processing from big data storage through hpc nodes to user interface.

a vital resource for bioinformatics and genomics, offering several advantages. Cloud computing reduces the costs associated with data storage and computational resources, which is especially beneficial for smaller research groups or institutions. It allows for the easy scaling of resources as the data volume grows. Cloud platforms provide easy access to data and computational resources from anywhere, anytime. The technology of cloud computing and its applications in biology and bioinformatics have enormously increased over recent years, providing a platform for the analysis of biological data that would not be possible without significant computational resources [83]. Resources such as NSF XSEDE, Google Cloud, and Amazon AWS have become more available, and a growing community of academicians are working on teaching the utility of HPC resources in genomics and big data analyses [84].

9.5.6 GPGPU (general-purpose computing on graphics processing units)

GPGPU stands for General-Purpose computing on Graphics Processing Units. It represents an innovative approach in which the powerful processing capabilities of graphics processing units (GPUs) are employed for general computing tasks beyond just rendering graphics. In bioinformatics, GPGPU has shown significant promise in accelerating various computationally intensive tasks. The utilization of GPGPU in bioinformatics is primarily facilitated through libraries such as Nvidia's CUDA (Compute Unified Device Architecture). CUDA is a widely used library for developing GPU-based tools in bioinformatics, computational biology, and systems biology. It is specifically tailored to use Nvidia GPUs, although alternative solutions like Microsoft DirectCompute also exist. The adoption of GPGPU in bioinformatics has been driven by the need to reduce the running time required by standard CPU-based software, allowing for more intensive investigations of biological systems. GPGPU offers computational power comparable to a small computer cluster but at a significantly lower cost, around $400. This advantage, coupled with the developing of specific algorithms tailored for GPU computing, has led to a growing interest in GPGPU within the scientific community [85].

A collection of GPU tools has been developed to perform computational analyses in life science disciplines, emphasizing the advantages and drawbacks of these parallel architectures. GPUs can considerably reduce the running time, enabling more efficient data processing and analysis in bioinformatics [86].

9.5.7 Big data analytics in bioinformatics

Big data analytics in bioinformatics refers to applying advanced analytic techniques on extensive and complex biological datasets. The emergence of high-throughput technologies, like NGS, has led to the generation of massive amounts of biological and genomic data. Big data analytics is crucial for extracting meaningful insights from these data, including discovering new knowledge, identifying patterns, and making informed decisions. Several primary approaches are used in data analysis to derive meaning from large datasets. Data mining is a fundamental approach, utilizing algorithms to filter through large datasets and reveal hidden patterns and relationships. ML takes center stage, as complex algorithms are applied to develop predictive models that can estimate future events based on the existing data. Statistical analysis is crucial to drawing meaningful conclusions from data, which uses statistical techniques to analyze the data, identify patterns, and rigorously test hypotheses. To better grasp a dataset, visualization methods are often used to construct visual representations of the data, providing a more transparent picture of the underlying patterns and connections. Several tools and frameworks have been built expressly for big data analytics in bioinformatics to manage the absolute volume and variety of biological data. Accelerating research in the biological sciences, these tools improve data processing, visualization, and interpretation [87].

9.5.8 Systems biology modelling

Systems biology modeling uses computer models to assess biological data and predict system behavior to comprehend the complicated relationships within biological systems. Network analysis and metabolic pathway analysis are essential analytical techniques in system biology. In systems biology, network analysis often involves the examination of biological networks to clarify the intricate relationships between diverse biological entities, including proteins, metabolites, and genes. This method helps to comprehend the fundamental design and operation of biological systems. Building and analyzing networks using molecular data is known as molecular networking. Vital biological insights can be made by studying the relationships between molecules, such as finding crucial regulatory molecules or comprehending the processes behind the disease. Networks are inferred from experimental data using a variety of instruments and techniques, and these networks are then analyzed to determine their topological characteristics, dynamics, and functional consequences [88]. Metabolic pathway analysis includes the study of metabolic pathways to understand the movement of materials and information inside biological systems. Flux-based analysis is carried out to learn more about how metabolic pathways are controlled and how they contribute to cellular function, which entails the use of computer models to evaluate the flow of metabolites via metabolic networks [89]. To offer a thorough knowledge of biological systems, systems biology analysis is a more complete approach that includes metabolic pathway analysis, among other techniques. It analyzes and interprets the behavior of complex biological systems, such as metabolic networks, using computer models and experimental data [88].

9.5.9 Systems pharmacology

An interdisciplinary field called systems pharmacology combines computational and experimental methods to study how medications interact with biological networks and disease states. The goal of system pharmacology is to create mechanistic, quantitative knowledge that can estimate medication reactions and direct the development of novel treatment approaches. Quantitative systems pharmacology (QSP) is a mechanistic platform in pharmacology that models the interplay between medications, biological networks, and disease states to foretell optimal therapy responses. Small molecules, nucleic acids, proteins, pathways, cells, organs, and disease processes are all explored regarding medication interactions. Step-by-step enhancement of the modeling process to make it more effective and repeatable is essential to creating and validating QSP models. These models are flexible and ever-evolving, so they can easily absorb newly available data and insights [90]. Multiscale modeling in systems pharmacology, especially in disease situations, links the cellular responses to protein or drug interactions in the context of animal or human physiology. When it comes to converting preclinical scientific discoveries into useful clinical applications, these models are essential [91]. In addition, discovering combination therapy treatments, particularly those targeting the immune system, might benefit from multiscale systems pharmacology modeling techniques [92].

9.5.10 Multiscale modeling

The goal of multiscale modeling is to combine data from different scales and different physics in order to determine the processes behind the formation of function in biological systems. It includes analyses of biological and medical phenomena at several levels of organization, from the molecular to the organismal. ML methods are rapidly being included in multiscale modeling because of the valuable tools they provide for the robust management of challenging issues and the handling of sparse and noisy data. When multiscale modeling is combined with ML, the resulting models can better capture the nuanced details of biological systems [93]. Recently, ML has found its way into the multiscale modeling of hierarchical engineering materials and the solution of high-dimensional partial differential equations, unveiling its interdisciplinary relevance across various fields [94]. Constructing computational and mathematical models based on experimental data is a common approach to comprehending and predicting the behavior of complex biological systems. Simple modeling techniques like differential equations or Boolean networks benefit from incorporating multiscale modeling, enabling a more comprehensive representation of these intricate systems [95]. Multiscale modeling is emerging as a significant discipline within computational biomedicine. While numerous promising multiscale models are in existence and are currently under development, it is worth noting the need for a unified multiscale modeling methodology, indicating a potential area for further research and development to enhance the multiscale modeling foundation [96].

9.5.11 Computational genomics

Computational genomics is a field that utilizes computational and statistical techniques to deduce biological information from genomic data. With the advent of high-throughput sequencing technologies, there has been an exponential increase in genomic data available, necessitating the development of computational methods to analyze this data effectively. In the field of genomics, various essential processes and techniques are employed for data handling and analysis. Database construction and management involve creating and maintaining databases to store, organize, and manage genomic data efficiently. Data retrieval systems are developed to facilitate the swift retrieval of data from these genomic databases. Sequence alignment techniques are crucial in aligning DNA, RNA, or protein sequences to pinpoint regions of similarity. Methods for detecting motifs and domains are used to locate regions of DNA or RNA that are conserved. Prediction of 3D structures is a computer approach for predicting the 3D structures of proteins and nucleic acids. Structural elements are assigned biological roles based on their 3D structures using the functional annotation of structural elements. One may create phylogenetic trees showing evolutionary links between different species using phylogenetic analysis. To understand evolutionary linkages and processes, molecular evolutionary analysis examines molecular sequences. Genome-wide association studies (GWAS) use statistical methods to find gene variations linked to certain diseases. This information may then be used to understand the underlying biology of such conditions better. Biological consequences may be predicted with the help of predictive models generated using ML algorithms from genetic data. Deep learning techniques are used to examine large genetic datasets and discover hidden patterns and correlations [97]. Essential for controling gene expression, regulatory elements are the subject of regulatory element identification. These elements include promoters, enhancers, and silencers. Building and analyzing regulatory networks to learn more about how genes are controlled is the goal of regulatory network construction. Understanding DNA methylation and histone modifications, two examples of epigenetic marks may be gained by the computational process known as epigenetic mark identification. In order to analyze the effects of gene regulation on cellular processes, it is necessary to combine genomic and transcriptomic data with epigenetic data [98].

9.5.12 Functional genomics

The goal of functional genomics is to determine how genetics affects behavior. Methods from several disciplines are used to show the complete process of how genes function in living organisms. When we talk about sequencing, we mean doing a whole-genome sequence from scratch [99]. In order to find variants in a genome that has previously been sequenced, genome resequencing is used. Pan-genomic analyses take into account all of a species or a set of related species' genomic information, which helps to understand the functional components and evolutionary dynamics of the genomes [99]. The RNA-seq and metabolomics analyses cover the RNA-seq which is utilized for transcriptome profiling to determine the continuously altering cellular transcriptome. Metabolomics provides a more comprehensive picture of the organism's metabolic profile by analyzing all of the substrates and metabolites in a biological sample. Uncovering the molecular pathways that underlie different biological activities requires a thorough knowledge of novel genes, including their roles and interactions [99, 100].

9.5.13 Comparative genomics

Genomes from various species are analyzed and compared as part of comparative genomics. Comparative genomics uses principles of structure, function, and genomic evolution. Understanding gene function and evolution is aided by gene family analyses, which look at the evolution and function of gene families across many species. Genomic data from different plant species may be compared using plant evolutionary analyses, which can reveal hidden connections and histories between them [101]. Gene evolution and function may be better understood when orthologs and paralogs are identified and compared across species and within genomes, respectively. Understanding the evolution and function of genomes depends on the identification of conserved areas within genomes, which is made possible by the use of colinearity analysis in comparative genomics [102].

9.5.14 Epigenomics

Epigenomics explores modifications of genetic materials and associated proteins, affecting gene expression without altering the DNA sequence. It influences high-throughput technologies to map the epigenome, enhancing understanding of different genomic outputs [103]. Single-cell epigenomics focused on understanding non-coding disease-associated human variants, single-cell epigenomics provides detailed maps of candidate cis-regulatory elements in heterogeneous human tissues, aiding in interpreting the genetic basis of common traits and diseases [103, 104]. High-throughput technologies have propelled epigenomics into a multi-omics era, where powerful tools describe and record diverse layers of genomic output, allowing for a thorough interrogation of cellular components [104].

9.5.15 Metagenomics

Metagenomics encompasses the analysis of genetic material directly sourced from environmental samples, extending the scope of microbial genomics beyond cultured organisms [105]. In the field of metagenomics, two fundamental methodologies play a pivotal role in understanding microbial communities—marker gene studies and whole-genome shotgun (WGS) metagenomics. These approaches are the foundation of our understanding of diverse ecosystems. Marker gene studies focus on specific genes, often 16S ribosomal RNA genes, to provide insights into the taxonomic composition of microbial communities. Conversely, WGS metagenomics takes a comprehensive approach, searching through the entire genomic material present within a sample, offering a comprehensive snapshot of microbial diversity and potential functional capabilities. These methods, while distinct, work together to enhance our comprehension of microbial ecosystems [106]. Metagenomics empowered by NGS, has brought significant advancements in our ability to investigate this complex ecosystem. The gut microbiome exerts a profound influence on host health, and metagenomics provides us with the tools needed to interpret its role with unprecedented precision. By decoding the genetic makeup of the many microorganisms residing within our intestines, we gain valuable insights into their functional contributions to processes such as digestion, metabolism, and even immune system modulation. This novel understanding not only deepens our appreciation of the gut microbiome's significance but also paves the way for novel therapeutic interventions aimed at maintaining and restoring the delicate balance within this microbial community, ultimately boosting host health and well-being [107].

9.6 Bioinformatics in precision medicine

Bioinformatics plays a pivotal role in precision medicine, which aims to tailor medical treatment to individual characteristics of each patient. It is an interdisciplinary field that utilizes bioinformatics to analyze molecular data to identify genetic, epigenomic, and other molecular predictors of drug response and disease susceptibility. Genomic medicine is an emerging medical discipline that involves using genomic information about an individual as part of their clinical care and the health outcomes and policy implications of that clinical use. Pharmacogenomics is a crucial part of genomic medicine and precision medicine at large. It is the study of how genes affect a person's response to drugs. This field aims to develop rational means to optimize drug therapy, with respect to the patient's genotype, to ensure maximum efficacy with minimal adverse effects. By understanding an individual's genetic makeup, doctors can prescribe medications and doses personalized to the genetic profile of the individual [108, 109]. For instance, pharmacogenomics helps in predicting drug dose, like the dose of thiopurines based on variation in the thiopurine methyltransferase (TPMT). Despite its potential, the understanding of pharmacogenomic guidelines in clinical practice has been slow but is gradually improving. Genomic predictors of disease refer to genetic variants or patterns that are associated with the risk of developing particular diseases. Bioinformatics tools and techniques are employed to analyze large datasets to identify these predictors which can then be used for risk assessment, early detection, or personalized treatment plans. Genomic counseling extends beyond traditional genetic counseling to encompass a broader range of genetic and genomic information. It involves discussing with individuals or families about their genomic information and what it means for their health, disease risk, and other life aspects [110]. Key points in genomic counseling include:

- The number and/or type of diseases for which testing is available and discussed.
- The purpose of testing.
- Intervention and clinical utility.
- Access to testing [111].
- Transition from traditional genetic counseling to genomic counseling involves a move from reactive genetic testing for diagnosis of primarily single-gene diseases to proactive genome-based testing for multiple conditions [111].

Personal genomics pertains to the use of genomic information at an individual level to guide healthcare decisions includes:

- Advanced diagnostics.
- Tumor profiling.
- Genomic risk assessments [112].

Personal genomics has the potential to significantly influence healthcare by enabling personalized medicine, which tailors medical interventions to an individual's unique genomic profile. It is also a subject of genomics education, emphasizing the importance and benefits of understanding personal genomic information in society, including in classrooms, clinics, and the public sphere [113].

9.7 Translational bioinformatics

Translational bioinformatics (TBI) is a crucial field that bridges the gap between biomedical data science and informatics, determined for a seamless translation of scientific discoveries into clinical practice. TBI is in the forefront in areas like the clinical utility of polygenic risk scores, data integration, and using artificial intelligence (AI) and ML for enhanced healthcare delivery [114]. Clinical decision support systems (CDSSs) are integral tools in TBI that assist healthcare professionals in making informed clinical decisions. They analyze data from various sources to provide evidence-based recommendations tailored to individual patient conditions. By integrating with electronic health records (EHRs), these systems ensure a seamless flow of patient data, thereby facilitating better clinical decisions, improving patient outcomes, and reducing healthcare costs. The integration of EHRs is central to TBI as it facilitates the utilization of rich patient data for better clinical decision-making. By convoluting EHRs with clinical decision support, healthcare differences can be addressed more effectively, especially in low-resource settings, thereby improving health equity [115]. Moreover, the real-world integration of genomic data into EHRs is an effort to operationalize guidelines for precision medicine delivery, enhancing the EHR's capability for such advanced healthcare provision. A significant aspect of a CDSS is its integration or interoperability with EHRs to enhance healthcare for populations facing discrepancies. This integration facilitates the seamless flow of patient-specific information, enabling personalized clinical recommendations. Various studies have been conducted on clinicians facing CDSS integrated or interoperable with EHR, revealing that most of these were implemented in primary care outpatient settings for screening or treatment purposes. The types of clinical decision support (CDS) tools include point-of-care alerts, order facilitators, workflow support, relevant information display, expert systems, and medication dosing support. The potential of CDS tools lies in improving health equity and outcomes, especially for patients who face disparities. The user-centered design is crucial during the planning, development, and implementation phases of CDSS. It ensures that the system is adapted to meet the needs and preferences of its users, thereby enhancing its usability and effectiveness. Implementation strategies most frequently employed include education and consensus facilitation, which are vital for the successful deployment and adoption of CDSSs [115].

Patient stratification is a crucial process in personalized medicine, which involves categorizing patients into different subgroups based on their risk of developing certain medical conditions or their response to specific treatments. This process aids in tailoring medical treatment to individual patients or groups of patients, thereby enhancing the effectiveness and efficiency of healthcare delivery [116]. ML models play a significant role in patient risk stratification by predicting future disease states based on a patient's current clinical state and historical data. These models can help identify which applications of predictions will be sound by distinguishing between predictions based on physician behavior and those based on a constant representation of patient physiology [117]. Disease modeling is essential for understanding the dynamics of disease spread and the impact of various factors on disease outcomes. It is a multidimensional approach encompassing biological, social, and behavioral factors. The integration of social and behavioral dynamics in disease models is particularly significant as it influences the emergence, spread, and containment of diseases. Recent global health threats like the Ebola and COVID-19 pandemics have highlighted the importance of developing disease models that incorporate these dynamics for more effective response measures and policies [118]. Disease modeling makes use of a wide range of approaches, including computational systems biology and the creation of patient-specific cell lines from induced pluripotent stem cells (iPSCs), to highlight on disease causes, medication responses, and prospective therapeutic treatments [119, 120].

9.8 Bioinformatics in drug discovery and development

The field of bioinformatics has become more important in the creation of new medicines in recent years. It has several uses and is a major factor in the success of modern drug research. Understanding the molecular basis of diseases and therapeutic targets requires the management and analysis of massive volumes of biological data produced by fields such as genomics, transcriptomics, proteomics, population genetics, and molecular phylogenetics [121]. Predictive models may be developed to understand the behavior of bioactive chemicals using bioinformatics tools and methodologies, which can help in the design and development of novel medications. Bioinformatics can anticipate interactions between medications and proteins, examine the influence on biological processes and activities, and uncover genetic variations that may modify drug response. This is critical for comprehending the workings of possible medications and their side effects [122]. Bioinformatics may greatly speed up drug target selection, drug candidate screening, and refinement despite the difficulties involved in drug development. This helps to overcome the lengthy and costly nature of conventional drug discovery procedures [123]. Potential targets must successfully move from the discovery stage to clinical trials and ultimately the market, and bioinformatics plays a critical role in this process by assisting with the prediction, analysis, or interpretation of clinical data. To better understand and solve problems in drug discovery and development, chemoinformatics, combines chemistry and computer science. To better comprehend chemical characteristics and molecular interactions in biological systems, it uses computational methods to examine chemical data. When it comes to the computer study of molecules, molecular representation plays a crucial role by providing a means for the systematic storage and retrieval of chemical data in both 2D and 3D formats. Chemical databases are mined for relevant patterns and insights using data mining methods such structural similarity matrices, classification algorithms, and descriptor computations. Additionally, chemoinformatics and quantitative structure–activity relationship (QSAR) modeling work in combination to improve molecular design prediction modeling and provide insightful information about the behavior of bioactive substances. Together, these fundamental applications enhance our knowledge of chemical structures and how they interact, advancing materials research and medication development. Chemoinformatics supports the production of comprehensive databases, predictive models, and analytical tools required for current drug discovery procedures, expediting the journey from molecular idea to drug development [124].

New therapeutic indications for previously authorized or experimental medications may be found via a process known as drug repositioning, repurposing, redirecting, or reprofiling. Because of the high prices, severe hazards, and poor speed of conventional drug development techniques, this method is gaining popularity. A crucial component of pharmaceutical research is drug repositioning, which entails a number of essential components. In this process, computational techniques play a key role by analyzing current data to find novel potential uses for well-established medications. These methods use ML and computational tools to find correlations between medications and diseases based on chemical, genomic, or phenotypic data. In addition, drug repositioning is well-known for its financial viability, as it provides a cost-effective alternative to conventional drug discovery by making use of already-existing data and resources, thus shortening the time and lowering the costs normally associated with bringing drugs to market [125].

In the early phases of drug development, virtual screening (VS) is used to filter through chemical libraries in search of structures with the highest propensity to bind to therapeutic targets. It is crucial for cutting down on the time and money needed to find potential medication candidates. Consensus virtual screening (CVS) is a recent development in SBVS (structure-based virtual screening) with the goal of improving SBVS accuracy and decreasing false positives in these kinds of research. Having access to the 3D structure of the target protein is necessary for SBVS to be used. The process of predicting drug–target interactions (DTIs) is a cornerstone of the pharmaceutical industry. Drug mechanism of action, impact prediction, and side effect avoidance all rely on this process of discovering possible drug interactions with biological targets. Predicting DTIs is important for several reasons in the pharmaceutical industry, including virtual screening, drug repurposing, and the detection of adverse drug reactions. It has been reported that using deep learning and ML models in virtual screening might enhance DTI prediction, emphasizing the use of computational methods in contemporary drug development procedures [126].

9.8.1 Artificial intelligence (AI) and machine learning in bioinformatics

The use of deep learning, a type of ML and AI, in the analysis of big biological data, prediction, and the discovery of new biological insights has shown great promise in bioinformatics. The analysis of sequences, the identification of motifs, and the prediction of the function or structure of molecules have all been performed using deep learning models like CNNs and RNNs. Understanding the function of proteins and other biomolecules requires knowing their 3D structures, which may be predicted. Predicting molecular structures using deep learning, and in particular CNNs, has led to significant advances in the field, with tools like AlphaFold highlighting the potential of deep learning in structural biology. Learning how genes work and what influences their expression, such as epigenetics, is made easier with the help of deep learning. Deep learning may be used to investigate massive genomic datasets in order to better understand the regulatory networks that govern cellular activity. Deep learning aids in the comprehension of complex biological systems by combining data at many biological scales. Multi-omics analysis, which involves characterizing and quantifying groups of biological molecules, falls under this category [127]. Different methods used in AI are listed in figure 9.6.

9.8.2 AI-driven drug discovery

Modern drug development procedures greatly benefit from AI, especially ML and deep learning, which speed up the conversion of data into useful ideas. Big datasets of chemical substances may be processed by AI algorithms, which can then forecast their possible toxicity and effectiveness. This speeds up the drug development process's first screening step considerably. With the analysis of vast datasets, AI may discover novel therapeutic applications for already-approved medications and potentially connect pharmacological mechanisms with disease pathways. For pharmaceuticals to be safe, it is essential to anticipate how they may interact with one another or with diseases. AI may help in the creation of safer medications by analyzing large, complicated information to predict potential interactions. The identification of biomarkers is essential for tracking the effectiveness of treatments and making diagnosis. AI can select through massive biological datasets to uncover potential biomarkers. AI can help design more efficient clinical trials, predict outcomes, and identify the most suitable candidates for trials. These speed up the drug development process and bring new therapies to patients faster. Predictive modeling encompasses a variety of statistical and ML techniques to predict outcomes based on data. It is a crucial tool in bioinformatics and drug discovery,

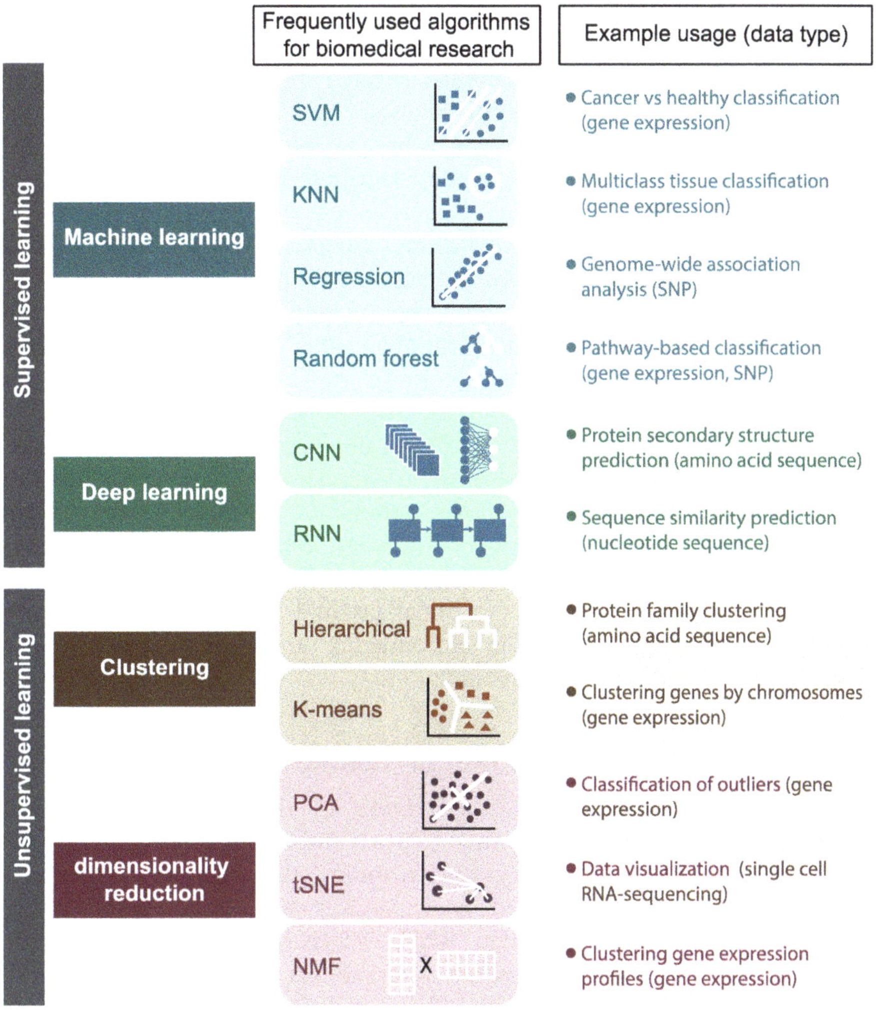

Figure 9.6. Commonly employed machine learning algorithms in bioinformatics investigations are outlined. Each algorithm is accompanied by an example of its application and the corresponding input data, as depicted on the right side. Abbreviations include SVM for support vector machines, KNN for K-nearest neighbors, CNN for convolutional neural networks, RNN for recurrent neural networks, PCA for principal component analysis, t-SNE for t-distributed stochastic neighbor embedding, and NMF for non-negative matrix factorization. Reproduced from [128] CC BY 4.0.

where it enables the forecasting of biological and chemical phenomena based on existing data [129]. Regression analysis is used to predict continuous outcomes. For instance, it can be used to predict the binding affinity of a drug to a particular target based on certain molecular descriptors. Classification techniques are used to predict categorical outcomes. In bioinformatics, it might be used to classify genes into different functional categories based on expression data. Time-series analysis can predict outcomes over time, essential in studying biological processes that change over time like cell growth or gene expression levels over a developmental timeline. Essential for handling high-dimensional data common in bioinformatics and drug discovery. It identifies the most informative features or reduces the dimensionality of the data without losing essential information, and ensures the reliability and robustness of predictive models through techniques like cross-validation [130].

Advancements in AI, particularly deep learning, have significantly impacted image analysis and microscopy in biological research, enabling automated and more accurate analysis. Deep learning algorithms, especially CNNs, have empowered automated image segmentation, object detection, and classification in biological and medical imaging. Deep learning can enhance the resolution of microscopy images through super-resolution techniques, enabling finer examination of biological structures. Analyzing time-lapse microscopy images using AI can reveal dynamic biological processes, tracking cells and understanding cellular dynamics over time. High-content screening (HCS) often involves analyzing large sets of microscopy images to understand cellular phenotypes. AI accelerates this analysis, identifying phenotypic changes in response to various treatments. 3D image analysis is crucial for understanding complex biological structures. Deep learning algorithms can segment, classify, and analyze 3D images, providing insights into 3D cellular structures and tissues. Comprehensive understanding of biological processes may be gained by combining data from several imaging modalities or picture data with other forms of data (such as genomic data) [131].

9.9 CRISPR and genome editing in bioinformatics

Genome editing has been given a major boost by the CRISPR-Cas (Clustered Regularly Interspaced Short Palindromic Repeats and CRISPR-associated proteins) technology. Bioinformatics' ability to streamline the planning, analysis, and interpretation of studies is crucial to expanding and directing CRISPR-Cas applications. Designing good guide RNAs (gRNAs) is critical for efficient CRISPR-Cas genome editing. In order to pick gRNA sequences with optimal on-target activity and minimal off-target effects, bioinformatics methods are useful. Using sequence similarity and other genetic markers, bioinformatics systems may identify probable off-target regions. Algorithms and ML models have been created to predict the on-target effectiveness of gRNAs, facilitating in the selection of the most successful gRNAs for genome editing. Numerous options for genome editing are made possible by the variety of CRISPR-Cas systems [132]. Bioinformatics aids in defining and cataloging these variations, understanding their causes, and predicting their genome-editing capabilities. The collection of data from CRISPR-Cas research has led to the formation of databases and libraries. These tools are useful for the community, allowing the exchange of gRNA sequences, efficiency ratings, and off-target predictions. Genes implicated in certain traits may be discovered using CRISPR screening. The high-throughput data produced by these screens, the identification of relevant hits, and the interpretation of the findings all need the use of bioinformatics tools. The integration of CRISPR-Cas bioinformatics tools with other bioinformatics resources may give more complete insights. The whole extent to which genome editing affects biological processes, for instance, may be shown by integrating data on genome editing with those on gene expression, proteomics, or pathway analysis [133].

Computational tools are essential in genome editing because they guarantee accuracy and productivity of the editing procedure. The development of guide RNAs (gRNAs), the anticipation of off-target effects, and the analysis of genome editing experiment results. Software tools like CRISPR Design and Benchling aid in designing gRNAs with high on-target efficiency and minimal off-target effects. They often provide a user-friendly interface for selecting target sequences and designing gRNAs. Tools like Cas-OFFinder and CRISPRscan help in predicting potential off-target sites based on sequence similarity, aiding in the design of gRNAs with higher specificity. Certain tools offer predictions on the efficiency of designed gRNAs, integrating factors like sequence composition and genomic context to provide a score indicative of the likely editing efficiency. For projects requiring multiplexed editing, tools that assist in designing multiple gRNAs and organizing complex editing strategies are crucial.

Genome editing, especially in the context of human genomes, brings out plenty of ethical considerations. Editing the germline potentially alters the genetic makeup of future generations, raising concerns about unintended consequences and the ethics of altering human evolution. Obtaining informed consent, especially in germline editing, is a complex issue, given the long-term and often unknown implications of genome editing. There is concern over genome editing technologies becoming a means of extending existing social inequalities if access is restricted to affluent individuals or communities. Establishing robust regulatory frameworks is crucial to ensure the responsible use of genome editing technologies [134].

Functional genomics aims to understand the relationship between the genome and the phenotype. CRISPR-based screens are powerful tools in functional genomics. Systematically interrogating gene function on a genome-wide scale by utilizing libraries of gRNAs targeting every gene in the genome. Following genome editing, phenotypic changes can be assessed using a variety of assays, elucidating the function of individual genes or gene networks. Bioinformatics tools are essential for analyzing the vast datasets generated from CRISPR screens, identifying significant genes, and interpreting the biological implications. Combining CRISPR screen data with other omics data (transcriptomics and proteomics) can provide a more broader understanding of gene function and cellular processes [135].

9.10 Integrative and multi-omics analysis

The advent of high-throughput technologies has facilitated the generation of large-scale biological data across different molecular levels. Integrative and multi-omics analyses seek to combine these data to provide a more comprehensive understanding of biological systems. Integrative genomics aims to combine data from different genomic datasets to elucidate the underlying genetic architectures of traits and diseases. Integrative genomics is the harmonization of different genomic datasets, ensuring data representation and analysis consistency. Meta-analysis techniques are used to aggregate information from various studies to identify common genetic traits. Integrative genomics often involves cross-species comparisons to identify conserved genetic elements and pathways [136]. Multi-omics integration aims to combine data across different 'omics' layers (genomics, transcriptomics, proteomics, metabolomics) to provide a more comprehensive understanding of biological systems. Techniques like matrix factorization and network integration are used to combine data across different omics layers, revealing relationships between molecular entities across these layers. Principal component analysis (PCA) and t-distributed stochastic neighbourhood embedding (t-SNE) are two dimensionality reduction methods that are used to handle the complexity of multi-omics data and find patterns within the data [137]. Single-cell multi-omics provides a high-resolution view of the cellular landscape by analyzing multiple omics layers at the single-cell level. At the single-cell level, multi-omics data is generated using technologies like single-cell RNA sequencing (scRNA-seq) and single-cell ATAC sequencing (scATAC-seq). Clustering methods are applied to identify cell kinds and states based on single-cell multi-omics data. Modeling interactions between molecular entities across many omics layers requires a network-based methodology. A framework for navigating multi-omics data is provided by networks built based on statistical correlations between molecular components. Modules inside networks, frequently corresponding to biological routes or functional groupings, are identified using community detection techniques. Methods for predicting the effects of disturbances on a network or locating key regulatory nodes are essential for understanding how changes in one part of the system can affect the entire network.

References

[1] Baxevanis A D, Bader G D and Wishart D S 2020 *Bioinformatics* (New York: Wiley)

[2] Gauthier J *et al* 2019 A brief history of bioinformatics *Brief. Bioinform.* **20** 1981–96

[3] Min S, Lee B and Yoon S 2017 Deep learning in bioinformatics *Brief. Bioinform.* **18** 851–69

[4] Zvelebil M J and Baum J O 2007 *Understanding Bioinformatics* (Garland Science)

[5] Mirsaydaliyevich Y 2022 History of bioinformatics *Int. J. Soc. Sci. Interdiscip. Res.* **11** 72–6

[6] Ouzounis C A and Valencia A 2003 Early bioinformatics: the birth of a discipline—a personal view *Bioinformatics* **19** 2176–90

[7] Jawdat D 2006 The era of bioinformatics 2nd Int. Conf. on Information & Communication Technologies (Piscataway, NJ: IEEE)

[8] Danchin A 2000 A brief history of genome research and bioinformatics in France *Bioinformatics* **16** 65–75

[9] Mardis E R 2017 DNA sequencing technologies: 2006–2016 *Nat. Protoc.* **12** 213–8

[10] Pearson W R *et al* 1997 Comparison of DNA sequences with protein sequences *Genomics* **46** 24–36

[11] Mizrachi I 2007 GenBank: the nucleotide sequence database *The NCBI Handbook [Internet], updated* (National Center for Biotechnology Information) 22

[12] Stoesser G *et al* 1999 The EMBL nucleotide sequence database *Nucleic Acids Res.* **27** 18–24

[13] Kulikova T *et al* 2004 The EMBL nucleotide sequence database *Nucleic Acids Res.* **32** D27–30

[14] Baker W *et al* 2000 The EMBL nucleotide sequence database *Nucleic Acids Res.* **28** 19–23

[15] Dunn J J *et al* 2002 Genomic signature tags (GSTs): a system for profiling genomic DNA *Genome Res.* **12** 1756–65
[16] van der Lelie D *et al* 2006 Use of single-point genome signature tags as a universal tagging method for microbial genome surveys *Appl. Environ. Microbiol.* **72** 2092–101
[17] Thareau V *et al* 2003 Automatic design of gene-specific sequence tags for genome-wide functional studies *Bioinformatics* **19** 2191–8
[18] Hilson P *et al* 2004 Versatile gene-specific sequence tags for *Arabidopsis* functional genomics: transcript profiling and reverse genetics applications *Genome Res.* **14** 2176–89
[19] Han W *et al* 2006 DNA methylation mapping by tag-modified bisulfite genomic sequencing *Anal. Biochem.* **355** 50–61
[20] Cochrane G *et al* 2016 The international nucleotide sequence database collaboration *Nucleic Acids Res.* **44** D48–50
[21] Apweiler R, Bairoch A and Wu C H 2004 Protein sequence databases *Curr. Opin. Chem. Biol.* **8** 76–80
[22] Xu D and Xu Y 2004 Protein databases on the internet *Curr. Protoc. Mol. Biol.* **68** 19.4. 1–19.4. 15
[23] Gasteiger E, Jung E and Bairoch A 2001 SWISS-PROT: connecting biomolecular knowledge via a protein database *Curr. Issues Mol. Biol.* **3** 47–55
[24] Radivojac P *et al* 2004 Classification and knowledge discovery in protein databases *J. Biomed. Inform.* **37** 224–39
[25] Cannataro M, Guzzi P H and Veltri P 2010 Protein-to-protein interactions: technologies, databases, and algorithms *ACM Comput. Surv. (CSUR)* **43** 1–36
[26] Lo Conte L *et al* 2000 SCOP: a structural classification of proteins database *Nucleic Acids Res.* **28** 257–9
[27] Altschul S F *et al* 2005 Protein database searches using compositionally adjusted substitution matrices *FEBS J.* **272** 5101–9
[28] Federhen S 2003 The taxonomy project *The NCBI Handbook* (National Center for Biotechnology Information)
[29] Federhen S 2011 *Entrez Taxonomy Quick Start. Taxonomy Help [Internet]* (Bethesda, MD: National Center for Biotechnology Information (US))
[30] Page R D 2005 A taxonomic search engine: federating taxonomic databases using web services *BMC Bioinf.* **6** 1–8
[31] Gibney G and Baxevanis A D 2011 Searching NCBI databases using Entrez *Curr. Protoc. Bioinform.* **34** 1.3. 1–1.3. 25
[32] Wheeler D L *et al* 2000 Database resources of the national center for biotechnology information *Nucleic Acids Res.* **28** 10–4
[33] Pruitt K D and Maglott D R 2001 RefSeq and LocusLink: NCBI gene-centered resources *Nucleic Acids Res.* **29** 137–40
[34] Pruitt K D *et al* 2000 Introducing RefSeq and LocusLink: curated human genome resources at the NCBI *Trends in Genet.* **16** 44–7
[35] Sherry S T *et al* 2001 dbSNP: the NCBI database of genetic variation *Nucleic Acids Res.* **29** 308–11
[36] Sherry S T, Ward M and Sirotkin K 2000 Use of molecular variation in the NCBI dbSNP database *Hum. Mutat.* **15** 68–75
[37] Pruitt K D, Tatusova T and Maglott D R 2003 NCBI reference sequence project: update and current status *Nucleic Acids Res.* **31** 34–7

[38] Wheeler D L *et al* 2003 Database resources of the national center for biotechnology *Nucleic Acids Res.* **31** 28–33
[39] Mehmood M A, Sehar U and Ahmad N 2014 Use of bioinformatics tools in different spheres of life sciences *J. Data Min. Genom. Proteomics* **5** 1
[40] Saraiya P, North C and Duca K 2005 An insight-based methodology for evaluating bioinformatics visualizations *IEEE Trans. Visual Comput. Graphics* **11** 443–56
[41] Gill S K *et al* 2016 Emerging role of bioinformatics tools and software in evolution of clinical research *Perspectives Clin. Res.* **7** 115
[42] Arabi Z and Sardari S 2010 An investigation into the antifungal property of fabaceae using bioinformatics tools *Avicenna J. Med. Biotechnol.* **2** 93
[43] Attwood T K and Miller C J 2001 Which craft is best in bioinformatics? *Comput. Chem.* **25** 329–39
[44] Gallagher L A, Shendure J and Manoil C 2011 Genome-scale identification of resistance functions in Pseudomonas aeruginosa using Tn-seq *MBio* **2** e00315–10
[45] Okuda T and Kondoh H 1999 Identification of new genes ndr2 and ndr3 which are related to Ndr1/RTP/Drg1 but show distinct tissue specificity and response to N-myc *Biochem. Biophys. Res. Commun.* **266** 208–15
[46] Verde F, Mata J and Nurse P 1995 Fission yeast cell morphogenesis: identification of new genes and analysis of their role during the cell cycle *J. Cell Biol.* **131** 1529–38
[47] Abifadel M *et al* 2014 Living the PCSK9 adventure: from the identification of a new gene in familial hypercholesterolemia towards a potential new class of anticholesterol drugs *Curr. Atheroscler. Rep.* **16** 1–23
[48] Lassmann T 2020 *Kalign 3: Multiple Sequence Alignment of Large Datasets* (Oxford: Oxford University Press)
[49] Clark C and Kalita J 2014 A comparison of algorithms for the pairwise alignment of biological networks *Bioinformatics* **30** 2351–9
[50] Jararweh Y *et al* 2019 Improving the performance of the needleman-wunsch algorithm using parallelization and vectorization techniques *Multimedia Tools Appl.* **78** 3961–77
[51] Khajeh-Saeed A, Poole S and Perot J B 2010 Acceleration of the Smith–Waterman algorithm using single and multiple graphics processors *J. Comput. Phys.* **229** 4247–58
[52] Edgar R C 2004 MUSCLE: multiple sequence alignment with high accuracy and high throughput *Nucleic Acids Res.* **32** 1792–7
[53] Thompson J D, Gibson T J and Higgins D G 2003 Multiple sequence alignment using ClustalW and ClustalX *Curr. Protoc. Bioinform.* 2.3. 1–2.3. 22s
[54] Marco-Sola S *et al* 2021 Fast gap-affine pairwise alignment using the wavefront algorithm *Bioinformatics* **37** 456–63
[55] Altschul S F *et al* 1990 Basic local alignment search tool *J. Mol. Biol.* **215** 403–10
[56] Pearson W R 1994 Using the FASTA program to search protein and DNA sequence databases *Computer Analysis of Sequence Data: Part* I (Springer) pp 307–31
[57] Li H *et al* 2020 Modern deep learning in bioinformatics *J. Mol. Cell. Biol.* **12** 823–7
[58] Challa S and Neelapu N R R 2019 Phylogenetic trees: applications, construction, and assessment *Essentials of Bioinformatics, Volume III: In Silico Life Sciences: Agriculture* (Springer) pp 167–92
[59] Gascuel O and Steel M 2006 Neighbor-joining revealed *Mol. Biol. Evol.* **23** 1997–2000
[60] Gronau I and Moran S 2007 Optimal implementations of UPGMA and other common clustering algorithms *Inf. Process. Lett.* **104** 205–10

[61] Segura-Alabart N *et al* 2022 Nonunique UPGMA clusterings of microsatellite markers *Brief. Bioinform.* **23** bbac312
[62] Yan Z *et al* 2022 Maximum parsimony inference of phylogenetic networks in the presence of polyploid complexes *Syst. Biol.* **71** 706–20
[63] Kleinbaum D G *et al* 2010 Maximum likelihood techniques: an overview *Logistic regression: A Self-learning Text* (Springer) pp 103–27
[64] Hassler G W *et al* 2023 Data integration in bayesian phylogenetics *Annu. Rev. Stat. Appl.* **10** 353–77
[65] Shastry K A and Sanjay H 2020 Machine learning for bioinformatics *Statistical Modelling and Machine Learning Principles for Bioinformatics Techniques, Tools, and Applications* (Springer) pp 25–39
[66] Chen Z *et al* 2020 Feature selection may improve deep neural networks for the bioinformatics problems *Bioinformatics* **36** 1542–52
[67] Dara S *et al* 2022 Machine learning in drug discovery: a review *Artif. Intell. Rev.* **55** 1947–99
[68] Patel B, Singh V and Patel D 2019 Structural bioinformatics *Essentials of Bioinformatics, Volume I: Understanding Bioinformatics: Genes to Proteins* (Springer) pp 169–99
[69] Webb B and Sali A 2021 *Protein Structure Modeling with Modeller* (Berlin: Springer)
[70] Fan J, Fu A and Zhang L 2019 Progress in molecular docking *Quant. Biol.* **7** 83–9
[71] Valdés-Tresanco M S *et al* 2020 AMDock: a versatile graphical tool for assisting molecular docking with Autodock Vina and Autodock4 *Biol. Direct* **15** 1 12
[72] Chivian D *et al* 2003 Ab initio methods *Struct. Bioinform.* **44** 547–57
[73] Wu S, Skolnick J and Zhang Y 2007 Ab initio modeling of small proteins by iterative TASSER simulations *BMC Biol.* **5** 1–10
[74] Moretti R *et al* 2018 Web-accessible molecular modeling with Rosetta: the Rosetta online server that includes everyone (ROSIE) *Protein Sci.* **27** 259–68
[75] Kuhlman B and Bradley P 2019 Advances in protein structure prediction and design *Nat. Rev. Mol. Cell Biol.* **20** 681–97
[76] Buchan D W and Jones D T 2019 The PSIPRED protein analysis workbench: 20 years on *Nucleic Acids Res.* **47** W402–7
[77] Castrignanò T *et al* 2020 ELIXIR-IT HPC@ CINECA: high performance computing resources for the bioinformatics community *BMC Bioinf.* **21** 1–17
[78] Li Y *et al* 2019 Deep learning in bioinformatics: Introduction, application, and perspective in the big data era *Methods* **166** 4–21
[79] Sangaiah A K 2019 *Deep Learning and Parallel Computing Environment for Bioengineering Systems* (New York: Academic)
[80] González-Domínguez J 2021 Fast and accurate multiple sequence alignment with msap-robs-MPI *Multiple Sequence Alignment: Methods and Protocols* (Springer) pp 39–47
[81] Das A and Huang X 2019 HPC: Hierarchical phylogeny construction *PLoS One* **14** e0221357
[82] Behzadi P and Bernabò N 2020 *Computational Biololgy and Chemistry* (BoD–Books on Demand)
[83] Hanussek M, Bartusch F and Krüger J 2021 Performance and scaling behavior of bioinformatic applications in virtualization environments to create awareness for the efficient use of compute resources *PLoS Comput. Biol.* **17** e1009244

[84] Sethuraman A 2022 Teaching computational genomics and bioinformatics on a high performance computing cluster—a primer *Biol. Methods Protoc.* **7** bpac032
[85] Maciá-Lillo A *et al* 2023 GPU cloud architectures for bioinformatic applications *Int. Work-Conf. on Bioinformatics and Biomedical Engineering* (Berlin: Springer)
[86] Tangherloni A *et al* 2021 FiCoS: a fine-grained and coarse-grained GPU-powered deterministic simulator for biochemical networks *PLoS Comput. Biol.* **17** e1009410
[87] Patel D T 2019 Big data analytics in bioinformatics *Biotechnology: Concepts, Methodologies, Tools, and Applications* (IGI Global) pp 1967–84
[88] Greenyer H 2022 Evaluation of network inference algorithms and their effects on network analysis for the study of small metabolomic data sets *PhD Thesis* University of Victoria
[89] Majumder E L-W *et al* 2021 Cognitive analysis of metabolomics data for systems biology *Nat. Protoc.* **16** 1376–418
[90] Helmlinger G *et al* 2019 Quantitative systems pharmacology: an exemplar model-building workflow with applications in cardiovascular, metabolic, and oncology drug development *CPT: Pharmacomet. Syst. Pharmacol.* **8** 380–95
[91] Schoeberl B 2019 Quantitative systems pharmacology models as a key to translational medicine *Curr. Opin. Syst. Biol.* **16** 25–31
[92] Van Hasselt J C and Iyengar R 2019 Systems pharmacology: defining the interactions of drug combinations *Annu. Rev. Pharmacol. Toxicol.* **59** 21–40
[93] Peng G C *et al* 2021 Multiscale modeling meets machine learning: what can we learn? *Arch. Comput. Meth. Eng.* **28** 1017–37
[94] Alber M *et al* 2019 Integrating machine learning and multiscale modeling—perspectives, challenges, and opportunities in the biological, biomedical, and behavioral sciences *NPJ Digit. Med.* **2** 115
[95] Millar-Wilson A *et al* 2022 *Multiscale Modelling in the Framework of Biological Systems and its Potential for Spaceflight Biology Studies* (Iscience)
[96] van der Kolk M *et al* 2021 Des-ist: a simulation framework to streamline event-based in silico trials *Int. Conf. on Computational Science* (Berlin: Springer)
[97] Torri F *et al* 2012 Next generation sequence analysis and computational genomics using graphical pipeline workflows *Genes* **3** 545–75
[98] Tao H *et al* 2021 Computational methods for the prediction of chromatin interaction and organization using sequence and epigenomic profiles *Brief. Bioinform.* **22** bbaa405
[99] Song X *et al* 2021 *Comparative Genomics and Functional Genomics Analyses in Plants* (Frontiers Media SA) p 687966
[100] Lee H H *et al* 2019 Functional genomics of the rapidly replicating bacterium *Vibrio natriegens* by CRISPRi *Nat. Microbiol.* **4** 1105–13
[101] Kumwenda B 2013 *Comparative Genomics Study of Completely Sequenced Thermus Sp. Strains to Enhance and Facilitate their Application in Biotechnology* (University of Pretoria)
[102] Koonin E and Galperin M Y 2002 *Sequence—Evolution—Function: Computational Approaches in Comparative Genomics* (Kluwer Academic)
[103] Wang K C and Chang H Y 2018 Epigenomics: technologies and applications *Circ. Res.* **122** 1191–9
[104] Koch L 2023 Epigenomes get personal *Nat. Rev. Genet.* **24** 1–3
[105] Zhang L *et al* 2021 Advances in metagenomics and its application in environmental microorganisms *Front. Microbiol.* **12** 766364

[106] Pérez-Cobas A E, Gomez-Valero L and Buchrieser C 2020 Metagenomic approaches in microbial ecology: an update on whole-genome and marker gene sequencing analyses *Microb. Genom.* **6** 1–22
[107] Yen S and Johnson J S 2021 Metagenomics: a path to understanding the gut microbiome *Mamm. Genome* **32** 282–96
[108] Ahmed S *et al* 2016 Pharmacogenomics of drug metabolizing enzymes and transporters: relevance to precision medicine *Genom. Proteom. Bioinform.* **14** 298–313
[109] Hasanzad M *et al* 2022 Genomic medicine on the frontier of precision medicine *J. Diabetes Metab. Disorders* **21** 853–61
[110] Pirmohamed M 2023 Pharmacogenomics: current status and future perspectives *Nat. Rev. Genet.* **24** 350–62
[111] Mills R and Haga S B 2014 Genomic counseling: next generation counseling *J. Genet. Couns.* **23** 689–92
[112] Rehm H L 2017 Evolving health care through personal genomics *Nat. Rev. Genet.* **18** 259–67
[113] Whitley K V, Tueller J A and Weber K S 2020 Genomics education in the era of personal genomics: academic, professional, and public considerations *Int. J. Mol. Sci.* **21** 768
[114] Kim D, Kim J H and Moore J H 2020 Translational bioinformatics: integrating electronic health record and omics data *Biocomputing 2021: Proc. Pacific Symp.* (Singapore: World Scientific)
[115] Stipelman C H *et al* 2022 Electronic health record-integrated clinical decision support for clinicians serving populations facing health care disparities: literature review *Yearb. Med. Inform.* **31** 184–98
[116] Girwar S A M *et al* 2021 A systematic review of risk stratification tools internationally used in primary care settings *Health Sci. Rep.* **4** e329
[117] Beaulieu-Jones B K *et al* 2021 Machine learning for patient risk stratification: standing on, or looking over, the shoulders of clinicians? *NPJ Digit. Med.* **4** 62
[118] Bedson J *et al* 2021 A review and agenda for integrated disease models including social and behavioural factors *Nat. Hum. Behav.* **5** 834–46
[119] Rowe R G and Daley G Q 2019 Induced pluripotent stem cells in disease modelling and drug discovery *Nat. Rev. Genet.* **20** 377–88
[120] Yue R and Dutta A 2022 Computational systems biology in disease modeling and control, review and perspectives *npj Syst. Biol. Appl.* **8** 37
[121] Xia X 2017 Bioinformatics and drug discovery *Curr. Top. Med. Chem.* **17** 1709–26
[122] Romano J D and Tatonetti N P 2019 Informatics and computational methods in natural product drug discovery: a review and perspectives *Front. Genet.* **10** 368
[123] Sharma R *et al* 2023 Bioinformatics paradigms in drug discovery and drug development *Curr. Top. Med. Chem.* **23** 579–88
[124] Niazi S K and Mariam Z 2023 Recent advances in machine-learning-based chemo-informatics: a comprehensive review *Int. J. Mol. Sci.* **24** 11488
[125] Wang Y *et al* 2022 DrugRepo: a novel approach to repurposing drugs based on chemical and genomic features *Sci. Rep.* **12** 21116
[126] Shi W *et al* 2023 A review on predicting drug target interactions based on machine learning *Int. Conf. on Health Information Science* (Berlin: Springer)
[127] Bhardwaj K K, Banyal S and Sharma D K 2019 Artificial intelligence based diagnostics, therapeutics and applications in biomedical engineering and bioinformatics *Internet of Things in Biomedical Engineering* (Amsterdam: Elsevier) pp 161–87

[128] Auslander N, Gussow A B and Koonin E V 2021 Incorporating machine learning into established bioinformatics frameworks *Int. J. Mol. Sci.* **22** 2903
[129] Kaushik A C and Raj U 2020 AI-driven drug discovery: a boon against COVID-19? *AI Open* **1** 1–4
[130] David L *et al* 2020 Molecular representations in AI-driven drug discovery: a review and practical guide *J. Cheminf.* **12** 1–22
[131] Mak K-K, Balijepalli M K and Pichika M R 2022 Success stories of AI in drug discovery-where do things stand? *Expert Opin. Drug Discov.* **17** 79–92
[132] Alkhnbashi O S *et al* 2020 CRISPR-Cas bioinformatics *Methods* **172** 3–11
[133] Liu H *et al* 2015 CRISPR-ERA: a comprehensive design tool for CRISPR-mediated gene editing, repression and activation *Bioinformatics* **31** 3676–8
[134] Choudhary S *et al* 2020 Application of bioinformatics tools in CRISPR/Cas *CRISPR/Cas Genome Editing: Strategies and Potential for Crop Improvement* (Springer) pp 31–52
[135] Javed M R *et al* 2021 Tricks and trends in CRISPR/Cas9-based genome editing and use of bioinformatics tools for improving on-target efficiency *CRISPR and RNAi Systems* (Amsterdam: Elsevier) pp 441–62
[136] Sun Y V and Hu Y-J 2016 Integrative analysis of multi-omics data for discovery and functional studies of complex human diseases *Adv. Genet.* **93** 147–90
[137] Anowar F, Sadaoui S and Selim B 2021 Conceptual and empirical comparison of dimensionality reduction algorithms (PCA, KPCA, LDA, MDS, SVD, LLE, ISOMAP, LE, ICA, t-SNE) *Comput. Sci. Rev.* **40** 100378

IOP Publishing

Introduction to Pharmaceutical Biotechnology, Volume 2
(Second Edition)
Enzymes, proteins and bioinformatics
Ahmed Al-Harrasi, Saurabh Bhatia and Ajmal Khan

Chapter 10

Protein and enzyme engineering

10.1 Protein and enzyme engineering

Protein engineering is the design of new enzymes or proteins with new or desirable functions. It is based on the use of recombinant DNA technology to change amino acid sequences. Many different protein engineering methods are available today, owing to the rapid development in biological sciences, more specifically, recombinant DNA technology. In an earlier chapter, we discussed the principles, uses and techniques of biocatalysis and enzyme technology. In the past, the industry was largely dependent on these naturally occurring enzymes. However, naturally occurring enzymes and their related bioprocesses are often limited by a set of conditions. With advancements in biotechnology, it has been possible to plan and engineer novel enzymes and other macromolecules with predicted characteristics. This field of research also gained more support from computer aided molecular modeling (CAMM), which has contributed considerably, not only to protein and enzyme engineering, but also to drug design. Different characteristics of protein and biocatalyst engineering will be discussed in this chapter. To advance the production of a particular macromolecule or to produce novel products, metabolic pathways are also being designed in different ways. The various steps involved in protein engineering are shown in figure 10.1.

10.2 Designing macromolecules

Proteins are versatile macromolecules with various important functions, including structural, catalytic, sensory and regulatory functions. The rational design of enzymes is a great challenge to our understanding of protein structure and physical chemistry and has numerous potential applications. Protein design algorithms have been useful to design or engineer proteins that fold, fold faster, catalyze, catalyze faster, signal and adopt preferred conformational states. The field of *de novo* protein

doi:10.1088/978-0-7503-5387-8ch10

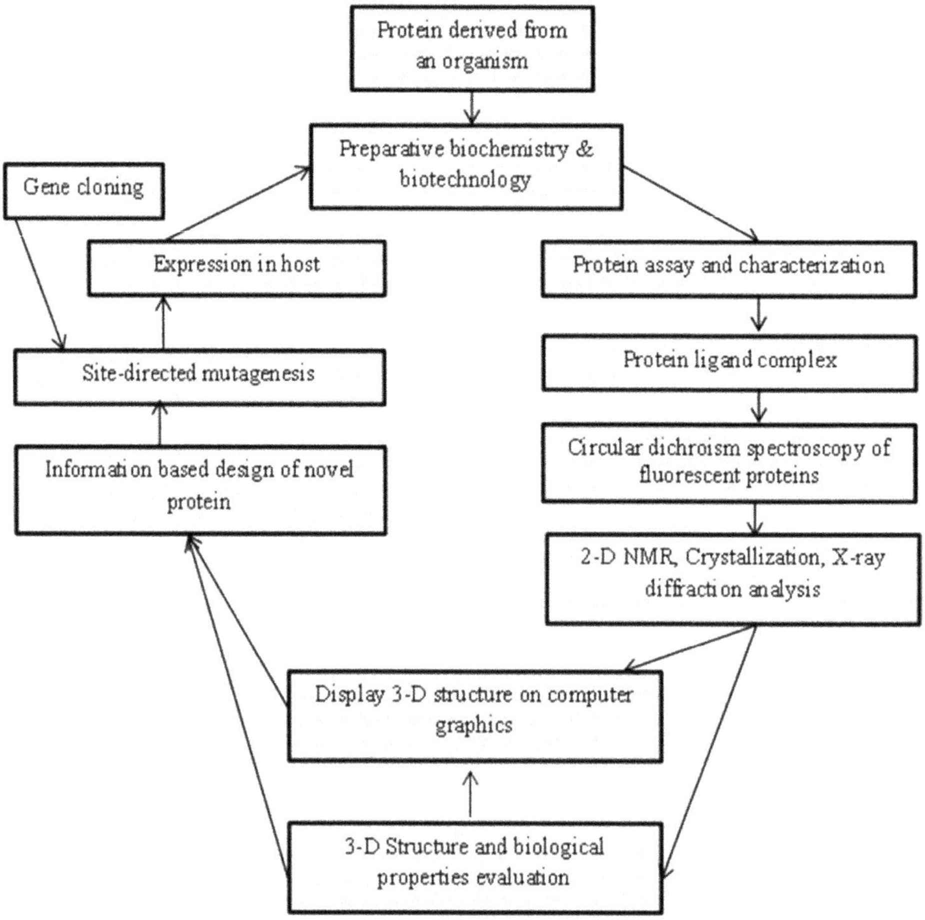

Figure 10.1. The various steps involved in protein engineering.

design, although only a few decades old, is beginning to produce exciting results. Advances in this field are already having a considerable influence on biotechnology and chemical biology. The application of powerful computational approaches for functional protein design has currently succeeded in engineering target activities [1].

In the last quarter of the twentieth century, various major discoveries have made it possible to modify/alter the structure of novel proteins/molecules/products in a deliberate way leading to a predicted functional role. Site-directed mutagenesis allows changes in sequences at identified sites, resulting in modification of proteins in a deliberate way. Moreover, computational and graphical developments have allowed access to the three-dimensional structure of proteins. These two developments allow us to understand protein–drug interactions more deeply. The steps involved in protein engineering are as follows:

- The protein sample is characterized with a ligand (drug, enzyme substrate, receptor hormone or antigen–antibody interaction).

- The three-dimensional structure is investigated using nuclear magnetic resonance (NMR) and x-ray diffraction patterns of crystals.
- The three-dimensional structure is displayed with interactive computer graphics and the available information is used to suggest a novel design suiting the requirements.
- The desired DNA sequence that is expected to give the novel designed protein is then either synthesized or obtained by site-directed mutagenesis of an available gene.
- The novel gene is incorporated into an appropriate expression system and the gene product is extracted, purified and characterized biochemically.
- If the biochemical profile does not fulfill the previously earlier anticipated structure, the cycle may be repeated again, until the anticipated structure is achieved.

It must be noted that the aforementioned steps of protein engineering share steps employed in the engineering of drugs, insecticides, herbicides and peptide vaccines, although there are other additional methods that are employed for drug discovery. The various cycles involved in genetic engineering and drug designing display common steps, as shown in figure 10.2.

Drug design and protein engineering are different from each other in the sense that drug design only concerns the ligand, which can be modified more efficiently by chemical synthesis, whereas in protein engineering rDNA technology is usually used. Three-dimensional structures for a small number of proteins that are interrelated to the novel protein of interest will usually be accessible to a protein engineer in developing a procedure for novel protein production as per the desired features.

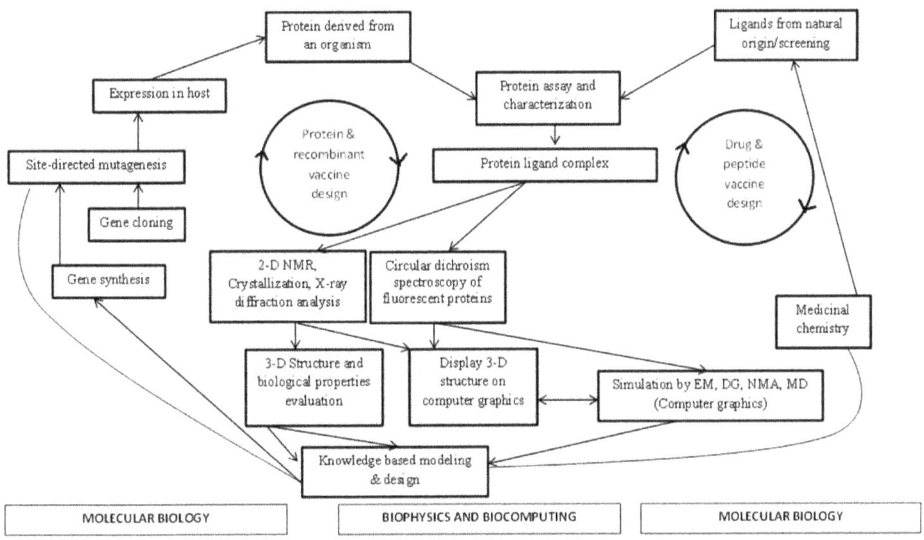

Figure 10.2. Various cycles involved in genetic engineering and drug design, demonstration the common steps of the two cycles.

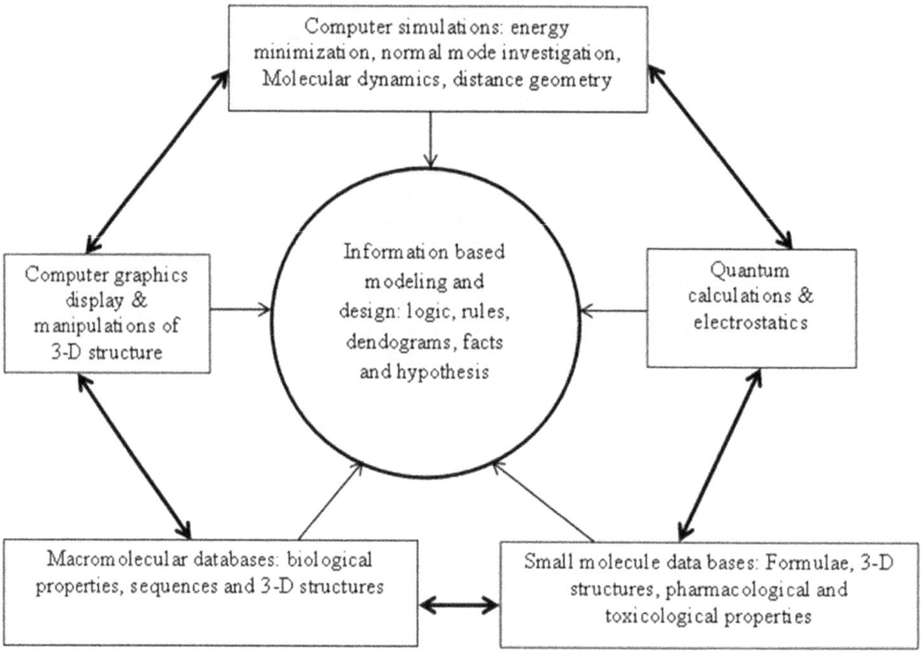

Figure 10.3. The various components of computer software used in knowledge based molecular modeling.

Consequently, a process is required for production of the three-dimensional structure of the protein of interest. This can be achieved *de novo* through modeling from homologous or analogous proteins, if they are accessible. This is defined as knowledge based modeling and involves design by means of computer software, comprising computer graphics, computer simulations and databases. Computer software comprises the complete set of methods and programmes used on the computer to rectify problems and provide operational aids. The various components of computer software used in knowledge based molecular modeling are illustrated in figure 10.3.

10.3 Protein engineering versus enzyme engineering

Protein engineering involves changing the structure of a protein to enhance or amend its properties. Protein engineers are progressively able to rely on structure–function insights, computational methods and deeper understanding of natural biosynthesis processes, to streamline the design and applications of enzymes [2, 3]. Enzyme engineering is experiencing the most intense and exciting transformation in its history. This promises extraordinary expansion in the scope and applications of modified or improved enzymes with the desired physical and catalytic properties. Two complementary approaches are currently available: rational redesign and directed evolution [4].

Although the terms protein engineering and enzyme engineering may often be used interchangeably, there is an indirect difference between the two. Protein engineering allows structural modifications of the function and selectivity of enzymes, mainly in an aqueous medium.

Enzyme engineering, in contrast, sometimes also includes engineering of the enzyme microenvironment, therefore offering applications in non-aqueous environments, as enzymes can function in organic solvents. Such non-aqueous environments offer benefits such as:

- higher substrate solubility;
- reversal of hydro reactions; and
- modified enzyme specificity.

These advantages offer new enzyme activities that can be achieved by means of genetic modifications or using complex multistep pathways within the cells.

10.4 Protein engineering

Protein engineering is the design of new enzymes or proteins with new or desired functions. It is based on the use of rDNA technology (to change amino acid sequences). The first report on protein engineering dates back to the early 1980s, in a publication by Ulmer (1983). Currently, due to the advancements in rDNA technology and high-throughput screening approaches, protein engineering methods and applications are becoming increasingly important and widespread [5].

In the last two decades rapid development has been made in the examination of protein structure and function. Amino acid sequences are now accessible for as many as 8000 proteins, however, the three-dimensional structures of only about 400 proteins have been determined using the x-ray crystallography technique. It has been observed that the investigation of protein structure and function has now reached the level which for DNA existed in the 1970s. Such an assessment is supported by the fact that only one center in the world is available for the procurement of protein data (the Brookhaven Data Bank), whereas a number of such centers are available for DNA sequence data. From the three-dimensional structure of the 400 proteins examined so far, it is likely that if two proteins are comparable in their amino acid sequence, they will be inclined to fold into similar three-dimensional structures, so that it will be possible for researchers to predict the three-dimensional structure of a protein and its amino acid sequence. This will then allow researchers to identify the perfect structure for a protein and forecast its function. This model can be further utilized for the production, identification and characterization of a gene that will give the anticipated sequence of amino acids, resulting in a three-dimensional structure for a specified protein. Another method of protein engineering may be to alter a protein by suitable reaction to make it more appropriate for desirable function. This area of protein research (which includes the modification/development of protein either by recombinant technology or by any chemical reaction) is currently growing considerably.

By means of rDNA technology, a gene can now be cloned in an expression vector and made to express in bacteria. During this procedure, using the considered cell containing the gene of interest cloned in a vector, a protein can be derived in sufficient quantity. As a gene can be artificially incorporated and altered by means of rDNA technology, novel proteins can be achieved. The field of protein engineering includes enzymes, synthetic peptides, storage proteins and drugs to be used in medicine, industry and agriculture. The goals of protein engineering are as follows:

- To generate superior enzymes to further catalyze the production of high value synthetic chemicals.
- To synthesize enzymes for large-scale use in the chemical industry and to produce biological compounds (including peptides, storage proteins and specific proteins) that are more therapeutically active/functional than natural ones.

10.5 Foundation of protein (enzyme) engineering

Many proteins have been characterized in prokaryotes and eukaryotes, but only a few have become commercially significant. This is because of the high cost of purifying enzymes in sufficient quantities. The cost factor can be overcome by producing an enzyme in sufficient quantities from bacteria, but for its commercial usage, an enzyme (under *in vitro* conditions) should also have some features in addition to those typical of enzymes in cells. These features are as follows:

- The enzyme should be vigorous with a long life.
- The enzyme should be able to use the substrate provided by industry even if it differs slightly from that in the cell.
- The enzyme should remain active under the conditions (e.g. extremes of pH, temperature and concentration) of the industry, even if these conditions differ from *in vivo* conditions.

As mentioned above, an enzyme should be designed to meet the specific needs. Thus, efforts have been made that modified the properties of enzymes. The following properties need to be modify to meet the requirements with the help of protein or enzyme engineering:

- allosteric regulation;
- cofactor requirements;
- the kinetic properties of enzyme-turnover and the Michaelis constant, K_M;
- the molecular weight and subunit structure;
- optimum pH;
- protease resistance;
- the stability and activity of the enzyme in non-aqueous solvents;
- substrate and reaction specificity; and
- thermostability and the optimum temperature for the enzyme.

For a specific category of enzymes, differences may be present for each of the above properties, so that one may like to combine the ideal characteristics to obtain the most effective form of enzyme. Occasionally, however, it may not be possible to obtain a combination of ideal properties [6]. For example, an enzyme with maximum activity may not be the most stable. Consequently, a compromise among properties might have to be made to produce an appropriate enzyme from the existing variability or even from inducing variability by mutagenesis. However, if the structure–function relationship of an enzyme is known, the structural properties for anticipated function may be combined and protein engineering procedures may then be employed to create a novel enzyme presenting a combination of all necessary functional properties. This part of protein engineering can be demonstrated by means of the example of glucose isomerases, which convert glucose into other isomers such as fructose, and is used to make high fructose corn syrup, which is vital for the soft drink industry. It displays wide variation in its properties [5]. Glucose isomerases from the TIM barrel family of enzymes look similar, with a highly characteristic domain called a TIM barrel with an active site for catalytic action at one end. This TIM barrel can be present in enzymes that may vary in sequence and may catalyze diverse reactions. As discussed, a resemblance in structure of a protein should suggest resemblance in function, thus the TIM barrel offers a challenge to this concept. However, it is interesting that certain enzymes in this family show similarity in their metabolic pathways, so that they catalyze two successive steps, consequently presenting coupling of their functions. As an example of two enzymes in the TIM barrel family, triose phosphate isomerase is one of the most efficient catalysts, while glucose isomerase is very inefficient. Consequently, if the glucose isomerase enzyme is restructured to use the highly effective domain of the TIM barrel family, it will be an extraordinary achievement for the soft drink industry [7].

10.6 Basic assumptions for protein engineering

In protein engineering, one should recognize the following characteristics of enzymes:

- Several amino acid substitutions, deletions or additions result in no enzyme activity, so they are silent mutations.
- Proteins have a limited number of basic structures and only minor changes need to be made to them to lead to variations.
- Related patterns of chain folding and domain structure can arise from different amino acid sequences, which show little or no homology (while similar amino acid sequences never give different folding or domain structures).

The above characteristics suggest that many base changes may occasionally result in modification in function; a number of modifications at particular positions may result in desired favorable modifications. For example, single amino acid replacement (glycine to aspartic acid) in *Escherichia coli* aspartate transcarbamylase results in:

- loss of activity, and
- a modification in the binding of catalytic and regulatory subunits.

Another example is the engineering of a single biosynthetic antibody binding site, which is only 1/6 of the size of the complete antibody but preserves its antigen-binding specificity. A heavy and light chain variable region present in this synthetic fragment is linked by a 15-amino acid linker. For this fragment, a synthetic gene has also been prepared, which is allowed to be expressed in *E. coli*. This fragment binds to digoxin, a cardiac glycoside. These types of single amino acid replacements in BABS fragments have occasionally resulted in major modifications in its binding affinity. Consequently it is essential to examine not only the crystal structure but also the active sites therein, so that the gene can be modified or artificially produced for protein engineering to meet the desired requirements [8].

10.7 Steps involved in protein engineering

Due to the rapid development in biological sciences, more specifically rDNA technology, different protein engineering methods are currently available. Figure 10.4 shows the steps involved in protein engineering.

10.7.1 Studying three-dimensional protein structure

Proteins are molecular devices (nanometer scale), where biological function is exercised [5]. There are 20 natural amino acids, whose occurrence is greater than that of other special ones with particular functions. These 20 amino acids can be grouped together forming polypeptide chains, or proteins, in different ways determined by the genetic code and limited by stereochemical properties. These proteins may have a constitutive or transient cell expression with regard to its functions. It is worth mentioning that efforts are underway to make proteins of unnatural amino acids as well [8].

An investigation of the three-dimensional structure of a protein (including examination of active sites) is the first and foremost step in any application of

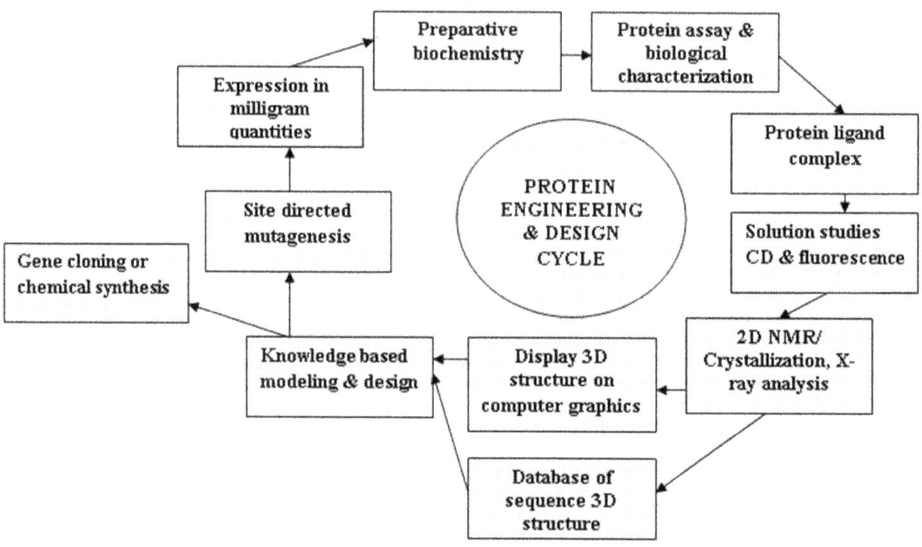

Figure 10.4. The steps involved in protein engineering.

protein engineering. For such an investigation, the protein should be present in crystal form. X-ray diffraction procedures have also been established to produce data at a rapid rate, to allow us to forecast the three-dimensional structure of proteins by means of model building. Experimental differences in the structures of various enzymes can be connected with the differences in their function, so that the information from such investigations can be further employed for protein engineering. X-ray diffraction information at altered temperatures also permits researchers to understand the modifications anticipated in protein structure due to changes in temperature, signifying that protein structure is dynamic. Likewise, the NMR method will permit researchers to understand the structure of enzymes in solution rather than in crystals, so that researchers can avoid the time-consuming process of crystallization, thus speeding up the study of protein structure. The information generated from all these techniques is utilized in protein modeling, which is then further employed for an exercise in protein engineering [9]. When crystals of a protein are not accessible for investigation, but amino acid sequence data exist, identical sequences in any two proteins are matched and the effects of substitution are studied. This is occasionally called 'sequence garing' and permits researchers to understand which amino acids are involved in catalytic binding at active sites.

10.7.2 Protein modeling

The tertiary structure of proteins can disclose information that is difficult to detect in a linear sequence. Understanding the tertiary structure is important when generating hypotheses and interpreting data. Unluckily, the gap between the number of known protein sequences and their associated structures is widening. One way to bridge this gap is to use computer-generated structure models of proteins [10]. By using information produced by x-ray diffraction and NMR investigations, models can be created with the help of computer graphics. Advanced computer programmes are available (interactive color graphics programmes) by means of which a protein structure can be fitted to the electron density map (obtained from x-ray diffraction) through simultaneous display on a computer monitor. Likewise, van der Waals surfaces for the specific protein can be presented and interaction between several molecules simulated. Other interactive molecular graphics can also be employed (with the help of computer software) to discover the perturbations (disturbances) in protein structure that will result from specific modifications of amino sequences. It was also observed that to a certain extent the three-dimensional structure of a protein can be anticipated from the amino acid sequence, however for more clarity researchers are still dependent on x-ray diffraction patterns for elucidating the three-dimensional structure. It is well known that accurate prediction of three-dimensional structure by amino acid sequences will rectify many problems in protein-based therapeutics, which may further result in long-term success in protein engineering. Once the three-dimensional structure is accessible, different protein models can be established to investigate the effect of amino acid sequence alterations on its structure–function relationships [11].

10.7.3 Perturbation theory

The theory of perturbation allows researchers to accurately calculate the effects of small changes in amino acid sequence. So, according to this theory, there will be no prerequisite to perform experiments at each step of the protein engineering process to evaluate the outcome (chat function) of recommended modifications [12]. Such a theory will result from protein refinement and calculation of the theoretical structure of a protein which will be homologous to other proteins of known structure. This theory can be tested by using families of monoclonal antibodies. When established for prediction, it can be used to engineer a variety of proteins [13].

10.8 Methods of protein engineering

Various different protein engineering approaches are available today, due to the rapid advancements in biological sciences, more specifically, rDNA technology. The most traditional approach in protein engineering is the so-called rational design approach, which encompasses site-directed mutagenesis of proteins [10]. Site-directed mutagenesis permits the introduction of specific amino acids into a target gene. The popular approach for site-directed mutagenesis is called the overlap extension approach. This approach includes two primer pairs, where one primer of each primer pair contains the mutant codon with a mismatched sequence [14].

Different methods have been introduced for future use in protein engineering (figure 10.5). In this context, mutagenesis, selection and recombinant DNA technology are being used and will be utilized more widely in the future.

10.9 Mutagenesis and selection of mutant enzymes

Mutagenesis is performed for the improvement of a specific property of an enzyme. The following are some examples of the selection of mutant enzymes:

- *Anthranilate synthetase*: Physiological studies were executed under nutritional stress and nonstress conditions to measure the relative importance of the various regulatory mechanisms that *E. coli* can use to modify its rate of tryptophan synthesis [15]. The enzyme *E. coli* anthranilate synthetase is normally sensitive to tryptophan inhibition due to feedback inhibition. After mutation, an MTR 2 mutation mutant strain of *E. coli* was found to possess a different form of anthranilate synthetase that is insensitive to tryptophan

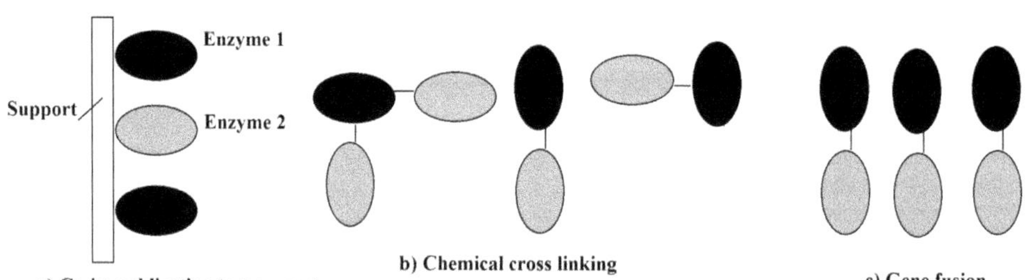

Figure 10.5. Basic methods for generating the proximity between two enzymes.

inhibition. This will allow the continuous synthesis of tryptophan without any inhibition accumulating as a product.

- Xanthine dehydrogenase: A point mutation in the structural gene for purine hydroxylase I (xanthine dehydrogenase) of *Aspergillus nidulans* results in several dramatic pleiotropic effects [16]. This enzyme oxidizes 2 hydroxypurine at position 8, but a mutant has been isolated which oxidizes 2 hydroxypurine at position 6.
- Lactate dehydrogenase: The mechanism of catalysis of malate dehydrogenase is similar to that of lactate dehydrogenase, an enzyme with which it shares a similar three-dimensional structure. This enzyme, present in bacteria, was altered to malate dehydrogenase by a natural mutation resulting in amino acid substitution. Substitution of a single amino acid residue of a lactate dehydrogenase changes the enzyme specificity to that of a malate dehydrogenase, but a similar substitution in a malate dehydrogenase resulted in relaxation of a high degree of specificity for oxaloacetate [17].

As mentioned above, single amino acid modification or addition/deletion is possible, however, if further improvement requires modifications in several amino acids, such a mutant will be rare or nonexistent and this type of alteration can only be achieved by gene modifications.

10.10 Gene modifications or gene synthesis for protein engineering

In gene modifications some oligonucleotides can be synthesized by means of automatic DNA synthesizers with solid supports or on microarrays. Two procedures are available for gene modification using synthetic oligonucleotides.

In vitro mutagenesis using synthetic oligonucleotides. In this procedure synthetic oligonucleotides can be employed for *in vitro* mutagenesis of genes of interest. This method involves synthesis of small synthetic oligonucleotide primers containing the desired modifications. Then it is hybridized to a suitable position in a cloned gene and the rest of the gene is then replicated by means of the polymerase enzyme, so that the rest of the gene remains intact. This strategy was employed to alter the active site of tyrosyl-tRNA synthetase, whose structure was already known. In this enzyme at position 35, cysteine was substituted by serine, with the expected effect of reducing K_M for adenosine triphosphate. In 1983, this was defined as the main step forward in protein engineering. Polymerase chain reaction (PCR) can also be employed for inducing mutations in known genes for the purposes of protein engineering [18].

The synthesis of complete modified genes (de novo). Complete genes can in some cases be chemically synthesized in the form of oligomers. For instance insulin, somatostatin and interferon are common examples in which complete genes have been synthesized in the form of oligomers. To introduce restriction enzyme sites at suitable positions, the sequence of the synthetic gene can be designed in a modular fashion. The cleaving gene at suitable positions allows the incorporation of desirable fragments, resulting in modification of function. As various oligomers are involved, modification can be incorporated in different oligomers and these oligomers can be further utilized in ligation mixtures for the synthesis of a complete gene, which will have a number of modifications [19]. This procedure can be employed for making extensive modifications in the amino acid sequence of the protein. For example, the interferon gene which was artificially synthesized opened the way to modify the portions of the interior so that a variety of artificial interferon genes can be prepared, which can be later allowed to express in *E. coli*.

10.11 Multi-enzyme systems

In biotechnological production, multi-enzyme systems have been artificially synthesized. These enzymes are capable of catalyzing sequential reactions. By using a number of techniques such as co-immobilization, chemical cross linking and gene fusion, the proximity of more enzymes can be achieved (figure 10.6). During gene fusion, the structural genes of two or more enzymes are joined together to prepare bi- and polyfunctional enzymes [20].

At the 3′-end the translational stop signal of the first gene is deleted and ligated in frame to the ATG start codon of the second gene. Short linkers can also be used for this purpose. A number of examples of multienzymes prepared by gene fusion *in vitro* are mentioned below:

- β-galactosidase–galactokinase (tetramer) for the sequential hydrolysis of lactose to glucose.
- β-galactosidase–galactose dehydrogenase (the hybrid enzyme is a dimeric enzyme) catalyzes the hydrolysis of lactose to galactose which is oxidized to galactolactone.
- β-galactosidase–galactose dehydrogenase–galactokinase (tetramer or an octamer).
- Galactose dehydrogenase–luciferase (a bifunctional enzyme).

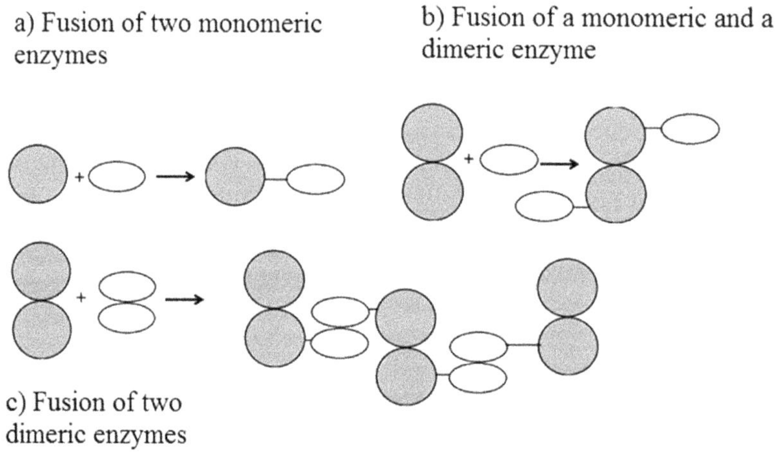

Figure 10.6. A fused polymer enzyme (multi-enzyme) system, showing interaction between component enzymes.

10.12 Chemical modification of enzyme

Proteins produced by genes undergo post-translational modifications which lead to stability, structural integrity, altered solubility and viscosity of individual proteins. This may also affect their chemical reactivity. These modifications can be achieved under laboratory conditions and occasionally it is even possible to produce entire new enzymes by exploring new active sites or altering old ones [21].

Enzyme–PEG conjugates. The enzyme called l-asparaginase is usually isolated from microbes and anti-cancer properties, however, its toxicity and half-life (less than 18 h) limit its utilization. It was observed that this enzyme can be modified by polyethylene glycol derivatives to form PEG-asparaginase conjugates. These conjugates differ from the native enzyme in the following characteristics:

It preserves only 52% of the catalytic activity of native enzyme.
It becomes resistant to proteolytic degradation.
It does not cause allergy.

Currently, these types of enzyme conjugates (e.g. uricase, catalase, etc) are prepared and utilized at the industrial scale to treat various types of tumors in rats and mice.

Modification of proteases into peptide ligases. To achieve high specificity and stereoselectivity, and to suppress side reactions, peptide ligation to the native enzyme is one of the best alternative procedures. Consequently, production of any enzyme that may catalyze peptide ligation will be most encouraged. Modification of protease subtilisin into thiol and selenolsubtilisin (two semisynthetic enzymes) can catalyze peptide ligation. Both of these modified proteases efficiently catalyze peptide ligases [22].

Production of site-specific nucleases. In this procedure chemical cleavage agents are used to combine DNA recognition and the binding properties of proteins.

Production of artificial semisynthetic oxidoreductases. By covalently attaching redox-active prosthetic groups to existing sites, artificial oxidoreductases can be prepared. Joining 10-methylisoalloxazine derivatives to specific sites of several proteins has been achieved. The ability of these semisynthetic enzymes compares favorably with that of naturally existing flavoenzymes [23].

10.13 Some early achievements of protein engineering

To determine the effects of site-specific mutagenesis involving substitution of one or more amino acids, a number of proteins have been examined. Attempts have also been made to examine the function of different regions of a protein [24]. Certain early achievements of protein engineering are mentioned as follows:

- *Acetylcholine receptor*: This protein is involved in delivery of acetylcholine across the membrane. The exact regions of this involved in acetylcholine binding and formation have been explored.
- *Cytochrome C*: A phenylalanine residue recognized to be non-essential for electron transfer, however, it is involved in determining the reduction potential of the protein.

- *Dihydrofolate reductase*: In this enzyme, substitution of a single amino acid, aspartic acid (Asp) by asparagine (Asn), results in a decrease in specific activity by a thousand fold, signifying that aspartic acid is significant for the active site. Other similar modifications were also examined.
- *Human-13 interferon*: Removal of the three cysteine residues led to an improvement in stability of the enzyme.
- *Insulin*: Contains A and B chains connected by a C-peptide of 35 amino acids. It was observed that a sequence of six amino C-peptides was satisfactory for the connecting function.
- *Lactose permease* (product of 'y' 'lac' operon): This enzyme is involved in delivery of lactose and, a cysteine to glycine replacement showed that this amino acid was vital for delivery. Further, of four histidine residues, two at positions 35 and 39 do not play any essential role in transport while the mutation in any of the other two at positions 208 and 322 result in a transport function.
- *T4 lysozyme*: A mutation of isoleucine to cysteine in this enzyme leads to formation of a disulfide bridge, leading to thermal stability and a 200-fold increase in enzyme activity even at 67 °C.
- *Trypsin*: This can be restructured to have modified substrate specificity.
- *β-lactamase*: This bacterial derived enzyme hydrolyzes and inactivates the β-lactam ring of penicillin derivatives and allows delivery across the inner membrane. In the course of transport a polypeptide (23 amino acids) is cleaved off. Comprehensive examination suggests that transport and processing are not influenced by this polypeptide of 23 amino acids alone. An active site comprising the amino acid serine has also been recognized, as its substitution by cysteine results in a reduction in the activity of this enzyme.
- λ repressor: This protein could be engineered to develop a specific site for cro-protein, since the alteration led to the development of a cro recognition site.
- *Subtilisin*: The serine protease subtilisin is an important industrial enzyme as well as a model for understanding the enormous rate enhancements effected by enzymes. Mutations in well over 50% of the 275 amino acids of subtilisin have been reported in the scientific literature. Most subtilisin engineering has involved catalytic amino acids, substrate binding regions and stabilizing mutations. Additional effective modification of substrate specificity includes the subtilisin.
- *Lactate dehydrogenase*: A lactate dehydrogenase isolated from *Bacillus stearothermophilus* was modified individually by each of the three substitutions of amino acids.

10.14 Computational approaches in protein engineering

Computational methods in protein engineering seek to interpret, design, and fine-tune proteins for several uses. This may be achieved by utilizing the power of computational tools and algorithms. These techniques enable the exploration of the vast protein design, which would be difficult to explore experimentally due to time and resource constraints [25].

10.14.1 Molecular dynamics simulations

An effective theoretical tool for examining the atomic-scale characteristics of proteins is a simulation of molecular dynamics (MD). MD simulations are critical for investigating the structure–function relationships of proteins, which is necessary to understand biological processes such as protein interactions and ligand binding. MD simulations may convert protein dynamics data into meaningful statistics, which can then be used to investigate thermodynamics and kinetics which are the two concepts crucial to understanding biological systems [26]. Moreover, recent improvements in simulation tools have allowed for the precise prediction and characterization of these processes, which, correctly used in structure-based drug design (SBDD) and are very helpful for accelerating the drug development process. Because of significant improvements in simulation speed, accuracy, and accessibility, simulations have become more important in molecular biology and drug development. The simulations capture the dynamics of proteins and other biomolecules with atomic precision at unprecedentedly high temporal resolutions. Furthermore, throughout time, the simulations' accessibility, accuracy, and speed have all experienced notable increases [25]. A workflow of MD simulation from preparation to analysis is shown in figure 10.7.

10.14.2 Quantum mechanical calculations

Quantum mechanical (QM) computations help understand and simulate protein activities at a deeper level. They thoroughly understand protein electronic structure. This is essential for a wide variety of uses, including ligand binding, protein–protein interactions, and enzyme catalysis. One efficient computational tool for modeling

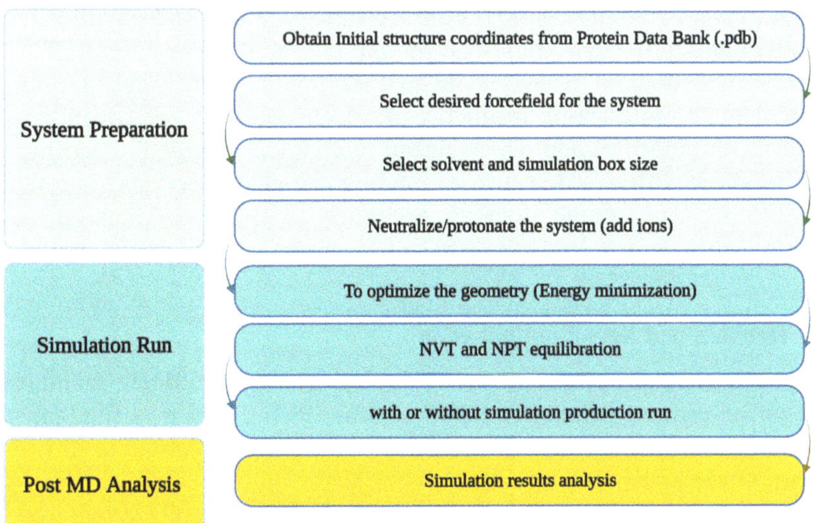

Figure 10.7. Molecular dynamics simulation process: setup, simulation, and analysis phases with detailed steps.

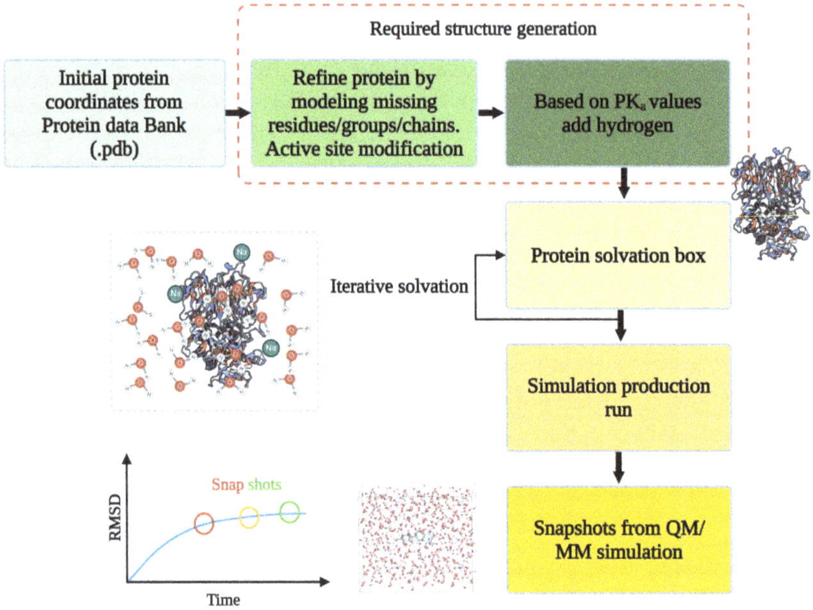

Figure 10.8. Flowchart illustrating the process of initiating a QM/MM calculation using crystal structure coordinates and producing MD snapshots.

protein electrostatics uses static point-charge model distributions based on a quantum mechanical technique termed electrostatically embedded generalized molecular fractionation with conjugate caps (EE-GMFCC) [27]. Compared to conventional molecular mechanics (MM) force fields, this method has shown a notable improvement in modeling the electrostatic potential and solvation energy of proteins by considering both polarization and charge transfer effects [27]. Correct scoring in protein docking relies heavily on quantum mechanical calculations, which are utilized to create docking protocols based on quantum mechanical/molecular mechanical computations and use quantum mechanical energy as a scoring metric. Several instances with a wide range of binding site characteristics have shown the effectiveness of this unique docking approach [28]. A workflow of QM/MM simulation including detailed steps is shown in figure 10.8.

10.14.3 Docking and ligand optimization

Docking and ligand optimization are crucial tools in SBDD, facilitating the elucidation of protein–ligand (PL) interactions (PLIs), which is fundamental for drug discovery and development. As a rapid and cheap alternative to traditional experimental methods, PL docking is essential for predicting the binding orientations and affinities of small molecules inside the binding site of a given protein [29]. Pose prediction and docking are both crucial in virtual high-throughput screening for optimizing leads. It has been noted that most docking systems pitched toward

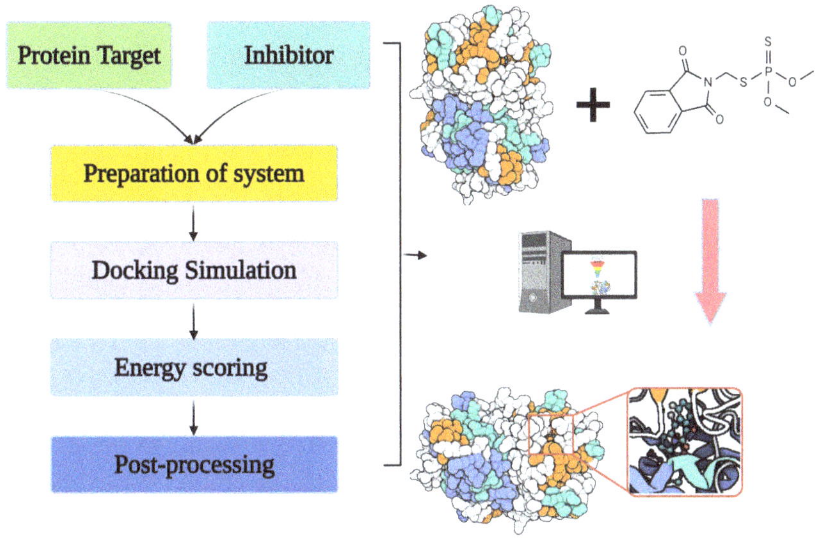

Figure 10.9. PL docking procedure: from target and ligand preparation to docking, scoring, and post-processing analysis.

pose prediction focus on redocking to a previously determined co-crystallized protein structure, while often overlooking structural flexibility [30]. Ligand optimization includes carefully creating or choosing ligands with optimum binding properties. The development of PL binding poses and the prediction of PL binding affinities rely heavily on this step [31]. Molecular optimization, also called ligand optimization, requires the examination of PL complex files to measure specific parameters that determine the relationship between protein structure and ligand. Tools like CABS-flex 2.0 have been utilized for efficient protein flexibility modeling in this domain [32]. The docking scheme having detailed steps is represented in figure 10.9.

10.14.4 Machine learning algorithms in protein design

The combination of machine learning (ML) and deep learning (DL) algorithms in protein design has significantly accelerated the optimization of protein functions by rendering a data-driven mapping of sequences to functions without requiring a detailed model of the underlying physics or biological pathways [33]. ML, particularly through directed evolution, has been involved in protein engineering, accurately predicting how sequence maps function [34]. DL is a subfield of ML that is igniting scientific revolution by making use of massive amounts of data and high-powered computers. Protein structural modeling is used for structure prediction from amino acid sequences and determined protein design [35]. The continuous protein design issue may be transformed into a discrete one by using ML-based algorithms, which may have an effect on the development of novel molecular therapeutics for human diseases [36]. Various ML algorithms have been extensively applied in pharmaceutical protein development, creating a significant development in therapeutic protein engineering [37].

10.15 Directed evolution techniques

Directed evolution is a robust methodology employed in protein engineering to enhance or modify the attributes of biomolecules for diverse applications. The process parallels natural evolution on a consolidated timescale, permitting rapid selection of biomolecule variants with desirable traits for specific applications [38]. There are two main phases to this method: creating genetic variety (library creation) and separating out interesting variations. Directed evolution is a powerful approach for creating new or better biological functionalities because it accelerates the natural evolution process of biological molecules and systems in a controlled setting via repeated rounds of gene diversification and library screening and selection [39].

10.15.1 Error-prone PCR

Error-prone PCR (epPCR) is a pivotal technique within directed evolution, utilized mainly to generate libraries of DNA molecules with a broad mutational spectrum, thus operating the genetic diversification required for directed evolution. epPCR introduces random mutations throughout a DNA sequence during the replication process. This method is particularly effective in directed evolution for creating diverse genetic variants from a given DNA sequence, which can then be screened or selected for desired traits or functionalities. The process of error-prone PCR represents the initial step in the directed evolution workflow, paving the way for the subsequent screening or selection processes to isolate promising variants. By employing epPCR, systematically exploring the genetic landscape and unveil novel or enhanced biomolecule functionalities, thereby driving innovation in protein engineering and other fields of molecular biology [25].

10.15.2 DNA shuffling

In directed evolution, DNA shuffling plays a crucial role by facilitating the *in vitro* recombination of a single gene or pools of homologous genes to generate new gene variants. The method involves cutting genes into pieces of varying sizes and then using PCR to reassemble the pieces back into functional genes. Recombination occurs as a result of this reassembly via self-priming because of PCR template switching [40]. DNA shuffling has been likened to 'sexual PCR', allowing for the recombination of homologous DNA sequences during *in vitro* molecular evolution, thereby generating a diverse set of genetic variants. Applications of DNA shuffling extend to enhancing metabolic pathways, modifying active site residues within enzymes to boost catalytic rates, and creating synthetic operons, all of which are essential for advancing molecular biology and protein engineering techniques [40]. Moreover, DNA shuffling has been utilized to develop new generation vaccines to counter rapidly evolving pathogens by overcoming natural selection and environmental pressures [41].

10.15.3 Saturation mutagenesis

The semi-rational protein engineering method known as saturation mutagenesis involves the whole or partial replacement of a target residue with any other naturally occurring amino acid. This method allows for the precise alteration of single or multiple amino acid residues, thereby generating a library of single-residue substitutions for further analysis and selection [42]. Saturation mutagenesis is used to identify sequence determinants of protein structure, stability, and function, particularly in situations where phenotypic readouts are easily accessible. A straightforward and productive approach to understanding protein structure and function is saturation mutagenesis coupled with deep sequencing [43].

10.15.4 Phage display

It is possible to study protein–protein, protein–peptide, and protein–DNA interactions with the use of a method called phage display. There is a direct link between the DNA that makes up the genotype and the phenotype that is expressed as a protein on the surface of bacteriophages via the expression of proteins or peptide sequences. Finding peptides and antibodies with high affinity and specificity for their target relies heavily on this link. Screening is performed by comparing a phage display library containing many different peptide or protein sequences to a target molecule [44]. Phages are selected based on the presence of peptides or proteins with a high affinity for the target. Next, we sequence the DNA of these phages to identify the peptide or protein sequences that exhibit the desired binding properties. After that, the phages are multiplied. Research into protein–protein and protein–ligand interactions, as well as drug discovery and vaccine development, has made extensive use of phage display. It is a useful technique in modern molecular biology and protein engineering, having been used to find and produce novel ligands, antibodies, and enzyme inhibitors, among other things [45].

10.16 Post-translational modifications

Proteins' functional characteristics are altered by a series of chemical reactions known as post-translational modifications (PTMs), which occur after proteins are synthesized. These modifications significantly influence proteins' behavior, activity, and interactions, thereby playing a vital role in regulating various biological processes [46].

10.16.1 Glycosylation engineering

Glycosylation engineering is a specialized domain focused on manipulating the glycosylation patterns of proteins to enhance or modify their functionalities. Glycosylation refers to the covalent attachment of glycans (sugars) to proteins, and it is a common PTM with profound implications on protein stability, solubility, immunogenicity, and bioactivity. The commercial demand for glycosylation engineering covers the biopharmaceutical sector, mainly for producing biological therapeutics with defined glycosylation patterns [47]. Glycoengineering methodologies are developed to modify glycan structures on proteins, thereby potentially improving their properties, such as enhancing the therapeutic efficacy of biopharmaceuticals [48].

10.16.2 Phosphorylation engineering

Phosphorylation is one of the most prevalent and new PTMs, regulating many cellular signaling pathways that control cell proliferation, survival, and differentiation. Enzymes called kinases (which add phosphate groups) and phosphatases (which remove phosphate groups) play essential roles in phosphorylation engineering (which remove phosphate groups). The phosphorylation state of proteins is altered by these enzymes, which affects the proteins' function and their interactions with other biomolecules [49]. Phosphorylation engineering comprehends techniques to analyze phosphorylation sites and their functional relevance, employing phosphoproteomic workflows to sove the complexities of phosphorylation networks within the cellular environment [50].

10.16.3 Methylation and acetylation

Methylation and acetylation are prominent PTMs impacting gene expression through epigenetic modifications. Histones may be methylated or acetylated, respectively, with methylation adding a methyl group to DNA or histones. Both acetylation and methylation are metabolically sensitive and may significantly impact how genes express themselves. Acetylation usually increases gene expression while methylation suppresses it [51]. Recently, studies have revealed that histone acetylation may operate as a DNA methylation target, suggesting a functional link between both systems. This functional connection might be significant in pathological conditions like atherosclerosis [51].

10.16.4 PEGylation for enzyme stability

PEGylation is the covalent attachment of polyethylene glycol (PEG) to proteins and is an essential strategy to increase the stability and solubility of therapeutic proteins. Enhancing the pharmacokinetic characteristics of protein therapeutics requires PEGylation since it has been associated with higher protein solubility, increased proteolysis resistance, lower toxicity, and decreased protein aggregation [52]. Significant progress has been made over the last three decades in addressing poor solubility, protein stability, shelf life, and bioactivity by developments in PEGylation procedures. Successful therapeutic uses of proteins rely on their desired qualities, which can only be guaranteed by preventing the formation of undesirable protein aggregates. Enzyme stability engineering benefits from the precision and efficacy of PEGylation conducted at specific sites on the protein [53].

10.17 Structural flexibility and allosteric regulation

The concepts of structural flexibility and allosteric regulation are closely related in protein study. Structural flexibility is the ability of a protein to undergo conformational changes. Conversely, the process by which a chemical interaction at one site on a protein may affect the function at another site is known as allostery [52, 54].

10.17.1 Intraprotein communication pathways

Intraprotein communication pathways are essential for proteins to function and be appropriately regulated. Information (in the form of structural modifications to the protein) may be sent from one part of the protein to another via these routes. The protein's structure may be altered in response to a stimulus, activating a functional reaction at a new place. Understanding these pathways is crucial for unraveling the complex mechanisms that run protein activity and regulation [55].

10.17.2 Allosteric site identification

One of the first steps in learning about and using allosteric control is identifying allosteric sites on a protein where small molecules or other proteins interact to create an allosteric response. Based on protein structure, approaches for predicting allosteric sites have been developed. For instance, allosteric interactions may be found in pockets and pathways that may be uncovered using computational methods. Allosteric regulation is defined as the process that begins when a small molecule effector or inhibitor binds to a location on a protein that is not the active site. Allosteric regulation is discussed in terms of its efficacy and robustness in controlling protein activity across various biological functions [56]. The relevance of changes in protein conformation in allosteric regulation and function emphasizes how crucial it is to think of proteins as conformational ensembles rather than static structures to comprehend allosteric pathways [57]. Allostery occurs when a protein's active or main site is modified by binding a ligand or another protein at a different position on the protein [58]. Govindara *et al* (2023) describe modern computational approaches applied to allosteric communication, which contribute to the finding and understanding of allosteric sites and pathways [58].

10.17.3 Modulator design

Modulator design, particularly allosteric modulators, is innovative in drug discovery and protein engineering. Allosteric modulators bind to allosteric sites on proteins to modulate their activity. Finding allosteric sites and creating compounds that can bind to them is crucial for developing allosteric modulators that can cause the required conformational changes in the target protein. Different methodologies have been employed for the identification of allosteric binding sites and modulators, including structure-based and ligand-based drug design methodologies [58]. There is also a method called a structure-based allosteric modulator design which is proposed to guide the design of allosteric modulators. Moreover, the discovery of allosteric modulators can transition from chance to a more structured approach through structure-based design [59].

10.17.4 Coupling allosteric regulation with catalytic function

The coupling of allosteric regulation with catalytic function is vital to many enzymes' operational efficiency and regulation. Allosteric regulation is a robust mechanism employed by proteins for regulating activity and adaptability during processes such as catalysis, signal transduction, and gene regulation. Allosteric regulation is responsible for the modifying of enzyme activity in living organisms, and it has also been used to construct artificial switchable catalysts by embedding catalytically active groups in allosteric scaffolds [60]. Allosteric crosstalk plays a significant role in activity modulation and function modification of proteins, and understanding allostery is crucial for advancing the discovery of allosteric drugs. Additionally, multistate models of enzyme catalysis and enzyme allostery have been developed to capture the large-scale conformational changes and the coupling between allosteric regulation and catalytic function in enzymes [61].

10.18 Protein–protein and protein–ligand interactions

Protein interactions with other proteins or ligands are fundamental to the functioning of biological systems. These interactions dictate a variety of cellular processes and understanding them is crucial in fields like drug discovery and molecular biology. Protein–protein interactions (PPIs) are essential in life processes and are associated with various diseases. Because of their association with cancer, infectious diseases, and neurological disorders, irregular PPIs are promising therapeutic development targets. PPI modulators, such as small compounds, peptides, and antibodies, have been developed recently, with some entering clinical trials and being licensed for sale [62].

10.18.1 Characterizing binding sites

Identifying and characterizing binding sites is critical for understanding protein interactions. Binding sites are the specific regions on a protein where another molecule, be it a protein or a ligand, interacts. Binding kinetics, thermodynamic principles, and driving forces of binding are only some of the methodologies and models created to comprehend the physicochemical processes underpinning PLIs [63]. Techniques such as ligand-based methods are used to anticipate possible PLIs. The conception is that chemically identical ligands are more likely to bind to chemically identical protein targets [64].

10.18.2 Fine-tuning affinity and specificity

Techniques like ligand-based methods are used to anticipate possible PLIs. The idea is that if two ligands are chemically similar, they will have a greater chance of binding to a protein with the same chemical make-up [65].

10.18.3 Interaction networks

The intricate interactions between proteins and other macromolecules in cells may be easier to understand within the context of an interaction network. These networks may be seen and investigated to provide insight on cellular processes and molecular dynamics. Biological networks, such those involving PPI, may be compared with the help of network alignment. It takes into account the topological similarity of the surrounding biological nodes across networks as well as the biological linkages between biological nodes. The behavior of molecular components may be better understood as a result. PPI networks incorporate a variety of technologies that might be used in drug development processes. These technologies consist of the yeast two-hybrid system, local and global network alignment, and alignment [66].

10.18.4 Biophysical methods for interaction studies

Biophysical approaches are critical for researching the interactions of macromolecules such as proteins. These approaches may offer quantitative data on binding affinity, kinetics, and other aspects of the interaction. The FRET (fluorescence resonance energy transfer) method is a strong tool for analyzing molecular interactions. It may give real-time data on the distance between interaction partners and how they are orientated in relation to one another. Surface plasmon resonance (SPR) is a technique often used to investigate molecular interactions. However, from the affinity of the interaction, it may give real-time information on the processes of binding and dissociation. The thermodynamics of binding interactions may be quantified using an isothermal titration calorimetry (ITC) technique [67]. It provides data on the energetics of interactions regarding enthalpy, entropy, and binding affinity. NMR spectroscopy and x-ray crystallography techniques are employed to get high-resolution structural data on protein complexes. They can provide thorough explanations of the chemical underpinnings of interactions. Protein interaction analysis and prediction may be done using various software programs and computational techniques. These techniques may give us a more profound knowledge of interaction networks and supplement experimental data [68].

10.19 Applications in synthetic biology

Synthetic biology expands the spectrum of created creatures and valuable results by applying engineering ideas to biological systems [69]. It demonstrates the field's adaptability by making possible situations outside of the laboratory, such as bioproduction, biosensing, and others [70].

10.19.1 Metabolic pathway engineering

Metabolic pathway engineering (MPE) is about modifying organisms' metabolic pathways to enhance the production of desired compounds. It is connected with synthetic biology, where it provides the necessary components and insights, and MPE applies this knowledge for optimization [71]. Techniques involve the selection of suitable host organisms, utilizing various genetic components and engineering tools for pathway modification. Whole-cell and cell-free systems, for instance, are used in bioproduction scenarios for the continuous and on-demand production of biochemical therapies. These systems need genetically and environmentally robust field-deployable platforms to keep metabolism going in a variety of environments [70].

10.19.2 Genetically encoded sensors

Dynamic regulation of genotype metabolism and evolution and screening of preferred phenotypes rely heavily on genetically encoded sensors (GES), making them indispensable in synthetic biology and metabolic engineering [72]. Their applications span the construction and management of biosynthetic pathways, enabling *in situ* monitoring with minimal interference, thereby revolutionizing synthetic biology and microbial cell factories [73]. Specific types of GES, like fluorescent biosensors, are promising for examining biochemical processes within complex cellular mechanisms, enabling targeted, long-term monitoring and control of cellular processes [72].

10.19.3 Protein-based logic gates

Protein-based logic gates are a promising field within synthetic biology, attempting to integrate computational logic into biological systems through protein interactions. Protein logic gates are designed to regulate protein association, mimicking electronic logic gates but utilizing biochemical interactions. Advances in protein design are pushing towards a nanoscale programming language where molecules serve as operands, facilitating computational operations within living cells [74]. Various forms like YES and AND gates have been developed, employing a range of reporter proteins to demonstrate their functionality. The dynamic ranges of these gates can be significantly large, indicating their potential for versatile applications. Protein logic gates can control cellular functions post-translationally, opening new avenues for modulating PPIs inside and outside cells. The *de novo* design of a wide range of logic gates using heterodimeric molecules signifies the potential for creating new protein-based control systems [75].

10.19.4 Gene circuits for dynamic control

The use of gene circuits to dynamically orchestrate cellular function is central to the field of synthetic biology. Genetic circuit design has evolved significantly with crucial works like the repressilator and the toggle switch setting a foundation. The design aims to program new biological behaviors, dynamics, and logic control, necessitating a structured approach for implementation [76]. The development of multilayer genetic circuits for dynamic regulation has allowed for more complex control of metabolic pathways in response to environmental factors and variations in gene expression. Gene circuits show promise as a means of dynamically regulating the redirection and balance of pathways in the production of useful compounds. They have the potential to replace conventional treatments, representing a major step toward the practice of customized and precision medicine [77]. A network-centric approach in designing gene circuits allows the engineering of increasingly complex Boolean logic circuits, which use transcriptional regulators for predefined cellular functions [78].

10.20 Engineering multi-functional proteins

Engineering multi-functional proteins is a dynamic field aimed at developing proteins with enhanced or novel functionalities. Through various engineering techniques, proteins can be tailored to exhibit multiple functionalities, which can be employed in numerous applications like drug development, material science, and synthetic biology [79].

10.20.1 Fusion proteins

Fusion protein engineering is a vital facet of synthetic biology and biotechnology, facilitating the creation of chimeric molecules with enhanced or diversified functionalities. Fusion proteins are often constructed by linking distinct gene fragments. The efficiency and functionality of the resultant chimeric protein can significantly be affected by the nature and length of the linkers used [80]. They find extensive application in therapeutics, for instance, in developing chimeric antigen receptor (CAR) T cell therapies. Domain-by-domain optimization strategies have been critical in enhancing the function of synthetic immunoreceptors through fusion protein engineering. The design and construction of fusion proteins come with challenges, like ensuring proper folding and functionality of the fused domains. Recent progress has been made in the structural prediction of fusion proteins, aiding in overcoming some of these challenges [81].

10.20.2 Protein scaffolds

Protein scaffolds are tools used in assembling multi-enzyme complexes, facilitating a high degree of specificity and efficiency in enzymatic reactions. Protein scaffolds can be constructed in various ways, with their components and construction methods significantly impacting enzyme kinetics. They play a crucial role in coordinating enzymatic complexes that power various metabolic pathways [82]. Better substrate channeling may result from the construction of multi-enzyme complexes on protein scaffolds, increasing the overall productivity of the enzymatic processes. Scaffold proteins play a critical role in the use of methods like compartmentalization and substrate channeling for the manipulation of multi-enzyme processes [83].

10.20.3 Modular protein design

Using known modules as building blocks, modular protein design is a method for designing proteins with certain properties. This method is useful for designing proteins with up to a particular number of amino acid residues in a single polypeptide chain and simplifying protein structures that incorporate them. Computational approaches that predict how these modules might be assembled to accomplish certain structural and functional goals have greatly assisted the concept of modularity in protein design. Designing modular architectures and developing new protein-building modules are crucial to investigating the vast array of potential topologies that evolution has not yet explored [84]. Computational protein design methods have been instrumental in advancing modular protein design, enabling the design of proteins with various structural motifs and functionalities. *De novo* design is a particular approach within modular protein design where proteins are designed from scratch without relying on existing protein templates [84].

10.20.4 Dual-enzyme systems

Dual-enzyme systems can be construed as systems where two enzymes work together either in tandem or synergistic manner to carry out a particular biochemical reaction or a set of reactions. Such systems are vital in metabolic pathways and can be engineered for biotechnological applications [85, 86].

10.21 Ethical and safety considerations

Like other fields of biotechnology, protein engineering presents a host of ethical and safety considerations that must be thoroughly examined to ensure responsible research and application [87].

10.21.1 Bioethics in protein engineering

Bioethics in protein engineering involves a range of considerations, including potential impacts on human health, the environment, and social norms. The ethical behavior in protein engineering research and applications is guided by the core concepts of bioethics, including autonomy, beneficence, nonmaleficence, and fairness. Therapeutic proteins and enzymes developed by protein engineering have great potential to improve human health. However, to ensure the subject's safety, it is necessary to thoroughly assess the potential risks to human health and their long-term consequences. The release of engineered proteins into Nature might have unexpected consequences. Evaluating these products for their ecological friendliness is crucial. Protein engineering advances may have far-reaching implications for social justice, including questions of equity and accessibility. It is crucial to build efficient regulatory frameworks to ensure that protein engineering is practiced ethically and that the benefits are shared fairly. Enzyme and therapeutic protein activity development is another area of protein engineering's purview. These features are exciting because they might bring improvements to current medical research and treatment ideas. These developments, however, need a careful assessment of ethical, safety, and social factors to guarantee the technology is created and used responsibly [88].

10.21.2 Biosafety and environmental concerns

In protein engineering, biosafety and environmental considerations are critical because they involve the possible dangers connected with the release and use of altered proteins and organisms. Protein engineering has the potential to endanger both human health and the environment. Unintended outcomes, such as developing dangerous byproducts or unintentionally manufacturing poisonous compounds, may pose concerns [89]. Advances in protein engineering and synthetic biology provide further biosecurity problems, particularly as technology becomes more widely available and complex. This covers the possibility of using genetically modified proteins improperly or harmfully. A strong regulatory structure is necessary to reduce these dangers. These principles incorporate confinement and supervision methods to promote practical applications while minimizing harm [90].

10.21.3 Intellectual property rights

Intellectual property rights (IPR) play a vital role in protein engineering and biotechnology by protecting discoveries and providing financial incentives for more studies. The patent system is an essential part of IPR, allowing creators to protect their innovations (IPR) legally. The changed proteins and the procedures used to create them are safeguarded alongside the results of genetic and proteomic studies [91, 92]. Open communication of scientific findings and the defense of inventors' rights to advance science and improve human health must coexist in a delicate balance. Maintaining this equilibrium is crucial to guarantee that the advantages of protein engineering are extensively obtainable while also stimulating creativity. The economic and legal components of intellectual property, including the costs and advantages of patents, are critical for comprehending the more significant influence of intellectual property on the diffusion of research tools and the advancement of the subject [93, 94].

10.21.4 Regulatory frameworks

It is essential to have regulatory frameworks in place to guarantee the development and deployment of protein engineering technologies safely. They encompass rules, guidelines, and procedures established by authorities to ensure safety, efficacy, and ethical practices in the field of protein engineering [95]. Regulatory frameworks worldwide have struggled to keep pace with new technologies, particularly in the field of genetic modification and genome editing, which are integral to protein engineering. The rapid advancement in these technologies exerts pressure on existing regulatory frameworks, necessitating their evolution to address the novel challenges and opportunities posed by these advancements. In a QbD-centered regulatory framework, the emphasis is on ensuring product quality through the design of the process itself. This approach is crucial in therapeutic protein product and process development, where the quality of the engineered proteins is vital. The regulatory pathway for therapeutic proteins, a significant aspect of protein engineering, often involves rigorous scrutiny by regulatory bodies like the U.S. Food and Drug Administration (FDA). The approval process examines therapeutic proteins' safety, efficacy, and quality, ensuring they meet the stringent regulatory standards before being introduced to the market [96].

10.22 Studies in protein engineering

The creation of therapeutic proteins is one area where protein engineering has become more important in the medical industry. The intricate design and engineering of proteins enable the treatment of various diseases, often surpassing the capabilities of traditional small-molecule drugs [96].

10.22.1 Therapeutic proteins

Protein-based therapies engineered in the lab have caused major changes in the way diseases are treated. By 2023, proteins are expected to make up half of the top ten selling pharmaceuticals, with effectiveness on par with or perhaps exceeding that of many currently used small molecule-based therapies [97]. After the first recombinant protein-based treatment, Humulin, was authorized by the FDA in 1982, the market for protein-based pharmaceuticals exploded to an estimated $400 billion with hundreds more candidates approved and in clinical studies. The potential of protein-based therapeutics lies in the versatility of proteins, which can act as catalysts, signaling molecules, transporters, and more. Their high specificity and potency are particularly advantageous, allowing them to execute complex functions owing to their intricate three-dimensional structures [97]. Strategic structural and chemical modifications directly made to protein structures have been crucial in overcoming challenges such as protein aggregation, degradation, and denaturation inherent to protein-based therapeutics. These design strategies have significantly improved *in vivo* stability, pharmacokinetics, cell permeability and reduced undesired immunogenicity. Protein engineering has enabled the development of various therapeutic proteins, including antibodies and enzymes. Antibodies, for instance, specifically target antigens, blocking specific signaling pathways or inducing cell death. They can also serve as transporters for targeted drug delivery, as seen in antibody–drug conjugates like trastuzumab emtansine. Enzyme-based drugs, conversely, can replace deficient or absent enzymes catalyzing the degradation or modification of therapeutically relevant targets, with examples including PEG-asparaginase and laronidase. A specific example of engineered therapeutic protein is Superoxide Dismutase, designed for effective diagnostics, biotherapeutics, and biocatalysts, highlighting the potential outcomes of protein engineering [88]. The field still faces challenges related to product heterogeneity, process monitoring, and analytics during the development and production of therapeutic proteins. Addressing these challenges is crucial for ensuring the efficacy and safety of protein-based therapeutics. Promising therapeutic protein techniques have been developed for the treatment of cancer, with a focus on the pharmacological profile and targeted therapy. The strengths and weaknesses of protein-based medicines for cancer therapy are highlighted, which also provides a thorough overview of the field's present state and prospective future possibilities. Continuous efforts have been invested to enhance the production and efficacy of protein therapeutics, addressing the demand for these potent biomolecules in modern medicine [98].

10.22.2 Industrial enzymes

The manufacturing of many useful goods for industry, such as drugs, animal feed, chemicals, cleaning agents, and biofuels, has been greatly facilitated by industrial enzymes. Protein engineering is a crucial part of making these enzymes more effective at their jobs. Post-translational enzyme modification, structure-assisted protein tailoring, and computational modeling approaches have all contributed to the development of methods for more effective biocatalyst manufacturing. Enzyme variations have been created via protein engineering that exhibit enhanced catalytic activity, widened or changed substrate specificity, and enhanced or reversed stereo-selectivity. The widespread interest in enzyme-based processing technologies stems from their potential for environmentally responsible product creation in a variety of industrial settings. The pharmaceutical, food and feed, chemical, detergent, and biofuel industries are just a few that are beginning to realize the vast industrial potential of enzymes as biocatalysts [99]. By demonstrating how easily the sequence of a protein can be modified to produce enzymes with improved functional properties like stability, specific activity, and inhibition, recent advances in protein engineering have had a significant impact on the development of commercially available enzymes into better industrial catalysts. The considerable progress achieved over the last three decades in recombinant DNA technology and the tools of protein engineering is producing solutions that answer the huge unmet demands of consumers and markets [100].

10.22.3 Diagnostic proteins

The engineering of diagnostic proteins is a pivotal application of protein engineering, enabling the development of robust diagnostic tools for various diseases. Reliable diagnostic tools have been developed using techniques from the area of protein engineering. These genetically engineered diagnostic proteins have shown remarkable potential in the pharmaceutical and enzyme industries, where they may help identify and manage several diseases [88]. Protein engineering aims to create diagnostically useful new proteins. Protein structural manipulation permits the development of diagnostic proteins, which may aid in diagnosing diseases earlier, leading to better health outcomes. Protein engineering that uses light to regulate the movement of kinesin and myosin motors along microtubules has potential diagnostic applications. Engineered diagnostic proteins have applications in various domains, including biotherapeutics and biocatalysts. Technologies such as created natural protein variations, Fc fusion protein, and antibody engineering, which also have diagnostic uses, have a major influence on the state of the art in protein treatments today. Protein engineering magnifies the already impressive range of molecular tasks performed by proteins that have evolved spontaneously. Proteins with optimized three-dimensional structures may be powerful diagnostic tools, offering a wide range of molecular functions that can be used in the detection, monitoring, and treatment of diseases [101].

10.23 Single-molecule techniques in protein engineering

Single-molecule techniques in protein engineering are vital for elucidating the intricate behaviors and properties of individual molecules which are often obscured in bulk measurements. Among these techniques, atomic force microscopy (AFM) stands out for its versatility and precision in characterizing molecular structures and interactions [102].

10.23.1 Atomic force microscopy

Providing three-dimensional topographic pictures and structural features of materials, AFM has emerged as a leading technology working at the single-molecule level. The atomic force microscope, which was developed in 1986, is a powerful instrument for studying things at the nanoscale. It uses a cantilever to scan surfaces. AFM has developed into a potent nanoscopic platform that makes it possible to characterize a wide variety of biointerfaces, both synthetic and biological. Such work has greatly benefitted the study of protein molecular and hierarchical assembly, especially of misfolded species that occur during protein aggregation, and the monitoring of their dynamics at the nanoscale [103]. AFM, along with its variants and hybrid techniques, offers molecular data to support studies in the biochemical area of protein engineering. The single-molecule statistical approach offered by AFM finds applications in the solving of molecular assemblages and the structural characteristics of functional nanomaterials inspired by amyloid. AFM-based single-molecule force spectroscopy (AFM-SMFS) research has been developed owing to contributions from a range of domains, including developments in surface chemistry, issues in protein engineering, and diverse data processing theories and methodologies. These improvements provide light on the growth of AFM methods, resulting in the instrument being a valuable resource for studying protein behaviors and interactions at the single-molecule level [104].

10.23.2 Single-molecule FRET

It is critical to investigate the dynamics of biomolecular structure using the single-molecule Forster Resonance Energy Transfer (smFRET) method. The basic idea behind smFRET is that energy may be transmitted between two fluorophore molecules that are near to each other. This allows for the monitoring of nanoscale distances as well as changes within them. The primary applications of this method are nanoscale examinations of the conformations and dynamics of biomolecular structures, which are often carried out in real time. Fluorescence microscopes are often employed in this procedure, and the molecules being studied may be surface-immobilized or allowed to spread freely. Individual FRET pairs are highlighted by lasers and other bright light sources, resulting in fluorescence signals strong enough for single-molecule detection [105].

10.23.3 Optical tweezers

In recent years, there has been a change in the focus of research into the alteration of single molecules toward the use of optical tweezers. This method makes use of light's ability to impose forces and torques on individual molecules in order to directly measure the forces and torques that are created by biological processes. Optical tweezers may be traced back to the work that Arthur Ashkin did in the 1970s and 1980s. In this study, light was used to capture and manipulate micron-sized latex spheres, bacteria, red blood cells, and organelles inside cells. This was the beginning of the development of optical tweezers. The versatility of optical tweezers is highlighted by their capability to measure not only forces and displacements but also torques and angles. A notable enhancement to the method includes integrating single-molecule fluorescence detection capabilities. Optical tweezers have a wide variety of uses, including but not limited to the investigation of protein–nucleic acid interactions, the folding of proteins and RNA, and the operation of molecular motors. The data from optical tweezer experiments offer vital insights, with data reproducibility and variability challenges across different laboratories. To transcend these challenges and optimize instrument operation, data extraction, and analysis indicates promising opportunities for future advancements in the field [106, 107].

10.23.4 Patch-clamp technique

The patch-clamp technique allows for precisely measuring ionic currents flowing through a cell's plasma membrane. It can either monitor currents passing through single ion channels or those traversing the entire plasma membrane. This method has been ideal in studying the functions and dysfunctions of electrically excitable cells and their networks [107]. Utilizing a glass electrode, the patch-clamp technique establishes a tight seal on a cell's surface, enabling the direct measurement of membrane potential and the amount of current passing across the cell membrane. It is the only technique that can reliably record electrical activity within a single neuron which make it as an exceptional resource. The precise observation and manipulation of ionic currents are only two of the many scientific uses for this technique [108]. Three decades ago, the patch-clamp method was developed, and it revolutionized the study of cellular physiology and biophysics. Researchers were able to get a better understanding of the physiological role of a single protein, in this instance an ion-permeable channel in the plasma membrane of a cell. This was a tremendous step forward for neurology and allied disciplines, as it opened the door to research of the cellular and molecular processes underlying neurological ailments. This approach may be used to study many other things; for example, ionic currents in the heart, the excitability of neurons, and the electrophysiological characteristics of different cell types [109]. Research into the biological basis of electrical signaling and the functional dynamics of ion channels would benefit greatly from these findings. Despite its widespread use, the patch-clamp method has certain limitations, such as the need for a high signal-to-noise ratio in recordings, the fabrication of electrodes, and the isolation of myocytes. Ongoing technical improvements, however, are helping to enhance the method's efficacy, broaden its applicability, and overcome its existing limitations [109].

10.24 High throughput screening methods

High throughput screening (HTS) allows for the quick evaluation of many compounds' biological or biochemical activity, making it an essential tool in the early stages of drug development. HTS aims to find promising compounds, or 'hits,' that may be further developed into helpful medicinal medicines [110]. To find potential ways for drug development screening large libraries of chemicals against a particular target or pathway of interest. Novel biomaterials and techniques for modifying them have proliferated in recent years intending to imitate the intricate microenvironments of genuine tissues, thereby improving the dependability and utility of HTS. The integration of NGS and ML is transforming the screening design and workflows, boosting the effectiveness of HTS [110].

10.24.1 Fluorescence-activated cell sorting (FACS)

Using physical and fluorescent properties, cells may be separated using a technique called fluorescence-activated cell sorting (FACS), which is a subset of flow cytometry. High-purity enrichment of certain cell populations is made possible by FACS's ability to sort a population of cells into subsets depending on the sum quantity of essential biomarkers produced by the cells [111]. It finds extensive application in separating and isolating antigen-specific B lymphocytes in a high-throughput manner, among other uses, thereby promoting the development of valuable reagents for immunological research. The technique utilizes fluorescent labeling of cells followed by their detection and sorting based on individual cellular characteristics, such as size and granularity, in addition to their fluorescence. FACS is often used in conjunction with other emerging technologies like droplet-based microfluidics to enhance its throughput and application scope [112].

10.24.2 Microfluidics-based assays

Microfluidics-based assays are instrumental in precision medicine, particularly in oncology, providing a more complex understanding of tumor behavior in response to treatments. Functional assays, which directly assess treatment responses on live cells while also taking into account parameters such as tissue of origin, tumor microenvironment, and immune response, are improved by microfluidic technology. In order to measure how well a therapy is working, functional assays might be used. They include a wide range of non-genomic cell-based tests. These assays aim to create an evolving system where the effect of molecular changes, as well as microenvironmental factors, can be captured over time, thus providing more robust predictors for optimal treatment identification [113]. Microfluidic models only need a small number of cells, therefore they may be used with small samples like those obtained from patient-derived biopsies. By simulating the complex tumor micro-environment, which includes elements impacting treatment response such as nutrition, waste products, chemokines, and diverse cell types, these tests have the potential to better predict treatment responses than conventional ones. Microphysiological systems and 'organs on a chip' are two recent developments that aim to replicate tissue/tumor function and therapy response. Multiple human diseases have been investigated using the technique, but recent years have seen particularly promising results in the study of cancer [114].

10.24.3 Yeast surface display

Yeast surface display (YSD) is a technology that displays recombinant proteins on the yeast cell surface, which finds applications across a broad spectrum of biotechnology and biomedical fields. YSD is favored due to several advantages, including its safety status by the FDA and the capability of yeast cells for PTMs, which is crucial for displaying complex proteins. The method includes joining recombinant proteins genetically to a protein found in high quantities in cell walls. This is very useful for protein engineering projects since it allows the proteins to be shown on the surface of yeast cells [115]. YSD has been used in various domains, including the creation of anti-cancer antibodies and the selection of binding proteins from scaffold protein combinatorial libraries. Research into creating carrier-free immobilized enzymes for biocatalysis includes several possibilities of inquiry into improving the efficiency of YSD systems for biotechnological applications [116].

10.24.4 Mass spectrometry-based methods

Methods based on mass spectrometry (MS-based methods) are essential for revealing details about biological and molecular mechanisms. Proteomic analysis based on MS is a significant method for finding novel disease biomarkers. It contributes to the molecular knowledge of diseases, essential for advancing customized treatment, particularly concerning complicated diseases like inflammatory bowel disease and diabetes [116]. Secondary ion mass spectrometry (SIMS), inductively coupled plasma mass spectrometry (ICP-MS), laser desorption ionization mass spectrometry (LDI-MS), and electrospray ionization mass spectrometry (ESI-MS) are all types of MS-based procedures (ESI-MS). These methods are used for studying individual cells. These techniques enable the investigation of single cells, expanding our understanding of the variety and functioning of biological systems [117]. Other technologies for improved characterization and analysis of complex materials such as lignin include matrix-aided laser desorption ionization and time-of-flight-secondary ion mass spectrometry. Profiling the metabolomic abundance of biological materials is an everyday use of MS-based approaches. Understanding the fluctuations in metabolite concentrations under various biological situations is essential for diagnosing and treating illness, and differential abundance analysis may assist with this. Over the years, advancements in MS-based technologies have made them well-suited for biomarker discovery. The specificity and sensitivity of MS have significantly contributed to the expansion of the proteomics field, supporting the discovery of biomarkers crucial for understanding disease pathology and developing new diagnostic and therapeutic strategies. While MS-based methods have the potential to advance biomarker discovery significantly, challenges such as improper experimental design, lack of standardized procedures, and quality control during sample collection and analyses can delay the reproducibility and clinical relevance of discovered biomarkers. Ensuring rigorous experimental design, proper sample collection, and validation of identified biomarkers are crucial for overcoming these challenges [118].

10.25 Protein engineering for nanotechnology

Protein engineering for nanotechnology explores the intersection of protein biology and nanotechnology, focusing on repurposing protein molecules as nanostructures and nanoscaffolds. This field enables the design and creation of protein-based nanomaterials and nanosystems (PNNS) with diverse properties offering various specialized applications owing to the unique characteristics of different proteins. By employing protein engineering, one can customize native enzymes, thereby generating enzyme variants with improved catalytic activity and broadened or altered substrate specificity. This trend significantly enhances the development and functionality of nanoscale materials and systems for many bio-applications [119].

10.25.1 Protein-based nanocarriers

Protein-based nanocarriers have emerged as a promising platform in the field of nanotechnology. Utilizing proteins as the fundamental building blocks, these nanocarriers are engineered to encapsulate or attach various therapeutic agents, including drugs, genes, or imaging agents, enabling their targeted delivery or controlled release within biological systems. The unique advantage of protein-based nanocarriers lies in the biocompatibility, biodegradability, and functional versatility of proteins, which can be engineered for specific interactions with biological entities or stimuli-responsive behaviors. One of the notable applications of protein-based nanocarriers is in the field of drug delivery, where they can significantly enhance the therapeutic efficacy and reduce the systemic toxicity of encapsulated drugs. For instance, utilizing genetically engineered cell membranes expressing specific anchors can further modulate the interaction of these nanocarriers with biological systems, thereby promoting immune evasion and prolonged circulation. Such modular approaches demonstrate the potential of protein engineering in advancing the design and functionality of protein-based nanocarriers for various biomedical applications [120].

10.25.2 Biosensors

To convert a biological reaction into an electrical signal, biosensors use integrated receptor–transducer devices. To identify pathogenic organisms, carcinogenic, mutagenic, or toxic compounds, or to report a biological impact, they are basically intended to integrate biological materials with appropriate platforms. Together, they make it possible to track and analyze a wide range of chemical and biological compounds in real time. Biosensors have been around since the 1960s, when they were first developed by Clark and Lyons. In 1967, the first enzyme-based sensor was described by Updike and Hicks [121]. Over the years, biosensor technology has witnessed substantial growth and progress, including the development of nanostructured materials-enabled biosensors, significantly enhancing their sensitivity and specificity [122]. Biosensors come in many forms, including those based on enzymes, tissues, immunosensors, DNA, heat, and piezoelectric forces [123]. The receptors and transducers may also be used to categorize them, with newer methods making use of nanomaterials such noble metal nanoparticles, metal oxide nanoparticles, nanowires, nanorods, carbon nanotubes, quantum dots, and dendrimers to advance biosensing technologies. Biosensors have found many of applications in medical fields for detecting pathogenic organisms and various hazardous chemicals. They are instrumental in reporting biological effects and pivotal for real-time monitoring and analysis in numerous bio-applications [123].

10.25.3 Protein nanowires and nanotubes

Protein nanowires and nanotubes are at the line of biotechnology and nanotechnology, using the inherent properties of proteins to create nanoscale structures with potential applications in various fields. Protein nanowires and nanotubes synthesized from multiple sources. Protein nanotubes are often constructed through a self-assembly process where peptides act as building blocks, forming the final nanotube structure. For example, α-lactalbumin is utilized in a mechanism where divalent cations act as bridging agents between peptides to create the final tubular structure. Proteins emerge as valuable biotemplates for nanomaterials due to their assembly under physiologically relevant conditions and ease of manipulation via protein engineering [124]. In comparison to conventional nanowire materials, protein nanowires may be extracted from microorganisms and provide benefits in terms of functionality and sustainability. New electronic devices are already being produced for neuromorphic memory and sustainable power generation. Protein nanotubes (PNTs) are being studied for usage as molecular imaging biosensors, conducting wires for microelectronics, fuel cells, and drug delivery systems because of their biocompatible and biodegradable properties. PNTs and their composites with carbon nanotubes (CNTs) are being studied extensively for their electrical and mechanical properties, despite concerns regarding CNT toxicity and biodegradability [124]. Protein nanowires have several potential uses in bioelectronics, including renewable energy generation and neuromorphic memory storage. As a bottom-up strategy for creating innovative bionanosystems, protein nanowires and PNTs are being investigated for use in biosensors due to their promising properties. Advances in synthetic biology have made it possible to encode synthetic chemistries in genes with monomeric precision, opening the door to the production of programmable materials with adjustable properties. This has enormous implications for the field of protein nanowires and PNTs. These materials open doors for groundbreaking applications in medicine, electronics, and other domains, reflecting the translational potential of protein nanowires and PNTs in modern nanobiotechnology [125].

10.25.4 DNA–protein hybrid structures

DNA–protein hybrid structures are fascinating constructs that influence the unique properties of both DNA and proteins. They have received attention in nanotechnology and molecular biology for various applications. Protein–DNA hybrid sequence-specific DNA-binding proteins may be used to build structures. DNA origami, in which small single-stranded ‘staples’ are used to fold a long single-stranded bacteriophage M13 ‘scaffold’ strand into specified forms, was described in 2017 by Dietz and Praetorius [126]. Potentially useful in simulating nucleoprotein complexes like those seen in viruses, transcription factors, and ribosomes, these hybrid structures offer great promise. Gene delivery systems and low-fidelity models of viruses made from viromic hybrid materials have been created for use in structural biology and biophysics research. Hybrid structures’ attachment may be done by either chemical conjugation or protein domains that bind specifically to DNA or RNA. Proteins have been conjugated to small strands of single-stranded

DNA using a variety of chemical techniques [127]. DNA is the genetic information carrier, while proteins are the functional components executing most biological processes. The hybrid complexes of DNA and proteins cooperatively and efficiently conduct sophisticated biological functions, demonstrating their potential in advancing molecular biology and bioengineering [128]. Over the last decade, several researchers have investigated the potential of artificial DNA–protein hybrid structures. Particularly, DNA nanotechnology has greatly increased nanoscale molecule manufacturing and led to the exact spatial organization of protein components, which in turn has allowed for the construction of innovative nano-architectures [129].

References

[1] Tiwari M K *et al* 2012 Computational approaches for rational design of proteins with novel functionalities *Comput. Struct. Biotechnol. J.* **2** e201204002

[2] Chen R 2001 Enzyme engineering: rational redesign versus directed evolution *Trends Biotechnol.* **19** 13–4

[3] Bernal C, Rodriguez K and Martinez R 2018 Integrating enzyme immobilization and protein engineering: an alternative path for the development of novel and improved industrial biocatalysts *Biotechnol. Adv.* **36** 1470–80

[4] Fersht A R *et al* 1984 Analysis of enzyme structure and activity by protein engineering *Angew. Chem. Int. Ed. Engl.* **23** 467–73

[5] Liu Q, Xun G and Feng Y 2019 The state-of-the-art strategies of protein engineering for enzyme stabilization *Biotechnol. Adv.* **37** 530–7

[6] Yoo Y J *et al* 2017 *Fundamentals of Enzyme Engineering* (Berlin: Springer)

[7] Huang J *et al* 2020 Enzymatic biofuel cells based on protein engineering: recent advances and future prospects *Biomater. Sci.* **8** 5230–40

[8] Fersht A R, Matouschek A and Serrano L 1992 The folding of an enzyme: I. Theory of protein engineering analysis of stability and pathway of protein folding *J. Mol. Biol.* **224** 771–82

[9] Sauer J *et al* 2000 Glucoamylase: structure/function relationships, and protein engineering *Biochim. Biophys. Acta (BBA)-Protein Struct. Mol. Enzymol.* **1543** 275–93

[10] Peitsch M C 1995 Protein modeling by e-mail *Bio/Technol.* **13** 658–60

[11] Šali A *et al* 1995 Evaluation of comparative protein modeling by modeller *Proteins Struct. Funct. Bioinf.* **23** 318–26

[12] Hirschfelder J O, Brown W B and Epstein S T 1964 Recent developments in perturbation theory *Adv. Quantum. Chem.* **1** 255–374

[13] Iliopoulos J, Itzykson C and Martin A 1975 Functional methods and perturbation theory *Rev. Mod. Phys.* **47** 165

[14] Muir T W, Sondhi D and Cole P A 1998 Expressed protein ligation: a general method for protein engineering *Proc. Natl Acad. Sci.* **95** 6705–10

[15] Estell D A, Graycar T P and Wells J A 1985 Engineering an enzyme by site-directed mutagenesis to be resistant to chemical oxidation *J. Biol. Chem.* **260** 6518–21

[16] Lai Y P *et al* 2004 A new approach to random mutagenesis *in vitro Biotechnol. Bioeng.* **86** 622–7

[17] Ly H D and Withers S G 1999 Mutagenesis of glycosidases *Annu. Rev. Biochem.* **68** 487–522

[18] Ulmer K M 1983 Protein engineering *Science* **219** 666–71
[19] Blackburn M C *et al* 2016 Integrating gene synthesis and microfluidic protein analysis for rapid protein engineering *Nucleic Acids Res.* **44** e68 e68
[20] Schoffelen S and van Hest J C 2012 Multi-enzyme systems: bringing enzymes together *in vitro Soft Matter* **8** 1736–46
[21] DeSantis G and Jones J B 1999 Chemical modification of enzymes for enhanced functionality *Curr. Opin. Biotechnol.* **10** 324–30
[22] Kaiser E T, Lawrence D S and Rokita S E 1985 The chemical modification of enzymatic specificity *Annu. Rev. Biochem.* **54** 565–95
[23] Cowan D A and Fernandez-Lafuente R 2011 Enhancing the functional properties of thermophilic enzymes by chemical modification and immobilization *Enzyme Microb. Technol.* **49** 326–46
[24] Carter P J 2011 Introduction to current and future protein therapeutics: a protein engineering perspective *Exp. Cell. Res.* **317** 1261–9
[25] Hollingsworth S A and Dror R O 2018 Molecular dynamics simulation for all *Neuron* **99** 1129–43
[26] Lazim R, Suh D and Choi S 2020 Advances in molecular dynamics simulations and enhanced sampling methods for the study of protein systems *Int. J. Mol. Sci.* **21** 6339
[27] Wang X *et al* 2018 A quantum mechanical computational method for modeling electrostatic and solvation effects of protein *Sci. Rep.* **8** 5475
[28] Cho A E *et al* 2009 Quantum mechanical scoring for protein docking *J. Chem. Phys.* **131** 134108
[29] Fu Y, Zhao J and Chen Z 2018 Insights into the molecular mechanisms of protein–ligand interactions by molecular docking and molecular dynamics simulation: a case of oligopeptide binding protein *Comput. Math. Methods Med.* **2018** 3502514
[30] Masters M R *et al* 2023 Deep learning model for efficient protein–ligand docking with implicit side-chain flexibility *J. Chem. Inf. Model.* **63** 1695–707
[31] Zhang X *et al* 2023 Efficient and accurate large library ligand docking with KarmaDock *Nat. Comput. Sci.* **3** 789–804
[32] Dey D *et al* 2021 Molecular optimization, docking, and dynamic simulation profiling of selective aromatic phytochemical ligands in blocking the SARS-CoV-2 S protein attachment to ACE2 receptor: an in silico approach of targeted drug designing *J. Adv. Vet. Anim. Res.* **8** 24
[33] Xu Y *et al* 2020 Deep dive into machine learning models for protein engineering *J. Chem. Inf. Model.* **60** 2773–90
[34] Yang K K, Wu Z and Arnold F H 2019 Machine-learning-guided directed evolution for protein engineering *Nat. Methods* **16** 687–94
[35] Gao W *et al* 2020 Deep learning in protein structural modeling and design *Patterns* **1** 100142
[36] Hallen M A and Donald B R 2019 Protein design by provable algorithms *Commun. ACM* **62** 76–84
[37] Kamerzell T J and Middaugh C R 2021 Prediction machines: applied machine learning for therapeutic protein design and development *J. Pharm. Sci.* **110** 665–81
[38] Vidal L S *et al* 2023 *A Primer to Directed Evolution: Current Methodologies and Future Directions* (RSC Chemical Biology)

[39] Wang Y *et al* 2021 Directed evolution: methodologies and applications *Chem. Rev.* **121** 12384–444
[40] Reid A J 2000 DNA shuffling: modifying the hand that nature dealt *In Vitro Cell. Dev. Biol. Plant* **36** 331–7
[41] Marshall S H 2002 DNA shuffling: induced molecular breeding to produce new generation long-lasting vaccines *Biotechnol. Adv.* **20** 229–38
[42] Siloto R M and Weselake R J 2012 Site saturation mutagenesis: methods and applications in protein engineering *Biocatal. Agric. Biotechnol.* **1** 181–9
[43] Ma L *et al* 2017 CRISPR-Cas9–mediated saturated mutagenesis screen predicts clinical drug resistance with improved accuracy *Proc. Natl Acad. Sci.* **114** 11751–6
[44] Jaroszewicz W *et al* 2022 Phage display and other peptide display technologies *FEMS Microbiol. Rev.* **46** fuab052
[45] Ledsgaard L *et al* 2022 Advances in antibody phage display technology *Drug Discov. Today* **27** 2151–69
[46] Ramazi S and Zahiri J 2021 Post-translational modifications in proteins: resources, tools and prediction methods *Database* **2021** baab012
[47] Jefferis R 2013 *Review of Glycosylation Engineering of Biopharmaceuticals: Methods and Protocols* (Springer)
[48] Ma B *et al* 2020 Protein glycoengineering: an approach for improving protein properties *Front. Chem.* **8** 622
[49] Esmaili F *et al* 2023 A review of machine learning and algorithmic methods for protein phosphorylation sites prediction *Genom. Proteom. Bioinform.* **21** 1266–85
[50] Urban J 2022 *A review on recent trends in the phosphoproteomics workflow*. From sample preparation to data analysis *Anal. Chim. Acta* **1199** 338857
[51] Millán-Zambrano G *et al* 2022 Histone post-translational modifications—cause and consequence of genome function *Nat. Rev. Genet.* **23** 563–80
[52] Zuma L K *et al* 2022 Protein PEGylation: navigating recombinant protein stability, aggregation, and bioactivity *BioMed Res. Int.* **2022** 8929715
[53] Lawrence P B and Price J L 2016 How PEGylation influences protein conformational stability *Curr. Opin. Chem. Biol.* **34** 88–94
[54] Chiu J and Hogg P J 2019 Allosteric disulfides: sophisticated molecular structures enabling flexible protein regulation *J. Biol. Chem.* **294** 2949–5908
[55] Lee A L 2009 Frameworks for understanding long-range intra-protein communication *Curr. Protein Pept. Sci.* **10** 116–27
[56] Verkhivker G M *et al* 2020 Allosteric regulation at the crossroads of new technologies: multiscale modeling networks, and machine learning *Front. Mol. Biosci.* **7** 136
[57] Wrabl J O *et al* 2011 The role of protein conformational fluctuations in allostery, function, and evolution *Biophys. Chem.* **159** 129–41
[58] Govindaraj R G, Thangapandian S, Schauperl M, Denny R A and Diller D J 2023 Recent applications of computational methods to allosteric drug discovery *Front. Mol. Biosci.* **9** 1070328
[59] Lu S *et al* 2019 Allosteric modulator discovery: from serendipity to structure-based design *J. Med. Chem.* **62** 6405–21
[60] Pan T *et al* 2022 Rational design of allosteric switchable catalysts *Exploration* (Wiley Online Library)
[61] Klem H, McCullagh M and Paton R S 2022 Modeling catalysis in allosteric enzymes: capturing conformational consequences *Top. Catal.* **65** 165–86

[62] Lu H *et al* 2020 Recent advances in the development of protein–protein interactions modulators: mechanisms and clinical trials *Signal Transduc. Target. Ther.* **5** 213
[63] Du X *et al* 2016 Insights into protein–ligand interactions: mechanisms, models, and methods *Int. J. Mol. Sci.* **17** 144
[64] Zhao L *et al* 2022 A brief review of protein–ligand interaction prediction *Comput. Struct. Biotechnol. J.* **20** 2831–8
[65] Chatterjee A *et al* 2023 Improving the generalizability of protein–ligand binding predictions with AI-Bind *Nat. Commun.* **14** 1989
[66] Athanasios A *et al* 2017 Protein-protein interaction (PPI) network: recent advances in drug discovery *Curr. Drug Metab.* **18** 5–10
[67] Ward T J, Farris III A B and Woodling K 2001 Synergistic chiral separations using the glycopeptides ristocetin a and vancomycin *J. Biochem. Bioph. Methods* **48** 163–74
[68] Bisen P S 2014 *Laboratory Protocols in Applied life Sciences* (Boca Raton, FL: CRC Press)
[69] Hanczyc M M 2020 Engineering life: a review of synthetic biology *Artif. life* **26** 260–73
[70] Brooks S M and Alper H S 2021 Applications, challenges, and needs for employing synthetic biology beyond the lab *Nat. Commun.* **12** 1390
[71] García-Granados R, Lerma-Escalera J A and Morones-Ramírez J R 2019 *Metabolic engineering and synthetic biology: synergies*, future, and challenges *Front. Bioeng. Biotechnol.* **7** 36
[72] Yu W *et al* 2022 Genetically encoded biosensors for microbial synthetic biology: from conceptual frameworks to practical applications *Biotechnol. Adv.* **62** 108077
[73] Michener J K *et al* 2012 Applications of genetically-encoded biosensors for the construction and control of biosynthetic pathways *Metab. Eng.* **14** 212–22
[74] Vishweshwaraiah Y L *et al* 2021 Two-input protein logic gate for computation in living cells *Nat. Commun.* **12** 6615
[75] Chen Z *et al* 2020 De novo design of protein logic gates *Science* **368** 78–84
[76] Slusarczyk A L, Lin A and Weiss R 2012 Foundations for the design and implementation of synthetic genetic circuits *Nat. Rev. Genet.* **13** 406–20
[77] Sedlmayer F, Aubel D and Fussenegger M 2018 Synthetic gene circuits for the detection, elimination and prevention of disease *Nat. Biomed. Eng.* **2** 399–415
[78] Crowther M, Wipat A and Goñi-Moreno Á 2022 A network approach to genetic circuit designs *ACS Synth. Biol.* **11** 3058–66
[79] Eisenstein M 2023 AI-enhanced protein design makes proteins that have never existed *Nat. Biotechnol.* **41** 303–5
[80] Patel D K *et al* 2022 Linkers: a synergistic way for the synthesis of chimeric proteins *Protein Expr. Purif.* **191** 106012
[81] Yu K *et al* 2015 Synthetic fusion protein design and applications *Biotechnol. Adv.* **33** 155–64
[82] Gad S and Ayakar S 2021 Protein scaffolds: a tool for multi-enzyme assembly *Biotechnol. Rep.* **32** e00670
[83] Wang X *et al* 2023 Research progress of multi-enzyme complexes based on the design of scaffold protein *Bioresour. Bioprocess.* **10** 72
[84] Lapenta F and Jerala R 2020 Design of novel protein building modules and modular architectures *Curr. Opin. Struct. Biol.* **63** 90–6
[85] Tarazona N A *et al* 2022 Rapid depolymerization of poly (ethylene terephthalate) thin films by a dual-enzyme system and its impact on material properties *Chem. Catal.* **2** 3573–89

[86] Barth M *et al* 2016 A dual enzyme system composed of a polyester hydrolase and a carboxylesterase enhances the biocatalytic degradation of polyethylene terephthalate films *Biotechnol. J.* **11** 1082–7
[87] Sengupta S, Sengupta L and Bisen P 2001 Bioengineered crops: the commercial and ethical considerations *Curr. Genom.* **2** 181–97
[88] Lakhawat S S *et al* 2023 Protein engineering, a robust tool to engineer novel functions in protein *Protein Pept. Lett.* **30** 541–51
[89] Wang F and Zhang W 2019 Synthetic biology: recent progress, biosafety and biosecurity concerns, and possible solutions *J. Biosafety Biosecurity* **1** 22–30
[90] Beeckman D S and Rüdelsheim P 2020 Biosafety and biosecurity in containment: a regulatory overview *Front. Bioeng. Biotechnol.* **8** 650
[91] Mann S P *et al* 2021 Ethical principles, constraints, and opportunities in clinical proteomics *Mol. Cell. Proteomics* **20** 100046
[92] Sariola S 2021 Intellectual property rights need to be subverted to ensure global vaccine access *BMJ Glob. Health* **6** e005656
[93] National Academies of Sciences, E. and Medicine 2021 *Biological Collections: Ensuring Critical Research and Education for the 21st Century* (National Academies Press)
[94] Richter J D and Zhao X 2021 The molecular biology of FMRP: new insights into fragile X syndrome *Nat. Rev. Neurosci.* **22** 209–22
[95] Engqvist M K and Rabe K S 2019 Applications of protein engineering and directed evolution in plant research *Plant Physiol.* **179** 907–17
[96] Alexaki A *et al* 2019 Effects of codon optimization on coagulation factor IX translation and structure: implications for protein and gene therapies *Sci. Rep.* **9** 15449
[97] Ebrahimi S B and Samanta D 2023 Engineering protein-based therapeutics through structural and chemical design *Nat. Commun.* **14** 2411
[98] Narad P *et al* 2023 Protein engineering methods to design protein therapeutics *Protein-based Therapeutics* (Berlin: Springer) pp 49–100
[99] Li C *et al* 2023 Biocatalysis and biotransformation guided by protein engineering *Front. Bioeng. Biotechnol.* **11** 1159555
[100] Arbige M V, Shetty J K and Chotani G K 2019 Industrial enzymology: the next chapter *Trends Biotechnol.* **37** 1355–66
[101] Kuhlman B and Bradley P 2019 Advances in protein structure prediction and design *Nat. Rev. Mol. Cell Biol.* **20** 681–97
[102] Mohapatra S *et al* 2019 Single-molecule analysis and engineering of DNA motors *Chem. Rev.* **120** 36–78
[103] Ruggeri F S *et al* 2019 Atomic force microscopy for single molecule characterisation of protein aggregation *Arch. Biochem. Biophys.* **664** 134–48
[104] Yang B *et al* 2020 Next generation methods for single-molecule force spectroscopy on polyproteins and receptor-ligand complexes *Front. Mol. Biosci.* **7** 85
[105] Hartmann A *et al* 2023 An automated single-molecule FRET platform for high-content, multiwell plate screening of biomolecular conformations and dynamics *Nat. Commun.* **14** 6511
[106] Pesce G *et al* 2020 Optical tweezers: theory and practice *Eur. Phys. J. Plus* **135** 1–38
[107] Gieseler J *et al* 2021 Optical tweezers—from calibration to applications: a tutorial *Adv. Opt. Photonics* **13** 74–241
[108] Noguchi A, Ikegaya Y and Matsumoto N 2021 In vivo whole-cell patch-clamp methods: recent technical progress and future perspectives *Sensors* **21** 1448

[109] Lovisolo D 2022 Patch clamp: the first four decades of a technique that revolutionized electrophysiology and beyond *Rev. Physiol. Biochem. Pharmacol.* 1–28
[110] Blay V *et al* 2020 High-throughput screening: today's biochemical and cell-based approaches *Drug Discov. Today* **25** 1807–21
[111] Li G, Cheng L and Su L 2021 Phenotypic and functional study of human plasmacytoid dendritic cells *Curr. Protoc.* **1** e50
[112] Fei C *et al* 2021 Potential applications of fluorescence-activated cell sorting (facs) and droplet-based microfluidics in promoting the discovery of specific antibodies for characterizations of fish immune cells *Front. Immunol.* **12** 771231
[113] Ayuso J M *et al* 2022 A role for microfluidic systems in precision medicine *Nat. Commun.* **13** 3086
[114] Rabiee N *et al* 2020 Nanotechnology-assisted microfluidic systems: from bench to bedside *Nanomedicine* **16** 237–58
[115] Sharma P, Procko E and Kranz D M 2022 Engineering proteins by combining deep mutational scanning deep mutational scanning and yeast display *Yeast Surface Display* (Berlin: Springer) pp 117–42
[116] Teymennet-Ramírez K, Martínez-Morales F and Trejo-Hernández M R 2022 Yeast surface display system: strategies for improvement and biotechnological applications *Front. Bioeng. Biotechnol.* **9** 794742
[117] Xu X *et al* 2023 Mass spectrometry-based techniques for single-cell analysis *Analyst* **148** 3690–707
[118] Rodrigues J E *et al* 2022 Systematic review and meta-analysis of mass spectrometry proteomics applied to human peripheral fluids to assess potential biomarkers of schizophrenia *Int. J. Mol. Sci.* **23** 4917
[119] White D W *et al* 2023 The hidden biocatalytic potential of the old yellow enzyme family *bioRxiv* 2023.07.10.548207v1
[120] Jain M *et al* 2023 Introduction to protein therapeutics *Protein-based Therapeutics* (Berlin: Springer) pp 1–22
[121] Mehrotra P 2016 Biosensors and their applications–a review *J. Oral Biol. Craniofac. Res.* **6** 153–9
[122] Chadha U *et al* 2022 Recent progress and growth in biosensors technology: a critical review *J. Ind. Eng. Chem.* **109** 21–51
[123] Haleem A *et al* 2021 Biosensors applications in medical field: a brief review *Sens. Int.* **2** 100100
[124] Audette G F *et al* 2019 Protein nanotubes: from bionanotech towards medical applications *Biomedicines* **7** 46
[125] Shapiro D M *et al* 2022 Protein nanowires with tunable functionality and programmable self-assembly using sequence-controlled synthesis *Nat. Commun.* **13** 829
[126] Stephanopoulos N 2020 Hybrid nanostructures from the self-assembly of proteins and DNA *Chem.* **6** 364–405
[127] Krissanaprasit A *et al* 2021 Self-assembling nucleic acid nanostructures functionalized with aptamers *Chem. Rev.* **121** 13797–868
[128] Li X *et al* 2020 Programmable assembly of DNA–protein hybrid structures *Chem. Res. Chin. Univ.* **36** 211–8
[129] Zhou K *et al* 2019 Toward precise manipulation of DNA–protein hybrid nanoarchitectures *Small* **15** 1804044

www.ingramcontent.com/pod-product-compliance
Ingram Content Group UK Ltd.
Pitfield, Milton Keynes, MK11 3LW, UK
UKHW051909100926
8556IPUK00005B/819

9 780750 353854